Williams OBSTETRICS STUDY GUIDE

25th Edition

Shivani Patel, MD
Assistant Professor
Department of Obstetrics and Gynecology
University of Texas Southwestern Medical Center
Parkland Health and Hospital System
Dallas, Texas

Scott Roberts, MD
Medical Director, High-Risk Obstetrical Unit Parkland Hospital
Professor
Department of Obstetrics and Gynecology
University of Texas Southwestern Medical Center
Parkland Health and Hospital System
Dallas, Texas

Vanessa Rogers, MD
Director, Obstetrics and Gynecology Residency Program
Associate Professor
Department of Obstetrics and Gynecology
University of Texas Southwestern Medical Center
Parkland Health and Hospital System
Dallas, Texas

Ashley Zink, MD
Assistant Professor
Department of Obstetrics and Gynecology
University of Texas Southwestern Medical Center
Parkland Health and Hospital System
Dallas, Texas

Elaine Duryea, MD
Medical Director, Maternal Fetal Medicine Clinic
Assistant Professor
Department of Obstetrics and Gynecology
University of Texas Southwestern Medical Center
Parkland Health and Hospital System
Dallas, Texas

Jamie Morgan, MD
Assistant Professor
Department of Obstetrics and Gynecology
University of Texas Southwestern Medical Center
Parkland Health and Hospital System
Dallas, Texas

Mc Graw Hill Education

New York Chicago San Francisco Athens London Madrid Mexico City
Milan New Delhi Singapore Sydney Toronto

Williams Obstetrics Study Guide, 25th Edition

1 2 3 4 5 6 7 8 9 DSS 23 22 21 20 19 18

ISBN: 978-1-259-64290-6
MHID: 1-259-64290-9

NOTICE

Medicine is an ever-changing science. As new research and clinical experience broaden our knowledge, changes in treatment and drug therapy are required. The authors and the publisher of this work have checked with sources believed to be reliable in their efforts to provide information that is complete and generally in accord with the standards accepted at the time of publication. However, in view of the possibility of human error or changes in medical sciences, neither the authors nor the publisher nor any other party who has been involved in the preparation or publication of this work warrants that the information contained herein is in every respect accurate or complete, and they disclaim all responsibility for any errors or omissions or for the results obtained from use of the information contained in this work. Readers are encouraged to confirm the information contained herein with other sources. For example and in particular, readers are advised to check the product information sheet included in the package of each drug they plan to administer to be certain that the information contained in this work is accurate and that changes have not been made in the recommended dose or in the contraindications for administration. This recommendation is of particular importance in connection with new or infrequently used drugs.

This book was set in Adobe Garamond Pro by Aptara, Inc.
The editors were Andrew Moyer and Regina Y. Brown.
The production supervisor was Rick Ruzycka.
Project management was provided by Indu Jawwad, Aptara, Inc.
The cover designer was W2 Design.

This book is printed on acid-free paper.

DEDICATION

At the same time I have endeavoured to present the more practical aspects of obstetrics in such a manner as to be of direct service to the obstetrician at the bedside.

—J. Whitridge Williams (1903)

We dedicate this edition of the study guide to perhaps the most important and oft-forgotten teachers of our profession, our patients. They permit us the unique privilege of caring for them and their unborn children, allow us the opportunity to hone our medical and surgical skills on a daily basis, stimulate our perpetual pursuit of knowledge, and inform future areas of investigation in the field of obstetrics. The many clinical images and case-based questions that fill this study guide are a tangible embodiment of their many contributions to our field and profession. We offer this dedication as a token symbol of our sincere gratitude.

Shivani Patel
Scott Roberts
Vanessa Rogers
Ashley Zink
Elaine Duryea
Jamie Morgan

CONTENTS

SECTION 1

OVERVIEW

SECTION 2

MATERNAL ANATOMY AND PHYSIOLOGY

SECTION 3

PLACENTATION, EMBRYOGENESIS, AND FETAL DEVELOPMENT

SECTION 4

PRECONCEPTIONAL AND PRENATAL CARE

SECTION 5

THE FETAL PATIENT

SECTION 6

EARLY PREGNANCY COMPLICATIONS

SECTION 7

LABOR

SECTION 8

DELIVERY

SECTION 9

THE NEWBORN

SECTION 10

THE PUERPERIUM

SECTION 11

OBSTETRICAL COMPLICATIONS

SECTION 12

MEDICAL AND SURGICAL COMPLICATIONS

PREFACE

The *Williams Obstetrics 25th Edition Study Guide* is designed to assess comprehension and retention of information presented in *Williams Obstetrics, 25th edition.* The questions for each section have been selected to emphasize the key points from each chapter. In total, nearly 2100 questions have been created from the 65 chapters. Questions are in a multiple-choice format, and one single best answer should be chosen for each. With this edition, we have also included more than 400 full-color and ultrasound images as question material. In addition, clinical case questions have been added to test implementation of content learned. At the end of each chapter, answers are found, and a page guide directs readers to the section of text that contains the answer. We hope that our clinical approach to this guide translates into a more accurate test of important clinical knowledge.

Shivani Patel
Scott Roberts
Vanessa Rogers
Ashley Zink
Elaine Duryea
Jamie Morgan

SECTION 1

OVERVIEW

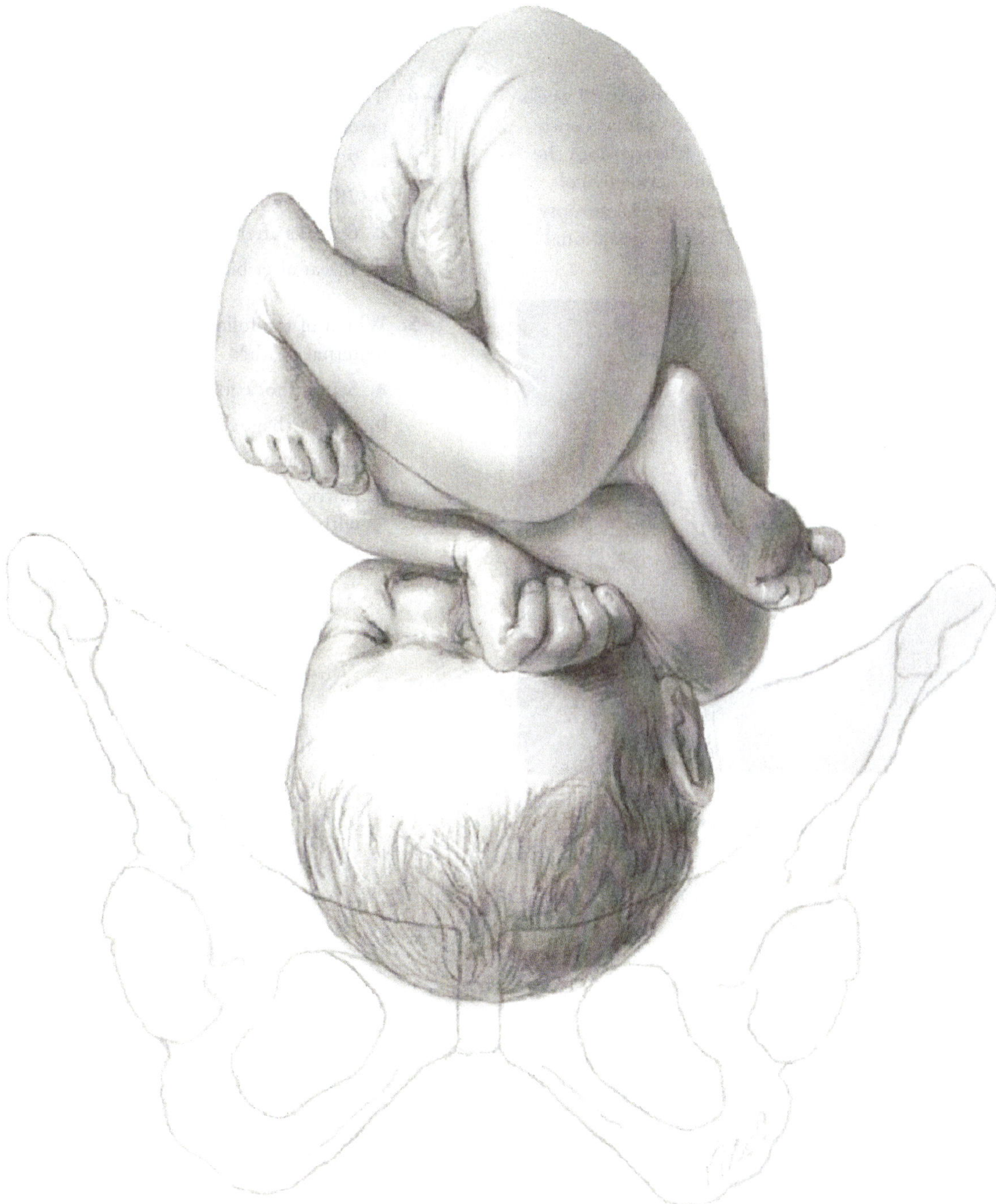

CHAPTER 1

Overview of Obstetrics

1–1. Which of the following is defined as the sum of stillbirths and neonatal deaths per 1000 total births?

a. Fetal death rate

b. Infant mortality rate

c. Perinatal mortality rate

d. Neonatal mortality rate

1–2. A patient presents with severe preeclampsia at 37 weeks' gestation. Labor is induced and she spontaneously delivers a 3260-g neonate. In the delivery room she complains of a severe headache and suddenly collapses. She is unable to be resuscitated. An autopsy reveals the following finding. Based on gestational age, how would her neonate be classified?

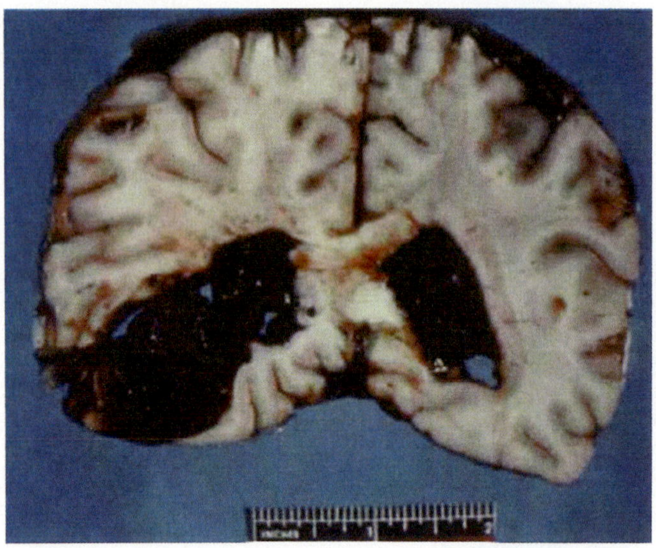

Reproduced with permission from Cunningham FG, Leveno KJ, Bloom SL, et al (eds): Hypertensive disorders. In Williams Obstetrics, 25th ed. New York, McGraw-Hill, 2018, Figure 40-10.

a. Postterm

b. Full term

c. Post dates

d. Early term

1–3. How would the maternal death in Question 1–2 be classified?

a. Perinatal death

b. Nonmaternal death

c. Direct maternal death

d. Indirect maternal death

1–4. The perinatal period starts after delivery at 20 weeks' gestation or older. When does it end?

a. 7 days after birth

b. 28 days after birth

c. 6 weeks after birth

d. 1 year after birth

1–5. Which of the following is an example of an indirect maternal death?

a. Septic shock following an abortion

b. Hemorrhage following uterine atony

c. Aspiration following an eclamptic seizure

d. Aortic rupture at 36 weeks' gestation in a patient with Marfan syndrome

1–6. A 30-year-old multigravida presents with ruptured membranes at term but without labor. Following induction with misoprostol, her labor progresses rapidly, and she spontaneously delivers a liveborn 3300-g neonate. Immediately after delivery, she complains of dyspnea. She becomes apneic and pulseless and is unable to be resuscitated. Photomicrographs from her autopsy reveal fetal squames (*arrows*) within the pulmonary vasculature. How would her death be classified?

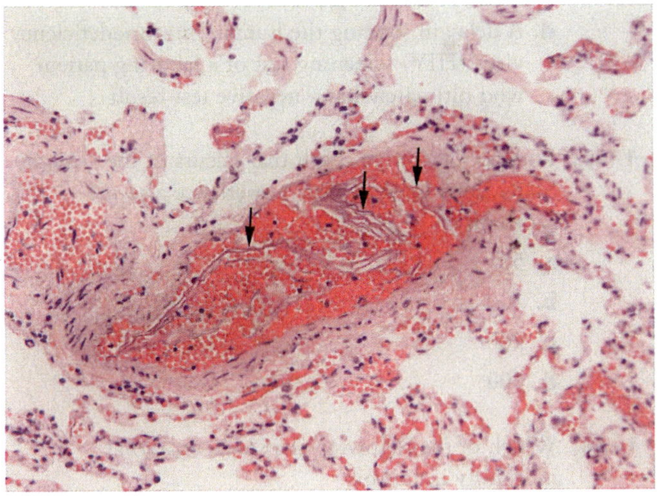

- **a.** Perinatal death
- **b.** Nonmaternal death
- **c.** Direct maternal death
- **d.** Indirect maternal death

1–7. A patient presents at 22 weeks' gestation with spontaneous rupture of membranes and delivers a 489-g male infant who dies at 4 hours of life. Her last menstrual period and early sonographic evaluation confirm her gestational dating. All except which of the following definitions accurately apply to this delivery?

- **a.** Abortus
- **b.** Preterm neonate
- **c.** Early neonatal death
- **d.** Extremely low birthweight

1–8. Which of the following is accurate regarding pregnancy rates in the United states?

- **a.** The fertility rate has been stable since 1990.
- **b.** The lowest birth rate ever was recorded in 2015.
- **c.** The birth rate increased for adolescents in 2015.
- **d.** More than half of births in the United States are unintended at the time of conception.

1–9. Which of the following is defined as the number of maternal deaths that result from the reproductive process per 100,000 live births?

- **a.** Maternal mortality rate
- **b.** Maternal mortality ratio
- **c.** Direct maternal death rate
- **d.** Pregnancy-related death rate

1–10. A 26-year-old woman is brought to the emergency department with abdominal pain and dizziness. On exam she is found to be pale and tachycardic. Her urine pregnancy test is positive and her hemoglobin is 5 g/dL. Bedside ultrasound reveals a left adnexal mass and free fluid. She is taken to the operating room for a ruptured ectopic pregnancy. While in the operating room she arrests and is unable to be resuscitated. How would her death be classified?

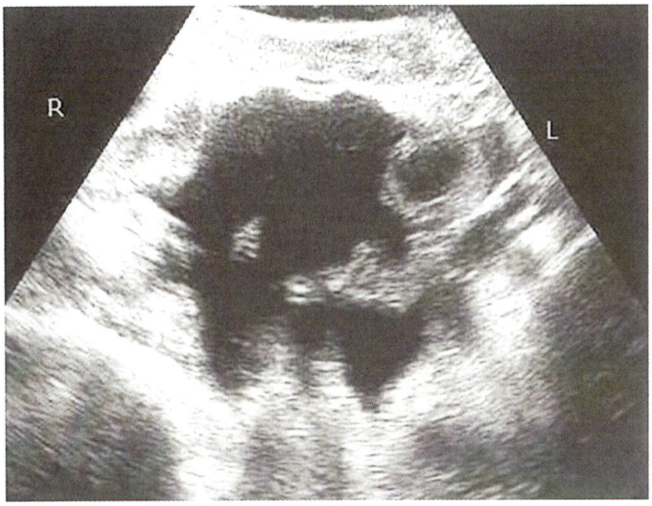

- **a.** Perinatal death
- **b.** Nonmaternal death
- **c.** Indirect maternal death
- **d.** Pregnancy-related death

1–11. Most infant deaths occur in which of the following groups?

- **a.** Low-birthweight infants
- **b.** Infants of diabetic mothers
- **c.** Infants with congenital anomalies
- **d.** Infants with chromosome abnormalities

1–12. Which of the following is the most common cause of pregnancy-related deaths in the United States?

a. Sepsis

b. Hemorrhage

c. Cardiovascular

d. Thromboembolism

1–13. Which of the following explains the trend on this graph?

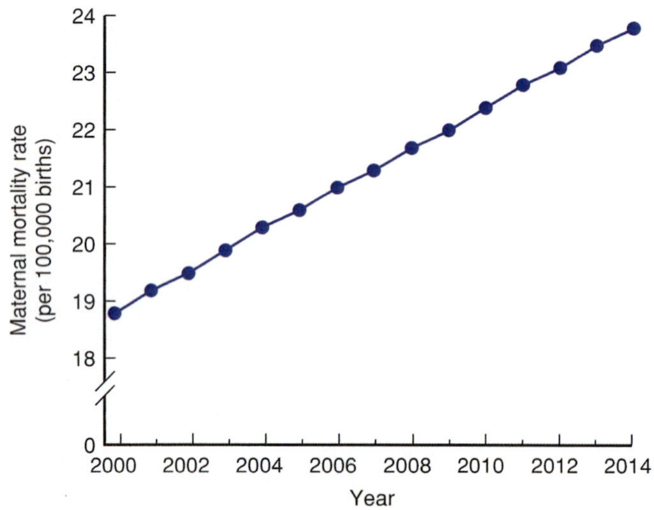

Data from MacDorman MF, Declercq E: Trends and characteristics of United States out-of-hospital births 2004–2014: new information on risk status and access to care. Birth 43(2):116, 2016a. MacDorman MF, Declercq E, Cabral H, et al: Recent increases in the U.S. maternal mortality rate: disentangling trends from measurement issues. Obstet Gynecol 128(3):447, 2016b.

a. An increase in maternal deaths

b. Improved reporting of maternal deaths

c. More pregnant women suffer from severe chronic health conditions

d. All of the above

1–14. Which of the following obstetrical complications contributes the least to the pregnancy-related death rate in the United States?

a. Infection

b. Preeclampsia

c. Amniotic fluid embolus

d. Anesthetic complications

1–15. Which racial group has the highest maternal mortality rate?

a. White

b. Black

c. Asian

d. Hispanic

1–16. All except which of the following is an example of a "near miss"?

a. A postpartum patient who falls in the shower without injury

b. High spinal anesthesia resulting in intubation, admission to the intensive-care-unit, and a ventilator-associated pneumonia

c. Failure to give Rh immunoglobulin to a Rh-negative postpartum patient who ultimately has no change in antibody screen

d. A delay in sending the human immunodeficiency virus (HIV) screening test of a laboring patient who ultimately has a negative test result

1–17. For every maternal death that occurs in the United States, how many women experience a severe morbidity?

a. 50

b. 100

c. 200

d. 500

1–18. Which of the following is a severe maternal morbidity indicator?

a. Hypertension

b. Cystic fibrosis

c. Sickle cell crisis

d. Systemic lupus erythematosus

1–19. Which of the following is a lesson from former President Barack Obama's summary of the Affordable Care Act?

a. Pragmatism is important

b. Special interests pose an obstacle to change

c. Change is difficult in the face of hyperpartisanship

d. All of the above

1–20. Medicaid insures approximately what percentage of the births in the United States?

a. 25%

b. 33%

c. 48%

d. 62%

1–21. What insurance type covered more than half of all hospital stays for preterm and low-birthweight infants?

a. Medicaid

b. Medicare

c. Private insurance

d. Health maintenance organizations

1–22. Which of the following is a cause of excessive health care costs in the United States?

a. Greater life expectancy

b. Better healthcare outcomes

c. Greater use of medical technology

d. All of the above

1–23. Which of the following best describes the primary role of the Ob/Gyn hospitalist?

a. Assist other obstetricians in procedures

b. Be a backup for physicians taking calls from home

c. Care for hospitalized patients who have no primary doctor

d. Care for hospitalized obstetrical patients and help manage their emergencies

1–24. What do some hospitals hope to gain by having an Ob/Gyn hospitalist?

a. Less cost

b. Fewer *near misses*

c. Improved quality and safety

d. Improved patient satisfaction

1–25. What percentage of home births are attended by nurse midwives certified by the American Midwife Certification Board?

a. 26%

b. 33%

c. 52%

d. 78%

1–26. Which of the following is accurate regarding home birth in the United States?

a. The American College of Obstetricians and Gynecologists endorses home births

b. They are associated with a higher perinatal mortality rate than births occurring in medical facilities

c. Randomized trials suggest their outcomes are equivalent to those of births occurring in medical facilities

d. None of the above

1–27. For which of the following purposes would fetal chromosomal microarray analysis be potentially beneficial?

a. Evaluating a stillborn fetus

b. Screening the fetus of an advanced-age mother

c. Evaluating the fetus with trisomy 21 and a double-outlet right ventricle

d. Screening the fetus at 12 weeks' gestation whose mother personally carries a balanced translocation

1–28. Which of the following contributes to the current health care fiscal crisis?

a. Prices for surgical procedures

b. Prices charged by health insurance companies

c. Expensive interventions without robust evidence

d. All of the above

1–29. What population is most affected by governmental interference with the reproductive rights of women?

a. Immigrants

b. Black women

c. Rural population

d. Indigent population

1–30. The increase in opioid abuse in pregnancy has led to which of the following?

a. A rise in neonatal abstinence syndrome

b. Increase in intrauterine growth restriction

c. Improvement in pain control during labor

d. Increase in neurologic anomalies diagnosed in utero

1–31. A 16-year-old G1 delivers an infant with a complex congenital heart defect. The death of the newborn at 5 days of life due to the congenital heart defect would be counted in which of the following rates?

a. Infant mortality rate

b. Perinatal mortality rate

c. Early neonatal death rate

d. All of the above

1–32. As the patient in Question 1–31 makes family planning decisions in the postpartum period, which of the following will cause her to be most affected by governmental interference with women's reproductive rights?

a. Age

b. Ethnicity

c. Pregnancy within the last year

d. Prior child with a congenital anomaly

CHAPTER 1 ANSWER KEY

Question number	Letter answer	Page cited	Header cited
1–1	**c**	p. 3	Definitions
1–2	**d**	p. 3	Definitions
1–3	**c**	p. 3	Definitions
1–4	**b**	p. 3	Definitions
1–5	**d**	p. 3	Definitions
1–6	**c**	p. 3	Definitions
1–7	**a**	p. 3	Definitions
1–8	**d**	p. 4	Pregnancy Rates in the United States
1–9	**b**	p. 4	Definitions
1–10	**d**	p. 4	Definitions
1–11	**a**	p. 5	Infant Deaths
1–12	**c**	p. 5	Maternal Mortality
1–13	**d**	p. 5	Maternal Mortality
1–14	**d**	p. 5	Maternal Mortality
1–15	**b**	p. 6	Maternal Mortality
1–16	**b**	p. 6	Severe Maternal Morbidity
1–17	**c**	p. 6	Severe Maternal Morbidity
1–18	**c**	p. 7	Table 1-3
1–19	**d**	p. 6	Obamacare and Medicaid
1–20	**c**	p. 7	Obamacare and Medicaid
1–21	**a**	p. 7	Obamacare and Medicaid
1–22	**c**	p. 7	Maternal and Infant Health Care Costs
1–23	**d**	p. 8	The Ob/Gyn Hospitalist
1–24	**c**	p. 8	The Ob/Gyn Hospitalist
1–25	**b**	p. 8	Home Births
1–26	**b**	p. 8	Home Births
1–27	**a**	p. 8	Genomic Technology
1–28	**d**	p. 8	Maternal and Infant Health Care Costs
1–29	**d**	p. 9	Family Planning Services
1–30	**a**	p. 9	Opioid Abuse in Pregnancy
1–31	**d**	p. 3	Definitions
1–32	**a**	p. 9	Family Planning Services

SECTION 2

MATERNAL ANATOMY AND PHYSIOLOGY

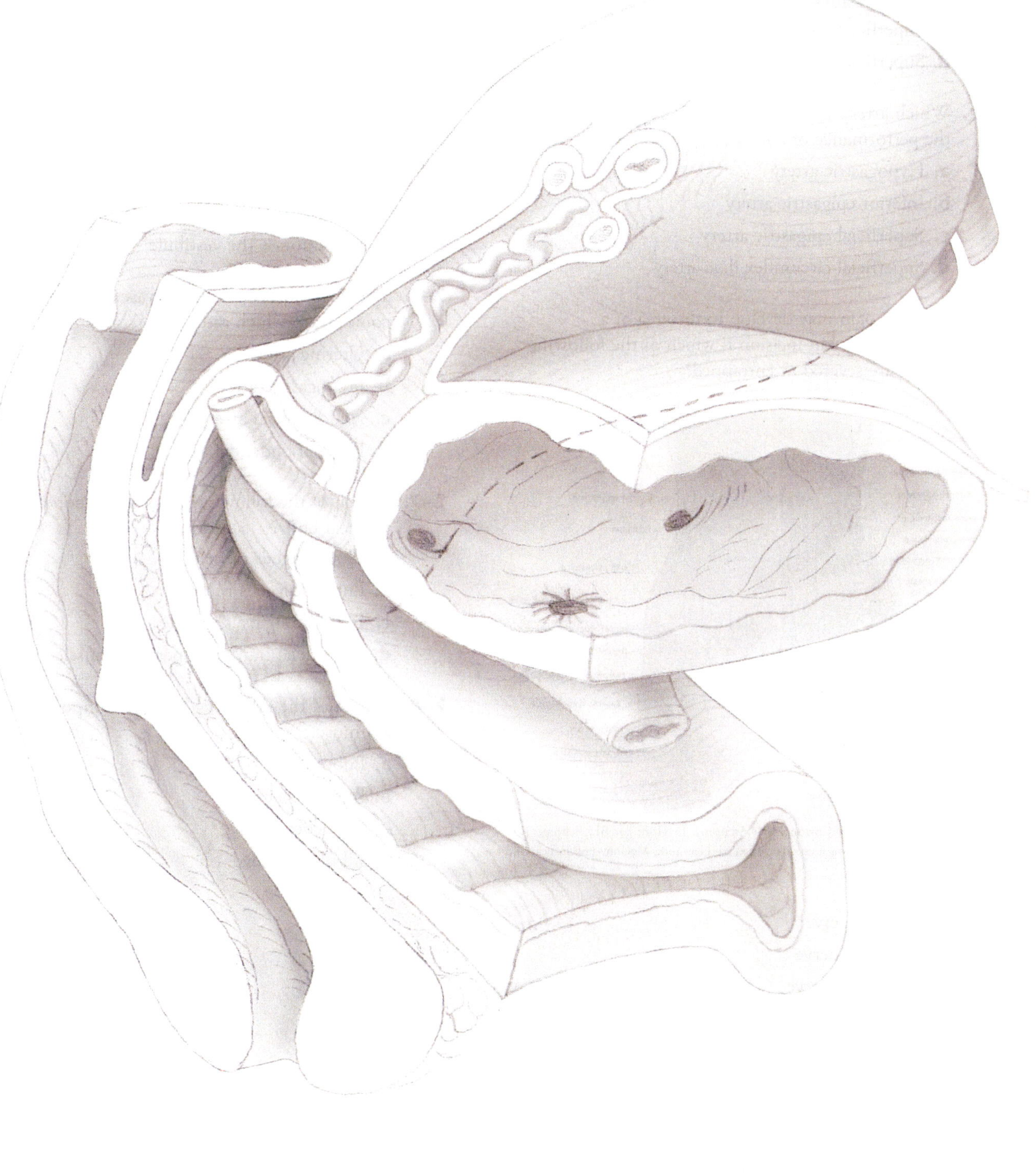

CHAPTER 2

Maternal Anatomy

2–1. Which artery is frequently encountered when a Pfannenstiel skin incision is performed during a cesarean delivery?

- **a.** Hypogastric artery
- **b.** Inferior epigastric artery
- **c.** Superficial epigastric artery
- **d.** Superficial circumflex iliac artery

2–2. Which artery should be found and ligated prior to the performance of a Maylard incision?

- **a.** Hypogastric artery
- **b.** Inferior epigastric artery
- **c.** Superficial epigastric artery
- **d.** Superficial circumflex iliac artery

2–3. Chronic pain may develop in the area of a Pfannenstiel skin incision if which of the following nerves are severed or entrapped?

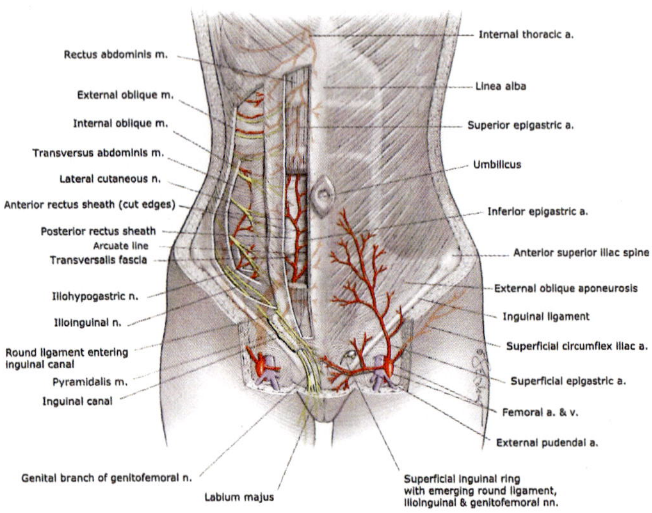

Modified with permission from Corton MM: Anatomy. In Hoffman BL, Schorge JO, Bradshaw KD, et al (eds): Williams Gynecology, 3rd ed. New York, McGraw-Hill Education, 2016, Figure 38-3.

- **a.** Femoral nerve
- **b.** Subcostal nerve
- **c.** Intercostal nerve
- **d.** Iliohypogastric nerve

2–4. The labia minora is invested by which of the following structures?

- **a.** Hair follicles
- **b.** Eccrine glands
- **c.** Apocrine glands
- **d.** Sebaceous glands

2–5. Which of the following does not perforate the vestibule?

- **a.** Urethra
- **b.** Skene glands
- **c.** Bartholin glands
- **d.** All perforate the vestibule

2–6. The posterior vaginal wall's vascular supply primarily comes from which artery?

- **a.** Uterine artery
- **b.** Hypogastric artery
- **c.** Middle rectal artery
- **d.** Internal pudendal artery

2–7. Which of the following is not a component of the perineal body?

- **a.** Iliococcygeus muscle
- **b.** Pubococcygeus muscle
- **c.** Bulbospongiosus muscle
- **d.** Superficial transverse perineal muscle

2–8. Which of the following muscles compose the levator ani muscle?

- **a.** Puborectalis
- **b.** Iliococcygeus
- **c.** Pubococcygeus
- **d.** All of the above

2–9. Which of the following statements regarding the borders of the ischiorectal fossae is incorrect?

a. Anterior border: inferior border of the posterior triangle

b. Medial border: anal sphincter complex and fascia of the levator ani

c. Lateral border: obturator internus muscle fascia and ischial tuberosity

d. Posterior border: gluteus maximus muscle and sacrotuberous ligament

2–10. Which combination of structures provides support for fecal continence?

a. Internal and external anal sphincter

b. External anal sphincter and levator ani muscle

c. Puborectalis muscle and internal anal sphincter

d. Puborectalis muscle and external anal sphincter

2–11. A 33-year-old nulligravida undergoing labor without anesthesia arrests at +2 station. You decide to perform an outlet forceps delivery with a pudendal nerve block. What is the landmark you use to perform the nerve block?

a. Ischial spine

b. Sacrospinous ligament

c. Sacrotuberous ligament

d. All of the above

2–12. Which of the following statements is accurate in regard to the uterus?

a. It is made up of two equal parts.

b. The bulk of uterine tissue is fibroelastic tissue.

c. Visceral peritoneum covers the anterior surface.

d. Pregnancy stimulates uterine growth through hyperplasia.

2–13. Which of the following refers to the blue tint of the cervix that is due to increased cervical vascularity in pregnancy?

a. Hegar sign

b. Goodell sign

c. Chadwick sign

d. All of the above

2–14. During a postpartum hysterectomy for intractable bleeding, a Heaney clamp is placed on the uterine artery near its insertion to the uterus. What is the relationship between the ureter and uterine artery at this point?

a. The ureter is 2 cm medial to the uterine artery at this location.

b. The ureter is 2 cm medial to the uterine artery and crosses under it.

c. The ureter is 2 cm lateral to the cervix and crosses over the uterine artery.

d. The ureter is 2 cm lateral to the cervix and crosses under the uterine artery.

2–15. The vascular supply of the uterus comes from which of the follow arteries?

a. Uterine artery

b. Sampson artery

c. Middle sacral artery

d. Middle rectal artery

2–16. Which of the following arteries comes off the posterior division of the internal iliac artery?

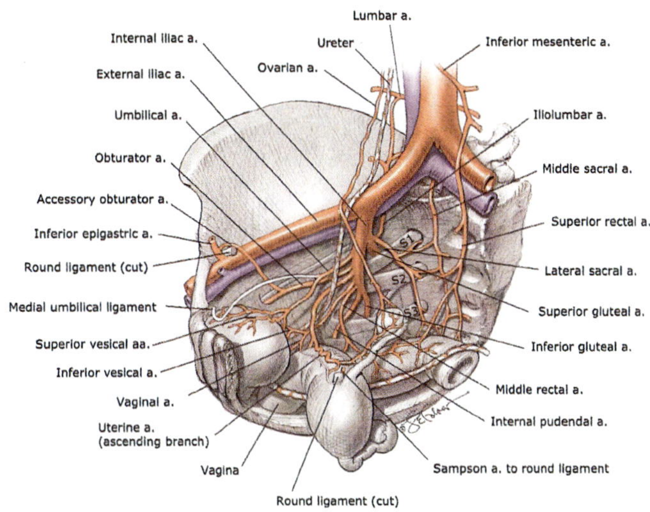

Reproduced with permission from Corton MM: Anatomy. In Hoffman BL, Schorge JO, Bradshaw KD, et al (eds): Williams Gynecology, 3rd ed. New York, McGraw-Hill Education, 2016, Figure 38-12.

a. Uterine artery

b. Obturator artery

c. Superior vesical artery

d. Superior gluteal artery

2–17. Which of the following statements regarding the pelvic visceral innervation is inaccurate?

a. Parasympathetic innervation is from L4–S1.

b. Origins of sympathetic innervation is from T10–L2.

c. The superior hypogastric plexus is also known as the presacral nerve.

d. The pelvic plexus is the result of blending of the sympathetic and parasympathetic nerves.

2–18. Which of the following is the correct anatomic progression of the fallopian tube from proximal to distal?

a. Isthmus, ampulla, infundibulum

b. Ampulla, infundibulum, isthmus

c. Infundibulum, ampulla, isthmus

d. Ampulla, isthmus, infundibulum

2–19. A cross-section of the extrauterine fallopian tube contains which of the following?

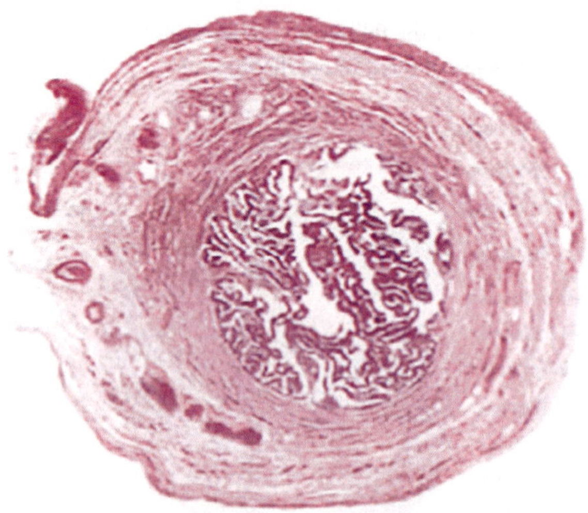

Reproduced with permission from Cunningham FG, Leveno KJ, Bloom SL, et al (eds): Maternal anatomy. In William Obstetrics, 25th ed. New York, McGraw-Hill, 2018, Figure 2-14. Photo contributor: Dr. Kelley S. Carrick.

a. Myosalpinx

b. Mesosalpinx

c. Endosalpinx

d. All of the above

2–20. Which bones make up the pelvis?

a. Sacrum

b. Coccyx

c. Innominate

d. All of the above

2–21. The mobility of which joint aids in the delivery of the obstructed shoulder in the case of a shoulder dystocia?

a. Sacroiliac

b. Sacrococcygeal

c. Pubic symphysis

d. All of the above

2–22. Which of the following is the correct anatomical description of the ureter?

a. Passes just lateral to the ovarian vessels

b. Lies inferolateral to the uterosacral ligaments

c. Crosses underneath the bifurcation of the common iliac artery

d. Lies medial to the anterior branches of the internal iliac artery as it descends in the pelvis

2–23. The pelvic ureter receives blood supply from which of the following blood vessels?

a. Uterine

b. Internal iliac

c. Common iliac

d. All of the above

2–24. Which plane is the plane of least pelvic dimensions?

a. The plane of the midpelvis

b. The plane of the pelvic inlet

c. The plane of the pelvic outlet

d. None of the above

2–25. The pelvic inlet is bounded by which of the following?

a. Posteriorly by the promontory

b. Laterally by the linea terminalis

c. Anteriorly by horizontal pubic rami

d. All of the above

2–26. Which of the following does not characterize the obstetric conjugate?

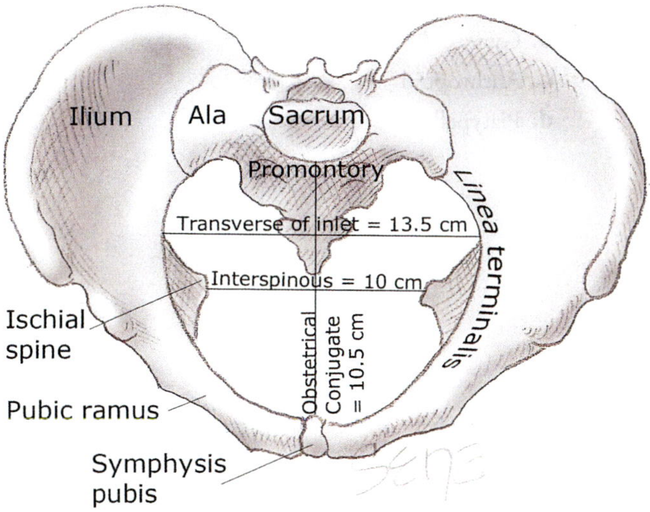

Reproduced with permission from Cunningham FG, Leveno KJ, Bloom SL, et al (eds): Maternal anatomy. In William Obstetrics, 25th ed. New York, McGraw-Hill, 2018, Figure 2-16.

- **a.** It cannot be directly measured.
- **b.** It normally measures 11 cm or more.
- **c.** It is the least clinically important diameter of the pelvic inlet.
- **d.** It is the shortest distance from the sacral promontory and the symphysis pubis.

2–27. Which of the following is accurate regarding the midpelvis?

- **a.** Contains the smallest pelvic diameter
- **b.** Serves as the point to measure station
- **c.** Is marked by the interspinous diameter
- **d.** All of the above

2–28. What is the most common Caldwell-Moloy anatomical pelvis?

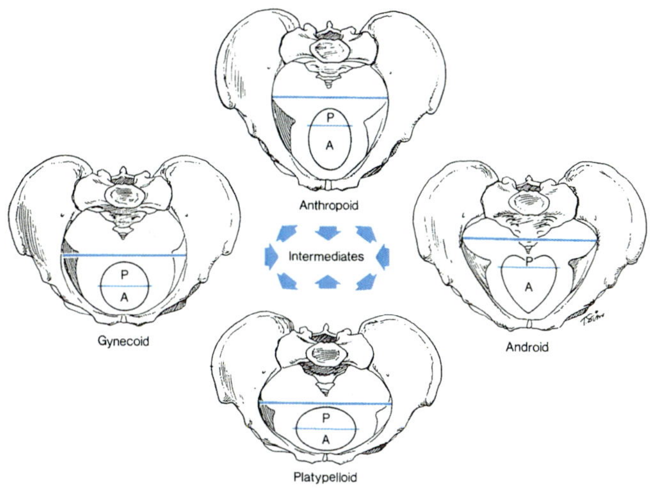

Reproduced with permission from Cunningham FG, Leveno KJ, Bloom SL, et al (eds): Maternal anatomy. In William Obstetrics, 25th ed. New York, McGraw-Hill, 2018, Figure 2-17.

- **a.** Android
- **b.** Gynecoid
- **c.** Anthropoid
- **d.** Platypelloid

2–29. A 22-year-old primigravida presents in active labor at 5 cm and −2 station. Which of the following is true?

- **a.** The fetal head is engaged.
- **b.** The biparietal diameter has reached the level of the midpelvis.
- **c.** The biparietal diameter has reached the level of the pelvic inlet.
- **d.** None of the above

2–30. Regarding the patient in Question 2–29, 2 hours later she is 8 cm dilated and the fetal head is noted to be at 0 station. Which of the following is true?

- **a.** The fetus is too big to fit through her pelvis.
- **b.** Internal rotation of the fetal head to transverse should be occurring.
- **c.** The top of the fetal head is noted at the level of the midpelvic interspinous diameter.
- **d.** None of the above

2–31. After three more hours the patient in Question 2–29 is completely dilated and the head is at +5 station. Which of the following is true?

a. The caput may be visualized at the level of the introitus.

b. The caput is now 5 cm distal to the midpelvic interspinous diameter.

c. The fetal head has most likely internally rotated into an occiput anterior presentation.

d. All of the above

2–32. The fetal head presents at +5 station in a transverse diameter. What is the most likely pelvic shape?

a. Android

b. Gynecoid

c. Anthropoid

d. Platypelloid

CHAPTER 2 ANSWER KEY

Question number	Letter answer	Page cited	Header cited
2–1	**c**	p. 15	Blood Supply
2–2	**b**	p. 15	Blood Supply
2–3	**d**	p. 16	Innervation
2–4	**d**	p. 17	Mons Pubis, Labia, and Clitoris
2–5	**d**	p. 17	Vestibule
2–6	**c**	p. 19	Vagina and Hymen
2–7	**a**	p. 19	Perineum
2–8	**d**	p. 19	Perineum
2–9	**a**	p. 21	Ischioanal Fossae
2–10	**a**	p. 22	Anal Sphincter Complex
2–11	**a**	p. 22	Pudendal Nerve
2–12	**c**	p. 23	Uterus
2–13	**c**	p. 24	Cervix
2–14	**d**	p. 25	Pelvic Blood Supply
2–15	**a**	p. 26	Pelvic Blood Supply
2–16	**d**	p. 26	Figure 2-12
2–17	**a**	p. 27	Pelvic innervation
2–18	**a**	p. 28	Fallopian Tubes
2–19	**d**	p. 28	Fallopian Tubes
2–20	**d**	p. 29	Pelvic Bones
2–21	**a**	p. 29	Pelvic Joints
2–22	**d**	p. 29	Ureter
2–23	**d**	p. 29	Ureter
2–24	**a**	p. 30	Planes and Diameters of the Pelvis
2–25	**d**	p. 30	Pelvic Inlet
2–26	**b**	p. 30	Pelvic Inlet
2–27	**d**	p. 30	Midpelvis and Pelvic Outlet
2–28	**b**	p. 31	Pelvic Shapes
2–29	**d**	p. 30	Pelvic Inlet
2–30	**c**	p. 30	Pelvic Inlet and Midpelvis and Pelvic Outlet
2–31	**d**	p. 30	Midpelvis and Pelvic Outlet
2–32	**b**	p. 31	Pelvic Shapes

CHAPTER 3

Congenital Genitourinary Abnormalities

3–1. Which structure arises from the urogenital sinus?

a. Uterus
b. Distal vagina
c. Fallopian tubes
d. Proximal vagina

3–2. Which uterine anomaly shown below is least likely to be associated with a renal abnormality?

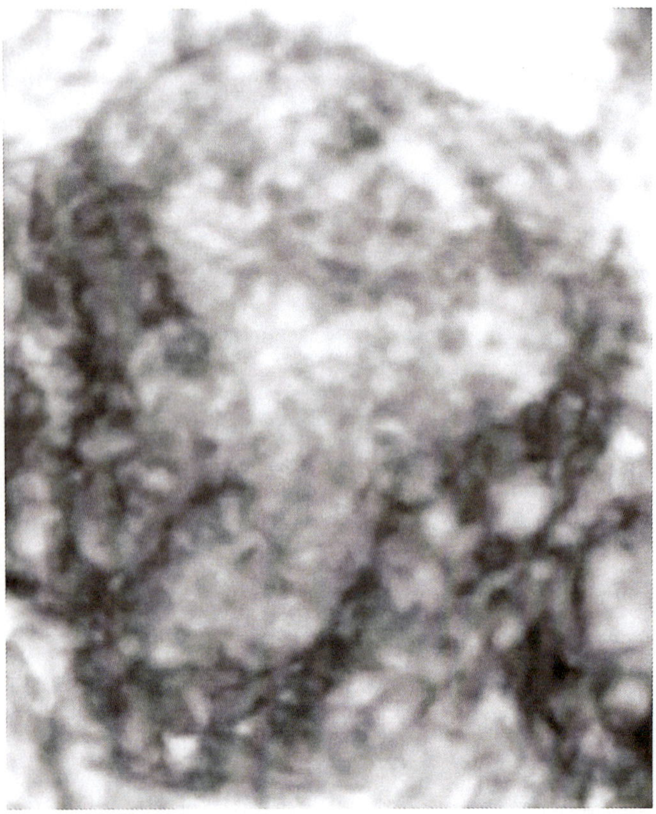

a. Arcuate uterus
b. Uterine didelphys
c. Unicornuate uterus
d. Müllerian agenesis

3–3. Which is a remnant of mesonephric tissue?

a. Urachus
b. Bartholin cyst
c. Gartner duct cyst
d. Urethral diverticulum

3–4. At what gestational age is it possible to visually differentiate between male and female external genitalia?

a. 10 weeks' gestation
b. 12 weeks' gestation
c. 14 weeks' gestation
d. 16 weeks' gestation

3–5. Where is fetal antimüllerian hormone produced?

a. Theca cells
b. Leydig cells
c. Sertoli cells
d. Granulosa cells

3–6. Which complication is associated with Turner syndrome?

a. Diabetes mellitus
b. Hashimoto thyroiditis
c. Coarctation of the aorta
d. All of the above

3–7. A 30-year-old woman presents to your office at 18 weeks' gestation with a large ovarian mass and complaints of hirsutism and new-onset clitoromegaly. You make a presumptive diagnosis of Sertoli-Leydig cell tumor based on her clinical presentation and elevated levels of androstenedione and testosterone. The action of which of the following placental enzymes allows you to reassure her that her fetus is unlikely to be affected by her elevated androgen levels?

a. Sulfatase
b. Aromatase
c. 5-alpha reductase
d. 17-alpha hydroxylase

3–8. A woman with Mayer-Rokitansky-Küster-Hauser syndrome presents to your office for a consult to discuss her reproductive options as she would like to start a family. Which of the following is her best option for producing a biological child?

a. Timed intercourse
b. Uterine transplant
c. In vitro fertilization
d. In vitro fertilization with a surrogate

3–9. Which imaging modality has the highest accuracy for the diagnosis of uterine anomalies?

a. Hysterosalpingography
b. Magnetic resonance imaging
c. Transvaginal 2-dimensional sonography
d. Transvaginal 3-dimensional sonography

3–10. A woman with a unicornuate uterus is at increased risk for which obstetrical complication?

a. Miscarriage
b. Malpresentation
c. Preterm delivery
d. All of the above

3–11. For which uterine anomaly would a surgical procedure be recommended prior to attempting pregnancy?

a. Arcuate uterus
b. Bicornuate uterus
c. Uterine didelphys
d. Unicornuate uterus with a communicating horn

3–12. Which uterine anomaly arises from a complete lack of fusion of the müllerian ducts?

a. Arcuate uterus
b. Bicornuate uterus
c. Uterine didelphys
d. Unicornuate uterus

3–13. Which finding on 3-dimensional sonography is most consistent with a septate uterus?

a. Two cervices
b. Intrafundal downward cleft measuring <1 cm
c. Intrafundal downward cleft measuring ≥1 cm
d. Inter-cornual angle greater than 105 degrees

3–14. Which uterine anomaly is associated with the highest risk of obstetrical complications?

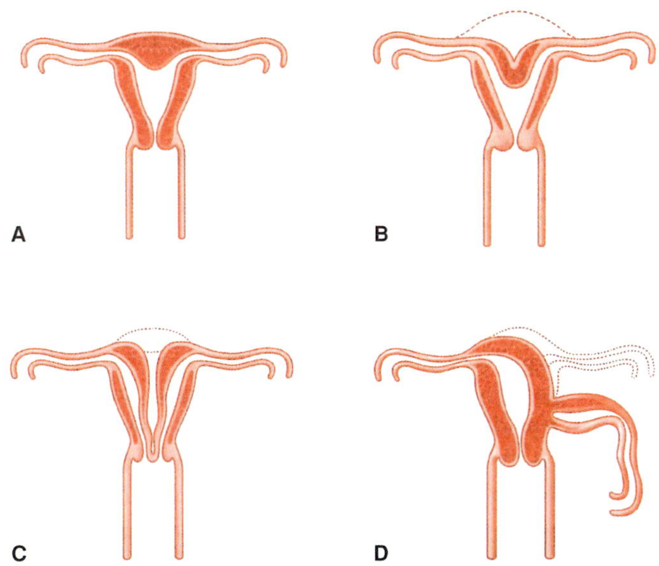

3–15. A woman presents for evaluation of recurrent spontaneous abortions. She undergoes 3-dimensional sonography with the finding below. What intervention may be recommended to decrease her risk of recurrent pregnancy loss?

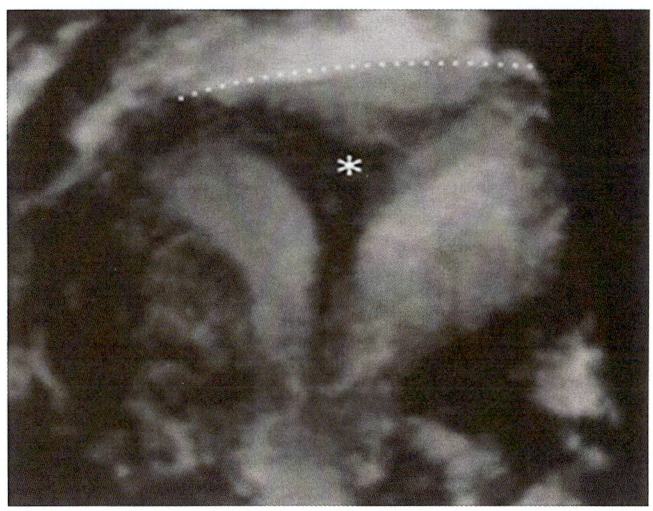

Reproduced with permission from Cunningham FG, Leveno KJ, Bloom SL, et al (eds): Congenital genitourinary abnormalities. In William Obstetrics, 25th ed. New York, McGraw-Hill, 2018, Figure 3-6b.

a. Metroplasty
b. Uterine septum resection
c. Resection of a uterine horn
d. Prophylactic anticoagulation

3–16. A 23-year-old G3P2 woman at 12 weeks' gestation with a uterine anomaly presents asking if she should undergo cerclage placement to prevent preterm birth. The decision to place a cerclage should be based on which of the following?

a. The type of müllerian anomaly
b. Cervical length at 14 weeks' gestation
c. The same criteria used for women without uterine anomalies
d. All of the above

3–17. A woman, whose sonogram at 6 weeks' gestation is pictured below, calls your office at 13 weeks' gestation complaining of abdominal pain and urinary retention. You examine her and suspect uterine incarceration. Which is the most appropriate first step in treatment?

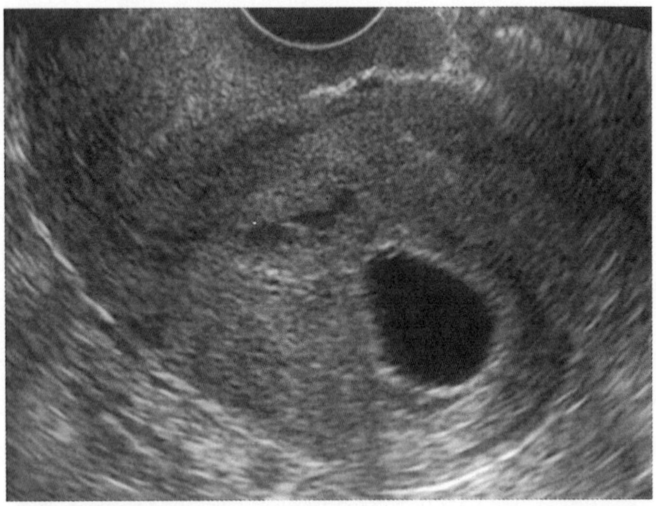

a. General anesthesia
b. Expectant management
c. Urinary catheter placement
d. Attempt manual replacement

3–18. Which category of unicornuate uterus poses the greatest risk for ectopic pregnancy?

a. Agenesis of one horn
b. Communicating noncavitary rudimentary horn
c. Noncommunicating cavitary rudimentary horn
d. Noncommunicating noncavitary rudimentary horn

3–19. A longitudinal vaginal septum is least likely to be seen with which müllerian anomaly?

a. Septate uterus
b. Bicornuate uterus
c. Uterine didelphys
d. Unicornuate uterus

3–20. A 22-year-old G1 presents to your office for prenatal care. During transvaginal 2-dimensional sonography a müllerian anomaly is suspected, so a 3-dimensional study is performed (shown below). This shows an arcuate uterus containing a gestational sac with a fetal pole and cardiac motion. Which of the following outcomes is most likely?

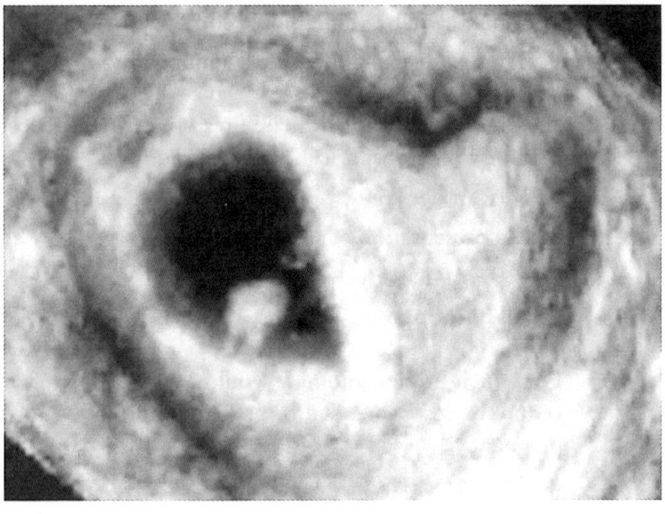

Reproduced with permission from Cunningham FG, Leveno KJ, Bloom SL, et al (eds): Congenital genitourinary abnormalities. In William Obstetrics, 25th ed. New York, McGraw-Hill, 2018, Figure 3-6c.

a. Preterm birth
b. First trimester loss
c. Second trimester loss
d. Uncomplicated term delivery

3–21. Which of the following is a disadvantage of hysterosalpingography for the diagnosis of müllerian anomalies?

a. Dye will not fill noncavitary horns
b. No outer uterine fundal contour seen
c. Dye will not fill noncommunicating horns
d. All of the above

3–22. With magnetic resonance imaging, a septate uterus is displayed here. For diagnosing müllerian anomalies, which of the following are advantages of this modality?

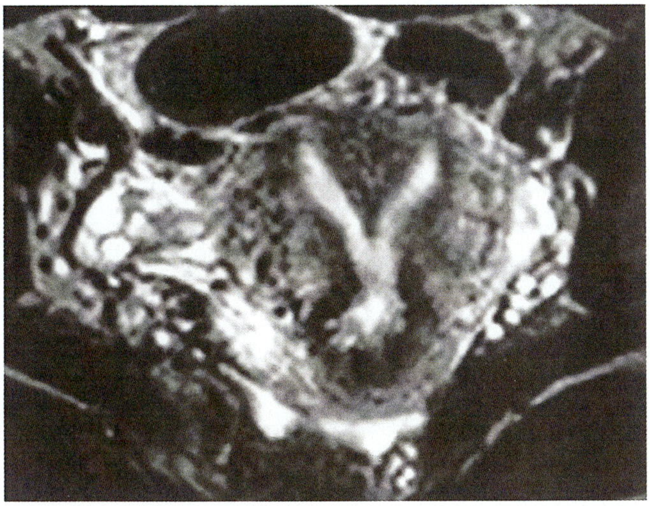

Reproduced with permission from Moschos E, Twickler DM: Techniques used for imaging in gynecology. In Schorge JO, Schaffer JI, Halvorson LM, et al (eds): Williams Gynecology. New York, McGraw-Hill, 2008, Figure 2-27. Photo contributor: Dr. Diane Twickler.

a. Is nearly 100% accurate
b. Displays fundal, myometrial, and endometrial contours
c. Permits identification of concurrent skeletal or renal anomalies
d. All of the above

3–23. In females, what does the metanephros ultimately form?

a. Uterus
b. Kidney
c. Vagina
d. Embryonic remnants

3–24. Your patient presents with vaginal spotting in the first trimester. During transvaginal 2-dimensional sonography an intrauterine pregnancy is seen, and a uterine anomaly is suspected. 3-dimensional sonography is performed and shows a banana-shaped uterus containing a gestational sac. What is the next best step in the care of this pregnancy?

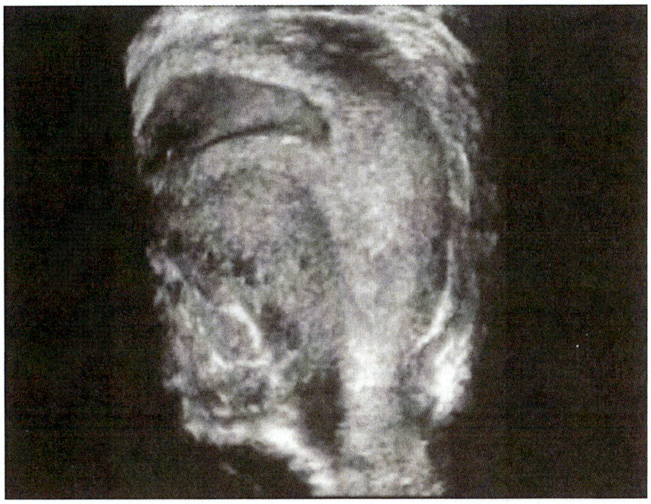

Reproduced with permission from Moschos E, Bailey AA: Techniques used for imaging in gynecology. In Hoffman BL, Schorge JO, Bradshaw KD (eds): Williams Gynecology, 3rd ed. New York, McGraw-Hill, 2016, Figure 2-26.

a. Schedule renal sonographic evaluation
b. Schedule computed tomography with contrast
c. Perform prophylactic cerclage placement at 14 weeks' gestation
d. Recommend pregnancy termination due to high rate of uterine horn rupture

3–25. Which uterine anomaly is seen in this hysterosalpingogram?

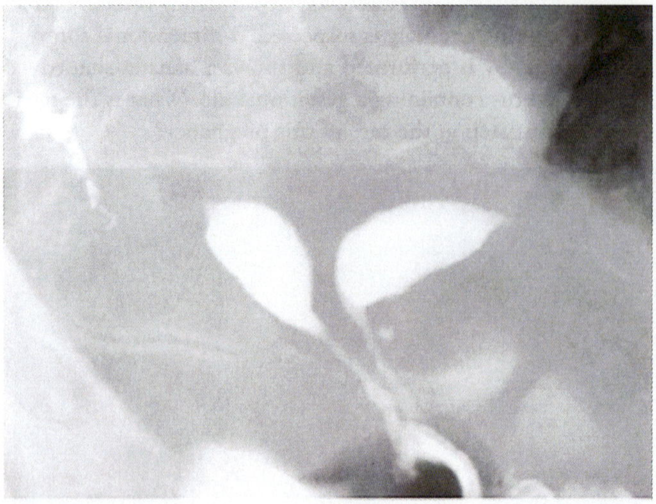

Reproduced with permission from Halvorson LM: Evaluation of the infertile couple. In Schorge JO, Schaffer JI, Halvorson LM, et al (eds): Williams Gynecology. New York, McGraw-Hill, 2008, Figure 19-7C. Photo contributor: Dr. Diane Twickler.

a. Arcuate uterus
b. Septate uterus
c. Uterine didelphys
d. Bicornuate uterus

3–26. Which of the following is the most common uterine anomaly?

a. Uterine agenesis
b. Bicornuate uterus
c. Uterine didelphys
d. Unicornuate uterus

3–27. Local production of which hormone is necessary for the virilization of male genitalia in the fetus?

a. Testosterone
b. Androstenedione
c. Dihydrotestosterone
d. Antimüllerian hormone

3–28. When is this patient most likely to present?

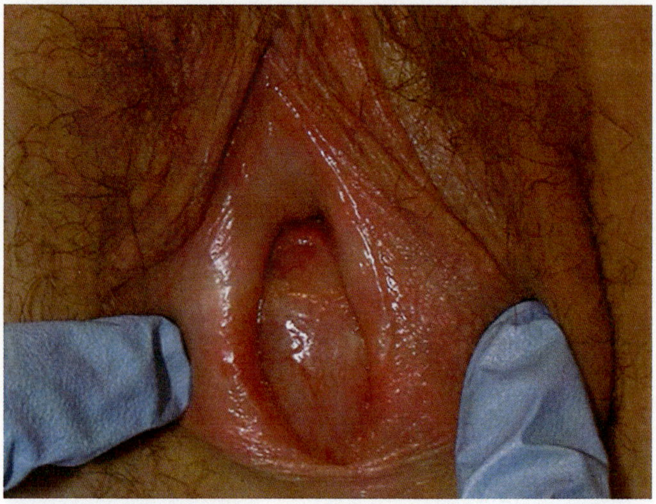

Reproduced with permission from Hoffman BL, Schorge JO, Schaffer JI, et al (eds): Williams Gynecology, 2nd ed. New York, McGraw-Hill, 2012, Figure 18-11. Photo contributor: Dr. Ellen Wilson.

a. In utero with polyhydramnios
b. Perimenarche with amenorrhea
c. Neonatal period with urinary retention
d. Reproductive age with primary infertility

3–29. A sonogram at 24 weeks' gestation demonstrates a mass anterior to the fetal abdomen and the bladder is not seen. The fetus is later confirmed to have bladder exstrophy. This anomaly originates from premature rupture of which of the following?

a. Yolk sac
b. Mesonephros
c. Müllerian duct
d. Cloacal membrane

3–30. Which of the following pairs of female and male structures share a common origin?

a. Ovary and glans penis
b. Labia minora and scrotum
c. Granulosa cells and Leydig cells
d. Paraurethral glands and prostate glands

3–31. A married couple presents with primary infertility. Their work-up is remarkable for azoospermia. The husband is tall, with gynecomastia; you suspect Klinefelter syndrome, which is diagnosed by karyotype. You explain he is at risk for which of the following as compared to other men?

a. Breast cancer

d. Hypothyroidism

c. Diabetes mellitus

d. All of the above

3–32. Which hormone acts locally to prevent the formation of the uterus, fallopian tube, and upper vagina?

a. Testosterone

b. Androstenedione

c. Dihydrotestosterone

d. Antimüllerian hormone

3–33. A 67-year-old woman presents for pelvic sonogram with the findings as shown below. She reports an obstetrical history of multiple first-trimester miscarriages with no live births. What is the most likely uterine anomaly present?

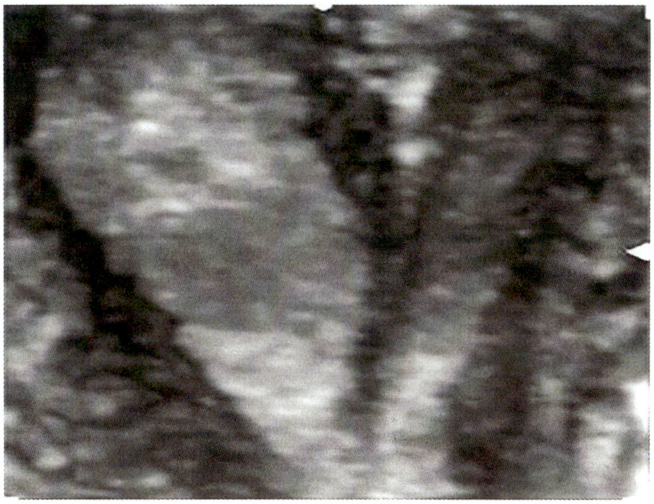

a. Arcuate uterus

b. Septate uterus

c. Bicornuate uterus

d. Uterine didelphys

CHAPTER 3 ANSWER KEY

Question number	Letter answer	Page cited	Header cited
3–1	**b**	p. 33	Embryology of the Genital Tract
3–2	**a**	p. 35	Embryology of the Genital Tract
3–3	**c**	p. 35	Embryology of the Genital Tract
3–4	**b**	p. 35	Embryology of the External Genitalia
3–5	**c**	p. 38	Sexual Differentiation
3–6	**d**	p. 39	Sex Chromosome Disorders of Sex Development
3–7	**b**	p. 40	Androgen Excess
3–8	**d**	p. 42	Vaginal Abnormalities
3–9	**b**	p. 44	Uterine Abnormalities
3–10	**d**	p. 44	Uterine Abnormalities
3–11	**d**	p. 44	Uterine Abnormalities
3–12	**c**	p. 44	Uterine Abnormalities
3–13	**b**	p. 45	Uterine Abnormalities
3–14	**d**	p. 44	Uterine Abnormalities
3–15	**b**	p. 45	Uterine Abnormalities
3–16	**c**	p. 45	Uterine Abnormalities
3–17	**c**	p. 46	Uterine Flexion
3–18	**c**	p. 44	Uterine Abnormalities
3–19	**d**	p. 44	Uterine Abnormalities
3–20	**d**	p. 45	Uterine Abnormalities
3–21	**d**	p. 43	Uterine Abnormalities
3–22	**d**	p. 43	Uterine Abnormalities
3–23	**b**	p. 34	Embryology of the Genital Tract
3–24	**a**	p. 44	Uterine Abnormalities
3–25	**c**	p. 45	Uterine Abnormalities
3–26	**b**	p. 43	Uterine Abnormalities
3–27	**c**	p. 38	Sexual Differentiation
3–28	**b**	p. 42	Bladder and Perineal Abnormalities
3–29	**d**	p. 34	Embryology of the Urinary System
3–30	**d**	p. 38	Disorders of Sexual Development
3–31	**d**	p. 39	Sex Chromosome Disorders of Sex Development
3–32	**d**	p. 38	Sexual Differentiation
3–33	**b**	p. 44	Uterine Abnormalities

CHAPTER 4

Maternal Physiology

4–1. Which of the following accurately characterize Braxton Hicks contractions?

a. Are usually non-rhythmic

b. Have an intensity of 5–25 mmHg

c. Can be detected by bimanual examination

d. All the above

4–2. Which of the following soluble receptors attenuates vascular endothelial and placental growth factor in vivo?

a. PIGF

b. sFlt-1

c. VEGF

d. Estrogen

4–3. A 23-year-old presents for her initial prenatal care visit. She undergoes an ultrasound and the findings are shown below. What is the adnexal mass seen below?

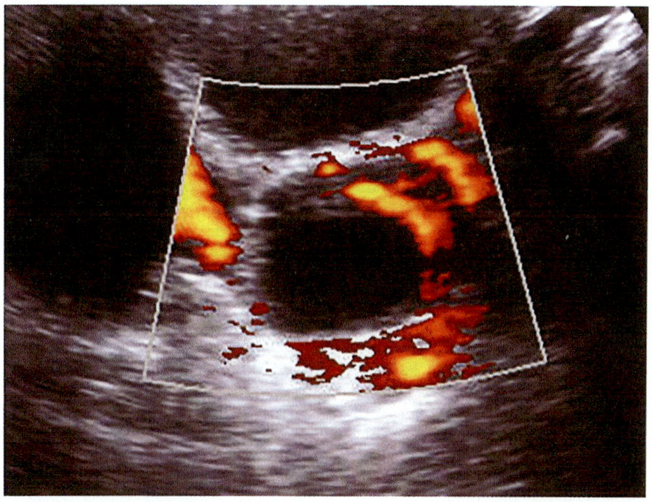

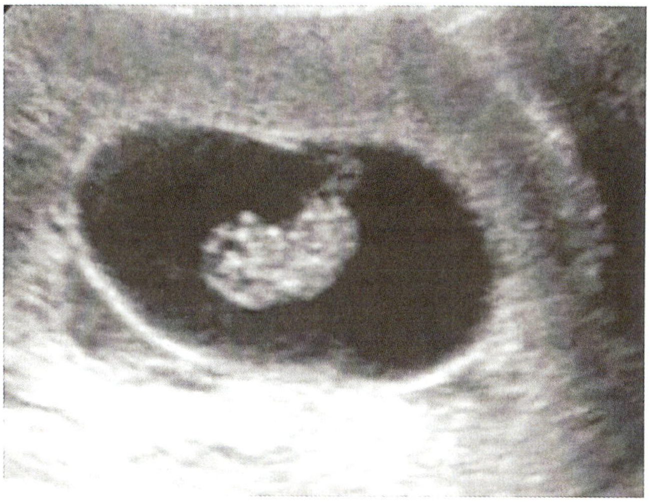

a. Teratoma

b. Hydrosalpinx

c. Corpus luteum

d. Hemorrhagic cyst

4–4. The patient in Question 4–3 reports that she had a cyst on her right ovary removed 3 years earlier and asks if the cyst below needs to be removed as well. You explain the function of the cyst and that excision of this cyst before what gestational age would lead to loss of the pregnancy?

a. 5–6 weeks' gestation
b. 8–9 weeks' gestation
c. 10–12 weeks' gestation
d. 14 weeks' gestation

4–5. A 32-year-old multigravida presents to triage complaining of increasing vaginal discharge for the last 24 hours. You perform a microscopic examination of the discharge and see the image pictured below under the slide. What is the diagnosis?

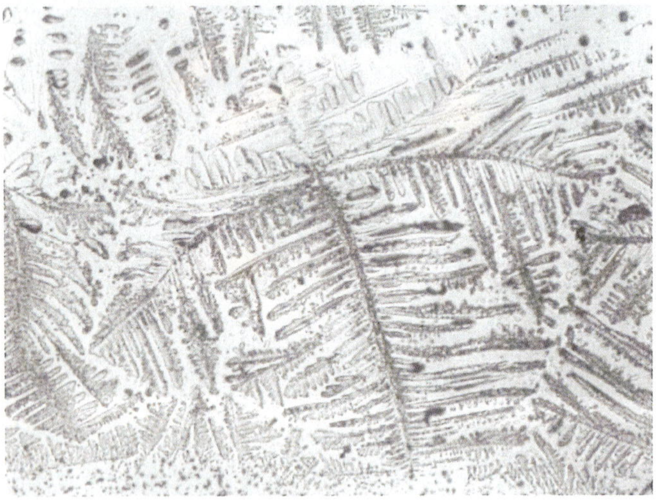

Used with permission from Dr. Barbara Hoffman.

a. Bacterial vaginosis
b. Cervical shortening
c. Rupture of membranes
d. Normal physiologic discharge

4–6. A 26-year-old primigravida is in your office for a prenatal care visit at 34 weeks' gestation. Her abdomen is pictured below. She comments that her 36-year-old friend does not have these marks and wants to know why she does. Which of the following is not a strong risk factor associated with the development of striae gravidarum?

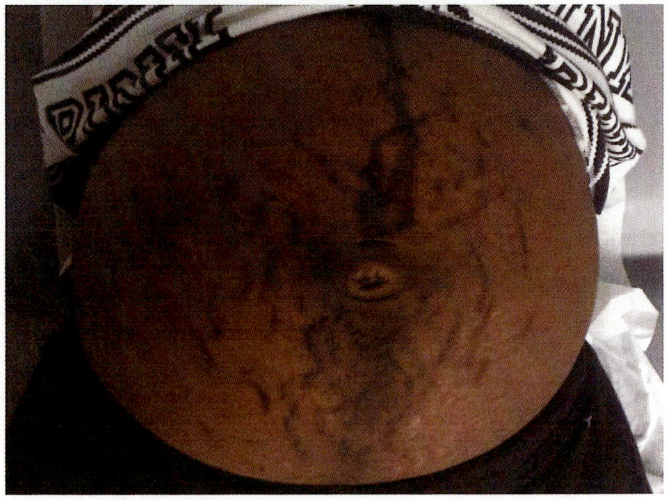

Used with permission from Amber Portley.

a. Family history
b. Prepregnancy weight
c. Younger maternal age
d. Class II maternal obesity

4–7. Which of the following statements is consistent with findings published by the World Health Organization?

a. Protein deposition is highest per day in the third trimester.
b. Fat deposition is highest per day in the third trimester.
c. The total energy cost of pregnancy is about 50,000 kcal.
d. Maternal weight gain is highest per day in the third trimester.

4-8. Which of the following is true about the patient in the following picture?

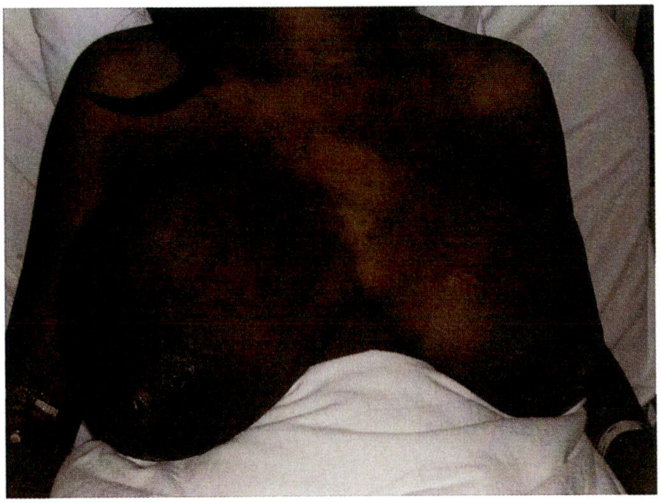

a. This is probably bilateral mastitis.
b. This is classic inflammatory breast carcinoma.
c. The patient should receive antepartum parlodel.
d. Surgery may be required postpartum for reduction.

4-9. Which of the following is not a consequence of vascular changes in women during pregnancy?

a. Angiomas
b. Palmar erythema
c. Melasma gravidarum
d. Dissipate excess heat generated by increased metabolism

4-10. The fetus gains the most weight proportionately during which time period in pregnancy?

a. 10–20 weeks' gestation
b. 20–30 weeks' gestation
c. 30–40 weeks' gestation
d. 40–42 weeks' gestation

4-11. Based on the graph below, which of the following is true?

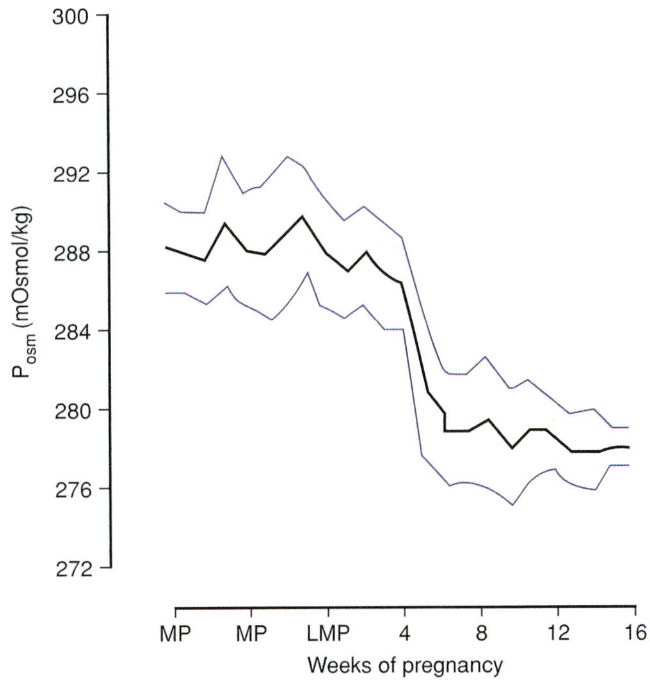

a. Blood osmolality increases after 4–6 weeks' gestation.
b. Blood osmolality decreases after 4–6 weeks' gestation.
c. Plasma osmolality stays about the same during pregnancy.
d. Plasma osmolality decreases by about 10 mOsm/kg during pregnancy.

4-12. Which of the following statements regarding amino acid concentration is accurate?

a. It is highest in fetal compartment.
b. It is highest in maternal compartment.
c. The placenta is not involved with oxidation of amino acids.
d. The placenta does not concentrate amino acids into the fetal circulation.

4-13. Which of the following statements is true regarding glucose and insulin levels in pregnant and nonpregnant women?

a. Insulin levels decrease after meals in pregnancy.
b. Glucose levels decrease after meals in nonpregnant women.
c. Glucose concentrations increase after meals in pregnancy.
d. Insulin levels increase prior to meals in non-pregnant women.

4–14. Which of the following is a safeguard provided by pregnancy-induced hypervolemia?

a. Provides abundant nutrients and elements to support the rapidly growing fetus and placenta.

b. Meets the metabolic demands of the enlarged uterus and its greatly hypertrophied vascular system.

c. Protects the mother, and in turn the fetus, from deleterious effects of impaired venous return in the supine and erect positions.

d. All the above

4–15. When are maternal iron stores used in pregnancy?

a. First trimester

b. Second trimester

c. Third trimester

d. Latter half of pregnancy

4–16. Which of the following inflammatory markers are unaltered in pregnancy?

a. Procalcitonin

b. Erythrocyte sedimentation rate

c. Leukocyte alkaline phosphatase levels

d. All of the above are altered in pregnancy

4–17. Levels of which of the following coagulation factors are unchanged in pregnancy?

a. Protein C

b. Fibrinogen

c. Factor VII

d. Antithrombin III

4–18. What is the relationship between stroke volume and position in the pregnant woman when compared to the nonpregnant woman?

a. Compared to the nonpregnant state, stroke volume is increased when in the supine position at all gestational ages.

b. Compared to the nonpregnant state, stroke volume is increased when in the lateral position at all gestational ages.

c. At 26–30 weeks' gestation, stroke volume in the supine position is equivalent to that of the nonpregnant woman in the lateral position.

d. All of the above

4–19. Which of the following statements regarding hemodynamic changes from the third trimester to the postpartum period is not accurate?

a. Heart rate decreases in the postpartum period.

b. Serum colloid oncotic pressure is lower during pregnancy.

c. Pulmonary capillary wedge pressure is higher during pregnancy.

d. Systemic vascular resistance decreases in the postpartum period.

4–20. This graphic suggests which of the following?

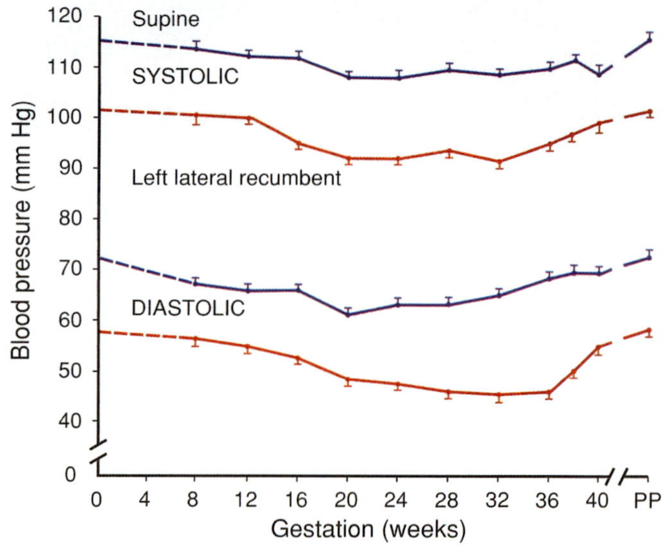

Adapted with permission from Wilson M, Morganti AA, Zervoudakis I, et al: Blood pressure, the renin-aldosterone system and sex steroids throughout normal pregnancy, Am J Med 1980 Jan;68(1):97–104.

a. Diastolic pressures decrease more than systolic pressures.

b. Arterial pressure usually declines to a nadir at 24–26 weeks' gestation.

c. Brachial artery pressure when supine is higher than that when in the lateral recumbent position.

d. All the above

4–21. Which of the following statements are true?

a. Angiotensinogen is produced in the maternal kidney.

b. Vascular refractoriness to angiotensin II may be estrogen related.

c. Refractoriness to angiotensin II is characteristic of mothers who develop preeclampsia.

d. None of the above

4–22. Which statement accurately describes the changes in respiratory physiology during pregnancy?

a. Respiratory rate increases.

b. Tidal volume remains the same.

c. Inspiratory capacity rises by 5–10%.

d. Functional residual capacity decreases by approximately 50%.

4–23. Concerning acid–base equilibrium during pregnancy, which of the following statements is true?

a. Bicarbonate levels are decreased to compensate for the resulting alkalosis.

b. A physiological dyspnea results from greater tidal volume that lowers the blood PCO_2.

c. Progesterone acts centrally, where it lowers the threshold and raises the sensitivity of the chemoreflex to CO_2.

d. All of the above

4–24. A 32-year-old multigravida presents to you at 8 weeks' gestation. Her baseline serum creatinine is 1.0 mg/dL, and her blood pressure is 145/105 mmHg. Which test might you consider next?

a. Kidney ultrasound

b. 50-gram glucose screen

c. 24-hour total urine protein

d. Serum anti-double-stranded DNA

4–25. The following scatter plot depicting 24-hour total urinary protein excretion by gestational age illustrates which of the following changes concerning renal function in pregnancy?

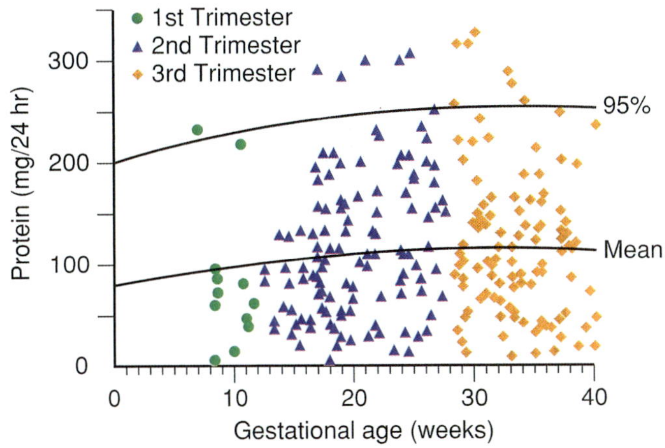

Modified with permission from Higby K, Suiter CR, Phelps JY, et al: Normal values of urinary albumin and total protein excretion during pregnancy, Am J Obstet Gynecol 1994 Oct;171(4):984–989.

a. Proteinuria remains the same throughout pregnancy.

b. Excretion of more than 200 mg/24 hours is abnormal in the third trimester.

c. Excretion of more than 300 mg/24 hours is abnormal in the second trimester.

d. None of the above

4–26. Which of the following statements is true regarding ureteral dilation in pregnancy?

a. Left-sided dilation is seen more often.

b. β-hCG is responsible for the ureteral dilation seen in pregnancy.

c. Unequal dilation results from right ureteral compression by the dextrorotated uterus.

d. None of the above

4–27. Concerning bladder function in pregnancy, which of the following is true?

a. Urethral length increases to compensate for decreased bladder capacity.

b. In primigravidas bladder pressure increases from 8 cm H_2O to 20 cm H_2O at term.

c. Maximal urethral pressure increases from 70 cm H_2O to 93 cm H_2O to maintain continence.

d. All of the above

4–28. Concerning the gastrointestinal tract during pregnancy, which of the following is correct?

a. Gastric emptying time increases during pregnancy.
b. Intraesophageal pressures are lower during pregnancy.
c. Lower esophageal sphincter tone is increased during pregnancy.
d. None of the above

4–29. Which of the following hepatic enzymes is increased in normal pregnancy?

a. Alkaline phosphatase
b. Alanine transaminase
c. Aspartate transaminase
d. γ-Glutamyl transpeptidase

4–30. During normal pregnancy, which of the following is true regarding gallbladder physiology and function?

a. Gallbladder contractility is increased
b. Decreased cholesterol saturation of bile
c. Impaired emptying and increased stasis
d. None of the above

4–31. Your patient with previous diagnosis of pituitary microadenoma presents at 15 weeks' gestation complaining of impaired vision. You suspect pituitary enlargement. What is your next course of action?

a. Initiate bromocriptine
b. Collect a 24-hour urine collection
c. Refer to neurosurgery for excision
d. Refer to ophthalmology for visual field testing

4–32. Which statement accurately reflects placental growth hormone secretion in pregnancy?

a. After 20 weeks' gestation the placenta is the main source.
b. Primary source throughout pregnancy is the maternal pituitary gland.
c. It influences fetal growth by downregulation of insulin-like growth factor 1.
d. Placental and maternally secreted growth hormone have the same amino acid composition.

4–33. Which of the following is true regarding the pituitary gland?

a. Oxytocin is secreted from the anterior pituitary gland.
b. Prolactin is secreted from the posterior pituitary gland.
c. Antidiuretic hormone is secreted from the anterior pituitary gland.
d. Oxytocin and antidiuretic hormone are secreted from the posterior pituitary gland.

4–34. Regarding the thyroid gland during pregnancy, which of the following is true?

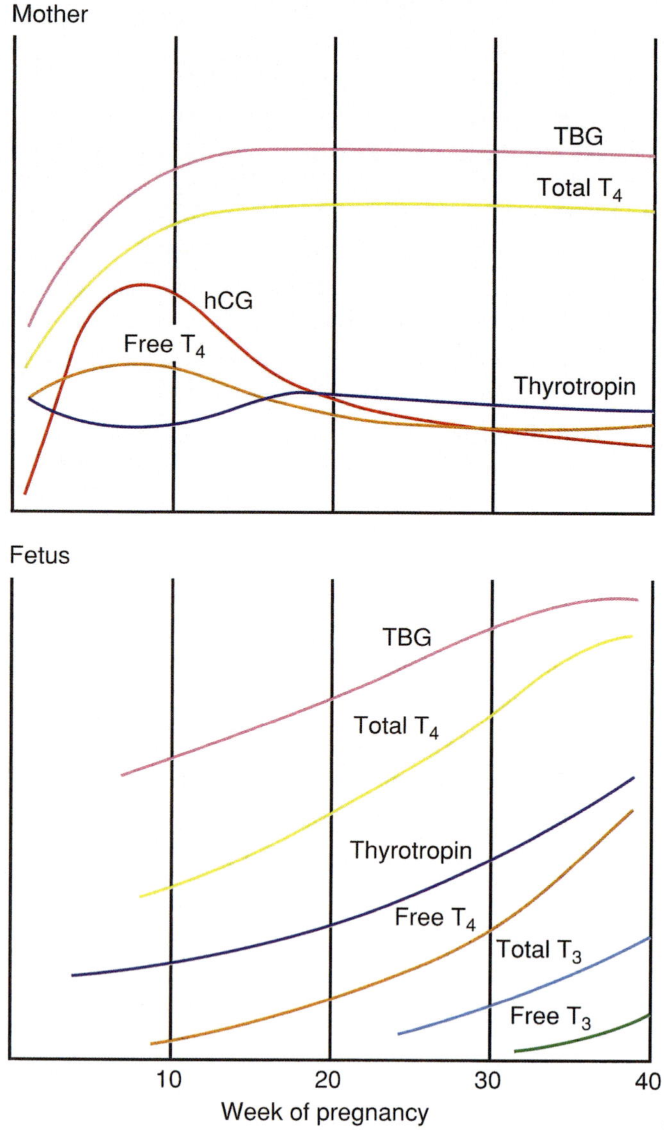

Modified with permission from Burrow GN, Fisher DA, Larsen PR: Maternal and fetal thyroid function, N Engl J Med 1994 Oct 20;331(16):1072–1078.

a. The highest concentration of maternal free T_4 is early in gestation.
b. Fetal concentration of thyroxine-binding globulin increases throughout pregnancy.
c. Maternal concentration of thyroid-stimulating hormone reaches a plateau by the mid-second trimester.
d. All the above

4–35. Which of the following is inaccurate concerning fetal and maternal skeletal metabolism?

a. All markers of bone turnover decrease during pregnancy.

b. Fetal skeletal mineralization requires approximately 30 grams of calcium.

c. Prevention of possible pregnancy-related maternal osteoporosis is difficult.

d. Greater maternal calcium absorption occurs and is mediated by elevated maternal 1,25-dihydroxyvitamin D concentrations.

4–36. Which of the following is true about hormone physiology during pregnancy?

a. Fetal levels of testosterone correlate with maternal levels.

b. The trophoblast incompletely converts testosterone to 17β-estradiol.

c. Maternal plasma levels of androstenedione and testosterone are increased.

d. The source of production of androstenedione and testosterone is the placenta.

4–37. Concerning the musculoskeletal system, which of the following is not true?

a. Most relaxation takes place during the second half of pregnancy.

b. Symphyseal separation greater than 1 cm may cause significant pain.

c. Progressive lordosis is a characteristic feature of normal pregnancy.

d. Sacroiliac, sacrococcygeal, and pubic joints have increased mobility during pregnancy.

4–38. A 33-year-old multigravida at 21 weeks' gestation presents for her prenatal care visit. She reports that she is having difficulties at work doing her secretarial and administrative duties. She is experiencing aching, numbness, and weakness in her upper extremities. What is the likely diagnosis?

a. Rheumatoid arthritis

b. Carpal tunnel syndrome

c. Early-onset preeclampsia

d. Traction on the median and ulnar nerves from lordosis

4–39. Pregnancy-related memory decline is limited to which period in pregnancy?

a. First trimester

b. Second trimester

c. Third trimester

d. Postpartum

4–40. Which of the following is true regarding difficulties in sleep patterns in pregnancy?

a. Include difficulty awakening

b. Last up to 8 weeks postpartum

c. Begin as early as 6 weeks' gestation

d. Are more common in multiparous women

CHAPTER 4 ANSWER KEY

Question number	Letter answer	Page cited	Header cited
4–1	d	p. 50	Uterine Contractility
4–2	b	p. 51	Utero Placental Blood Flow Regulation
4–3	c	p. 51	Ovaries
4–4	a	p. 51	Ovaries
4–5	c	p. 51	Cervix
4–6	d	p. 53	Abdominal Wall
4–7	a	p. 54	Table 4-1
4–8	d	p. 53	Breasts
4–9	c	p. 54	Vascular Changes
4–10	a	p. 54	Table 4-2
4–11	d	p. 54	Water Metabolism
4–12	a	p. 55	Protein Metabolism
4–13	c	p. 55	Carbohydrate Metabolism
4–14	d	p. 57	Blood Volume
4–15	d	p. 58	Iron Requirements
4–16	d	p. 59	Inflammatory Markers
4–17	d	p. 60	Table 4-3
4–18	b	p. 61	Figure 4-7
4–19	d	p. 62	Table 4-4
4–20	d	p. 62	Figure 4-10
4–21	d	p. 63	Renin, Angiotensin II, and Plasma Volume
4–22	c	p. 64	Pulmonary Function
4–23	d	p. 65	Acid–Base Equilibrium
4–24	c	p. 67	Measuring Urine Protein
4–25	c	p. 67	Figure 4-14
4–26	c	p. 67	Ureters
4–27	a	p. 68	Bladder
4–28	b	p. 68	Gastrointestinal Tract
4–29	a	p. 68	Liver
4–30	c	p. 68	Gallbladder
4–31	d	p. 69	Pituitary Gland
4–32	a	p. 69	Growth Hormone
4–33	d	p. 69	Oxytocin and Antidiuretic Hormone
4–34	d	p. 70	Figure 4-16
4–35	a	p. 71	Parathyroid Hormone
4–36	c	p. 72	Androgens
4–37	a	p. 72	Musculoskeletal System
4–38	d	p. 72	Musculoskeletal System
4–39	c	p. 72	Memory
4–40	b	p. 73	Sleep

SECTION 3

PLACENTATION, EMBRYOGENESIS, AND FETAL DEVELOPMENT

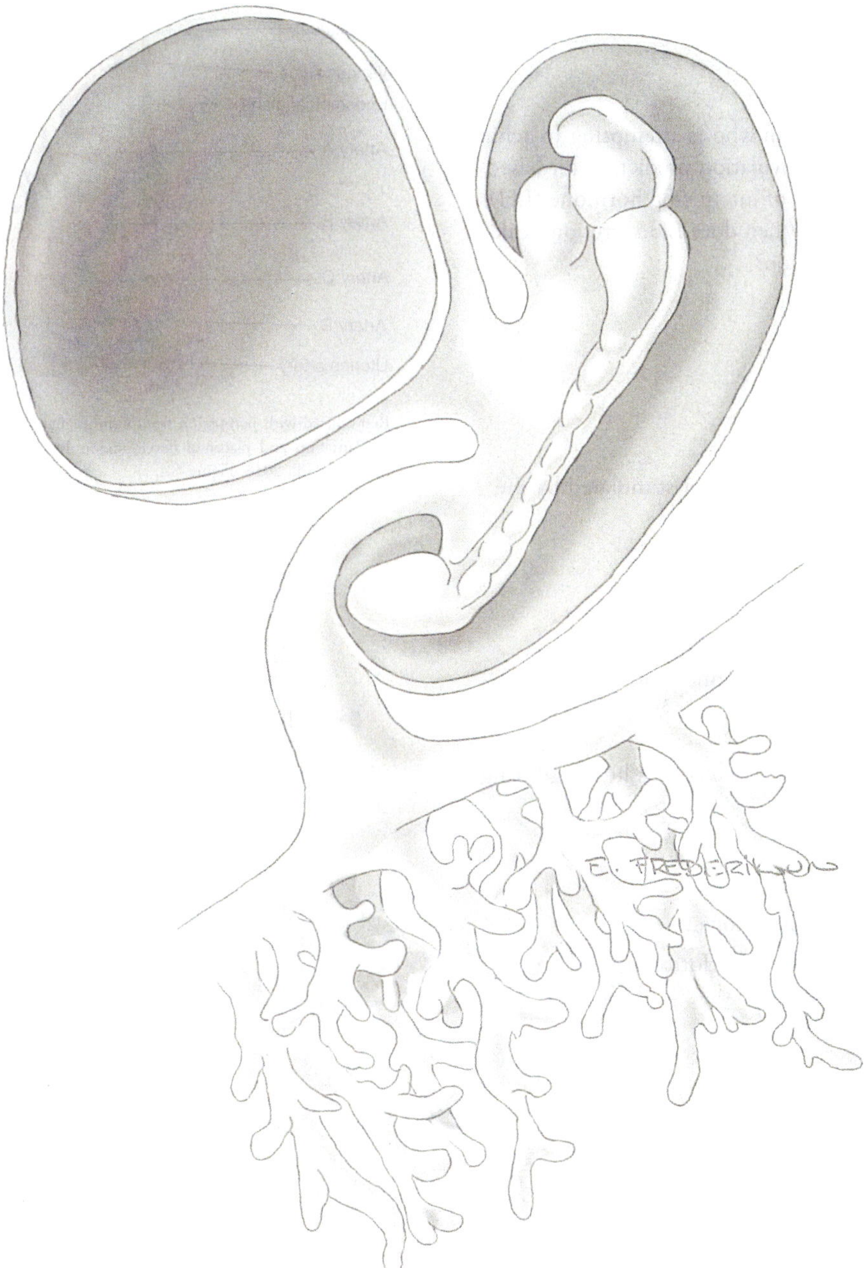

CHAPTER 5

Implantation and Placental Development

5–1. The average ovulatory menstrual cycle ranges from 25 to 32 days. Which phase of the cycle is most consistent in length?

a. Luteal
b. Antral
c. Follicular
d. Proliferative

5–2. A 30-year-old woman who is attempting to achieve pregnancy uses an ovulation prediction kit based on detecting the surge of luteinizing hormone (LH) to time intercourse. When does LH secretion peak in reference to ovulation?

a. 24 hours after
b. 24 hours before
c. 10–12 hours after
d. 10–12 hours before

5–3. Which of the following is not stimulated by the luteinizing hormone surge?

a. Release of first polar body
b. Expansion of the cumulus complex
c. Resumption of meiosis in the ovum
d. Inhibition of progesterone production by cumulus cells

5–4. What hormone rescues the corpus luteum during early pregnancy?

a. Progesterone
b. Androstenedione
c. Human placental lactogen
d. Human chorionic gonadotropin

5–5. The appearance of the endometrial gland in the image below is consistent with what phase of the menstrual cycle?

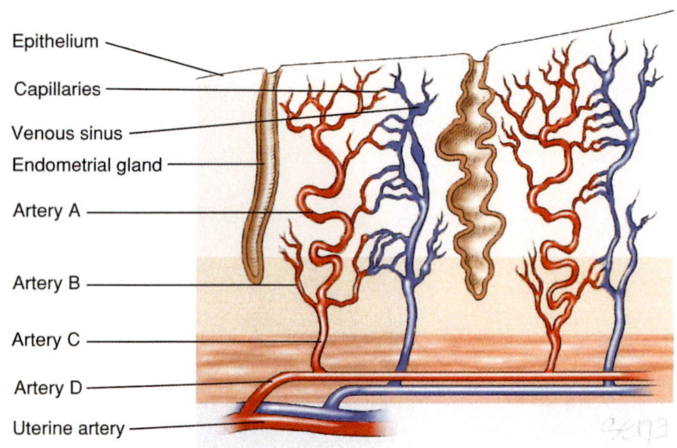

Reproduced with permission from Cunningham FG, Leveno KJ, Bloom SL, et al (eds): Implantation and placental development. In William Obstetrics, 25th ed. New York, McGraw-Hill, 2018, Figure 5-4.

a. Late secretory
b. Early secretory
c. Late proliferative
d. Early proliferative

5–6. In the image in Question 5–5, rupture of which blood vessel triggers menstrual bleeding?

a. Artery A
b. Artery C
c. Capillaries
d. Uterine artery

5–7. In the sequence from letters A to C, identify the three types of deciduas.

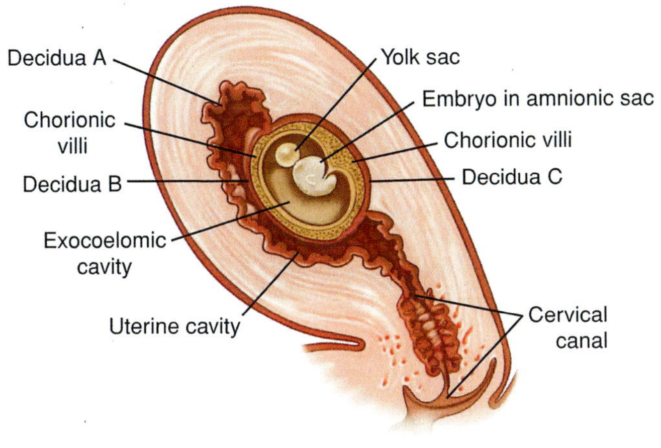

Reproduced with permission from Cunningham FG, Leveno KJ, Bloom SL, et al (eds): Implantation and placental development. In William Obstetrics, 25th ed. New York, McGraw-Hill, 2018, Figure 5-5.

a. Basalis, capsularis, parietalis
b. Parietalis, basalis, capsularis
c. Capsularis, basalis, parietalis
d. Parietalis, capsularis, basalis

5–8. A 23-year-old primigravida at 10 weeks' gestation presents with vaginal bleeding and undergoes uterine curettage for a spontaneous abortion. Necrotic decidua is present on the pathology report. Which of the following is accurate?

a. Decidual necrosis is normal in the first trimester of pregnancy.
b. Overactive decidual natural killer cells most likely contributed to the pregnancy loss.
c. A paucity of decidual lymphocytes may have caused reduced immunotolerance and pregnancy loss.
d. None of the above

5–9. Following ovulation, when is the latest time fertilization can occur for a successful pregnancy to ensue?

a. 6 hours
b. 12 hours
c. 24 hours
d. 48 hours

5–10. Which of the following gives rise to the chorionic structures that transport oxygen and nutrients between the fetus and mother?

a. Villous trophoblast
b. Interstitial trophoblast
c. Extravillous trophoblast
d. Endovascular trophoblast

5–11. In this drawing of implantation, which of the following labeled structures will eventually become the fetus?

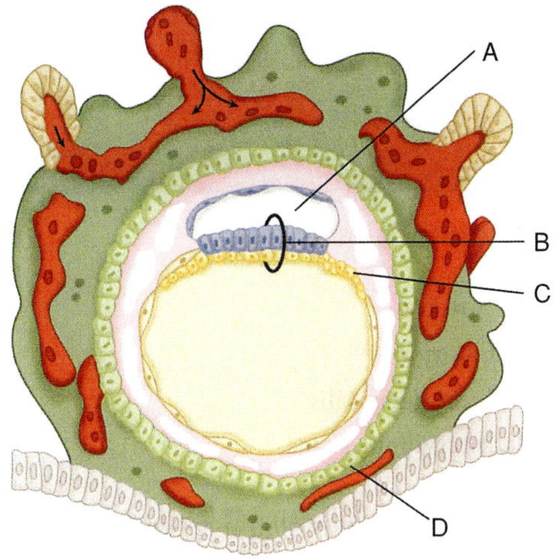

a. A
b. B
c. C
d. D

5–12. Which of the following is not a function of decidual natural killer cells?

a. Secrete cytotoxins
b. Promote decidual invasion
c. Produce placental growth factor
d. Regulate spiral artery remodeling

5–13. What structure is identified by the arrow in the image below?

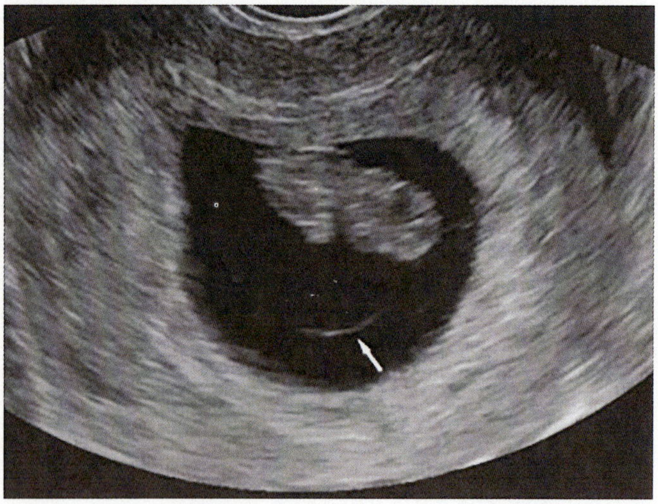

Used with permission from Dr. Robyn Horsager.

a. Amnion
b. Chorion
c. Decidua basalis
d. Intervillous space

5–14. Which of the following is a function of the structure identified by the arrow in Question 5–13?

a. Source of decidual natural killer cells
b. Produces human leukocyte antigens (HLA)
c. Provides tensile strength of the fetal membranes
d. Promotes oxygen exchange between fetal and maternal blood

5–15. Which of the following is a true statement about the structure indicated by the arrow?

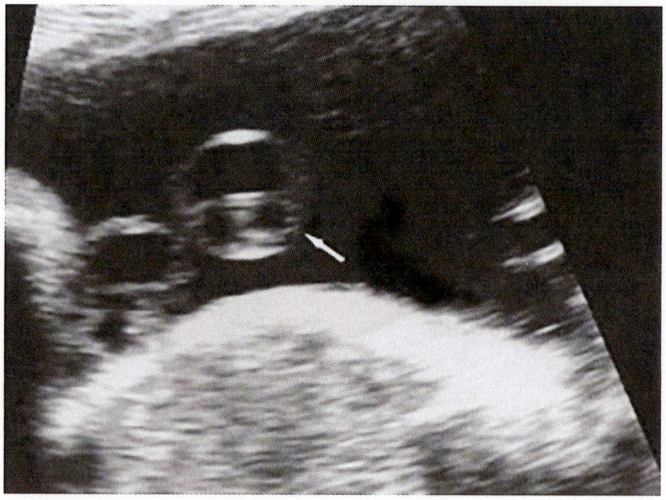

Used with permission from Dr. Robyn Horsager.

a. It carries oxygenated blood to the placenta.
b. It carries oxygenated maternal blood to the fetus.
c. It carries deoxygenated fetal blood to the placenta.
d. None of the above

5–16. Factors regulating blood flow in the intervillous space of the placenta do not include which of the following?

a. Intrauterine pressure
b. Arterial blood pressure
c. Maternal hemoglobin level
d. Uterine contraction pattern

5–17. The phenomenon that describes how fetal cells can become engrafted in the mother during pregnancy and then be identified decades later is called which of the following?

a. Microchimerism
b. Histocompatibility
c. Hemochorial invasion
d. Immunological neutrality

5–18. What is the composition of the membrane layers in this ultrasound image of an early twin pregnancy?

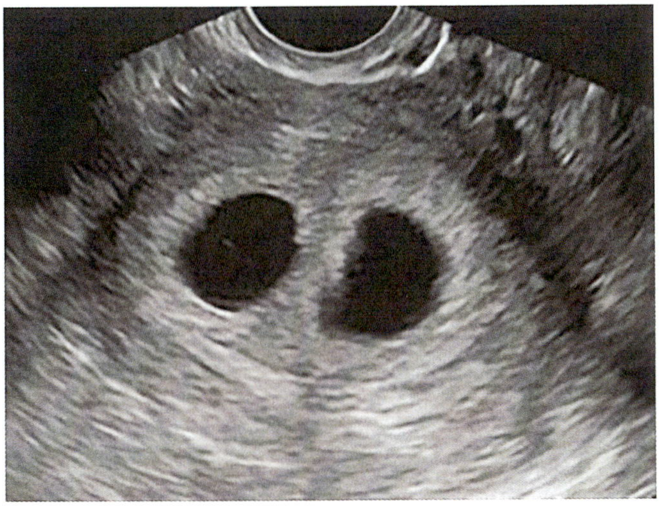

Used with permission from Dr. Robyn Horsager.

- **a.** Amnion, amnion
- **b.** Amnion, chorion, amnion
- **c.** Chorion, amnion, amnion, chorion
- **d.** Amnion, chorion, chorion, amnion

5–19. At what gestational age does the volume of the substance imaged below peak?

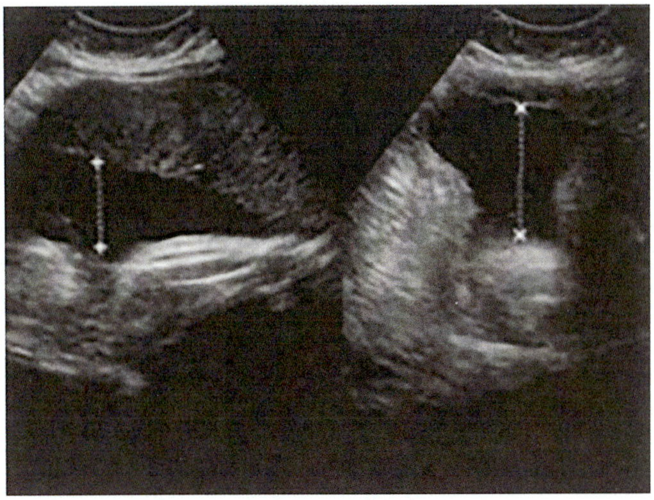

- **a.** 28 weeks
- **b.** 34 weeks
- **c.** 38 weeks
- **d.** 42 weeks

5–20. At term, what is the average amnionic fluid volume?

- **a.** 200 mL
- **b.** 500 mL
- **c.** 1000 mL
- **d.** 2000 mL

5-21. As shown in this figure, blood coming from the placenta to the fetus travels first from the umbilical vein into which of the following structures?

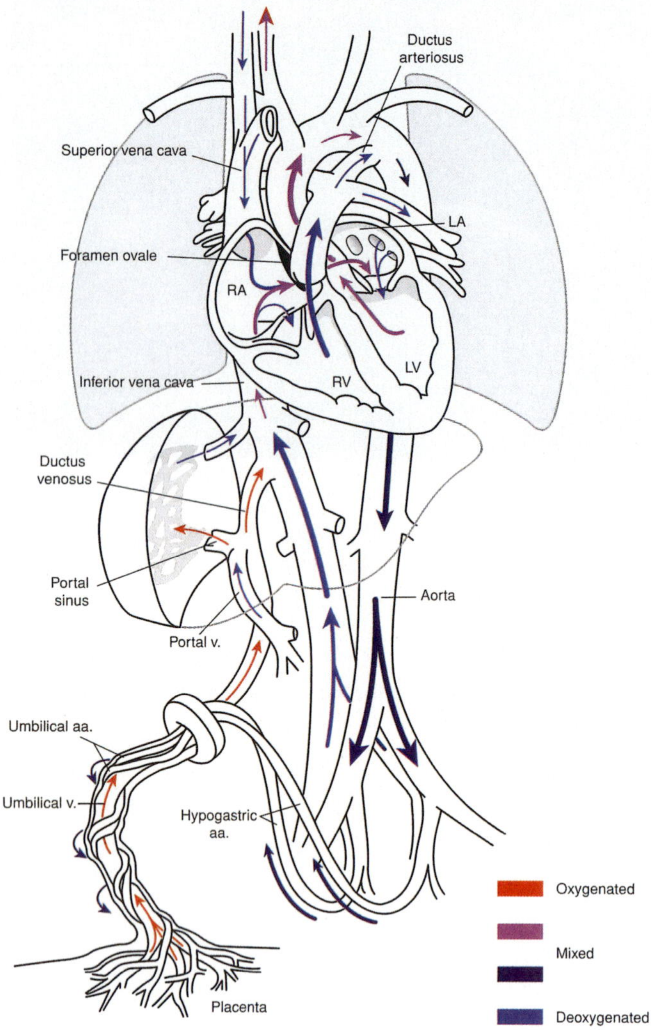

Reproduced with permission from Cunningham FG, Leveno KJ, Bloom SL, et al (eds): Embryogenesis and fetal development. In William Obstetrics, 25th ed. New York, McGraw-Hill, 2018, Figure 7-9.

a. The portal vein
b. The hepatic vein
c. The ductus venosus
d. The inferior vena cava

5-22 After birth, these vessels become which of the following structures?

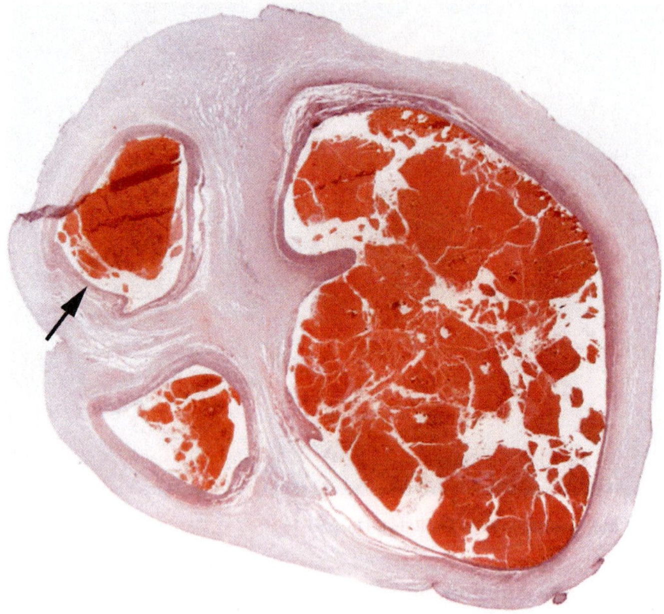

Reproduced with permission from Cunningham FG, Leveno KJ, Bloom SL, et al (eds): Implantation and placental development. In William Obstetrics, 25th ed. New York, McGraw-Hill, 2018, Figure 5-17. Photo contributor: Dr. Mandolin S. Ziadie.

a. Mesenteric cysts
b. Umbilical arteries
c. Hypogastric arteries
d. Medial umbilical ligaments

5-23. An 18-year-old woman with no contraception has intercourse mid-cycle. If pregnancy ensues, when is β-hCG detectable in her bloodstream?

a. 7 days after a missed period
b. 7–9 days following ovulation
c. 7–9 days following luteinizing hormone surge
d. None of the above

5-24. One week after her missed period, the patient's plasma β-hCG level is 1305 mIU/mL. Approximately how long will it take to reach 2500 mIU/mL?

a. 2 days
b. 4 days
c. 1 week
d. 2 weeks

5-25. At what gestational age are peak maternal β-hCG levels reached?

a. 10 weeks
b. 20 weeks
c. 28 weeks
d. 38 weeks

5–26. Which of the following is not a biological function of human chorionic gonadotropin?

a. Corpus luteum maintenance
b. Uterine vasculature vasoconstriction
c. Sexual differentiation in male fetuses
d. Smooth muscle relaxation of myometrial contractions

5–27. What is the half-life of human placental lactogen?

a. 10–30 minutes
b. 2 hours
c. 1 day
d. 1 week

5–28. What is the biological function of human placental lactogen?

a. Increases angiogenesis
b. Increases maternal lipolysis
c. Increases maternal insulin resistance
d. All of the above

5–29 A patient presents to the emergency room with right-sided pain. An ultrasound is performed and a 6-week pregnancy with the finding below is diagnosed. Operative removal of the structure increases the risk of which of the following?

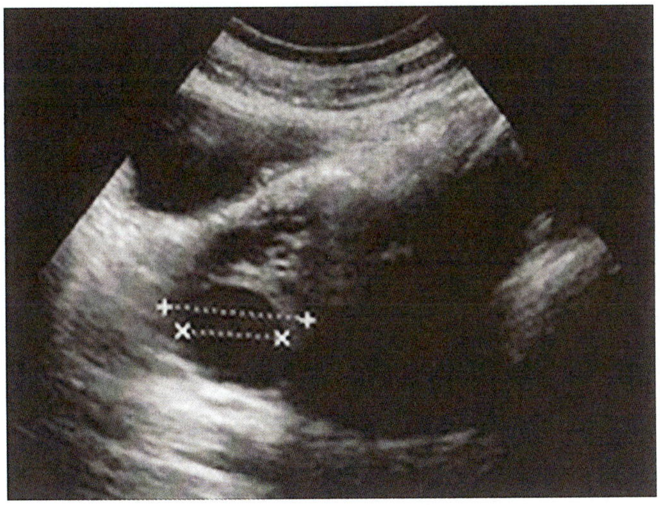

a. Spontaneous abortion
b. Fetal open neural-tube defect
c. Second trimester fetal growth restriction
d. None of the above

5–30. What is the primary hormone produced by the structure in the figure in Question 5–29?

a. Progesterone
b. α-Fetoprotein
c. Human placental lactogen
d. Human chorionic gonadotropin

5–31. What is the source of the precursor for progesterone production by the syncytiotrophoblast?

a. Maternal estrogen
b. Maternal cholesterol
c. Fetal LDL cholesterol
d. Fetal dehydroepiandrosterone

5–32. All of the following conditions except which are associated with reduced estrogen production secondary to diminished availability of C_{19} steroid precursors?

a. Anencephaly
b. Fetal demise
c. Fetal trisomy 21
d. Fetal–placental sulfatase deficiency

CHAPTER 5 ANSWER KEY

Question number	Letter answer	Page cited	Header cited
5–1	**a**	p. 81	Ovarian–Endometrial Cycle
5–2	**d**	p. 82	Ovulation
5–3	**d**	p. 82	Ovulation
5–4	**d**	p. 82	Figure 5-2
5–5	**d**	p. 84	Proliferative Phase
5–6	**a**	p. 85	Menstruation
5–7	**d**	p. 86	Decidual Structure
5–8	**a**	p. 86	Decidual Histology
5–9	**c**	p. 87	Fertilization
5–10	**a**	p. 88	Trophoblast Development
5–11	**b**	p. 89	Figure 5-9
5–12	**a**	p. 91	Regulators of Trophoblast Invasion
5–13	**a**	p. 93	Figure 5-13
5–14	**c**	p. 95	Amnion
5–15	**c**	p. 94	Fetal Circulation
5–16	**c**	p. 94	Maternal Circulation
5–17	**a**	p. 95	Breaks in the Placental "Barrier"
5–18	**d**	p. 96	Amnion Development
5–19	**b**	p. 96	Amnion Development
5–20	**c**	p. 96	Amnion Development
5–21	**c**	p. 97	Umbilical Cord
5–22	**d**	p. 97	Umbilical Cord
5–23	**c**	p. 99	Concentrations in Serum and Urine
5–24	**a**	p. 99	Concentrations in Serum and Urine
5–25	**a**	p. 99	Concentrations in Serum and Urine
5–26	**b**	p. 100	Biological Functions
5–27	**a**	p. 101	Biosynthesis
5–28	**d**	p. 101	Metabolic Actions
5–29	**a**	p. 103	Placental Progesterone Production
5–30	**a**	p. 102	Placental Progesterone Production
5–31	**b**	p. 103	Placental Progesterone Production
5–32	**d**	p. 105	Fetal Conditions Affecting Estrogen Production

CHAPTER 6

Placental Abnormalities

6–1. Which of the following statements use correct terminology to describe the maternal/uterine surface and fetal surface of the placenta?

a. Maternal surface: basal plate, fetal surface: amnionic plate

b. Maternal surface: basal plate, fetal surface: chorionic plate

c. Maternal surface: decidual plate, fetal surface: chorionic plate

d. Maternal surface: chorionic plate, fetal surface: amnionic plate

6–2. In their 2013 recommendations, the American Institute of Ultrasound in Medicine states that which of the following should be imaged during prenatal ultrasound examination?

a. Number of vessels contained in umbilical cord

b. Umbilical cord at both fetal and placental insertion sites

c. Placental location and relationship to internal cervical os

d. All of the above

6–3. Which of the following is true regarding placental measurements?

a. Normal placenta weighs approximately 500 grams at term.

b. Normal placenta is approximately 2 to 4 cm thick as visualized on ultrasound.

c. Normal placenta increases in thickness at a rate of approximately 1 mm per week.

d. All of the above

6–4. The image below is best described as which placental variant?

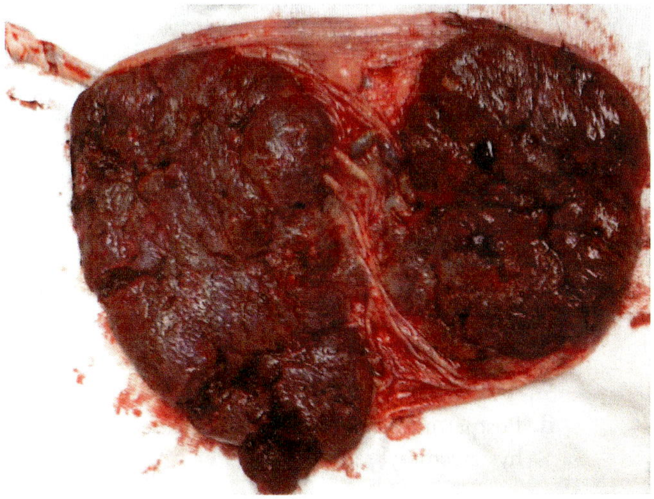

Used with permission from Dr. Lindsey Jackson.

a. Bilobate placenta

b. Succenturiate lobe

c. Placenta membranacea

d. Circumvallate placenta

6–5. For which situation is submission of the placenta for pathological examination the most informative and cost effective?

a. After cesarean delivery for arrest of descent

b. Cholestasis complicating the third trimester

c. Oligohydramnios complicating the third trimester

d. All of the above

6–6. The placental variant demonstrated in this ultrasound image is most likely to be associated with which of the following?

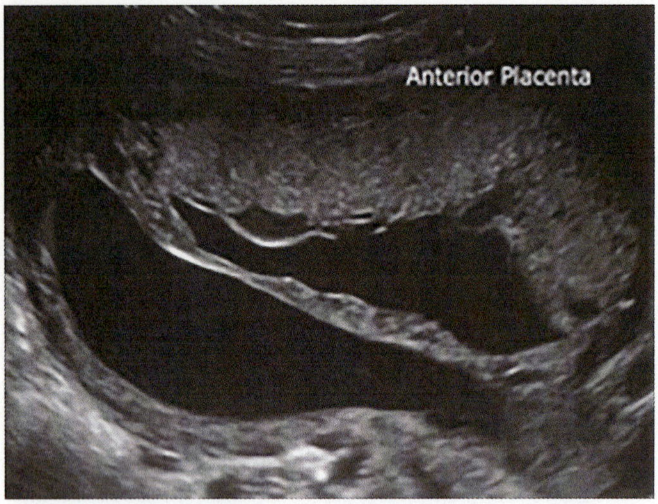

Used with permission from Dr. Robert Stewart.

a. Stillbirth
b. Normal pregnancy outcome
c. Asymmetric fetal extremity amputation
d. Postpartum hemorrhage and increased risk for hysterectomy

6–7. It has been estimated that up to what percentage of placental villi can be lost without resulting in adverse impact to the fetus?

a. 5%
b. 10%
c. 20%
d. 30%

6–8. A 28-year-old G4P2 at 20 weeks' gestation presents for her fetal anatomical survey. There have been no pregnancy complications to date. The placenta is imaged with the findings shown below. What do you document on the ultrasound report?

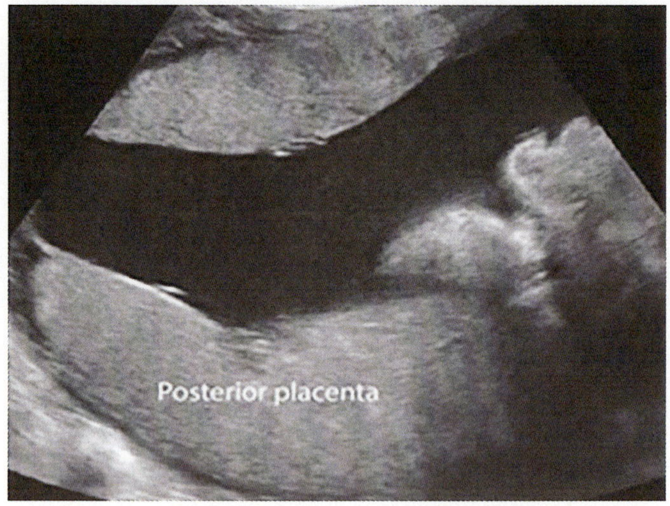

a. Posterior placenta
b. Posterior placenta with chorioangioma
c. Posterior placenta with succenturiate lobe
d. Posterior placenta with remote subchorionic hematoma

6–9. As the primary obstetrician of the patient in Question 6–8, which of the following is a note you make in her chart?

a. Follow with serial growth ultrasounds
b. Schedule her delivery at 39 weeks in the absence of a prior indication.
c. Closely examine the placenta after delivery to account for all portions and perform a manual sweep of the uterine cavity if she has postpartum hemorrhage.
d. All of the above

6–10. A 16-year-old primigravida presents at 19 weeks' gestation for a prenatal visit followed by her fetal anatomical survey. During her ultrasound the finding seen below is found. After reviewing the images, you also order which of the following?

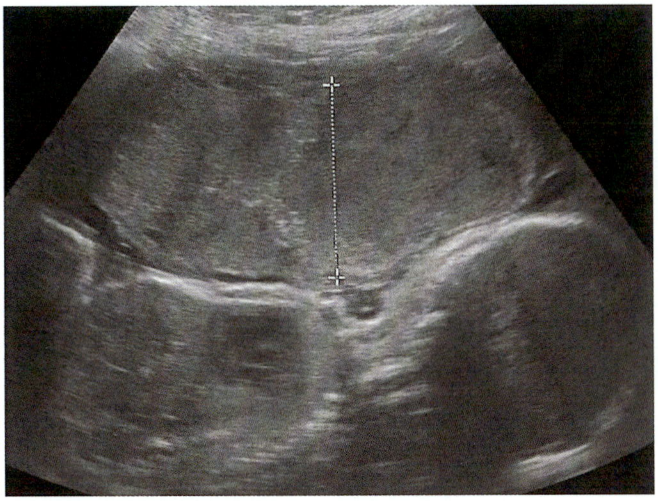

Used with permission from Dr. Jodi Dashe.

- **a.** Additional maternal lab studies
- **b.** Middle cerebral artery Doppler of the fetus
- **c.** Detailed fetal anatomical survey and fetal echo
- **d.** All of the above

6–11. A 37-year-old G1P0100 presents to you for preconception consultation after her recent stillbirth at 27 weeks' gestation. Her pregnancy had progressed without complication until fetal demise was diagnosed at a routine prenatal visit. They elected for autopsy, which was unremarkable. She had undergone amniocentesis after diagnosis of the fetal demise with negative infectious studies and normal fetal microarray. She has the placental pathology report with her, and it states "massive perivillous fibrin deposition." How does this impact your counseling?

- **a.** You recommend antiphospholipid antibody lab panel.
- **b.** You recommend antihypertensive therapy in her next pregnancy.
- **c.** You recommend prophylactic anticoagulation in her next pregnancy.
- **d.** None of the above.

6–12. A 24-year-old G3P2 presents at 11 weeks' gestation because she had some light bleeding 3 days prior that she now describes as scant dark spotting. The following is seen during the study. What is the most appropriate way to counsel this patient?

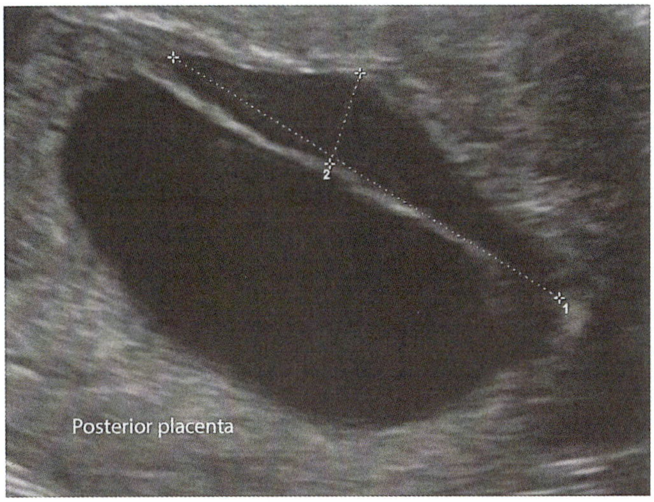

- **a.** No atypical findings are seen on ultrasound today. I would like to do a speculum exam to evaluate your cervix.
- **b.** A small subamnionic hematoma is seen today, which does not explain your recent bleeding, so I would like to do a speculum exam to evaluate your cervix.
- **c.** A small retroplacental hematoma is seen today, which likely explains your recent bleeding. You may have further dark spotting, but even if the spotting stops this is associated with an increased risk for miscarriage.
- **d.** A small marginal hematoma is seen today, which likely explains your recent bleeding. You may have further dark spotting for a few more days, but this finding is not likely to result in adverse impact to your pregnancy.

6–13. The following is an ultrasound image noted during the routine fetal anatomical survey of a 31-year-old G3P1 at 20 weeks' gestation. Your recently hired sonographer calls you in to review the finding (asterisk) and asks whether you are concerned or not. Because you recognize this as an intervillous thrombus, you tell your sonographer which of the following?

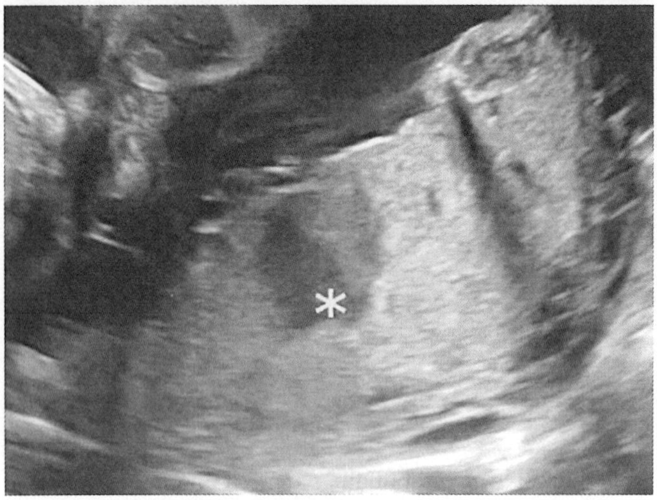

a. These are fairly common and not typically associated with adverse fetal sequelae.

b. If you use color Doppler on the area during ultrasound, you will see high-velocity flow.

c. I will make a note of this in her chart in case the patient's maternal serum estradiol is elevated on her maternal serum screen.

d. All of the above

6–14. Which of the following scenarios is an indication for a screen for fetal–maternal bleed?

a. Chorioangioma noted during a routine 22-week ultrasound

b. Marginal hematoma noted during a routine 10-week ultrasound

c. Retroplacental hematoma noted during a 28-week ultrasound performed for lagging fundal height

d. Subamnionic hematoma noted on visual inspection of the placenta after manual extraction of the placenta secondary to a prolonged third stage

6–15. Which of the following is true regarding calcium deposits in the placenta and the Grannum grading scale?

a. A grade 3 placenta at 38 weeks should prompt delivery.

b. A grade 3 placenta at 36 weeks is associated with fetal lung maturity.

c. A grade 3 placenta at 26 weeks suggests need for maternal calcium supplementation.

d. A grade 3 placenta at 30 weeks is associated with increased risk for adverse pregnancy outcome.

6–16. A 23-year-old multigravida presents for routine fetal anatomical survey at 20 weeks' gestation. The placental finding seen below was found during the study. What modality is best used as a next step in narrowing the differential of this placental mass?

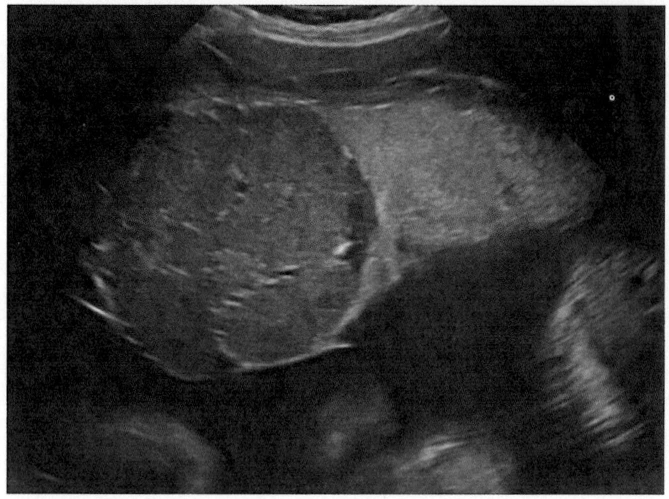

Used with permission from Dr. Robert Stewart.

a. Placental biopsy

b. Color Doppler ultrasound

c. Magnetic resonance imaging

d. Three-dimensional ultrasound

6–17. The patient in Question 6–16 is seen for counseling regarding the ultrasound finding. You do not recommend which of the following?

a. Serial middle cerebral artery Doppler of the fetus.

b. Serial ultrasound for observation of fetal growth and fluid.

c. Submission of the placenta for pathological examination after delivery.

d. Maternal serum alpha-fetoprotein for open neural-tube defect screening.

6–18. Which of the following maternal malignancies is least likely to metastasize to the placenta?

a. Melanoma

b. Lymphoma

c. Breast cancer

d. Cervical cancer

6–19. Which of the following serve as avenues of bacterial inoculation that may lead to chorioamnionitis?

a. Ascension from lower reproductive tract

b. Hematogenous spread from maternal circulation

c. Direct inoculation during needle-based intraamnionic procedures

d. All of the above

6–20. Which of the following leads to the majority of chorioamnionitis cases?

a. Maternal smoking
b. Maternal immunosuppression
c. Prolonged rupture of membranes
d. Pregnancies complicated by gestational diabetes

6–21. What is least likely to be the initial finding in a pregnancy complicated by amnionic band sequence?

a. Amnionic band
b. Atypical facial cleft
c. Limb reduction defect
d. Frontoparietal encephalocele

6–22. A pathology report states that the umbilical cord is 59 cm in length. Which of the following statements is true regarding this finding?

a. It is within normal range for a typical umbilical cord.
b. It is associated with an increased risk for cord entanglement.
c. It is associated with an increased risk for cord avulsion during third stage.
d. All of the above

6–23. The umbilical cord coiling index is determined by the number of complete coils per centimeter of umbilical cord length. Which of the following is true of umbilical cord coiling?

a. Hypocoiling has not been associated with adverse fetal outcome.
b. Hypercoiling has been consistently associated with fetal macrosomia.
c. A normal coiling index in a visually inspected postpartum cord is 1.4.
d. None of the above

6–24 A healthy 21-year-old primigravida presents at 19 weeks' gestation for basic fetal anatomical survey and a common umbilical cord vessel anomaly is found, as shown below. Which of the following is not a reasonable subsequent management recommendation?

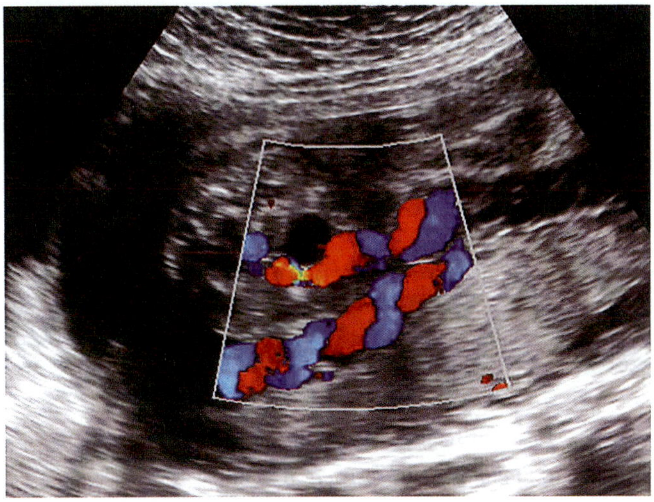

a. Serial surveillance of fetal growth
b. Detailed fetal anatomical survey and fetal echo
c. Pursuing delivery at 39–40 weeks in the absence of a prior indication
d. Counseling regarding increased risk for aneuploidy, even when seen in isolation

6–25. A single umbilical cord cyst is found during a first trimester ultrasound performed for assessment of vaginal bleeding. No other remarkable findings were noted during the study. What is the most reasonable next step?

a. No alteration of routine care is indicated
b. Ultrasound-guided needle aspiration of the cyst
c. Schedule follow-up ultrasound at 16–18 weeks' gestation
d. Counseling regarding increased aneuploidy risk and offering chorionic villus sampling

6–26. The umbilical cord variant shown here is associated with of the following?

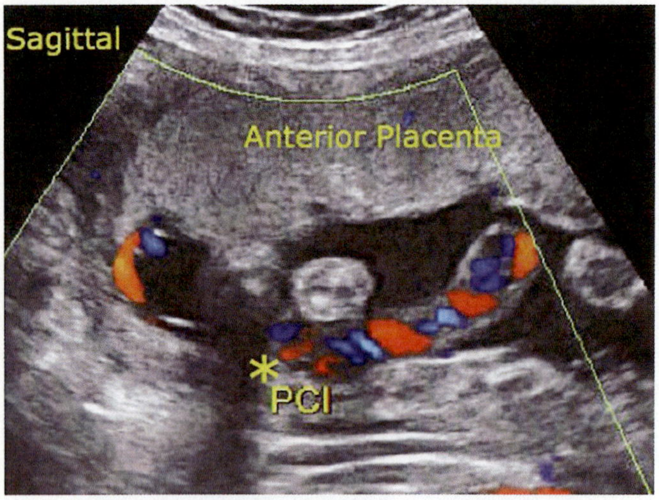

a. Vasa previa

b. Multifetal gestation

c. Fetal growth restriction

d. All of the above

6–27 The umbilical cord insertion variant seen here is most commonly associated with a higher rate of which of the following?

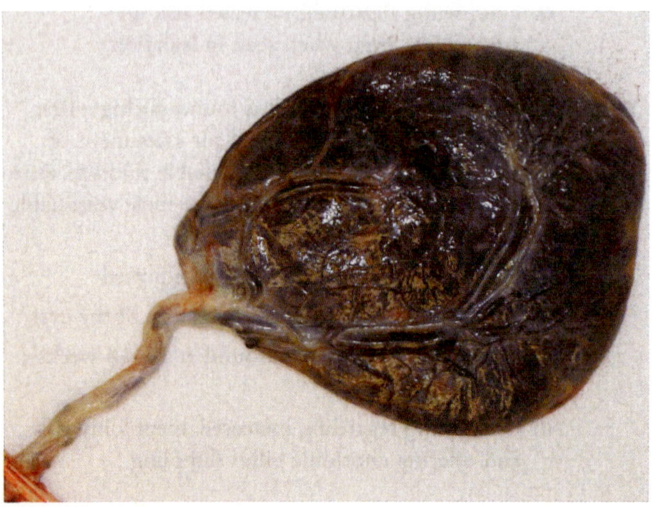

a. Cord avulsion

b. Fetal anomalies

c. Uterine inversion

d. Single umbilical artery

6–28. A 26-year-old primigravida presents for fetal anatomical survey at 20 weeks' gestation. Based on the finding shown below, which of the following would you recommend?

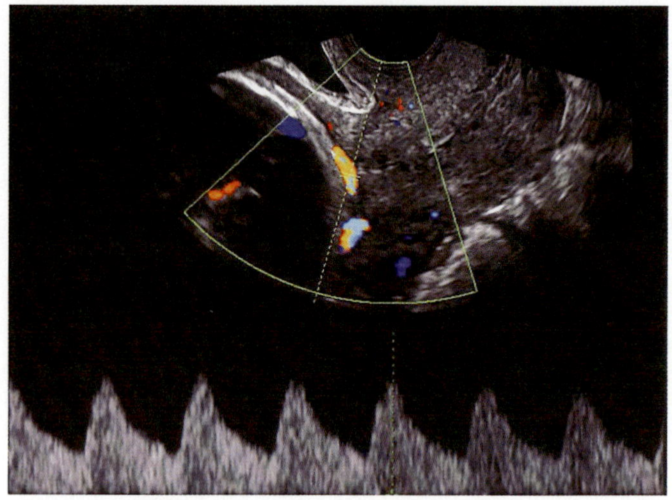

a. Initiating nightly vaginal progesterone suppository

b. Preparations for a cesarean hysterectomy at 39 weeks

c. Continuing routine prenatal care in the absence of bleeding

d. Scheduling serial follow-up with transvaginal ultrasound for reassessment of the lower uterine segment with color Doppler

6–29. A true knot in the umbilical cord is associated with which of the following?

a. Stillbirth

b. Polyhydramnios

c. Monoamnionic twin gestation

d. All of the above

6–30. Which of the following is true regarding the ultrasound finding highlighted with the asterisk?

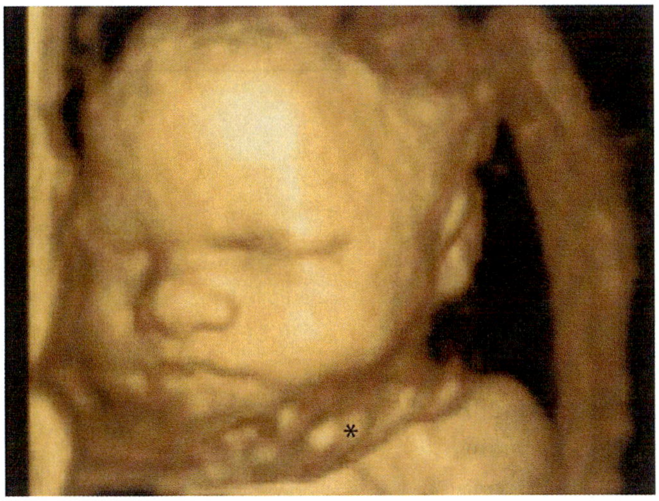

a. A single loop is present in 20–34% of deliveries.

b. A nuchal cord is associated with late fetal heart rate decelerations in labor.

c. Cesarean delivery is indicated when found incidentally on ultrasound.

d. All of the above

6–31. A 32-year-old G2P1 at 38 weeks' gestation with one prior cesarean delivery presents for growth ultrasound. On ultrasound the fetus is footling breech, with appropriate growth for gestational age, and an amnionic fluid index of 21 cm. No anomalies are seen. Which of the following is an appropriate next step in her management?

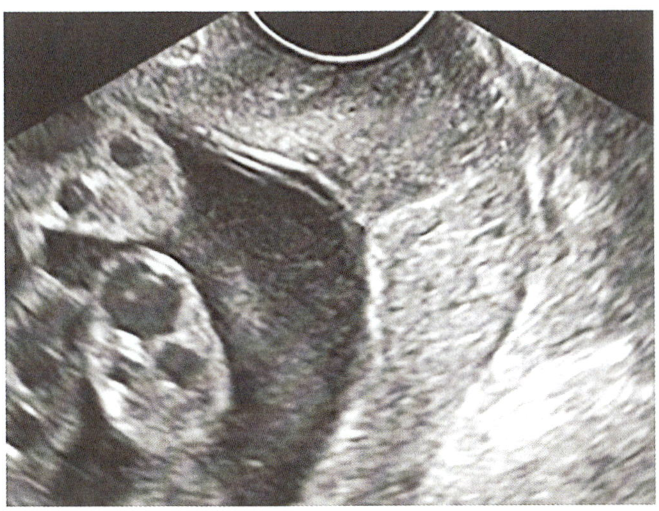

a. Schedule a follow-up prenatal appointment in 1 week if undelivered.

b. Counsel the patient about the findings and send her to labor and delivery for repeat cesarean delivery.

c. Counsel the patient about the findings and send to labor and delivery for amniotomy induction for trial of labor after cesarean.

d. All of the above are reasonable options

6–32. A healthy 31-year-old multigravida is seen for ultrasound at 26 weeks' gestation for assessment of fetal growth. Biometrics are consistent with her menstrual dating and amnionic fluid volume is normal. Which of the following is an appropriate modification to her prenatal course after the following is seen during the study?

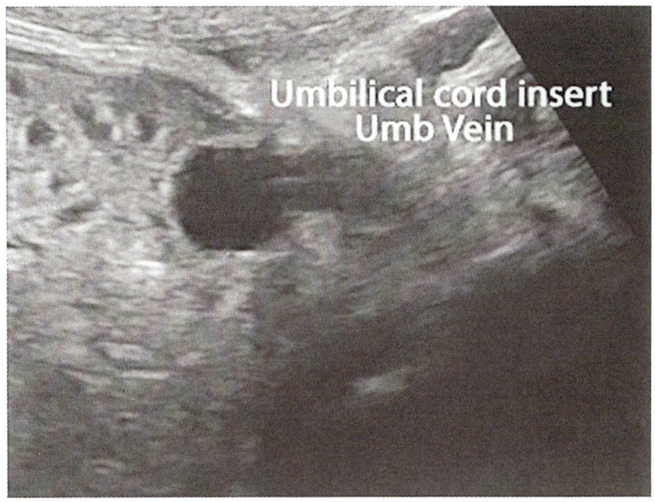

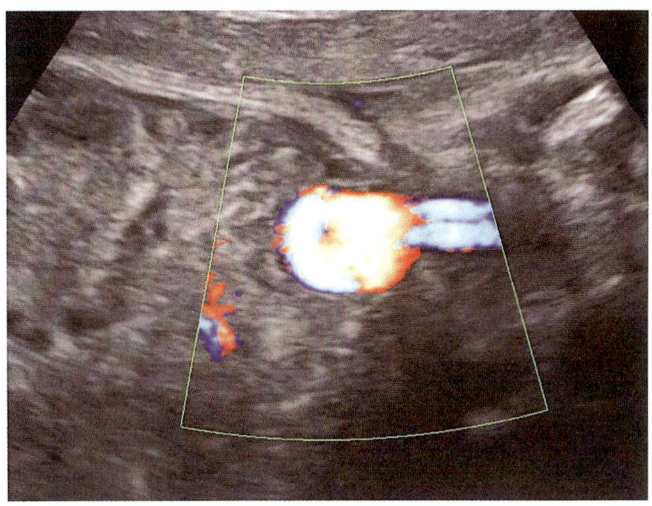

a. No alteration to routine care

b. Referral for fetal echocardiogram

c. Consideration of delivery at 38–39 weeks

d. Genetic counseling and offering of amniocentesis for fetal karyotype

CHAPTER 6

CHAPTER 6 ANSWER KEY

Question number	Letter answer	Page cited	Header cited
6–1	b	p. 111	Normal Placenta
6–2	d	p. 111	Normal Placenta
6–3	d	p. 111 p. 113	Normal Placenta Shape and Size Variants
6–4	a	p. 112	Shape and Size Variants
6–5	c	p. 112	Table 6-1
6–6	b	p. 113	Extrachorial Placentation
6–7	d	p. 113	Circulatory Disturbances
6–8	c	p. 112	Shape and Size Variants
6–9	c	p. 113	Shape and Size Variants
6–10	d	p. 113	Shape and Size Variants
6–11	a	p. 114	Maternal Floor Infarction
6–12	d	p. 114–115	Hematoma
6–13	a	p. 114	Intervillous Thrombus
6–14	c	p. 114 p. 115	Hematoma Subamnionic Hematoma
6–15	d	p. 115	Placental Calcification
6–16	b	p. 115	Chorioangioma
6–17	d	p. 115	Chorioangioma
6–18	d	p. 116	Metastatic Tumors
6–19	d	p. 116	Chorioamnionitis
6–20	c	p. 116	Chorioamnionitis
6–21	a	p. 117	Other Membrane Abnormalities
6–22	a	p. 117	Length
6–23	d	p. 117	Coiling
6–24	d	p. 117	Vessel Number
6–25	c	p. 118	Remnants and Cysts
6–26	d	p. 118	Insertion
6–27	a	p. 118	Insertion
6–28	d	p. 119	Vasa Previa
6–29	d	p. 119	Knots, Strictures, and Loops
6–30	a	p. 119	Knots, Strictures, and Loops
6–31	b	p. 119	Knots, Strictures, and Loops
6–32	c	p. 120	Vascular

CHAPTER 7

Embryogenesis and Fetal Development

7–1. Which of the following is assumed when using the first day of the last menstrual period for dating?

- **a.** The patient has a 36-day cycle.
- **b.** The patient became pregnant on that day.
- **c.** The patient ovulated approximately two weeks later.
- **d.** The first day of the last menstrual period was implantation bleeding.

7–2. What is the accuracy of an ultrasound measurement shown below?

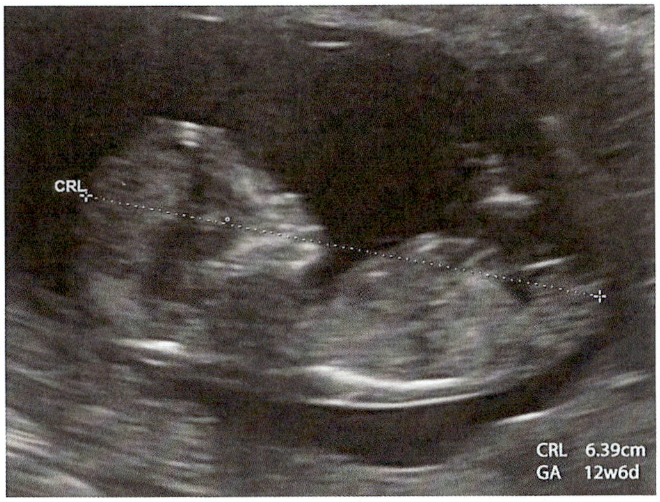

- **a.** ±2–3 days
- **b.** ±5–7 days
- **c.** ±8–10 days
- **d.** ±12–14 days

7–3. Approximately how long is each trimester of pregnancy?

- **a.** 12 weeks
- **b.** 13 weeks
- **c.** 14 weeks
- **d.** 15 weeks

7–4. When is a conceptus termed an embryo?

- **a.** Third week from the last menstrual period
- **b.** Fifth week from the last menstrual period
- **c.** Sixth week from the last menstrual period
- **d.** Twelfth week from the last menstrual period

7–5. A 20-year-old primigravida presents to your office to start prenatal care. She reports having an ultrasound performed last week at another facility. She shows you an ultrasound image which is provided below. Interested in science, the patient would like to know what is happening to the fetus at this gestational age. Which of the following statements would be incorrect?

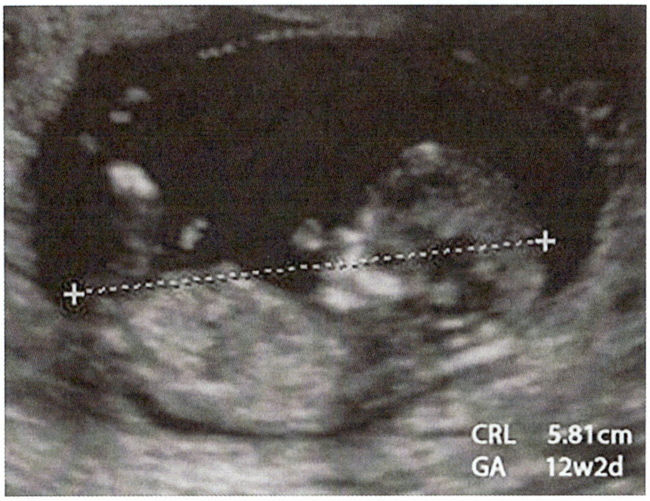

- **a.** The fetus has fingers and toes.
- **b.** Skins and nails are developing.
- **c.** The eyes are moving, and there is blinking.
- **d.** The fetus is beginning to make spontaneous movements.

7–6. A 29-year-old multigravida presents at 15 weeks' gestation to establish prenatal care. The patient's first child had a neural-tube defect. The patient did not know she was pregnant until this week, so she asks you about starting folic acid as she was counseled in her last pregnancy that she needed a higher dose because of her first child's condition. Which of the following statements should be covered in your counseling?

a. Starting folic acid is just as beneficial now as ever, so she should start today but at a dose of 8 mg per day.

b. The neural-tube does not close until 21 weeks' gestation, so she should start folic acid 4 mg daily within the next 1–2 weeks.

c. The neural-tube closes by 6 weeks' gestation, so she would have needed to start the folic acid before then for it to be efficacious.

d. Having a prior child with a neural-tube defect does not increase the risk of a neural-tube defect in this pregnancy, so she does not need to worry about that.

7–7. The diencephalon, pictured below, gives rise to what part of the brain?

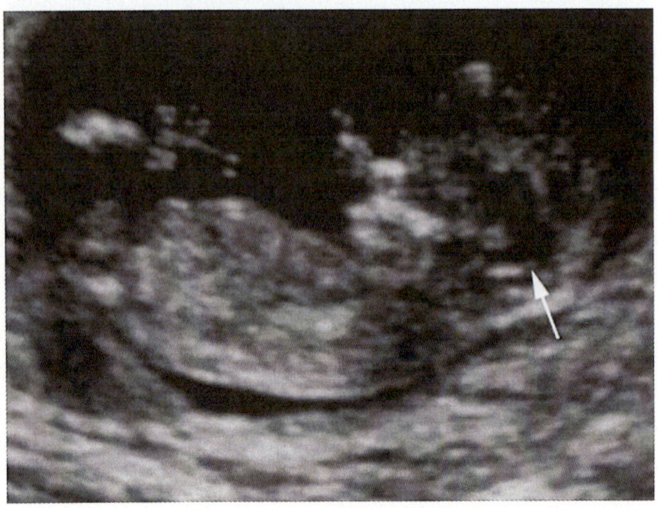

a. Thalami

b. Medulla

c. Midbrain

d. Cerebral hemispheres

7–8. How does the oxygen content of the blood coming to the heart from the inferior vena cava compare to the oxygen content of the blood leaving the placenta?

a. Equal

b. Lower

c. Higher

d. Varies depending on fetal activity

7–9. After birth, the intraabdominal remnants of the umbilical vein become which of the following?

a. Ligamentum teres

b. Umbilical ligaments

c. Ligamentum venosum

d. Ligamentum vascularum

7–10. Which value defines anemia in the fetus?

a. 20%

b. 25%

c. 30%

d. 40%

7–11. Approximately what percentage of the total hemoglobin is hemoglobin F in a term fetus?

a. 25%

b. 40%

c. 50%

d. 75%

7–12. The last stage of fetal lung development starts late in the fetal period and continues into childhood. What is this stage called?

a. Alveolar stage

b. Canalicular stage

c. Terminal sac stage

d. Pseudoglandular stage

7–13. Where does biosynthesis of surfactant take place?

a. Type I pneumocytes

b. Type II pneumocytes

c. Type III pneumocytes

d. Type IV pneumocytes

7–14. Starting at what gestational age does the fetus engage in respiratory movements that are intense enough to move amnionic fluid in and out of the respiratory tract?

a. 4 months

b. 5 months

c. 6 months

d. 7 months

7–15. The foregut gives rise to all except which of the following?

a. Liver

b. Stomach

c. Pancreas

d. Appendix

7–16. At what gestational age does swallowing begin?

a. 6–8 weeks' gestation
b. 10–12 weeks' gestation
c. 16–18 weeks' gestation
d. 20–22 weeks' gestation

7–17. How much amnionic fluid do term fetuses swallow per day?

a. 50–100 mL per day
b. 100–200 mL per day
c. 200–760 mL per day
d. 1500–2000 mL per day

7–18. Which of the following gives meconium its greenish-black color?

a. Vernix
b. Biliverdin
c. Scalp hair
d. Hydrochloric acid

7–19. At what gestational age do the fetal kidneys start producing urine?

a. 6 weeks' gestation
b. 8 weeks' gestation
c. 12 weeks' gestation
d. 16 weeks' gestation

7–20. How much urine does a fetus make at term?

a. 10 mL per day
b. 50 mL per day
c. 200 mL per day
d. 650 mL per day

7–21. Which of the following increases fetal urine formation?

a. Urethral obstruction
b. Fetal growth restriction
c. Uteroplacental insufficiency
d. Maternally administered furosemide

7–22. Which of the following hormones is not produced by the anterior lobe of the fetal pituitary gland?

a. Vasopressin
b. Growth hormone
c. Follicle-stimulating hormone
d. Thyroid-stimulating hormone

7–23. Which of the following statements about the fetal thyroid gland is true?

a. The fetal thyroid starts to make hormones starting at 36 weeks' gestation.
b. By 12 weeks' gestation, the fetal thyroid is concentrating iodide more avidly than the maternal thyroid.
c. With congenital fetal hypothyroidism, the fetus will develop a large goiter in addition to hepatosplenomegaly.
d. After birth, cooling to room temperature causes a sudden and marked decrease in the secretion of thyroid-stimulating hormone, which results in less serum T_4 with a nadir at 24–36 hours of life.

7–24. Where is fetal immunoglobulin M (IgM) produced?

a. Fetus
b. Mother
c. Mother and fetus
d. The fetus does not have IgM

7–25. Which immunoglobulin in colostrum provides mucosal protection against enteric infections?

a. IgA
b. IgE
c. IgG
d. IgM

7–26. Which of the following statements about leptin is true?

a. It is produced exclusively by the placenta.
b. Concentrations peak in amnionic fluid at term.
c. 95% of placental production enters the fetal circulation.
d. Abnormal levels have been associated with fetal growth disorders, gestational diabetes, and preeclampsia.

7–27. Which of the following is found in greater concentrations in maternal plasma compared to fetal plasma?

a. Zinc
b. Iodide
c. Copper
d. Vitamin A

7–28. Which of the following does not affect immunoglobulin G (IgG) transfer across the placenta?

a. Gestational age
b. Placental integrity
c. Maternal levels of IgG
d. Maternal levels of IgM and IgA

7–29. What is uteroplacental blood flow at term?

a. 200–400 mL/min
b. 400–600 mL/min
c. 700–900 mL/min
d. 1200–1400 mL/min

7–30. How does immunoglobulin G (IgG) cross the placenta?

a. Simple diffusion
b. It does not cross the placenta
c. Trophoblast receptor-mediated transfer
d. Facilitated diffusion involving calcium-binding protein

7–31. What is the average oxygen saturation of intervillous blood?

a. 25–35%
b. 45–55%
c. 65–75%
d. 85–95%

7–32. At term, what is the average PCO_2 in the umbilical arteries?

a. 30 mmHg
b. 50 mmHg
c. 60 mmHg
d. 100 mmHg

CHAPTER 7 ANSWER KEY

Question number	Letter answer	Page cited	Header cited
7–1	**c**	p. 124	Gestational Age
7–2	**b**	p. 125	Gestational Age
7–3	**c**	p. 126	Gestational Age
7–4	**a**	p. 126	Embryonic Period
7–5	**c**	p. 128	Fetal Period Epochs
7–6	**c**	p. 129	Central Nervous System Development
7–7	**a**	p. 129	Central Nervous System Development
7–8	**b**	p. 129	Cardiovascular System
7–9	**a**	p. 131	Cardiovascular System
7–10	**c**	p. 131	Hemopoiesis
7–11	**d**	p. 132	Hemopoiesis
7–12	**a**	p. 133	Respiratory System
7–13	**b**	p. 134	Respiratory System
7–14	**a**	p. 134	Respiratory System
7–15	**d**	p. 134	Digestive System
7–16	**b**	p. 134	Digestive System
7–17	**c**	p. 135	Digestive System
7–18	**b**	p. 135	Digestive System
7–19	**c**	p. 136	Urinary System
7–20	**d**	p. 136	Urinary System
7–21	**d**	p. 136	Urinary System
7–22	**a**	p. 136	Endocrine Gland Development
7–23	**b**	p. 136–137	Endocrine Gland Development
7–24	**a**	p. 137	Immunological System
7–25	**a**	p. 137	Immunological System
7–26	**d**	p. 138	Leptin
7–27	**c**	p. 139	Ions and Trace Metals
7–28	**d**	p. 139	Proteins
7–29	**c**	p. 140	The Intervillous Space
7–30	**c**	p. 140	Placental Transfer
7–31	**c**	p. 140	Placental Transfer
7–32	**b**	p. 141	Placental Transfer

SECTION 4

PRECONCEPTIONAL AND PRENATAL CARE

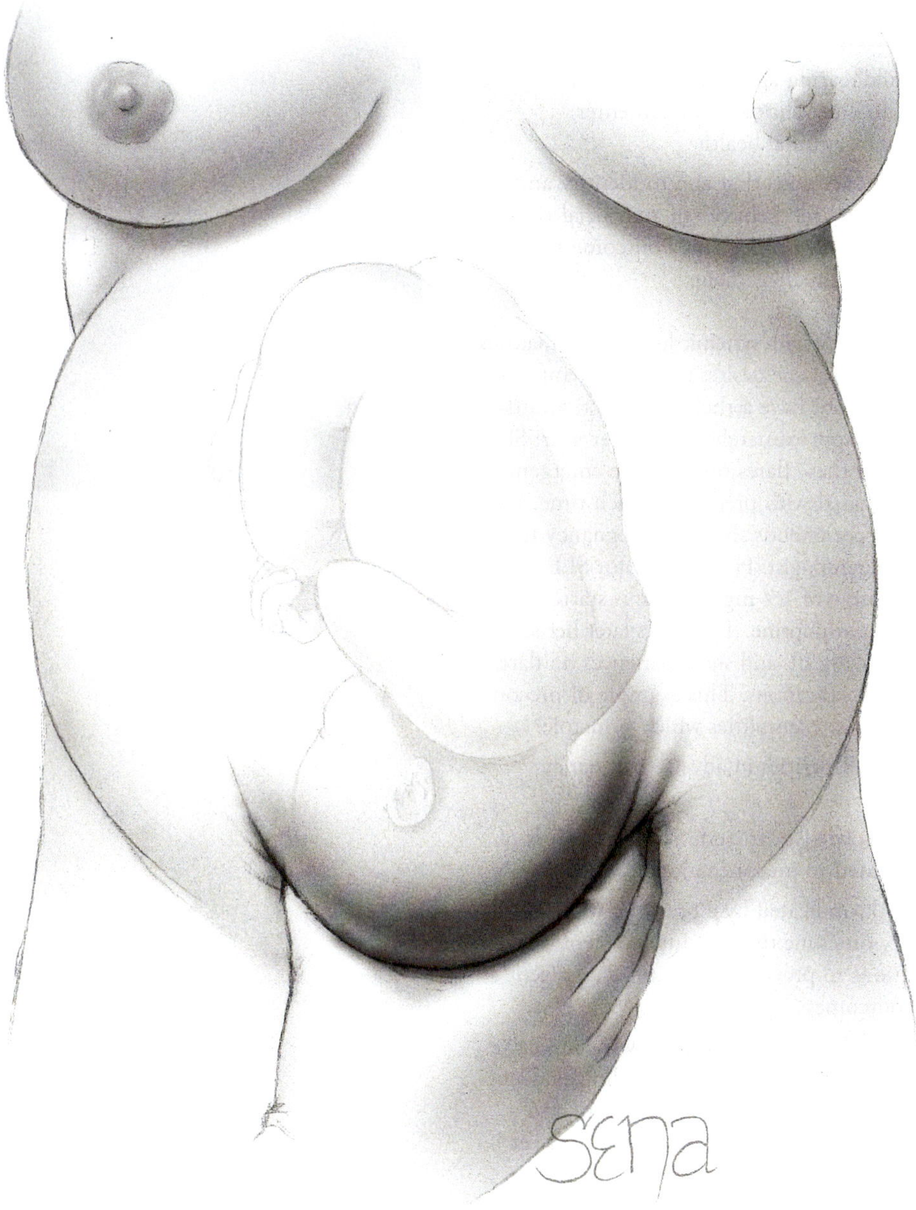

CHAPTER 8

Preconceptional Care

8–1. Which of the following is the most accurate definition of preconceptional care as defined by the Centers for Disease Control and Prevention?

- **a.** Implement strategies that mitigate potential pregnancy risks before conception
- **b.** Reduce risks of adverse pregnancy outcomes through preconceptional interventions
- **c.** Assure childbearing-aged women that with appropriate interventions they can enter pregnancy in optimal health
- **d.** A set of interventions that aim to identify and modify biomedical, behavioral, and social risks to a woman's health or pregnancy outcome through prevention and management

8–2. A 27-year-old patient with systemic lupus erythematosus tells her gynecologist she desires to get pregnant. She reports she does not have a rheumatologist, and that she experiences approximately 4 flares per year. She receives care for these flares through the emergency room and is treated with prednisone each time. Her gynecologist recommends she defer pregnancy until she sees a rheumatologist. Her workup for SLE reveals a serum creatinine of 1.2 mg/dL. She is started on plaquenil and azathioprine. Two years later her serum creatinine is 0.7 mg/dL and she experiences no flares while on these medications. This example of preconceptional care best exemplifies which principle?

- **a.** Reduce the disparities in adverse pregnancy outcomes
- **b.** Improve knowledge, attitudes, and behaviors of women related to preconceptional health
- **c.** Reduce risks indicated by a previous adverse pregnancy outcome through interconceptional interventions to prevent or minimize recurrent adverse outcomes
- **d.** Ensure that all childbearing-aged women receive preconceptional care services—including evidence-based risk screening, health promotion, and interventions—that will enable them to enter pregnancy in optimal health.

8–3. A 29-year-old with no prenatal care presents for her screening ultrasound at 28 weeks' gestation. Evaluation of the fetal head reveals the abnormality pictured below. What percentage of fetuses with this condition are born to women at low risk for the anomaly?

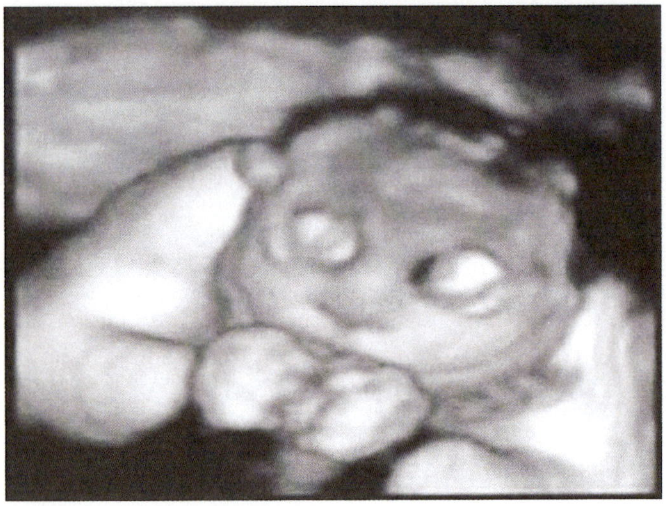

Used with permission from Lesly Sherman.

- **a.** 10%
- **b.** 33%
- **c.** 60%
- **d.** 90%

8–4. One year later you see the patient in Question 1–3 for an annual exam. You counsel her that the she can reduce her recurrence risk of having another baby with a neural-tube defect by supplementing with folic acid. This counseling is an example of which objective of preconceptional care?

a. Reduce the disparities in adverse pregnancy outcomes

b. Improve knowledge, attitudes, and behaviors of women related to preconceptional health

c. Reduce risks indicated by a previous adverse pregnancy outcome through interconceptional interventions to prevent or minimize recurrent adverse outcomes

d. Ensure that all childbearing-aged women receive preconceptional care services—including evidence-based risk screening, health promotion, and interventions—that will enable them to enter pregnancy in optimal health

8–5. Preconceptional folic acid supplementation can reduce the recurrence risk of having a child with a neural-tube defect by what percentage?

a. 11%

b. 26%

c. 72%

d. 90%

8–6. Preconceptional counseling has been shown to do which of the following?

a. Result in more intended pregnancies

b. Decrease the number of perinatal deaths

c. Decrease the number of infants born with birth defects

d. Improve pregnancy outcomes for women with preexisting medical conditions

8–7. When is the best opportunity to provide preconceptional counseling?

a. During the 6-week postpartum visit

b. During a hospitalization for an acute illness

c. During a periodic health maintenance examination

d. At the time an adverse pregnancy outcome is diagnosed

8–8. Preconceptional counseling involves collection of information regarding previous pregnancy outcomes, medical conditions, and family history. What is the optimal method of collecting this information?

a. Nurse visit

b. Paper intake form

c. Online questionnaire

d. Combined questionnaire plus interview

8–9. Hemoglobin A_{1C} measurement provides an assessment of which of the following?

a. Risk of stillbirth

b. Risk for major fetal anomalies

c. Risk for maternal end-organ damage

d. Diabetic control during the preceding 12 weeks

8–10. A 32-year-old woman with diabetes presents for her screening ultrasound and is found to have the fetal abnormality pictured below. Her hemoglobin A_{1C} was 10.9% at conception. What was her risk for developing this major congenital anomaly?

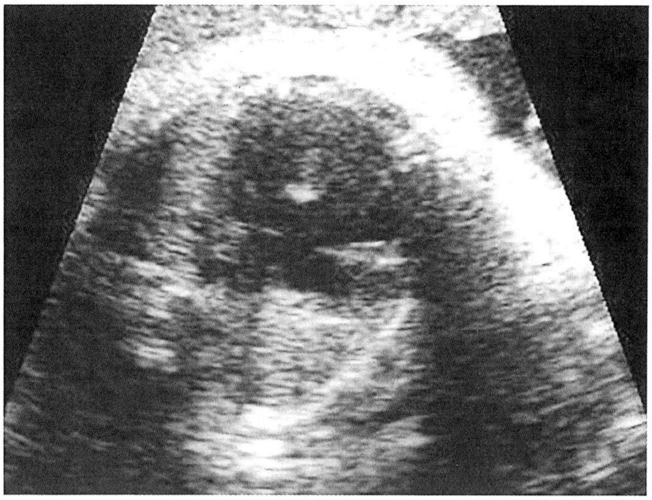

a. 3–5%

b. 25%

c. 30%

d. None of the above

8–11. The patient in Question 8–10 should undergo preconceptional counseling prior to her next pregnancy. Preconceptional counseling in the setting of diabetes has been associated with which of the following?

a. Lower perinatal death rate

b. Improved preconceptional folic acid use

c. Improved glycemic control before pregnancy and in the first trimester

d. All of the above

8–12. Women with epilepsy are at increased risk for which of the following?

a. Stillbirth

b. Miscarriage

c. Congenital anomalies

d. None of the above

8–13. A 27-year-old patient presents to her neurologist to discuss discontinuing her levetiracetam prior to attempting pregnancy. Which of the following characteristics make her a candidate for discontinuation?

- **a.** She has tonic-clonic seizures
- **b.** She is compliant with her medications
- **c.** She has been seizure free for 18 months
- **d.** She has not required an electroencephalogram in 18 months

8–14. What supplement should the patient in Question 8–13 initiate prior to attempting pregnancy?

- **a.** Iron
- **b.** Niacin
- **c.** Folate 1 mg
- **d.** Folate 4 mg

8–15. Which of the following is not an example of a killed bacterial or viral vaccine and therefore should not be administered during pregnancy?

- **a.** Rabies
- **b.** Tetanus
- **c.** Meningococcus
- **d.** Varicella-zoster

8–16. All except which of the following are true regarding vaccinations and pregnancy?

- **a.** Vaccines that contain toxoids may be administered during pregnancy
- **b.** The hepatitis B vaccine series may be administered during pregnancy
- **c.** Receiving the varicella vaccine is indication for pregnancy termination
- **d.** Conception should be delayed by 1 month after receiving the rubella vaccine

8–17. Birth defects are responsible for what percentage of infant mortality?

- **a.** 2%
- **b.** 5%
- **c.** 10%
- **d.** 20%

8–18. What is the most thorough way to obtain a family history?

- **a.** Patient interview
- **b.** Patient questionnaire
- **c.** Constructing a pedigree
- **d.** Interviewing all family members

8–19. What is the recommended daily dose of folic acid that all women who may become pregnant should take?

- **a.** 1 mg
- **b.** 4 mg
- **c.** 400 mg
- **d.** None of the above

8–20. Which fetal tissues are most susceptible to damage by high blood phenylalanine levels?

- **a.** Renal and hepatic
- **b.** Renal and cardiac
- **c.** Cardiac and neural
- **d.** Neural and hepatic

8–21. A 31-year-old woman with phenylketonuria wants to know what is the best way to prevent damage to a fetus when she gets pregnant.

- **a.** Use a donor egg to get pregnant
- **b.** Make sure her phenylalanine levels are normal 3 months prior to conception
- **c.** Adhere to a phenylalanine-restricted diet once she has a positive pregnancy test
- **d.** Undergo chorionic villus sampling in the first trimester to determine if the fetus inherited the defect

8–22. Worldwide, what are the most common single-gene disorders?

- **a.** Hemoglobinopathies
- **b.** Cystic fibrosis mutations
- **c.** Glycogen-storage diseases
- **d.** Phenylketonuria mutations

8–23. All except which of the following diseases are inherited in the manner demonstrated by this pedigree?

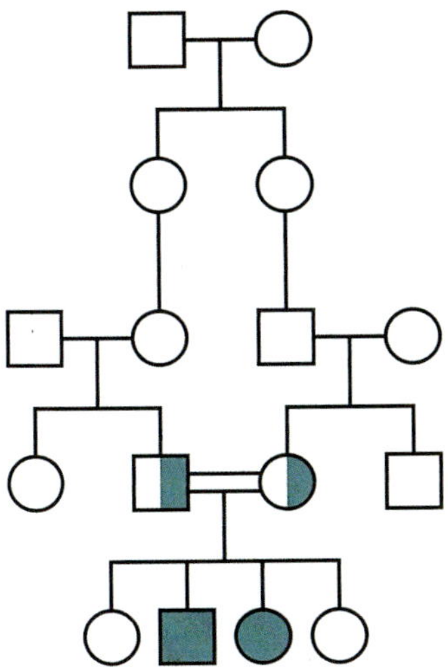

a. Cystic fibrosis
b. Bloom syndrome
c. Tay-Sachs disease
d. Huntington disease

8–24. What is the best way to identify a genetic abnormality in a stillborn fetus?

a. Autopsy
b. Karyotype
c. Maternal cell-free DNA testing
d. Chromosomal microarray analysis

8–25. Which of the following are important aspects of reproductive history that aid in preconceptional counseling?

a. Length of prior labor
b. Prior child's birthweight
c. History of preterm delivery
d. Prenatal screening results from prior pregnancy

8–26. Ashkenazi Jewish individuals should be offered preconceptional carrier screening for all except which of the following?

a. Cystic fibrosis
b. β-thalassemia
c. Canavan disease
d. Tay-Sachs disease

8–27. Which of the following obstetrical complications is increased in adolescent pregnancies compared with women aged 20 to 35 years?

a. Anemia
b. Aneuploidy
c. Cesarean delivery
d. Postpartum hemorrhage

8–28. Which of the following is the most common pregnancy complication in women older than 35 years according to the figure below?

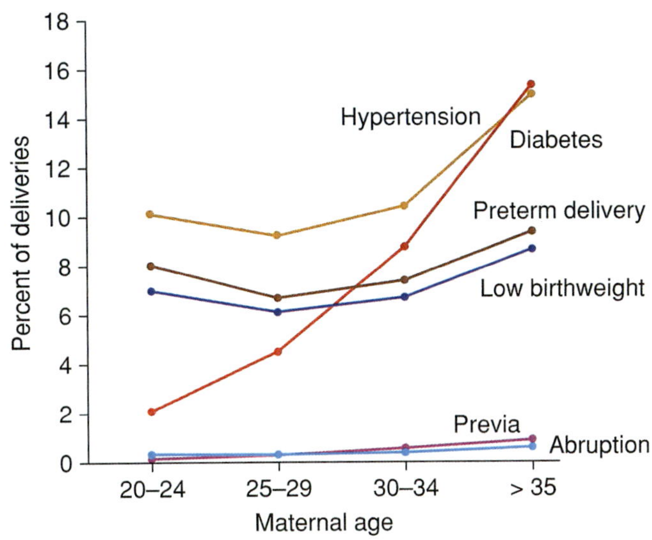

Reproduced with permission from Cunningham FG, Leveno KJ, Bloom SL, et al (eds): Preconceptional Care. In Williams Obstetrics, 25th ed. New York, McGraw-Hill, 2018, Figure 8-3.

a. Diabetes
b. Aneuploidy
c. Preeclampsia
d. Placenta previa

8–29. Fetal risks related to maternal age include which of the following?

a. Aneuploidy
b. Preterm birth
c. Growth disorders
d. All of the above

8–30. A 30-year-old patient presents for her first prenatal care visit and an initial ultrasound reveals the finding below. Morbidity and mortality related to this type of gestation result from which of the following?

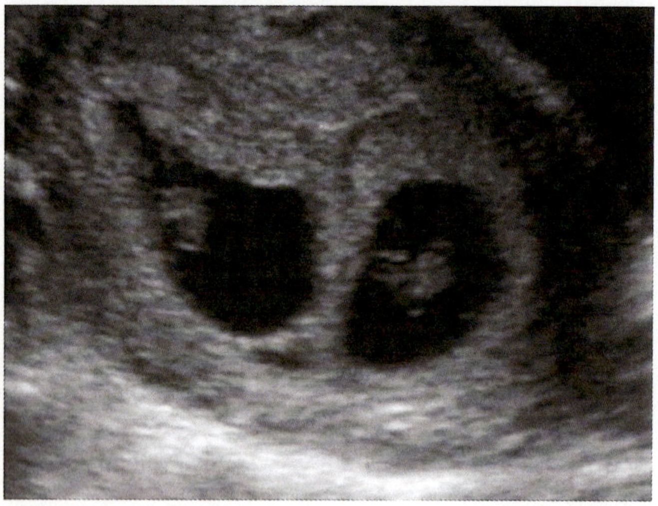

Used with permission from Dr. Tiffany Woodus.

a. Bed rest
b. Vaginal delivery
c. Cesarean section
d. Preterm delivery

8–31. A 40-year-old woman starts displaying poor coordination, involuntary jerking movements, and irritability. Family history reveals the pedigree below. The patient is represented with an arrow. What factor is most likely related to her genetic condition?

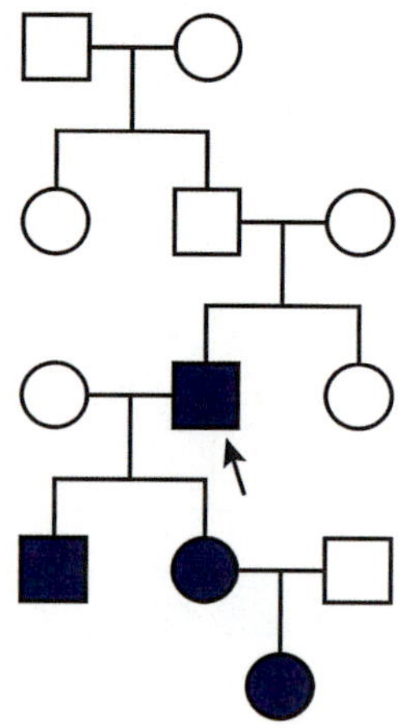

a. Her father was 51 years old when she was born.
b. Her mother was 42 years old when she was born.
c. Her mother was diagnosed with diabetes a few months prior to conception.
d. She was conceived with the use of assisted reproductive technologies.

8–32. Maternal obesity is associated with all except which of the following maternal complications?

a. Preeclampsia
b. Cesarean delivery
c. Gestational diabetes
d. Spontaneous preterm delivery

CHAPTER 8 ANSWER KEY

Question number	Letter answer	Page cited	Header cited
8–1	d	p. 146	Preconceptional Care and Counseling
8–2	d	p. 146	Preconceptional Care and Counseling
8–3	d	p. 149	Neural-tube Defects
8–4	c	p. 146	Preconceptional Care and Counseling
8–5	c	p. 147	Neural-tube Defects
8–6	a	p. 146	Preconceptional Care and Counseling
8–7	c	p. 147	Preconceptional Care and Counseling
8–8	d	p. 147	Counseling Session
8–9	b	p. 147	Diabetes Mellitus
8–10	b	p. 148	Figure 8-1
8–11	d	p. 148	Diabetes Mellitus
8–12	d	p. 148	Epilepsy
8–13	a	p. 148	Epilepsy
8–14	d	p. 148	Epilepsy
8–15	d	p. 149	Immunizations
8–16	c	p. 149	Immunizations
8–17	d	p. 149	Genetic Diseases
8–18	c	p. 149	Family History
8–19	c	p. 149	Neural-tube Defects
8–20	c	p. 149	Phenylketonuria
8–21	b	p. 150	Phenylketonuria
8–22	a	p. 150	Thalassemias
8–23	d	p. 151	Individuals of Eastern European Jewish Descent
8–24	d	p. 151	Reproductive History
8–25	c	p. 151	Reproductive History
8–26	b	p. 151	Individuals of Eastern European Jewish Descent
8–27	a	p. 151	Maternal Age
8–28	a	p. 151	Figure 8-3
8–29	d	p. 151	Maternal Age
8–30	d	p. 151	Assisted Reproductive Technologies
8–31	a	p. 152	Paternal Age
8–32	d	p. 152	Diet

CHAPTER 9

Prenatal Care

9–1. A 32-year-old nulligravida patient with no prenatal care presents in labor. You realize lack of prenatal care increases her risk of a poor outcome. Specifically, what is the increased risk of mortality for women who do not receive prenatal care as compared to women who do?

a. Risk unchanged

b. Twofold risk

c. Fourfold risk

d. Fivefold risk

9–2. Which of the following is more common when women do not obtain prenatal care?

a. Stillbirth

b. Preterm birth

c. Neonatal death

d. All of the above

9–3. A schematic of β-hCG levels in pregnancy is shown below. When do β-hCG levels peak in pregnancy?

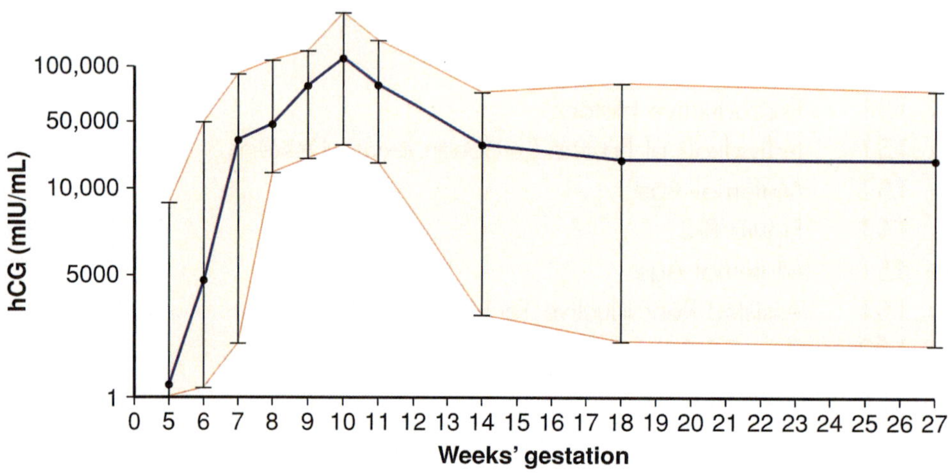

Reproduced with permission from Cunningham FG, Leveno KJ, Bloom SL, et al (eds): Prenatal care. In William Obstetrics, 25th ed. New York, McGraw-Hill, 2018, Figure 9-2.

a. 40–50 days after last menstrual period

b. 60–70 days after last menstrual period

c. 80–90 days after last menstrual period

d. 120–140 days after last menstrual period

9–4. Which possible cause of a "false-positive" β-hCG is most common?

a. Malignancy

b. Heterophilic antibodies

c. Exogenous β-hCG use for weight loss

d. β-hCG produced in the pituitary gland

9–5. Which sign confirming an early intrauterine pregnancy is best demonstrated in the image below?

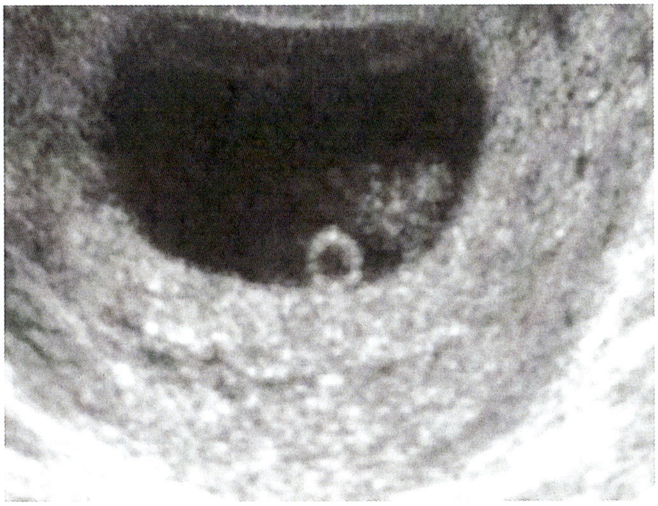

a. Yolk sac
b. Fetal pole
c. Intradecidual sign
d. Double decidual sign

9–6. A 33-year-old woman who presents for prenatal care is described as a G5P2-1-1-3. From this information you recognize she needs counseling regarding the risks of which of the following?

a. Grand multiparity
b. Advanced maternal age
c. Recurrent preterm birth
d. Recurrent pregnancy loss

9–7. A 26-year-old G1 presents to your office for prenatal care at 12 weeks' gestation. She denies any past medical or surgical history, but does report smoking 1 pack of cigarettes every 2–3 days. Which of the following statements regarding her tobacco use in pregnancy is not yet proven?

a. Smoking increases the risk of preterm birth.
b. Smoking increases the risk of placental abruption.
c. Use of a nicotine patch can improve perinatal outcomes.
d. Smoking cessation at any stage of pregnancy can improve perinatal outcomes.

9–8. A 24-year-old woman presents for prenatal care at 14 weeks' gestation. During your initial interview she reports that for the last year she has consistently consumed 8–10 alcoholic beverages per day. Which of the following fetal abnormalities is she at increased risk of experiencing? (An affected infant is pictured below.)

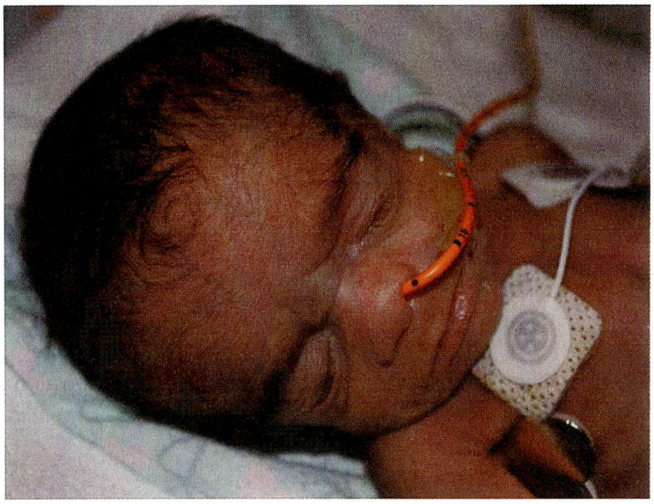

a. Facial abnormalities
b. Fetal growth restriction
c. Central nervous system dysfunction
d. All of the above

9–9. What is the prevalence of domestic violence in pregnancy?

a. <0.5%
b. 0.5%
c. 1–2%
d. 4–8%

9–10. For a routine low-risk woman with no complaints, which laboratory test should not be offered as part of her first prenatal visit?

a. Hepatitis B testing
b. Chlamydia screening
c. Blood type and screen
d. Thyroid function testing

9–11. A 29-year-old G2P1 at 8 weeks' gestation presents for her first prenatal care visit. She is 64 inches tall and weighs 160 pounds, making her body mass index 27 kg/m^2. What amount of total weight gain should you recommend for her pregnancy?

a. 0–10 pounds
b. 11–20 pounds
c. 15–25 pounds
d. 25–35 pounds

9–12. For an obese woman, the risk of preeclampsia and cesarean delivery is lowest with what amount of gestational weight gain?

a. 0–14 pounds
b. 11–20 pounds
c. 15–25 pounds
d. 25–35 pounds

9–13. Among women with a normal body mass index prior to pregnancy who have less than 25 pounds of gestational weight gain, which complication is increased?

a. Preeclampsia
b. Cesarean delivery
c. Large-for-gestational-age infant
d. Small-for-gestational-age infant

9–14. There is substantial evidence that severe undernutrition during pregnancy can result in a higher rate of which of the following?

a. Preterm birth
b. Perinatal mortality
c. Small-for-gestational-age infants
d. All of the above

9–15. For a woman with a normal prepregnancy body mass index, approximately how many additional kilocalories per day are recommended in the three trimesters of pregnancy, respectively?

a. 0, 340, 450
b. 0, 250, 500
c. 100, 200, 300
d. 200, 300, 400

9–16. Which food is the most complete source of nutrients for pregnant women?

a. Dairy
b. Fruit
c. Poultry
d. Leafy vegetables

9–17. Which mineral is least likely to be supplied in quantities sufficient for pregnancy when ingesting a normal diet?

a. Iron
b. Calcium
c. Vitamin D
d. Vitamin B_6

9–18. A 23-year-old G2P1 presents for her postpartum visit after delivering an infant with an encephalocele, as pictured below. You counsel her that next time she should initiate 4 mg of folic acid daily at least 4 weeks prior to conception. This will decrease her risk of a similar birth defect by what percentage?

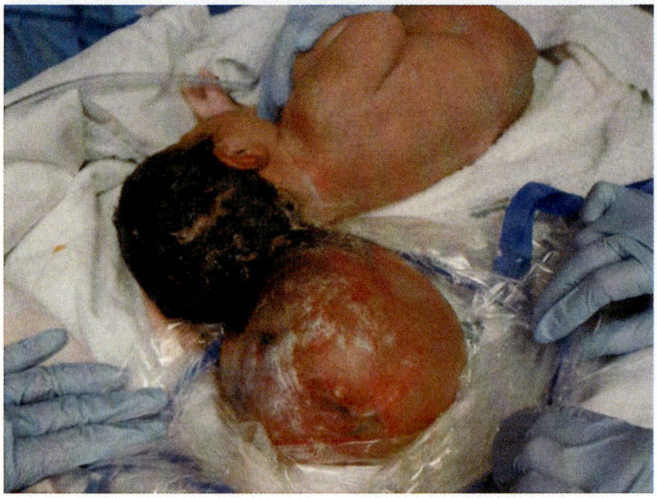

a. 30%
b. 50%
c. 70%
d. 90%

9–19. Which vitamin, when ingested in large quantities, causes a well-described constellation of birth defects?

a. Vitamin A
b. Vitamin C
c. Vitamin B_6
d. Vitamin B_{12}

9–20. A 27-year-old woman at 16 weeks' gestation reports a long history of regular aerobic exercise including cycling, running, swimming, and low-impact aerobics. Which of those activities do you recommend she forego during pregnancy?

a. Cycling
b. Running
c. Swimming
d. Low-impact aerobics

9–21. Which type of fish contains a level of methylmercury low enough to be safe for consumption during pregnancy?

a. Shark
b. Salmon
c. Tile fish
b. Swordfish

9–22. A 28-year-old G2P1 presents for a prenatal appointment and reports that recently her toddler was screened for lead exposure and had an elevated level, though he did not require treatment. They reside in a home built in 1950. You draw a maternal lead level, which is 10 μg/dL. What is the most appropriate recommendation?

a. No intervention

b. Chelation therapy

c. Relocate her family for the duration of the pregnancy.

d. Identify the source of lead in her environment and remove it.

9–23. At least how much elemental iron should be given as a supplement daily to a pregnant woman?

a. 15 mg

b. 27 mg

c. 42 mg

d. 60 mg

9–24. A 29-year-old primigravida with an unknown last menstrual period presents complaining of vaginal spotting and cramping. Transvaginal sonographic examination is performed as part of her evaluation. One image is shown here. Physical exam identifies a closed cervical os and no bleeding. Bimanual examination is benign. What is the most appropriate management plan?

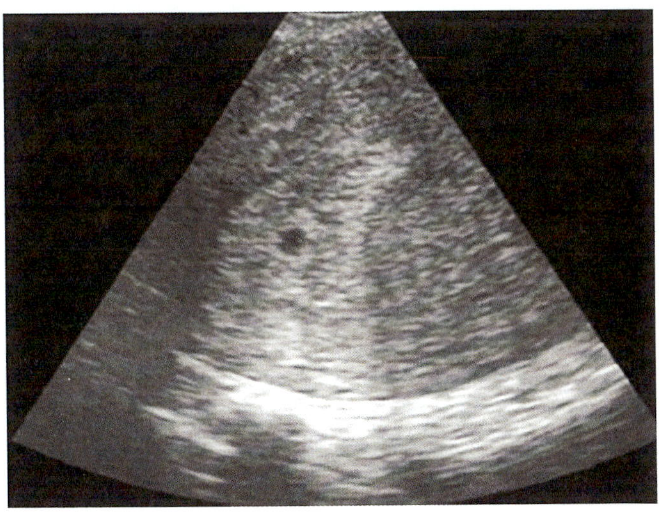

a. Dilation and curettage

b. Methotrexate administration

c. Obtain serial serum β-hCG levels

d. Repeat sonographic examination in 48 hours

9–25. Maternal deficiency of vitamin D has been associated with which of the following complications in the offspring?

a. Anemia

b. Seizures

c. Jaundice

d. Congenital rickets

9–26. Air travel is not recommended after which gestational age?

a. 14 weeks

b. 20 weeks

c. 30 weeks

d. 36 weeks

9–27. Which of the following statements regarding vaccinations in pregnancy is true?

a. All pregnant women should be offered influenza vaccine during the appropriate season.

b. The Tdap vaccine should be given to all pregnant women between 16 and 20 weeks' gestation.

c. Varicella vaccine should be offered to all women who are exposed to chicken pox during pregnancy.

d. The measles-mumps-rubella vaccine should be given to all pregnant women who are not immune.

9–28. When instructing a pregnant woman on proper safety restraints when operating an automobile, which statement is true?

a. A two-point restraint system is ideal.

b. Airbags should be disabled in the third trimester.

c. The lap belt should be under her abdomen and across her thighs.

d. The shoulder belt should be across her chest above the level of her breasts.

9–29. Which of the following concerns regarding international air travel during the third trimester cannot be mitigated with frequent ambulation?

a. Radiation exposure

b. Venous thromboembolism

c. Cabin air pressure changes

d. Development of complications remote from health resources

9–30. Sexual intercourse during pregnancy is associated with which of the following pregnancy complications?

a. Miscarriage

b. Preterm birth

c. Spontaneous rupture of membranes

d. None of the above

9–31. Which of the following is the only vaccine with proven fetal harm?

a. Varicella
b. Smallpox
c. Hepatitis B
d. Measles-mumps-rubella

9–32. As demonstrated in the image below, fundal height measurements in centimeters correlate closely with gestational age between 20 and 34 weeks. Which of the following can introduce error into this measurement?

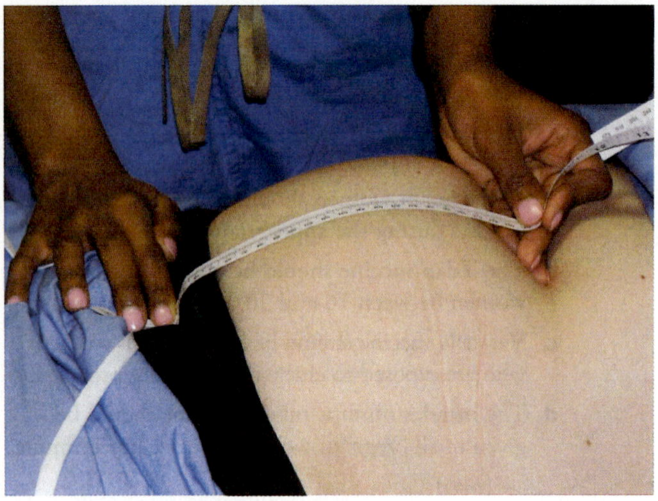

Used with permission from Dr. Elizabeth Swartout.

a. Obesity
b. Full bladder
c. Uterine leiomyomata
d. All of the above

9–33. What is the recommended amount of caffeine consumption in pregnancy according to the American College of Obstetricians and Gynecologists?

a. 0 mg/day
b. <100 mg/day
c. <200 mg/day
d. <500 mg/day

9–34. Over 70% of women experience lower back pain in pregnancy. Which treatment is contraindicated during pregnancy?

a. Baclofen 10 mg every 8 hours as needed
b. Ibuprofen 800 mg every 8 hours as needed
c. Cyclobenzaprine 5 mg every 8 hours as needed
d. Acetaminophen 650 mg every 6 hours as needed

CHAPTER 9 ANSWER KEY

Question number	Letter answer	Page cited	Header cited
9–1	d	p. 158	Prenatal Care in the United States
9–2	d	p. 158	Prenatal Care in the United States
9–3	b	p. 158	Diagnosis of Pregnancy
9–4	b	p. 159	Diagnosis of Pregnancy
9–5	a	p. 159	Diagnosis of Pregnancy
9–6	c	p. 161	Initial Prenatal Evaluation
9–7	c	p. 162	Initial Prenatal Evaluation
9–8	d	p. 162	Initial Prenatal Evaluation
9–9	d	p. 163	Initial Prenatal Evaluation
9–10	d	p. 163	Initial Prenatal Evaluation
9–11	c	p. 166	Nutritional Counseling
9–12	a	p. 166	Nutritional Counseling
9–13	d	p. 166	Nutritional Counseling
9–14	c	p. 166	Nutritional Counseling
9–15	a	p. 168	Nutritional Counseling
9–16	a	p. 168	Nutritional Counseling
9–17	a	p. 168	Nutritional Counseling
9–18	c	p. 169	Nutritional Counseling
9–19	a	p. 169	Nutritional Counseling
9–20	a	p. 170	Common Concerns
9–21	b	p. 170	Common Concerns
9–22	d	p. 171	Common Concerns
9–23	b	p. 168	Nutritional Counseling
9–24	c	p. 159	Diagnosis of Pregnancy
9–25	d	p. 169	Nutritional Counseling
9–26	d	p. 171	Common Concerns
9–27	a	p. 172	Common Concerns
9–28	c	p. 171	Common Concerns
9–29	d	p. 171	Common Concerns
9–30	d	p. 171	Common Concerns
9–31	b	p. 172	Common Concerns
9–32	d	p. 165	Subsequent Prenatal Visits
9–33	c	p. 173	Common Concerns
9–34	b	p. 173	Common Concerns

SECTION 5

THE FETAL PATIENT

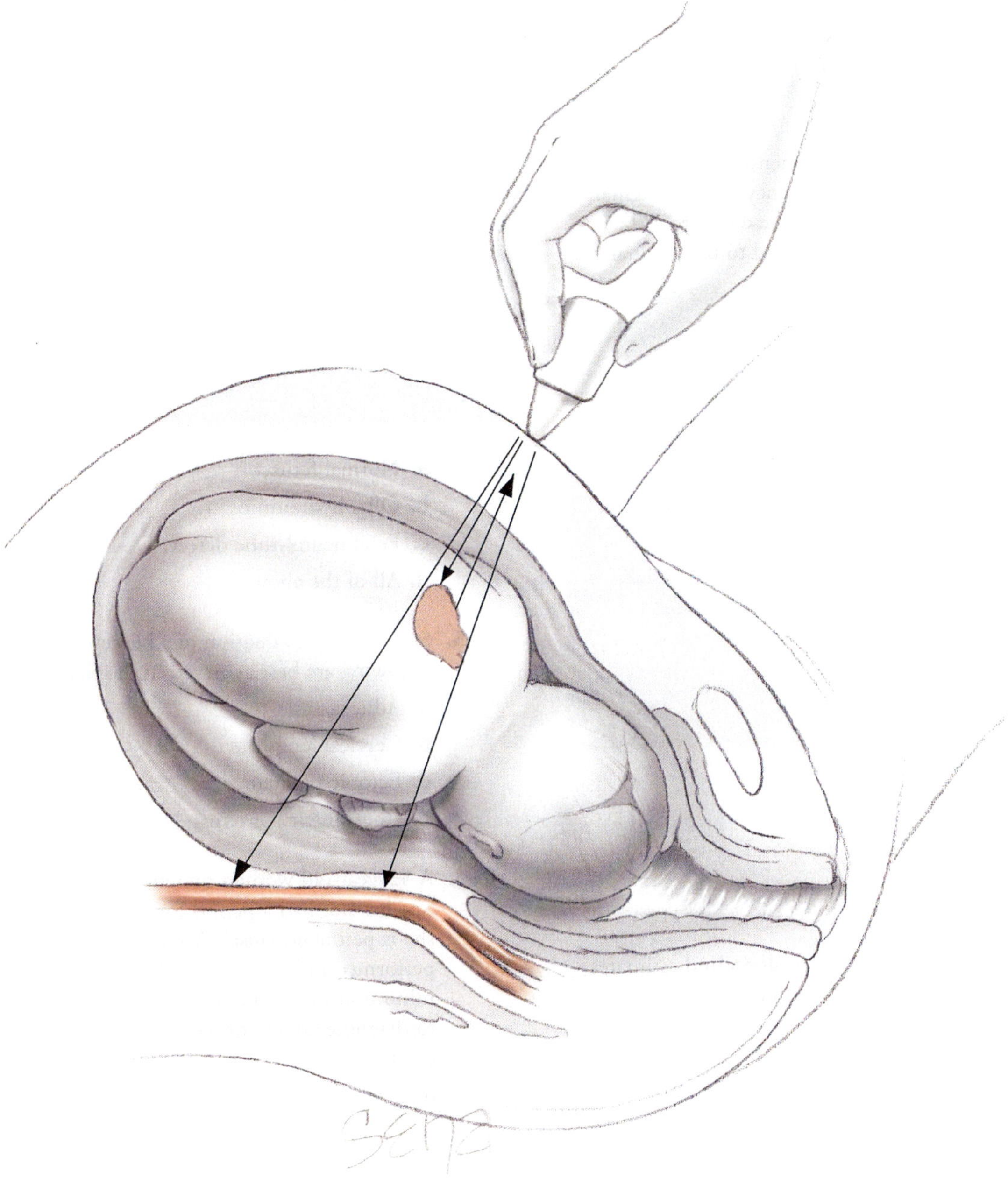

CHAPTER 10

Fetal Imaging

10–1. The thermal index, the temperature elevation that potentially can induce fetal injury, is increased in which of the following?

a. Pulsed Doppler imaging
b. Longer examination time
c. Locations near fetal bone
d. All of the above

10–2. A 25-year-old with irregular menstrual periods presents with a suspicion of pregnancy. A transvaginal ultrasound is performed with these results. What gestational age should be assigned to the pregnancy?

Composite Data

LMP		11/21/2017	
Clinical Age		23w 6d	EDC 8/28/2018
US Age	Hadlock (BPD, HC, AC, FL)		US EDC
EFW	Hadlock (BPD, HC, AC, FL)		
EFW%	Hadlock		

OB Gestational Age Measurements

	Author	w	d	2SD(d)			Growth Author	%
CRL	Hadlock	8	0	5	15.8	(mm)	Hadlock	
GSD	Rempen	7	4	12	24.6	(mm)	Hellman	

a. 7 weeks 4 days
b. 8 weeks 0 days
c. 8 weeks 6 days
d. None of the above

10–3. What is the standard error for ultrasound estimates of fetal weight after the first trimester?

a. 5%
b. 10%
c. 20%
d. 33%

10–4. What fetal conditions might explain the head measurements seen below?

LMP		10/29/2017		
Clinical Age		27w 1d	EDC	8/5/2018
US Age	Hadlock (BPD, HC, AC, FL)	26w 5d +/- 13d	US EDC	8/8/2018
EFW	Hadlock (BPD, HC, AC, FL)	973g +/- 144g(2 lb 2oz +/- 5oz)		
EFW%	Hadlock 22%			

OB Gestational Age Measurements

	Author	w	d	2SD(d)			Growth Author	%
BPD	Hadlock	26	3	15	65.3	(mm)	Hadlock	16
HC	Hadlock	27	5	14	255.5	(mm)	Hadlock	41
AC	Hadlock	26	1	15	216.7	(mm)	Hadlock	15
FL	Hadlock	27	2	15	50.9	(mm)	Hadlock	39
EFW	Osaka	25	5		973	(g)	Hadlock	22

a. Normal fetus
b. Oligohydramnios
c. Fetal neural-tube defect
d. All of the above

10–5. Sonographic evaluation of all except which of the following are best achieved in the first trimester?

a. Adnexa
b. Cervical length
c. Ectopic pregnancy
d. Chorionicity of twins

10–6. A 42-year-old woman presents with vaginal spotting. She has not had a period for 2 months and believes she is perimenopausal. A transvaginal ultrasound is performed in her gynecologist's office. What is the minimum mean sac diameter measurement necessary to diagnose an anembryonic pregnancy with certainty?

a. 7 mm
b. 10 mm
c. 20 mm
d. 25 mm

10–7. A 40-year-old multigravida presents at 12 weeks' gestation for a first-trimester ultrasound evaluation. The nuchal translucency is measured as shown in the image and is noted to be increased at 4.6 mm. She subsequently undergoes chorionic villus sampling and the fetal karyotype is 46,XY. Her fetus still needs to be evaluated in the second trimester for which of the following?

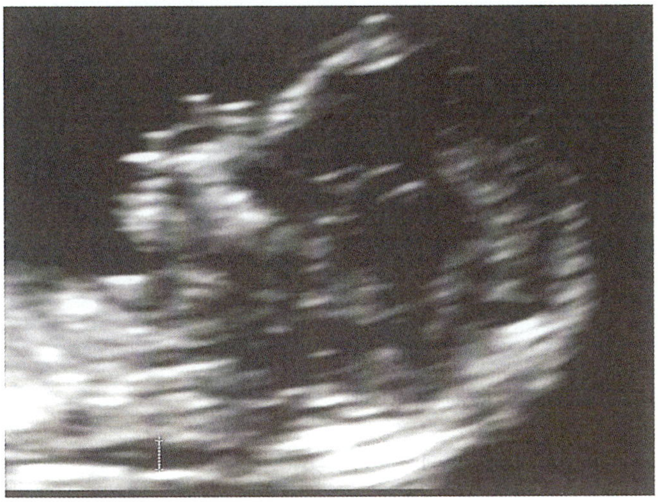

Used with permission from Dr. Deana Hussamy.

- **a.** Aneuploidy
- **b.** Cardiac defects
- **c.** Duodenal atresia
- **d.** Cleft lip and palate

10–8. The following measurement of the single deepest vertical pocket is taken from a pregnancy in which polyhydramnios is suspected. The distance between the two calipers must exceed what value to confirm this diagnosis?

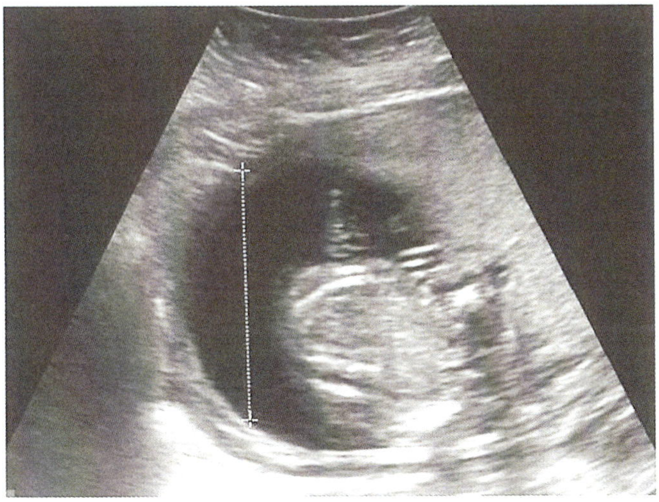

- **a.** 6 cm
- **b.** 8 cm
- **c.** 10 cm
- **d.** 12 cm

10–9. During a transabdominal ultrasound performed at 20 weeks' gestation to evaluate fetal anatomy, the following image is obtained. What is the appropriate next step in the care of this patient?

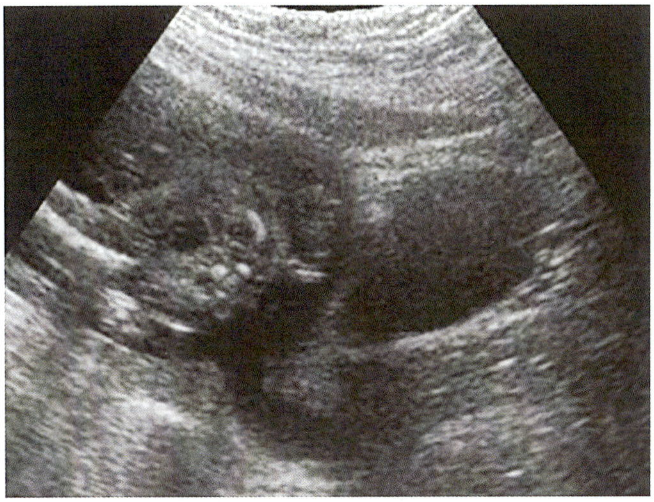

- **a.** Cerclage placement
- **b.** Transvaginal ultrasound
- **c.** Test for cervical infections
- **d.** Nothing as this is a normal finding

10–10. What additional ultrasound measurement should be taken in the same image that the cerebellum and cisterna magna are evaluated?

- **a.** Nuchal fold
- **b.** Lateral ventricle
- **c.** Nuchal translucency
- **d.** Cavum septum pellucidum

10–11. The image below is obtained when a primigravida has her first ultrasound. Targeted sonography is performed, and the finding is isolated. What is her recurrence risk in a subsequent pregnancy if she does not take periconceptional folic acid?

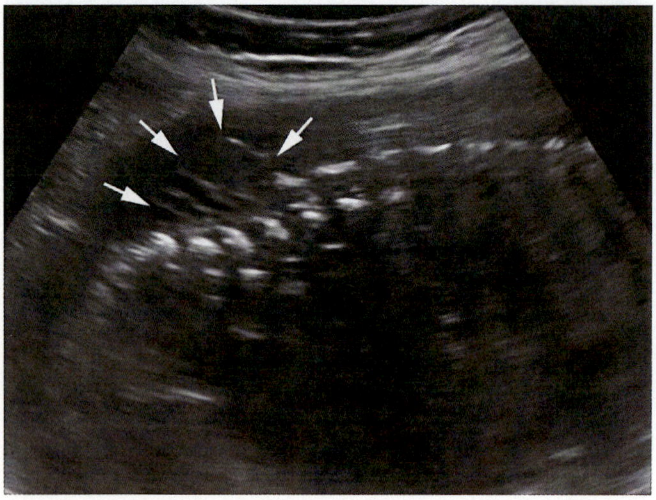

a. 0%
b. 1–2%
c. 3–5%
d. 10%

10–12. What other sonographic findings may be seen with the lesion seen in the Question 10–11?

a. Ventriculomegaly
b. Scalloping of the frontal bones
c. Effacement of the cisterna magna
d. All of the above

10–13. What is the upper limit of normal after 15 weeks' gestation for the lateral ventricle?

a. 5 mm
b. 10 mm
c. 15 mm
d. 20 mm

10–14. What condition should be suspected when a "tear-drop" shaped lateral ventricle is seen on prenatal sonography?

a. Holoprosencephaly
b. Arnold-Chiari malformation
c. Dandy-Walker malformation
d. Agenesis of the corpus callosum

10–15. Shown in the image below are the intracranial findings of alobar holoprosencephaly (V = ventricle, Th = thalami). Fetal karyotyping is most likely to identify which aneuploidy?

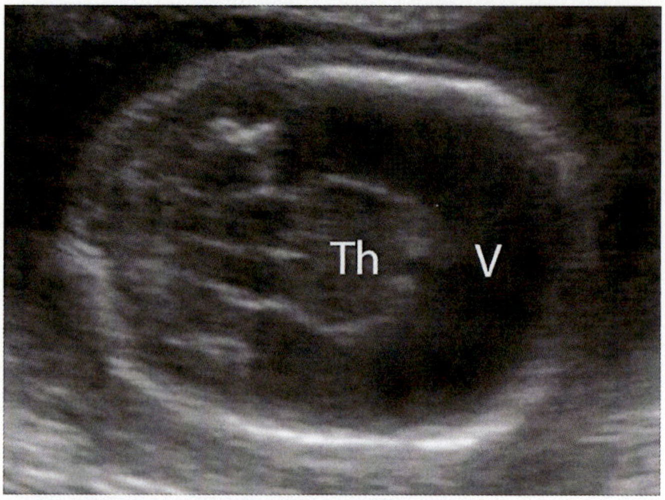

Used with permission from Dr. Jodi Dashe.

a. Trisomy 13
b. Trisomy 18
c. Trisomy 21
d. Monosomy X

10–16. Caudal regression sequence is increased in what maternal medical complication?

a. Seizure disorder
b. Diabetes mellitus
c. Advanced maternal age
d. Systemic lupus erythematosus

10–17. All of the following except which are true statements regarding the diagnosis seen in the image?

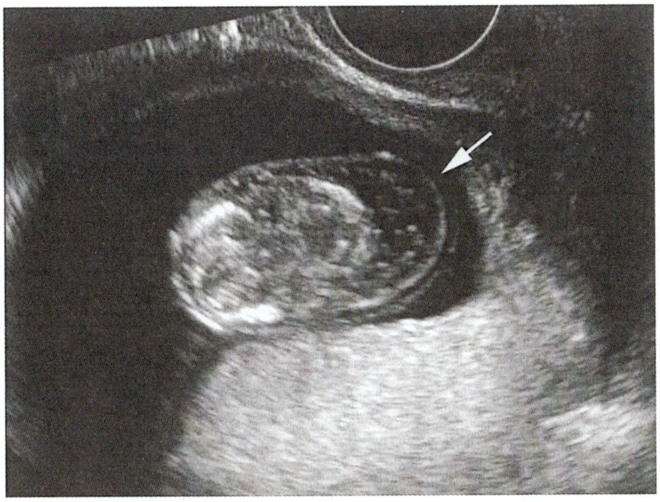

a. The incidence in the first trimester is 1/300.
b. Large lesions frequently resolve by the second trimester.
c. The finding portends a higher risk for aneuploidy than does a thickened nuchal translucency.
d. Trisomy 21 is the most common aneuploidy when the diagnosis is made in the first trimester.

10–18. Which of the following is not of prognostic significance in the evaluation of congenital diaphragmatic hernias?

a. Presence of fetal swallowing
b. Degree of liver herniation in the chest
c. Sonographic lung-to-head measurement
d. Magnetic resonance imaging of lung volumes

10–19. What is the most common class of congenital anomalies?

a. Spine
b. Renal
c. Cardiac
d. Gastrointestinal

10–20. All of the following except which are an indication for fetal echocardiographic evaluation?

a. Dizygotic twin gestation
b. Maternal phenylketonuria
c. Fetal arrhythmia heard on Doppler
d. Paternal history of ventricular septal defect

10–21. The finding below is present on an ultrasound performed at 24 weeks' gestation. What is the likelihood this fetus has trisomy 21?

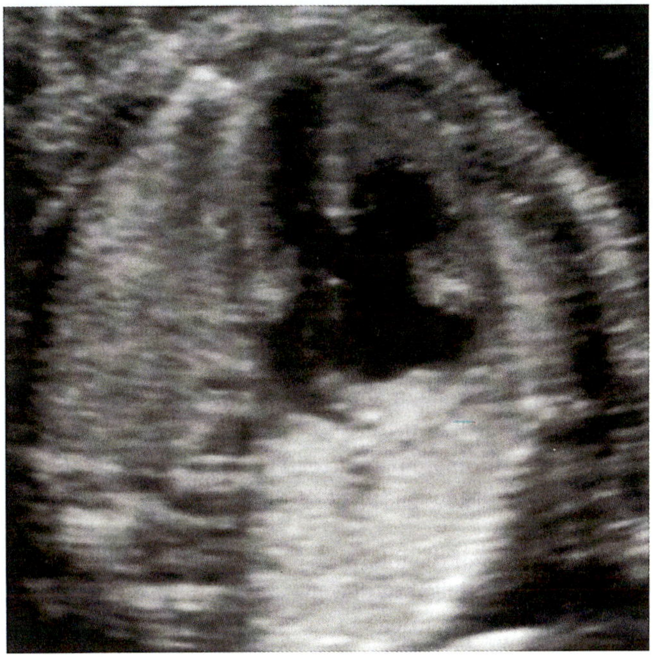

Reproduced with permission from Cunningham FG, Leveno KJ, Bloom SL, et al (eds): Fetal imaging. In William Obstetrics, 25th ed. New York, McGraw-Hill, 2018, Figure 10-30b.

a. 10%
b. 25%
c. 50%
d. 75%

10–22. At 20 weeks' gestation, the finding below is detected on ultrasound. All of the following except which are true statements about this condition?

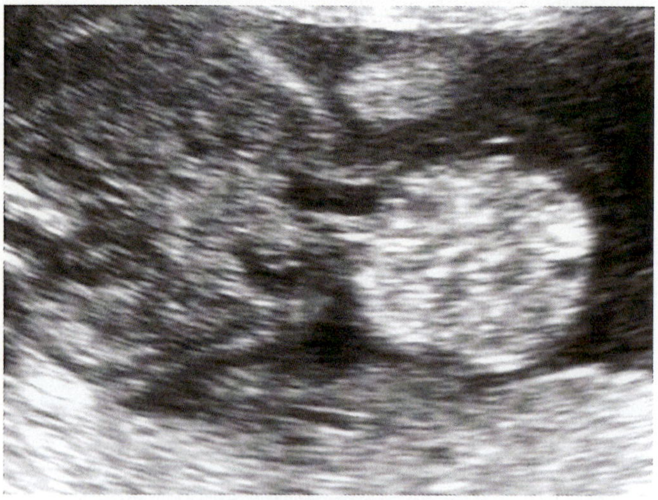

a. The defect is covered by amnion.

b. Large defects are associated with an increased risk of aneuploidy.

c. Other major anomalies or aneuploidy are present in half of these cases.

d. Chromosomal microarray should be offered when a diagnosis is made of this condition.

10–23. Which of the following is not associated with impaired fetal swallowing and non-visualization of the fetal stomach?

a. Hydrops fetalis

b. Duodenal atresia

c. Esophageal atresia

d. Craniofacial abnormalities

10–24. What is the primary source of amnionic fluid in the late second trimester?

a. Fetal urine production

b. Fetal pulmonary exudates

c. Secretions from syncytiotrophoblast

d. Transudate across the amnion mesenchyme

10–25. At 33 weeks' gestation the finding below is detected on an ultrasound performed for fetal growth. The anterior-posterior measurement of the renal pelvis is 6.5 mm bilaterally. What is the appropriate next step in the management of the patient?

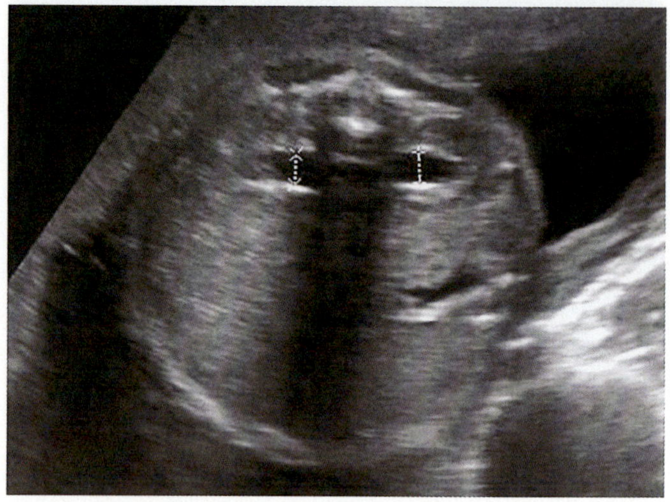

a. Repeat ultrasound in 1 week

b. No further evaluation necessary

c. Notify the pediatrician so postnatal evaluation can be arranged.

d. Schedule a consultation with a pediatric urologist prior to delivery.

10–26. If the measurement of the renal pelvis in Question 10–25 is 16 mm, what is the likelihood that a postnatal abnormality will be diagnosed?

a. 5%

b. 25%

c. 50%

d. 90%

10–27. What is a normal S/D ratio after 30 weeks' gestation?

a. 2.0

b. <3.0

c. 4.0

d. None of the above

10–28. Reversal of end-diastolic blood flow in the umbilical artery is present in which of the following situations?

a. Large-for-gestational-age fetal size

b. When placental impedance has fallen

c. When there is 50% obliteration of small arteries in the villi

d. None of the above

10–29. What is the normal volume of blood flow to the gravid uterus at term?

a. 50 mL/min

b. 100 mL/min

c. 500 mL/min

d. 1000 mL/min

10–30. Why is middle cerebral artery peak systolic velocity increased in fetal anemia?

a. Decreased blood viscosity

b. Decreased fetal cardiac output

c. Fetal pulmonary vasoconstriction

d. Increased maternal uterine artery resistance

10–31. Which of the following fetal malformations is least likely to benefit from prenatal magnetic resonance imaging?

a. Teratoma

b. Cardiac anomaly

c. Neural-tube defect

d. Suspected bowel obstruction

10–32. A patient is scheduled for fetal magnetic resonance imaging following the diagnosis of a fetal intracranial mass on ultrasound. Which of the following is a true statement about the use of magnetic resonance imaging during pregnancy?

a. Maternal anxiety prevents completion of the study in approximately 10% of women.

b. Gadolinium-based contrast agents are contraindicated because of the potential for fetal toxicity.

c. Cochlear function testing is abnormal in about 2% of neonates who underwent magnetic resonance imaging as a fetus.

d. Sonography provides better assessment of central nervous system migrational abnormalities than magnetic resonance imaging.

SECTION 5

CHAPTER 10 ANSWER KEY

Question number	Letter answer	Page cited	Header cited
10–1	**d**	p. 183	Fetal Safety
10–2	**b**	p. 183	Table 10-1
10–3	**c**	p. 183	Gestational Age Assessment
10–4	**d**	p. 185	Gestational Age Assessment
10–5	**b**	p. 185	First-Trimester Sonography
10–6	**d**	p. 186	First-Trimester Sonography
10–7	**b**	p. 186	Nuchal Translucency
10–8	**b**	p. 189	Amnionic Fluid Volume
10–9	**b**	p. 190	Cervical Length Assessment
10–10	**a**	p. 191	Brain and Spine
10–11	**c**	p. 192	Neural-Tube Defects
10–12	**d**	p. 193	Neural-Tube Defects
10–13	**b**	p. 193	Ventriculomegaly
10–14	**d**	p. 194	Agenesis of the Corpus Callosum
10–15	**a**	p. 194	Holoprosencephaly
10–16	**b**	p. 195	Caudal Regression Sequence—Sacral Agenesis
10–17	**b**	p. 197	Cystic Hygroma
10–18	**a**	p. 198	Congenital Diaphragmatic Hernia
10–19	**c**	p. 200	Heart
10–20	**a**	p. 201	Fetal Echocardiography
10–21	**c**	p. 203	Endocardial Cushion Defect
10–22	**b**	p. 206	Abdominal Wall
10–23	**b**	p. 206	Gastrointestinal Tract
10–24	**a**	p. 207	Kidneys and Urinary Tract
10–25	**b**	p. 208	Renal Pelvis Dilatation
10–26	**d**	p. 208	Table 10-10
10–27	**a**	p. 213	Umbilical Artery
10–28	**d**	p. 213	Umbilical Artery
10–29	**c**	p. 214	Uterine Artery
10–30	**a**	p. 214	Middle Cerebral Artery
10–31	**b**	p. 216	Table 10-11
10–32	**b**	p. 217	Technique

CHAPTER 11

Amnionic Fluid

11–1. Which of the following is correct regarding contribution to amnionic fluid volume in the second and third trimesters?

- **a.** Highest production is from fetal urination
- **b.** Highest resorption is into fetal respiratory tract
- **c.** Least resorption is across fetal vessels on placental surface
- **d.** All of the above are correct

11–2. What is the normal amnionic fluid volume at term?

- **a.** 300–500 mL
- **b.** 750–800 mL
- **c.** 1200–1500 mL
- **d.** 1800–2000 mL

11–3. Which of the following is not a significant source for fluid in the amnionic cavity in the first trimester?

- **a.** Fetal skin
- **b.** Fetal urine
- **c.** Flow across amnion
- **d.** Flow across fetal vessels

11–4. Which of the following is not true regarding osmolality of fetal urine?

- **a.** Fetal urine is isotonic to amnionic fluid.
- **b.** Fetal urine is hypertonic to fetal plasma.
- **c.** Fetal urine is hypotonic to maternal plasma.
- **d.** All of the above are true

11–5. In a healthy pregnancy at term, which of the following is the best estimation of daily fetal urine volume?

- **a.** 250 mL
- **b.** 500 mL
- **c.** 750 mL
- **d.** 1000 mL

11–6. Which of the following is not an acceptable way to document amnionic fluid when reporting ultrasound findings?

- **a.** Amnionic fluid index of 12.2 cm
- **b.** Deepest vertical pocket of 4.1 cm
- **c.** Maximal vertical pocket of 5.2 cm
- **d.** Subjectively normal amnionic fluid volume

11–7. Which of the following demonstrates proper technique for measuring a pocket of amnionic fluid with ultrasound?

a.

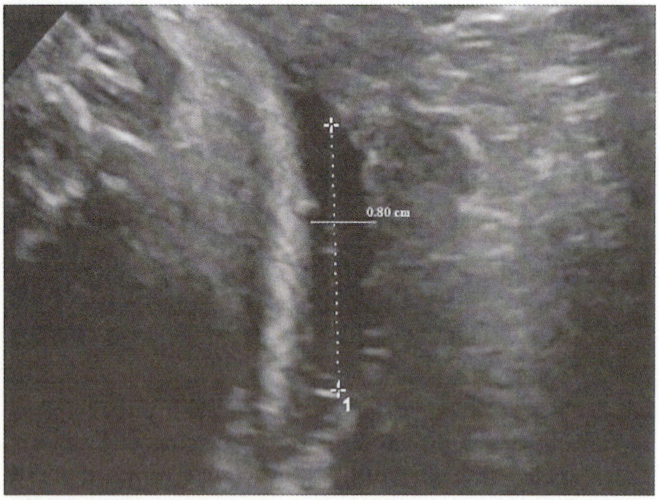

b.

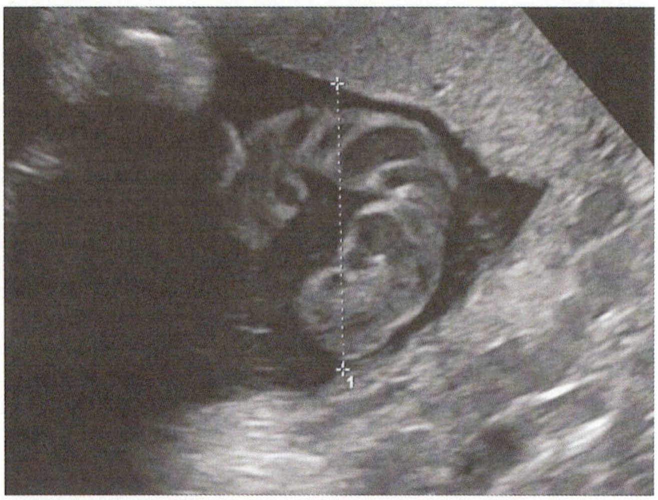

c.

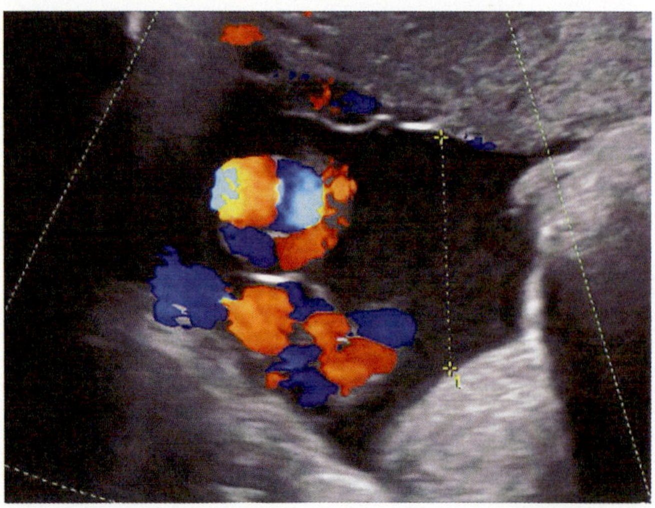

d. All of the above

11–8. Your sonographer performs a biophysical profile on a 32-week singleton fetus and obtains the following images to document the amnionic fluid. The fetus demonstrated flexion/extension movement, gross body movement, and fetal breathing during the study. How do you best report the findings?

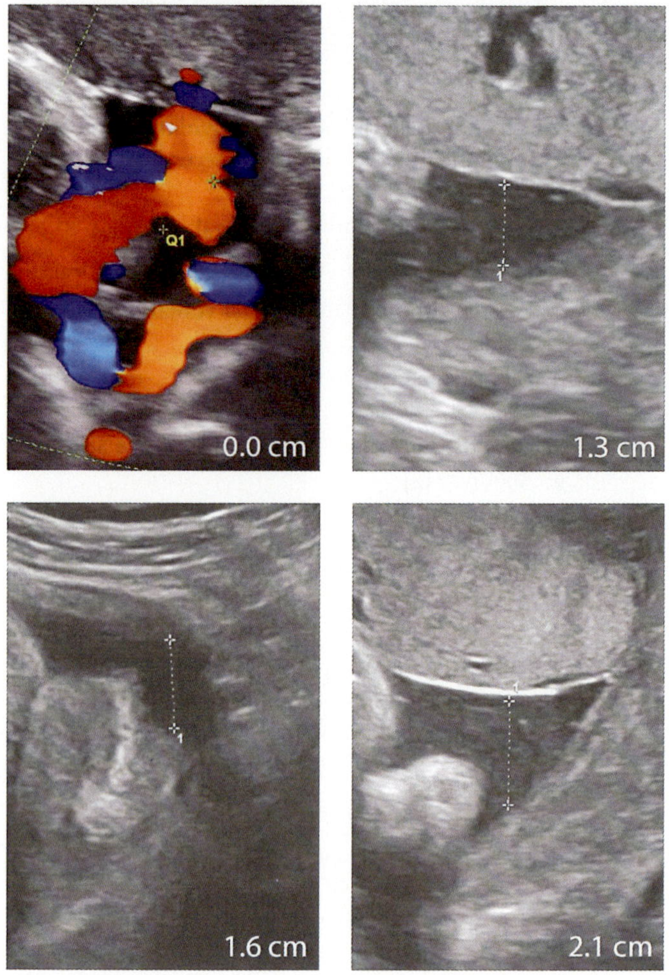

a. BPP 8/8 and normal amnionic fluid

b. BPP 8/8 and borderline oligohydramnios

c. BPP 8/8 and concern for oligohydramnios

d. BPP 6/8 and concern for oligohydramnios

11–9. A 28-year-old primigravida at 37 weeks' gestation presents with a 3-day history of fever, vomiting, and diarrhea. On your exam you notice her fundal height is lagging. Her blood pressure is at baseline and her pulse is 114, but otherwise her physical examination is unremarkable. An ultrasound is performed and shows appropriate fetal growth, but amnionic fluid index measures below the 5th percentile for gestational age. What is the most likely explanation?

- **a.** Placental insufficiency
- **b.** Decreased fetal urine output
- **c.** Increased maternal serum osmolality
- **d.** All of the above

11–10. Regarding the patient in Question 11–9, what would you recommend in addition to treating maternal symptoms?

- **a.** Maternal reassurance and resume routine obstetric care
- **b.** Proceed with delivery for oligohydramnios at term
- **c.** Amniocentesis for culture of fluid followed by amnioinfusion
- **d.** Intravenous hydration and reassess amnionic fluid index in 24 hours

11–11. Which of the following demonstrates the proper ultrasound technique to measure a pocket of amnionic fluid?

a.

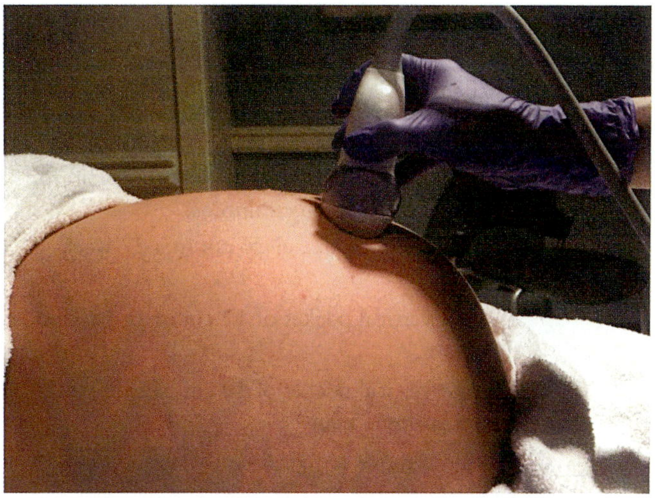

b.

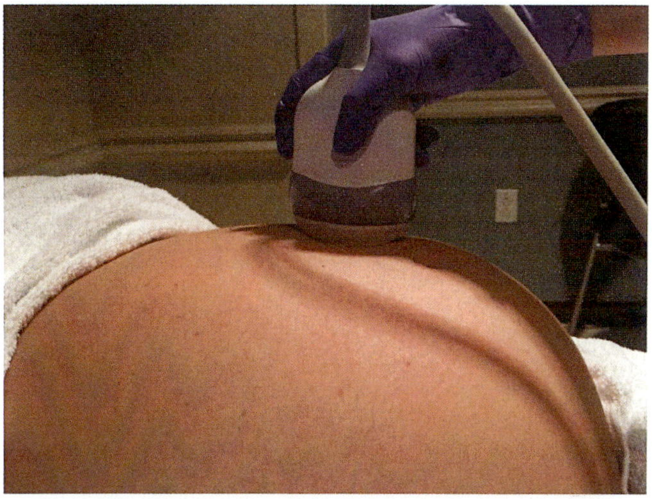

c.

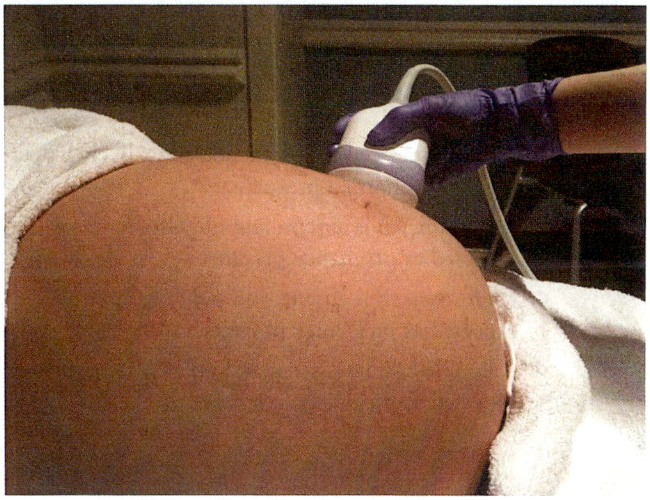

d. All of the above are acceptable techniques

11–12. Polyhydramnios is defined as which of the following?

a. Amnionic fluid index >25 cm

b. Single deepest vertical pocket >8 cm

c. Amnionic fluid index >97th percentile for gestational age

d. All of the above are consistent with polyhydramnios

11–13. In measuring amnionic fluid with ultrasound, which of the following meets the low threshold for diagnosis of severe polyhydramnios?

a. Amnionic fluid index of 26 cm in a 27-week singleton

b. Deepest vertical pocket of 12 cm in an 18-week singleton

c. Deepest vertical pocket of 10 cm in a 22-week monochorionic twin

d. All of the above are consistent with severe polyhydramnios

11–14. The images below are seen during a routine 20-week fetal anatomical survey in a young, healthy woman with low-risk aneuploidy screening and uncomplicated pregnancy to date. How do you counsel this family?

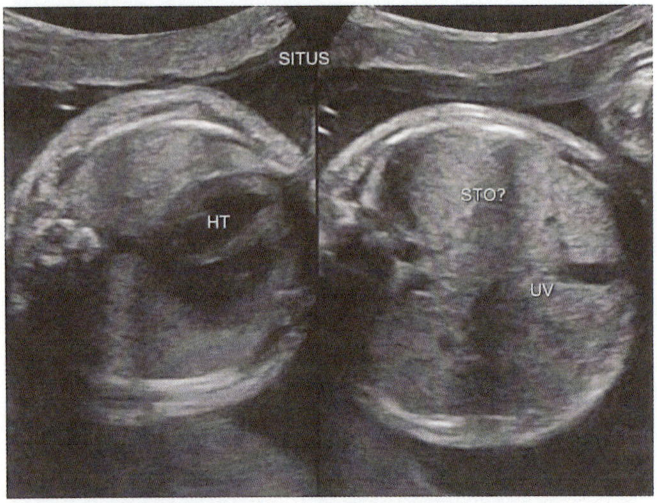

a. The finding seen is normal and most likely outcome is normal pregnancy

b. Fetal stomach is absent, and oligohydramnios is expected as pregnancy progresses

c. Fetal stomach is absent, and polyhydramnios is expected as pregnancy progresses

d. A double bubble is seen, and polyhydramnios is expected as pregnancy progresses

11–15. Which of the following conditions is not related to anhydramnios or severe oligohydramnios present from the early second trimester?

a. Fetal triploidy

b. Limb contractures

c. Pulmonary hypoplasia

d. Autosomal dominant polycystic kidney disease

11–16. A 23-year-old multigravida presents for establishment of prenatal care at 24 weeks' gestation. She denies any care elsewhere during this pregnancy aside from an 8-week ultrasound at an emergency room. On examination her fundal height is 38 cm. An ultrasound is performed, and images are shown below. Of the choices below, which test is least likely to reveal the underlying etiology of the ultrasound findings?

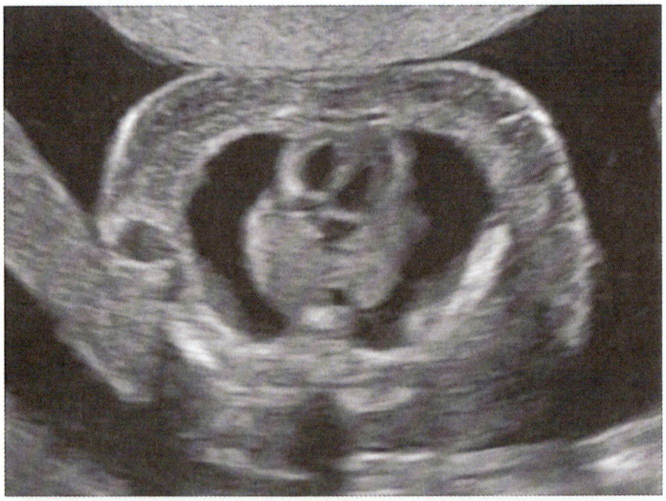

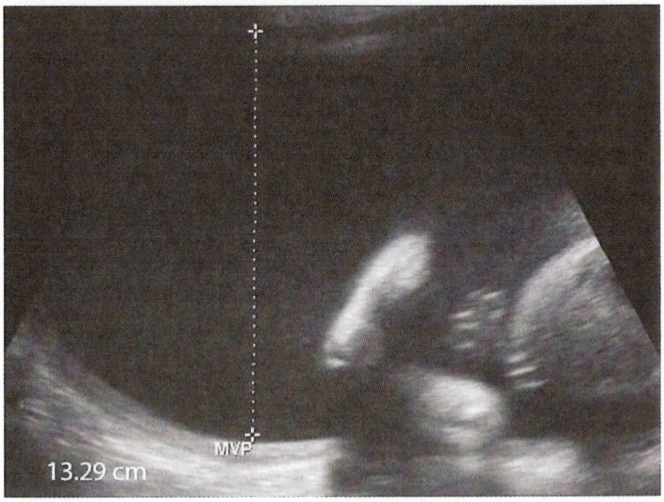

a. Maternal glucose screen

b. Amniocentesis for fetal karyotype

c. Fetal middle cerebral artery Doppler

d. Routine prenatal labs, which include RPR/reflex treponemal antibody test and indirect Coombs

11–17. When mild polyhydramnios is seen as an isolated finding on detailed fetal anatomical survey, with no fetal anatomical anomalies and an appropriately grown fetus, which of the following is most likely?

a. Maternal hyperglycemia

b. Intrauterine fetal demise

c. Idiopathic polyhydramnios

d. Undiagnosed fetal anomaly

11–18. A 28-year-old multigravida is referred to you for size >dates at 32 weeks, and you see moderate polyhydramnios on detailed fetal anatomical survey. The fetus is appropriately grown, and no fetal anomalies are visualized. Review of her prenatal record shows no abnormalities. What is the most appropriate way to counsel this family regarding the polyhydramnios?

a. No anomalies are seen today, so the polyhydramnios is idiopathic.

b. No anomalies are seen today, but she needs to repeat her glucose screen.

c. No anomalies are seen today, but the residual risk for a major fetal anomaly is at least 1% and may be as high as 28%.

d. No anomalies are seen today, but the residual risk for a major fetal anomaly is at least 14% and may be as high as 42%.

11–19. A 36-year-old G3P1 is seen at 32 weeks' gestation for suspected size >dates. The ultrasound shows fetal growth >97th percentile. Mild polyhydramnios is also noted. Review of her prenatal record shows she is obese and has thus far gained 32 lb this pregnancy. She had a normal fetal karyotype on elective amniocentesis, and her fetal anatomical survey did not show any anomalies. Her gestational diabetes screen was normal. She is at risk for which of the following complications due to polyhydramnios?

a. Oliguria

b. Preterm labor

c. Postpartum hemorrhage

d. All of the above

11–20. A 24-year-old G1 who is 16 weeks by known date of single embryo transfer presents for initial assessment of growth for her monochorionic/diamnionic twins. You see the following in addition to a 28% growth discordance. Your least urgent concern is which of the following?

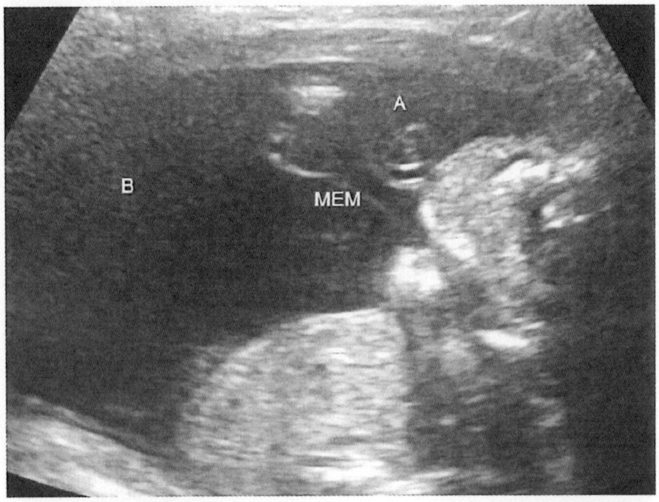

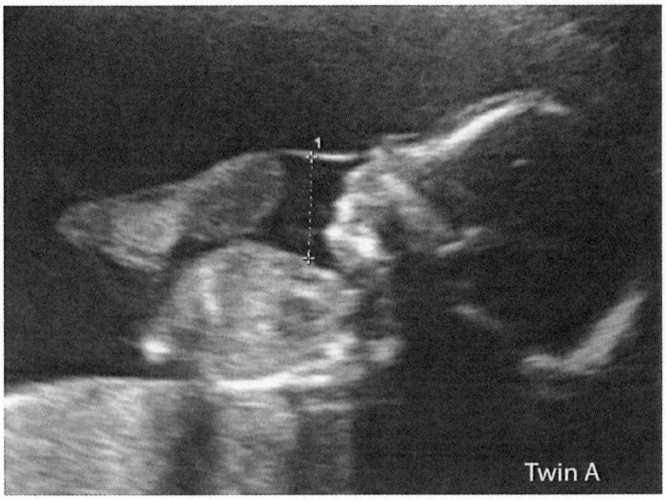

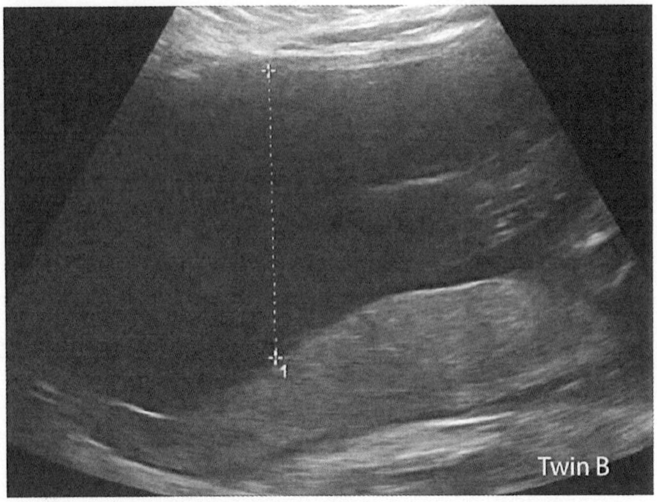

- **a.** Risk of infection in twin A because of early rupture of membranes.
- **b.** Aneuploidy in the smaller twin because of the known increased risk in monozygotic twins.
- **c.** Twin-twin transfusion syndrome because timely referral for selective fetoscopic laser ablation can be curative.
- **d.** Selective fetal growth restriction from placental share imbalance because timely referral for selective fetoscopic laser ablation can reduce complications in the larger twin.

11–21. A 24-year-old G1 is referred to you at 31 weeks' gestation for fundal height of 40 cm, early satiety, and inability to lie flat for the last week. On ultrasound you observe severe polyhydramnios and thus perform an amnioreduction. Her symptoms improve, and the fluid is sent for karyotype and reflex microarray. She returns 1 week later, and the karyotype is normal, but microarray is still pending. The amnionic fluid index is further increased and her symptoms have returned. She asks if it would make a difference that she and her husband, the father of the baby, are first cousins. What is your suspected diagnosis?

a. Fetal thyrotoxicosis
b. Fetal hemoglobinopathy
c. Microdeletion syndrome diagnosed via microarray
d. Autosomal recessive renal disease (i.e., Baarter syndrome)

11–22. The patient in Question 11–21 desires a repeat amnioreduction. Which of the following is not recommended in this setting?

a. Awaiting microarray results, as this is anticipated to provide the diagnosis.
b. Anticipated need for repetitive amnioreduction procedures until delivery is indicated.
c. Delivery planning to allow for delivery at a hospital with adequate neonatal intensive care unit capacity.
d. Submission of amnionic fluid for potassium, chloride, sodium levels to aid in diagnosing etiology of severe polyhydramnios.

11–23. Fetal growth restriction with polyhydramnios is most classically associated with which of the following chromosomal abnormalities?

a. 45,XO
b. 47,XXY
c. Trisomy 21
d. Trisomy 18

11–24. Maternal intake of which of the following is associated with oligohydramnios from direct fetal renal effect?

a. Angiotensin-receptor blockers
b. Nonsteroidal antiinflammatory drugs
c. Angiotensin-converting enzyme inhibitors
d. All of the above can be associated with oligohydramnios

11–25. A 35-year-old presents at 18 weeks' gestation for fetal anatomical survey. She has no pertinent medical, obstetric, or family history, and she takes only prenatal vitamins. She had low-risk cell-free DNA result around 12 weeks. Anhydramnios is readily apparent upon starting her ultrasound. She has not observed any leakage of fluid. What considerations do you have as you move through the ultrasound?

a. Identification of the bladder and external genitalia to rule out posterior urethral valve
b. Identification of fetal kidneys to rule out bilateral renal agenesis or bilateral multicystic dysplastic kidneys
c. Ensuring appropriate fetal growth and normal umbilical artery Doppler studies to rule out placental insufficiency
d. All of the above should be carefully assessed

11–26. A 24-year-old G1 at 35 weeks' gestation presents to labor and delivery with complaints of decreased fetal movement. She consistently drinks 2 liters of water per day. A variable deceleration is noted on her non-stress test, which was reactive. An ultrasound is performed, and an amnionic fluid index of 4.1 cm is found. What is the most appropriate next step?

a. Assessment of maternal blood pressure
b. Detailed patient history and sterile speculum exam
c. Umbilical artery Doppler study if fetal growth restriction is suspected
d. All of the above should be completed

11–27. In the patient in Question 11–26, her evaluation is otherwise normal, extended fetal monitoring remains category 1, and she now observes active fetal movement. Her cervix is closed. Which of the following is most appropriate in managing her late preterm oligohydramnios?

a. Proceed with cesarean delivery now.
b. Discharge home to resume routine obstetric care and instruct her on observing fetal kick counts.
c. Admit, administer antenatal corticosteroids, and plan delivery in 48 hours if not indicated prior.
d. Admit, observe closely, and plan delivery at 36–37 weeks if not indicated prior.

11–28. Oligohydramnios in the third trimester is associated with all except which of the following?

a. Preterm birth
b. Cesarean delivery
c. Intrauterine fetal demise
d. Amnionic fluid embolism

11–29. In which of the following scenarios is amnioinfusion currently considered an appropriate intervention?

- **a.** To improve neonatal outcome after rupture of membranes at 18 weeks' gestation
- **b.** To improve neonatal outcome after diagnosis of bilateral renal agenesis at 19 weeks
- **c.** To reduce intrapartum variable fetal heart rate decelerations after rupture of membranes
- **d.** To reduce meconium aspiration syndrome by diluting meconium noted intrapartum after artificial rupture of membranes

11–30. Anhydramnios or severe oligohydramnios prior to what gestational age is most likely to be associated with lethal pulmonary hypoplasia?

- **a.** Before 20 weeks
- **b.** Before 22 weeks
- **c.** Before 24 weeks
- **d.** Before 26 weeks

11–31. "Borderline" amnionic fluid index, considered to be between 5 cm and 8 cm, is not associated with increased rates of which of the following?

- **a.** Preterm birth
- **b.** Fetal growth restriction
- **c.** Intrauterine fetal demise
- **d.** Cesarean delivery for non-reassuring fetal heart rate pattern

11–32. A 39-year-old multigravida presents to labor and delivery at 37 weeks' gestation in early labor. Upon spontaneous rupture of membranes, the nurse calls out to ask for assistance because amnionic fluid volume is excessive and flowing over the bed onto the floor. When you come into the room, you consider which of the following?

- **a.** Sterile vaginal exam to rule out cord prolapse
- **b.** Close observation of the fetal monitoring to rule out abruption
- **c.** Sterile vaginal exam or ultrasound to confirm vertex presentation
- **d.** All of the above should be considered

CHAPTER 11 ANSWER KEY

Question number	Letter answer	Page cited	Header cited
11–1	**a**	p. 226	Physiology, Table 11-1
11–2	**b**	p. 225	Normal Amnionic Fluid Volume
11–3	**b**	p. 225	Physiology
11–4	**b**	p. 225	Physiology
11–5	**d**	p. 225	Physiology
11–6	**d**	p. 226	Sonographic Assessment
11–7	**c**	p. 226	Sonographic Assessment
11–8	**b**	p. 226 p. 232	Sonographic Assessment "Borderline" Oligohydramnios
11–9	**c**	p. 226	Physiology
11–10	**d**	p. 226	Physiology
11–11	**b**	p. 227	Amnionic Fluid Index
11–12	**d**	p. 227	Hydramnios
11–13	**b**	p. 228	Hydramnios
11–14	**c**	p. 228	Etiology
11–15	**d**	p. 231	Early Onset Oligohydramnios
11–16	**a**	p. 228	Etiology
11–17	**c**	p. 228	Etiology
11–18	**c**	p. 228	Etiology
11–19	**d**	p. 230	Complications
11–20	**a**	p. 229	Multifetal Gestation
11–21	**d**	p. 229 p. 230	Table 11-3 Management
11–22	**a**	p. 229	Table 11-3
11–23	**d**	p. 230	Pregnancy Outcomes
11–24	**d**	p. 231	Medication
11–25	**d**	p. 231	Early Onset Oligohydramnios
11–26	**d**	p. 231	Oligohydramnios after Midpregnancy
11–27	**d**	p. 231	Oligohydramnios after Midpregnancy
11–28	**c**	p. 232	Pregnancy Outcomes
11–29	**c**	p. 232	Management
11–30	**a**	p. 232	Pulmonary Hypoplasia
11–31	**c**	p. 232	"Borderline" Oligohydramnios
11–32	**d**	p. 230	Complications

CHAPTER 12

Teratology, Teratogens, and Fetotoxic Agents

12–1. What percentage of all newborns have a major congenital abnormality detected at birth?

- **a.** 2–3%
- **b.** 4%
- **c.** 5%
- **d.** 7%

12–2. The majority of birth defects with an identifiable etiology are caused by which of the following?

- **a.** Multiple gestations
- **b.** Medication exposure
- **c.** Environmental toxins
- **d.** Chromosome abnormality

12–3. What percentage of all birth defects are the result of medication exposure?

- **a.** 2%
- **b.** 6%
- **c.** 10%
- **d.** <1%

12–4. Approximately how many medications do women take while pregnant?

- **a.** 0
- **b.** 1
- **c.** 1–3
- **d.** 2–3

12–5. For what percentage of medications approved by the Food and Drug Administration is the pregnancy risk known?

- **a.** 75%
- **b.** 80%
- **c.** <5%
- **d.** <10%

12–6. Which of the following accurately defines a teratogen?

- **a.** An agent that alters growth
- **b.** An agent that interferes with normal maturation and function of an organ
- **c.** An agent that acts during embryonic or fetal development to produce a permanent alteration of form or function
- **d.** All of the above

12–7. All except which of the following are essential in the criteria for determining teratogenicity?

- **a.** Careful delineation of clinical cases
- **b.** Animal studies showing abnormalities with exposure
- **c.** Proof that exposure occurred at a critical time in development
- **d.** At least two epidemiological studies reporting similar findings

12–8. Which of the following factors affect transport of substances across the placenta?

- **a.** Molecular size
- **b.** Electrical charge
- **c.** Maternal metabolism
- **d.** All of the above

12–9. Folic acid is important in preventing the malformation pictured below. Initiation of folic acid prior to conception is important because major malformations of the central nervous system occur during what time period?

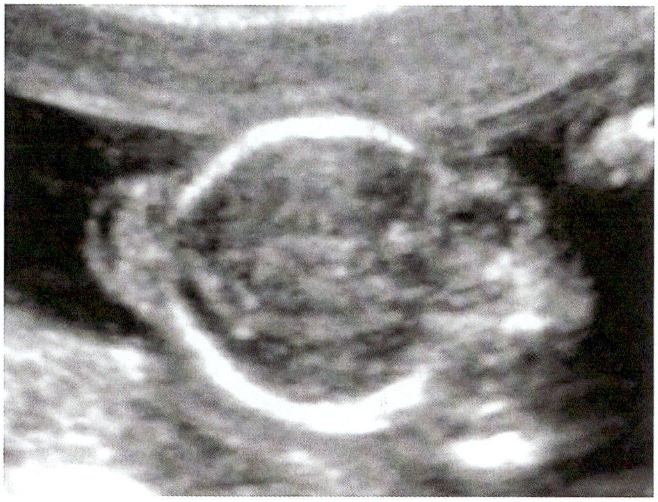

a. Fetal period
b. Pre-organogenesis
c. Embryonic period
d. Preimplantation period

12–10. A 38-year-old African American woman presents for a fetal growth ultrasound at 26 weeks' gestation. The fetal kidneys are found to have bilateral hyperechoic medullas *(arrows)*, and oligohydramnios is found. She denies rupture of membranes, but reports she is taking losartan for hypertension. Which of the following is the most likely etiology of the ultrasound findings?

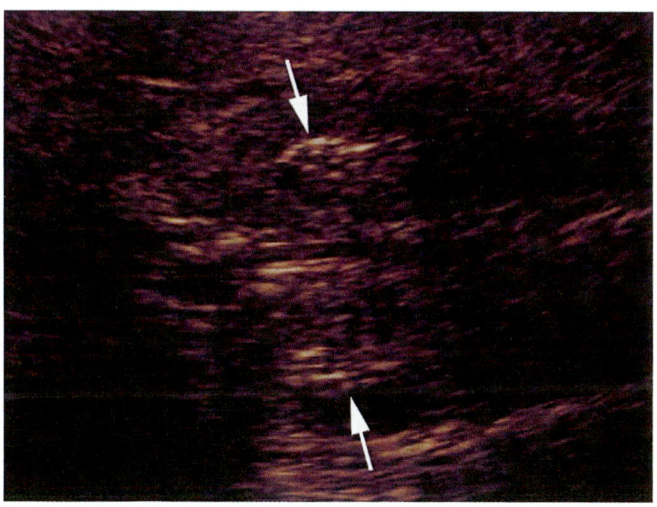

a. Losartan
b. Hypertension
c. Intrauterine growth restriction
d. Fetal multicystic dysplastic kidneys

12–11. The patient in Question 12–10 returns 4 weeks later for repeat ultrasound after having stopped the losartan. Her amnionic fluid index is normal as seen below. The reversible effects of losartan on fetal renal function may be due to exposure during what time period?

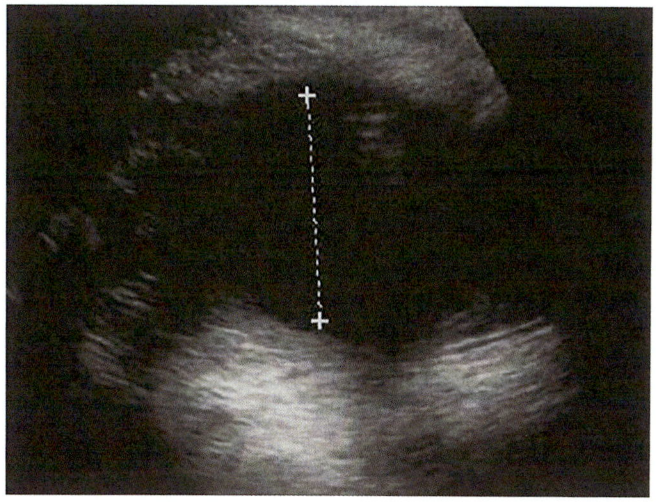

a. Fetal period
b. Embryonic period
c. Maturation period
d. Third trimester of pregnancy

12–12. Why are research studies regarding medication safety in pregnant women difficult to conduct?

a. Animal studies are considered sufficient.
b. Pregnant women are a special population usually excluded from studies.
c. The lowest dose possible should always be used in treating pregnant women.
d. The Food and Drug Administration gives priority to approving medications for pregnancy-related indications.

12–13. What of the following teratogens were discovered through case series?

a. Cocaine
b. Warfarin
c. Thalidomide
d. Beta-blockers

12–14. Which of the following drawbacks is typical of case-control studies when studying potential teratogens?

a. Recall bias
b. Lack of a control group
c. Only causality can be established
d. All of the above

12–15. All except which one of the following are limitations of the National Birth Defects Prevention Study?

a. Recall bias

b. Medical records were not reviewed

c. Differences in population characteristics between the cases and controls

d. All of the above

12–16. A recent earthquake leads to leakage of a pesticide into the soil and water supply of a rural community. The local health department wants to study the effects of the exposure on birth defects. What study design would best allow for this study?

a. Case series

b. Cohort studies

c. Pregnancy registry

d. Case-control study

12–17. Which of the following is true regarding the Food and Drug Administration's letter classification system for medications?

a. A higher letter grade signifies greater risk.

b. The classification system addresses inadvertent exposures.

c. Most medications demonstrated safety in human pregnancy.

d. Most medications have no safety data in human or animal studies.

12–18. The new Food and Drug Administration's labeling requirements include which of the following elements?

a. A lactation subsection

b. Summary of risks and clinical considerations

c. Potential risks in individuals with reproductive potential

d. All of the above

12–19. A 33-year-old woman with systemic lupus erythematosus (SLE) is at 18 weeks' gestation. At her screening ultrasound the fetal abnormality pictured below is found. What is the likely etiology of this congenital anomaly?

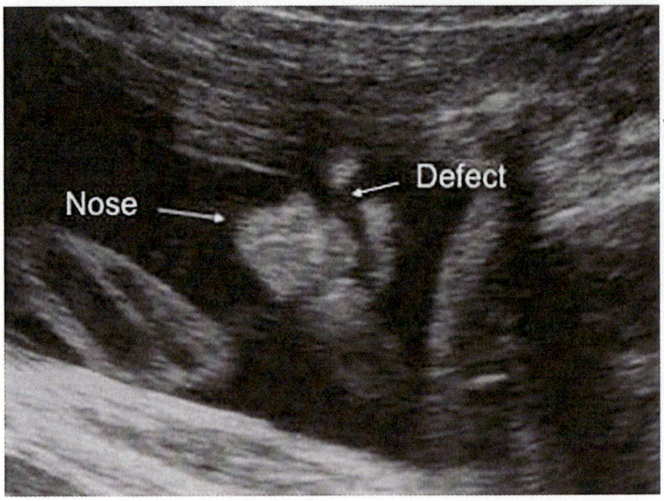

a. Idiopathic

b. Aneuploidy

c. Medication exposure

d. Systemic lupus erythematosus

12–20. What medication could the patient in Question 12–19 be taking that increases her risk for having a fetus with a cleft lip?

a. Prednisone

b. Leflunomide

c. Azathioprine

d. Hydroxychloroquine

12–21. The patient in Question 12–19 asks if prednisone increases the risk for this fetal anomaly. The best way to present the information to her is in which format?

a. Her risk is slightly increased

a. Her risk is triple that of the rest of the population

b. Her absolute risk increases from 1 per 1000 to 3 per 1000

d. She has a threefold increased risk for having a baby with a cleft lip

12–22. In addition to dysmorphic facial features and postnatal growth restriction, which of the following would have to be present for a diagnosis of fetal alcohol syndrome?

a. Scoliosis

b. Dysplastic kidney

c. Ventricular septal defect

d. Head size <10th percentile

12–23. Increased rates of which complication have been linked to binge drinking during pregnancy?

a. Stillbirth
b. Preterm birth
c. Postpartum depression
d. Fetal-growth restriction

12–24. Which of the following associations regarding anticonvulsants and their risk of birth defects has not been reported?

a. Hydantoin exposure can cause midfacial hypoplasia
b. Valproic acid exposure can cause neural-tube defects
c. Topiramate exposure increases the risk of orofacial clefts
d. Valproic acid exposure increases the risk of abdominal wall defects

12–25. What fetal complication is associated with indomethacin use?

a. Hydramnios
b. Pulmonary valve atresia
c. Bronchopulmonary dysplasia
d. Premature closure of the ductus arteriosus

12–26. Which of the following associations between first-trimester antibiotic exposure and the given birth defect is true?

a. Aminoglycosides and ototoxicity
b. Chloramphenicol and ashen-gray skin
c. Tetracyclines and deciduous teeth discoloration
d. Nitrofurantoin and hypoplastic left heart syndrome

12–27. Which antiviral agent is associated with skull, palate, eye, skeleton, and gastrointestinal abnormalities?

a. Ribavirin
b. Efavirenz
c. Zidovudine
d. Oseltamivir

12–28. All except which of the following is associated with in utero diethylstilbestrol exposure?

a. Hypospadias
b. Elongated fallopian tubes
c. Vaginal clear-cell adenocarcinoma
d. Hypoplastic, T-shaped uterine cavity

12–29. Which of the following statements is accurate?

a. The renal collecting system is susceptible to mercury.
b. Consumption of large fish is the primary source of mercury.
c. Prenatal lead exposure is only associated with childhood developmental delay.
d. Lead exposure is safe in pregnancy as long as serum levels are in the normal range.

12–30. A 32-year old woman has severe aortic stenosis. She is contemplating undergoing replacement with a mechanical valve versus balloon valvuloplasty. You counsel her that mechanical heart valves are at high risk for thrombosis, and therefore she will require warfarin therapy. What congenital abnormality pictured below is associated with first trimester warfarin exposure.

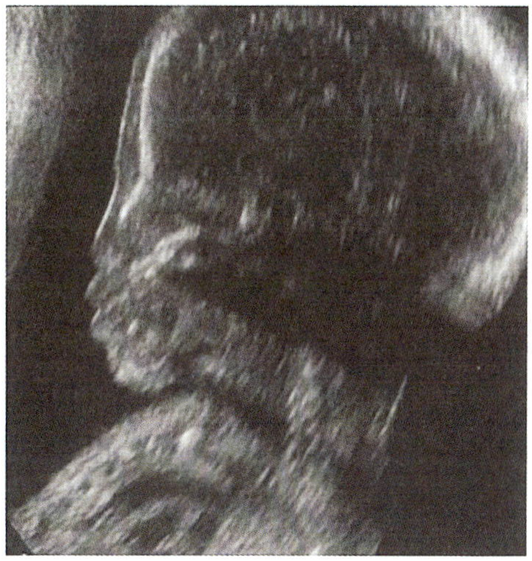

Reproduced with permission from Cunningham FG, Leveno KJ, Bloom SL, et al (eds): Teratology, teratogens, and fetotoxic agents. In William Obstetrics, 25th ed. New York, McGraw-Hill, 2018, Figure 12-6a.

a. Low-set ears
b. Micrognathia
c. Nasal hypoplasia
d. Prominent forehead

12–31. What can you tell the patient in Question 12–30 is the estimated prevalence of warfarin embryopathy?

a. 1%
b. 2–3%
c. 5%
d. 6%

12–32. Which drug is associated with the rare cardiac defect shown in this fetal sonogram?

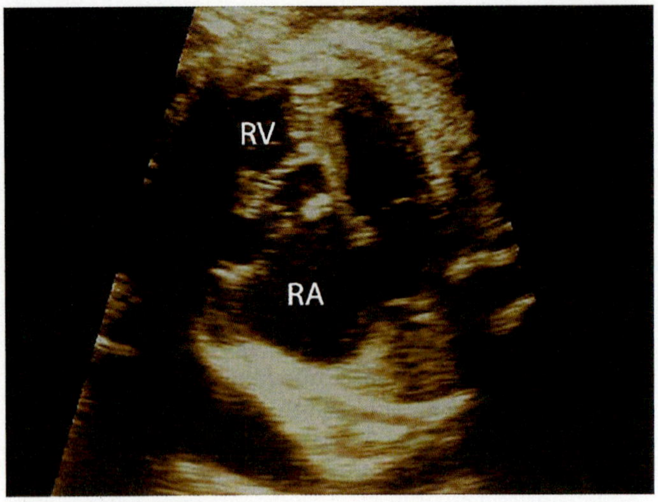

a. Lithium

b. Sertraline

c. Isotretinoin

d. Thalidomide

12–33. A 34-year-old woman presents for preconceptional counseling. Her medical history reveals a history of depression and a prior child with the cardiac defect shown below. She reports that she takes medication for depression but does not remember the name. Which of the medications listed below is associated with this cardiac defect?

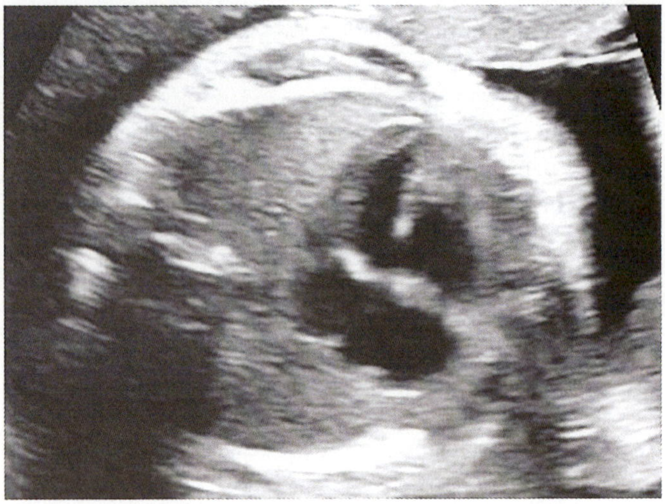

a. Sertraline

b. Paroxetine

c. Bupropion

d. Citalopram

CHAPTER 12 ANSWER KEY

Question number	Letter answer	Page cited	Header cited
12–1	a	p. 234	Teratology, Teratogens, and Fetotoxic Agents
12–2	d	p. 234	Teratology, Teratogens, and Fetotoxic Agents
12–3	d	p. 234	Teratology, Teratogens, and Fetotoxic Agents
12–4	d	p. 234	Teratology, Teratogens, and Fetotoxic Agents
12–5	c	p. 235	Teratology, Teratogens, and Fetotoxic Agents
12–6	c	p. 235	Teratology
12–7	b	p. 235	Table 12-2
12–8	d	p. 235	Criteria for Determining Teratogenicity
12–9	c	p. 236	Figure 12-2
12–10	a	p. 241	Angiotensin-Converting Enzyme Inhibitors and Angiotensin-receptor Blocking Drugs
12–11	a	p. 236	Figure 12-2
12–12	b	p. 236	Studies in Pregnant Women
12–13	c	p. 237	Case Reports and Series
12–14	a	p. 237	Case-control Studies
12–15	d	p. 237	Case-control Studies
12–16	b	p. 237	Cohort Studies
12–17	d	p. 238	The Food and Drug Administration: Letters and Labels
12–18	d	p. 238	The Food and Drug Administration: Letters and Labels
12–19	a	p. 239	Presenting Risk Information
12–20	a	p. 244	Corticosteroids
12–21	b	p. 239	Presenting Risk Information
12–22	d	p. 239	Table 12-4
12–23	a	p. 240	Alcohol
12–24	d	p. 240	Antiepileptic Medications
12–25	d	p. 241	Antiinflammatory Agents
12–26	d	p. 242	Antimicrobial Agents
12–27	a	p. 243	Antiviral Agents
12–28	b	p. 244	Sex Hormones
12–29	b	p. 244	Mercury
12–30	c	p. 247	Warfarin
12–31	d	p. 247	Warfarin
12–32	a	p. 244	Psychiatric Medications
12–33	b	p. 245	Psychiatric Medications

CHAPTER 13

Genetics

13–1. What percentage of newborns has a recognized structural defect?

a. 1–2%

b. 2–3%

c. 3–4%

d. 4–5%

13–2. A 40-year-old G2P1 presents at 36 weeks' gestation with decreased fetal movement. She is diagnosed with a stillbirth and undergoes induction. The stillborn infant is noted to have low-set ears, a high arched palate, and an imperforate anus. What is the chance that the fetus has an underlying genetic abnormality?

a. 6–8%

b. 10–12%

c. 13–15%

d. 18–20%

13–3. Which of the following abnormalities can be identified by chromosomal microarray analysis but not standard karyotype?

a. Microdeletions

b. Microduplications

c. Copy number variants

d. All of the above

13–4. In what phase of cell division are oocytes arrested between birth and ovulation?

a. Prophase I

b. Anaphase I

c. Metaphase I

d. Telophase I

13–5. A 30-year-old G1 undergoes cell-free DNA screening at 12 weeks' gestation, and the results indicate an increased risk of trisomy 18. She has an amniocentesis at 16 weeks' gestation which confirms the diagnosis. At 32 years old, she conceives again. What is her risk of an autosomal trisomy in this pregnancy?

a. 0.25%

b. 0.5%

c. 1.0%

d. 1.5%

13–6. When major and minor sonographic markers are considered, what percentage of fetuses with the karyotype shown can be detected sonographically?

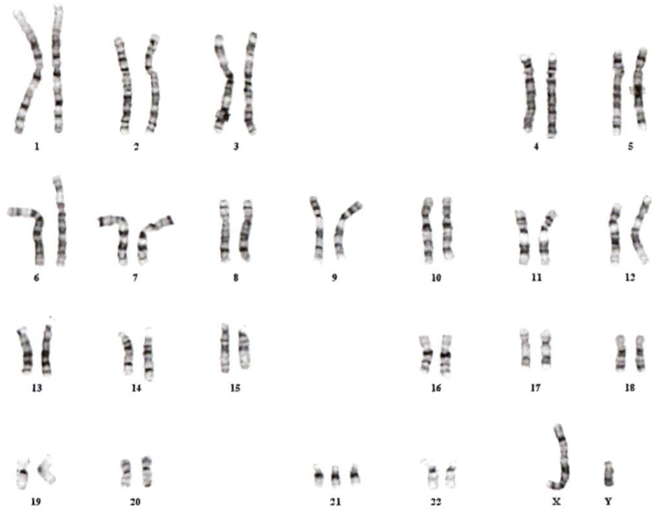

Reproduced with permission from Cunningham FG, Leveno KJ, Bloom SL, et al (eds): Genetic disorders. In William Obstetrics, 25th ed. New York, McGraw-Hill, 2018, Figure 13-3. Photo contributor: Dr. Frederick Elder.

a. 40–50%

b. 50–60%

c. 60–70%

d. 70–80%

13–7. You are seeing a 36-year-old G3P2 woman at 20 weeks' gestation for an anatomy scan. She did not have any genetic screening performed. You obtain the sonographic images, which are shown. Assuming the associated autosomal trisomy is confirmed on subsequent amniocentesis, which of the following would be accurate regarding the diagnosis?

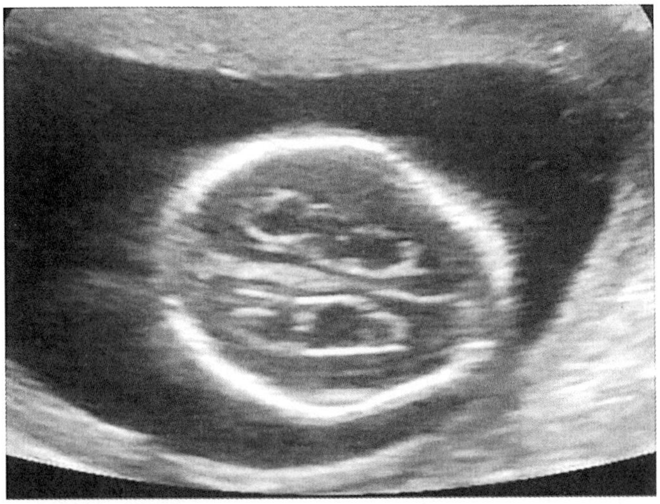

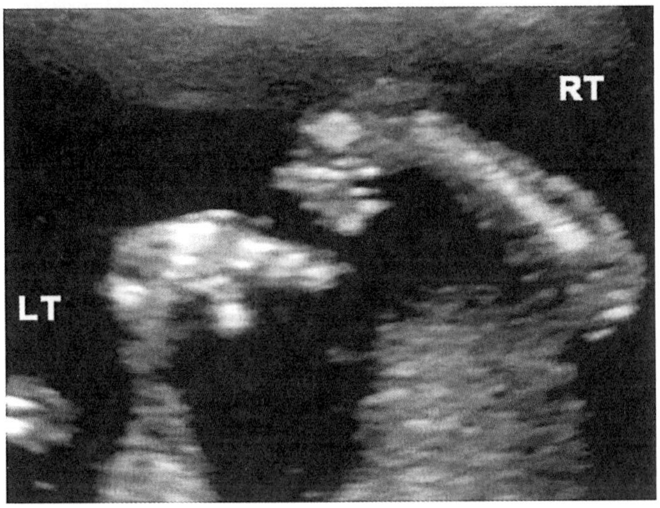

Reproduced with permission from Cunningham FG, Leveno KJ, Bloom SL, et al (eds): Genetic disorders. In William Obstetrics, 25th ed. New York, McGraw-Hill, 2018, Figures 13-5A and 13-5B.

- **a.** 90% of cases have a heart defect
- **b.** It can result from a robertsonian translocation
- **c.** Occurs in approximately 1 in 2,000 liveborn neonates
- **d.** None of the above

13–8. You are scanning a 34-year-old G2P1 woman at 19 weeks' gestation. You note the sonographic image shown. What syndrome are you most suspicious for based on the findings?

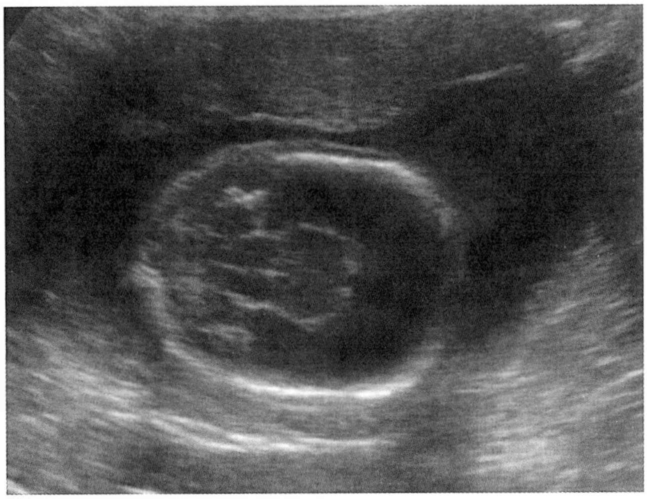

- **a.** Patau syndrome
- **b.** Edwards syndrome
- **c.** DiGeorge syndrome
- **d.** Angelman syndrome

13–9. A 38-year-old G1 is referred to you at 26 weeks' gestation. She had a normal cell-free DNA test in the first trimester. However, she was subsequently discovered to have a fetus with multiple anomalies including the defect shown in the sonographic image as well as hypertelorism, syndactyly, a ventricular septal defect, and a cleft lip and palate. Additionally, the placenta is small and there is asymmetric growth restriction. What is the most likely diagnosis based on her history and sonographic findings?

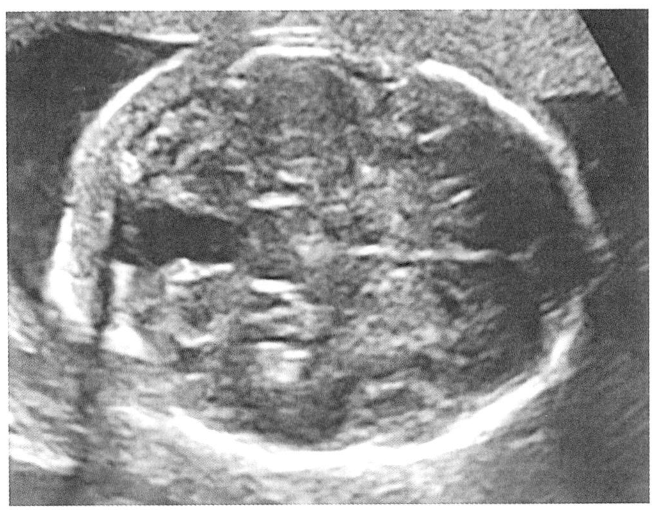

- **a.** Trisomy 13
- **b.** Monosomy X
- **c.** Digynic triploidy
- **d.** Diandric triploidy

13–10. Of the pregnancies that yield a liveborn infant with Turner syndrome, 25% have which of the following karyotypes?

a. 45,X

b. 46,X,i(Xq)

b. 45,X/46,XX

c. 45,X/47,XXY

13–11. Which of the following DNA deletion sizes would be detectable by standard cytogenetic karyotyping?

a. 1 million base pairs

b. 3 million base pairs

c. 5 million base pairs

d. None of the above

13–12. While performing an anatomical survey on a 24-year-old G2P1 in your office, you note the sonographic finding shown in the image. You also note unilateral renal agenesis, a likely cleft palate, and micrognathia. You suspect the most common microdeletion syndrome based on these findings. Which of the following is true regarding this syndrome?

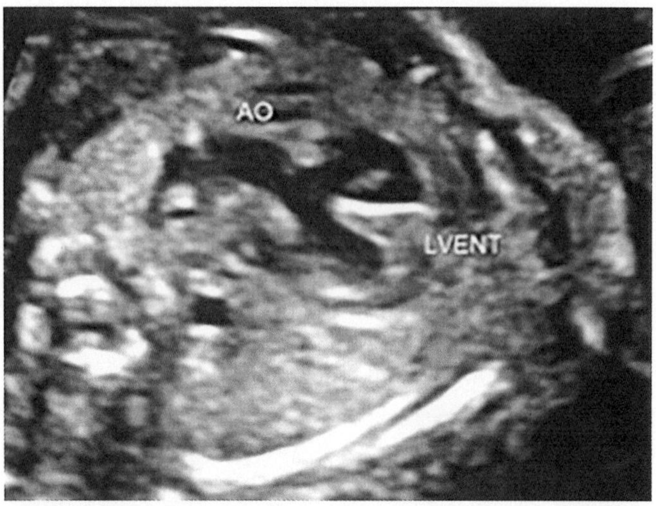

a. Has prevalence of 1 in 10,000 to 1 in 14,000

b. Is inherited in an autosomal recessive fashion

c. Is often accompanied by structural neurologic abnormalities

d. None of the above

13–13. What is the risk of a major structural or developmental abnormality for an individual with a balanced translocation?

a. 1%

b. 2%

c. 4%

d. 6%

13–14. A couple with a history of two prior first-trimester miscarriages presents to your office for evaluation. You perform parental karyotypes as a part of their workup and find that the man carries a robertsonian translocation. What is the couple's risk of producing an abnormal fetus related to the translocation?

a. 2%

b. 5%

c. 10%

d. 15%

13–15. You perform a chorionic villus sampling on a 40-year-old G3P2 at 11 weeks' gestation and the karyotype results indicate the presence of trisomy 16 mosaicism. How should you counsel the patient with regard to these findings?

a. No further workup is required.

b. Testing for uniparental disomy should be considered.

c. There is an increased risk for fetal growth restriction and stillbirth.

d. None of the above

13–16. Which of the following terms describes whether or not a dominant gene is phenotypically expressed?

a. Expressivity

b. Codominance

c. Penetrance

d. Heterogeneity

13–17. A couple with five normal children give birth to a sixth child who is diagnosed with cystic fibrosis. What is the chance that the phenotypically normal children are cystic fibrosis carriers?

a. 1/4

b. 1/2

c. 2/3

d. 3/4

13–18. You are caring for a pregnant patient with phenylketonuria. She has a 3-year-old boy who is a heterozygous carrier, but suffers from seizures and is developmentally delayed due to the patient's noncompliance during pregnancy. You counsel her that she should keep her phenylalanine concentration below what level to prevent recurrent problems for this infant?

a. 4 mg/dL

b. 6 mg/dL

c. 8 mg/dL

d. 10 mg/dL

13–19. You are caring for a pregnant patient who is a carrier of hemophilia A. She gives birth to a male infant who is diagnosed with hemophilia. What are the chances that he would produce a future son with hemophilia?

a. 0%
b. 25%
c. 50%
d. 100%

13–20. A patient presents to your office at 14 weeks' gestation. She reports a history of myoclonic epilepsy and would like to know the chance that her future child would also be affected. How do you counsel her?

a. Her future child has a 25% risk.
b. Her future child has a 50% risk.
c. Her future child has a 100% risk.
d. You are unable to estimate the risk.

13–21. Which of the following is true regarding the most common inherited form of intellectual disability?

a. The incidence is 1 in 6000 in males
b. It is inherited in an X-linked fashion
c. It is caused by a CCG trinucleotide repeat
d. All of the above

13–22. Which of the following is true regarding uniparental disomy?

a. Trisomic rescue is the most common cause
b. It often does not have clinical consequences
c. There is an increased risk of abnormality if chromosomes 6, 7, 11, 14, or 15 are involved.
d. All of the above

13–23. Which of the following defects or diseases is not caused by multifactorial inheritance?

a. Cleft lip
b. Diabetes
c. Sickle-cell disease
d. Neural-tube defect

13–24. You are caring for a patient whose first daughter had a neural-tube defect. She tells you that during that pregnancy, she did not realize she was pregnant until approximately 18 weeks and was not taking any multi- or prenatal vitamins during that time. You advise her daily folic acid supplementation of 4 mg during her next pregnancy will decrease her risk by how much?

a. 30%
b. 50%
c. 70%
d. 100%

13–25. Cytogenetic karyotype is performed on chromosomes arrested in what phase of replication?

a. Prophase
b. Anaphase
c. Metaphase
d. Telophase

13–26. You are performing an anatomy ultrasound on a 42-year-old G2P1 at 18 weeks' gestation. You note several abnormalities on ultrasound including choroid plexus cysts, clenched hands with overlapping digits, and a ventricular septal defect. She elects for amniocentesis, which is sent for fluorescence in situ hybridization testing. The result is pictured below. What is the diagnosis?

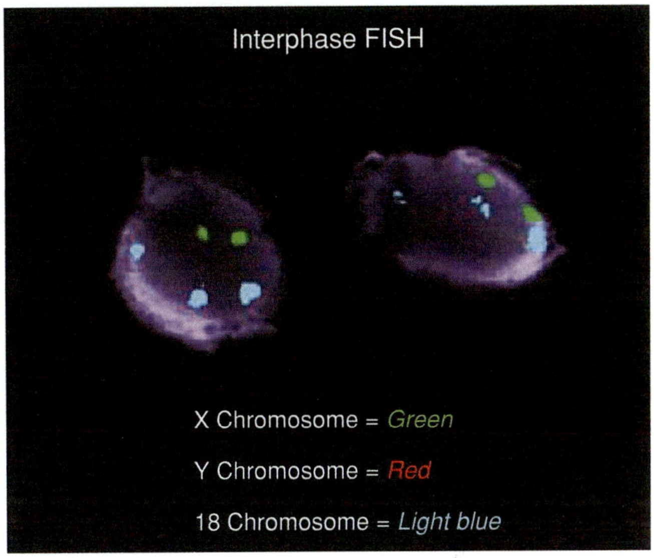

Reproduced with permission from Cunningham FG, Leveno KJ, Bloom SL, et al (eds): Genetic disorders. In William Obstetrics, 25th ed. New York, McGraw-Hill, 2018, Figure 13-12. Photo contributor: Dr. Frederick Elder.

a. Patau syndrome
b. Down syndrome
c. Edwards syndrome
d. DiGeorge syndrome

13–28. Which of the following cannot be detected using chromosomal microarray analysis?

a. Aneuploidy
b. Microdeletions
c. Balanced translocations
d. Unbalanced translocations

13–28. What percentage of chromosomal microarray samples yield clinically relevant copy number variants in the presence of fetal abnormalities and a normal karyotype?

a. 1–2%

b. 3–4%

c. 4–5%

d. 6–7%

13–29. Why is chromosomal microarray more likely than standard karyotyping to provide a genetic diagnosis in cases of stillbirth?

a. The assay is more sensitive

b. Dividing cells are not required

c. Genetic abnormalities are more common in cases of stillbirth

d. None of the above

13–30. When might whole genome sequencing be considered outside of a research context?

a. Cases of recurrent or lethal abnormalities

b. In the context of a normal karyotype analysis

c. In the context of a normal chromosomal microarray

d. All of the above

13–31. In general, what percentage of the total circulating cell-free DNA in maternal plasma is placental in origin?

a. 5%

b. 10%

c. 15%

d. 20%

13–32. For which of the following conditions would fetal sex determination using cell-free DNA analysis potentially impact clinical care in utero?

a. Hemophilia A

b. Sickle-cell disease

c. Duchenne muscular dystrophy

d. Congenital adrenal hyperplasia

CHAPTER 13 ANSWER KEY

Question number	Letter answer	Page cited	Header cited
13-1	**b**	p. 253	Introduction
13-2	**a**	p. 254	Chromosomal Abnormalities
13-3	**d**	p. 254	Standard Nomenclature
13-4	**a**	p. 255	Abnormalities of Chromosome Number
13-5	**c**	p. 256	Abnormalities of Chromosome Number
13-6	**b**	p. 256	Trisomy 21
13-7	**a**	p. 257	Trisomy 18
13-8	**a**	p. 258	Trisomy 13
13-9	**c**	p. 259	Polyploidy
13-10	**c**	p. 259	Sex Chromosome Abnormalities
13-11	**d**	p. 260	Microdeletions and Microduplications
13-12	**d**	p. 260	22q11.2 Microdeletion Syndrome
13-13	**d**	p. 261	Reciprocal Translocations
13-14	**a**	p. 262	Robertsonian Translocation
13-15	**c**	p. 263	Confined Placental Mosaicism
13-16	**c**	p. 265	Autosomal Dominant Inheritance
13-17	**c**	p. 265	Autosomal Recessive Inheritance
13-18	**b**	p. 266	Phenylketonuria
13-19	**a**	p. 266	X-Linked and Y-Linked Inheritance
13-20	**d**	p. 267	Mitochondrial Inheritance
13-21	**b**	p. 267	Fragile X Syndrome
13-22	**d**	p. 268	Uniparental Disomy
13-23	**c**	p. 268	Multifactorial Inheritance
13-24	**c**	p. 270	Neural-Tube Defects
13-25	**c**	p. 270	Cytogenetic Analysis
13-26	**c**	p. 270	Fluorescence In Situ Hybridization
13-27	**d**	p. 271	Chromosomal Microarray
13-28	**d**	p. 272	Chromosomal Microarray
13-29	**b**	p. 272	Chromosomal Microarray
13-30	**d**	p. 272	Whole genome sequencing
13-31	**b**	p. 273	Cell-free DNA
13-32	**d**	p. 274	Fetal Sex Determination

CHAPTER 14

Prenatal Diagnosis

14–1. The original designation of "advanced maternal age" in the 1970s was based on what?

a. The risk of having a fetus with aneuploidy increases sharply when a woman will be 35 at delivery.

b. The risk of having a fetus with an anomaly increases sharply when a woman will be 35 at delivery.

c. The fetal loss rate attributable to amniocentesis was equivalent to the risk of having a fetus with trisomy 21 at age 35.

d. All of the above

14–2. What is the closest approximation of aneuploidy prevalence using population-based registries?

a. 0.8 in 1000 births

b. 4 in 1000 births

c. 6 in 1000 births

d. 9 in 1000 births

14–3. A 33-year-old G0 presents for preconception consultation and inquires about risk factors for aneuploidy in a future pregnancy. Which of the following risk factors increases the risk for aneuploidy?

a. Increasing maternal age

b. Parental chromosomal rearrangement

c. Former pregnancy affected by aneuploidy

d. All of the above

14–4. A 32-year-old multigravida is in your office for a routine prenatal visit. She has a 10-week dichorionic twin gestation that is the result of in vitro fertilization with implantation of two embryos. What is it the most appropriate way to counsel her regarding aneuploidy screening?

a. You are still under age 35, so no screening is indicated

b. Cell-free DNA performs as well in a twin gestation as in a singleton.

c. If they would not terminate a pregnancy affected by aneuploidy, screening is not recommended.

d. With a dizygotic twin pregnancy, the risk for trisomy 21 in one of the fetuses approximates the risk of a singleton fetus in a mother who is 35 years old.

14–5. The patient in Question 14–4 did not desire aneuploidy screening after your discussion. She presents at 18 weeks' gestation for a detailed fetal anatomical survey. Twin B is found to have the abnormalities seen below. Which of the following is the appropriate next step?

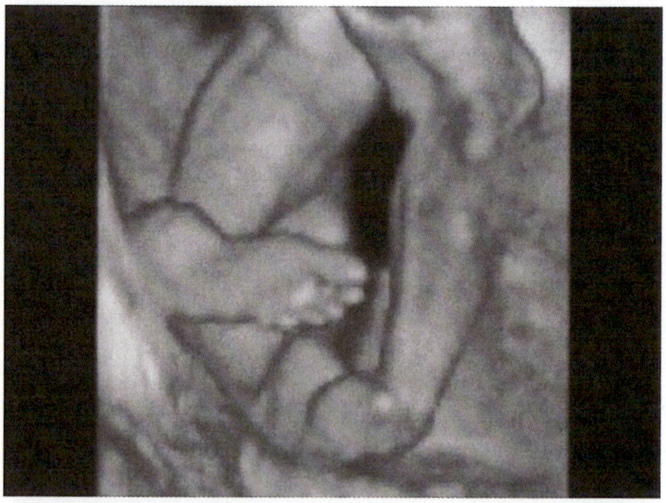

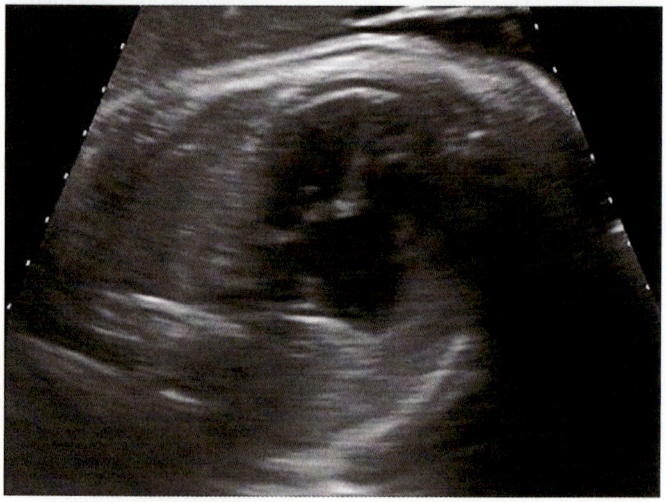

a. Discuss diagnostic testing

b. Referral to pediatric cardiology

c. Referral to pediatric orthopedics

d. Continue routine prenatal with no alterations at this time

14–6. A 24-year-old G4P0030 has had two first-trimester losses followed by a 16-week loss. Karyotype of the 16-week loss showed trisomy 15, and her husband was subsequently found to have a balanced translocation between chromosomes 9 and 15. She is now 8 weeks pregnant and inquires about aneuploidy testing with this pregnancy. What is the appropriate recommendation to this patient?

a. Screening with cell-free DNA

b. Chorionic villus sampling or amniocentesis

c. First-trimester nuchal translucency screening

d. Maternal serum screening in the second trimester to also assess for open neural-tube defect risk

14–7. Which of the following statements is correct regarding the statistical features of aneuploidy screening?

a. A test with a sensitivity of 99% will have a false-negative rate of 5%.

b. A test with a specificity of 95% will have a false-positive rate of 1%.

c. The positive predictive value is the proportion of those with a positive screen who are actually carrying an aneuploid fetus.

d. All of the above

14–8. Regarding screening for trisomy 21 in the general population, which of the following is true?

a. The positive predictive value of cell-free DNA screening varies with maternal age.

b. The positive predictive value of the quadruple screen is constant at 8%, regardless of maternal age.

c. The positive predictive value of first- and second-trimester integrated screen is constant at 11%, regardless of maternal age.

d. All of the above

14–9. Which of the following is not used to adjust maternal serum analytes?

a. Maternal age

b. Gestational age

c. Maternal weight

d. Maternal race and ethnicity

14–10. Which of the following statements is accurate?

a. Free β-hCG levels are lower with trisomy 21.

b. The sensitivity of nuchal translucency screening for trisomy 21 increases slightly from week 11 to week 13.

c. When the nuchal translucency measurement reaches ≥3.0 mm, nuchal translucency screening is not recommended.

d. All of the above

14–11. A 31-year-old G2P1 had a first-trimester nuchal translucency screen showing increased risk for trisomy 18, and a PAPP-A <5th percentile. She underwent chorionic villus sampling, which returned with normal karyotype. What is the significance of a PAPP-A <5th percentile?

a. There is none.

b. There is a high likelihood of oligohydramnios.

c. There is an increased risk for skeletal dysplasia.

d. There is an association with preeclampsia, fetal growth restriction, and fetal demise.

14–12. Which of the following statements regarding the second-trimester maternal serum quadruple screening test is accurate?

a. Has a higher false-positive rate for trisomy 18 than for trisomy 21.

b. Can be sent as a separate screen after the first-trimester screen to further improve aneuploidy detection.

c. Does not perform better than first-trimester screening for trisomy 21 or trisomy 18, but does include risk assessment for neural-tube defects.

d. All of the above

14–13. A 16-year-old G1 at 18 weeks' gestation presents for discussion of her maternal serum alpha-fetoprotein results, which were elevated at 3.0 MoM. What do you recommend as the next best step?

a. Magnetic resonance imaging

b. Basic fetal anatomical survey ultrasound

c. Targeted fetal anatomical survey ultrasound

d. Amniocentesis for amnionic fluid alpha-fetoprotein and acetylcholinesterase

14–14. An elevated maternal serum alpha-fetoprotein has been associated with which of the following?

a. Preeclampsia

b. Omphalocele

c. Maternal hepatoma

d. All of the above

14–15. Low levels of maternal serum estriol as part of a quadruple screen should prompt further investigation for which of the following?

a. Fetal triploidy

b. X-linked aqueductal stenosis

c. Smith-Lemli-Opitz syndrome

d. All of the above

14–16. When first- and second-trimester screens are combined, as in integrated or sequential screening, which of the following is the most accurate characterization?

a. Contingent sequential screening is the most cost effective.

b. Integrated screen has the highest detection rate for trisomy 21.

c. Serum integrated screening has the lowest trisomy 21 detection rate of the combined tests.

d. All of the above

14–17. A 27-year-old Japanese primigravida is seen for a fetal anatomical survey ultrasound at 18 weeks' gestation. The following is seen as an isolated finding. Which of the following is the most appropriate next step?

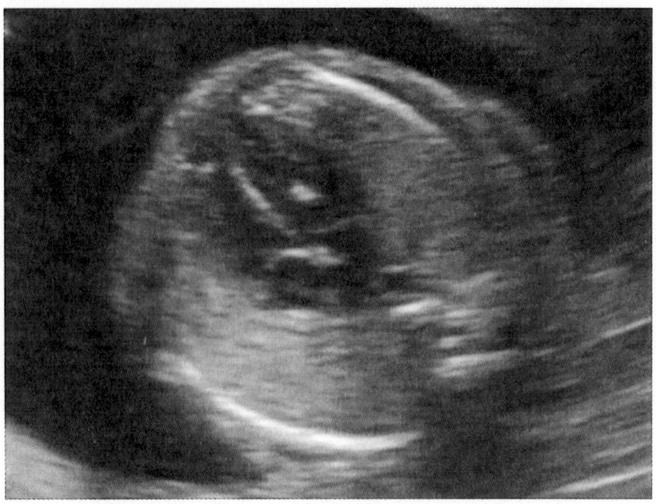

a. Cell-free DNA screening

b. Amniocentesis for microarray

c. Referral for fetal echocardiogram

d. Amniocentesis for tuberous sclerosis genetic testing

14–18. A 30-year-old G3P1 presents at 18 weeks' gestation for counseling regarding an increased risk for trisomy 21 on quadruple marker maternal serum screen. A targeted fetal anatomical survey shows no abnormalities. She understands the fetus may still have trisomy 21. What should she do next?

a. Cell-free DNA

b. Amniocentesis

c. Repeat anatomy scan in 4 weeks

d. Nothing—it is likely a false-positive result.

14–19. A 22-year-old primigravida at 11 weeks' gestation presents for nuchal translucency screening. Her only complication of pregnancy thus far is morbid obesity, as her body mass index is 48 kg/m^2. She inquires about the "DNA gender test" rather than first-trimester nuchal translucency screening. Which of the following counseling statements is accurate?

a. There is risk for a "no-call" result with cell-free DNA, and the risk is increased with early gestational age and increased maternal weight.

b. Nuchal translucency screening also allows for ultrasound visualization of the fetus and can detect some major anomalies, which would alter her risk.

c. With her age and the absence of a priori risk factors, first-trimester screening is more likely to identify any chromosomal abnormality that may be present.

d. All of the above

14–20. The patient in Question 14–19 actually left your office before testing was performed because she wanted to think about her options. She did not return until 16 weeks, and a maternal serum quadruple screen returned 1:1000 for trisomy 21. On ultrasound you find the "soft sign" seen below. Using likelihood ratios associated with the various "soft signs," what is her risk for having a fetus with trisomy 21?

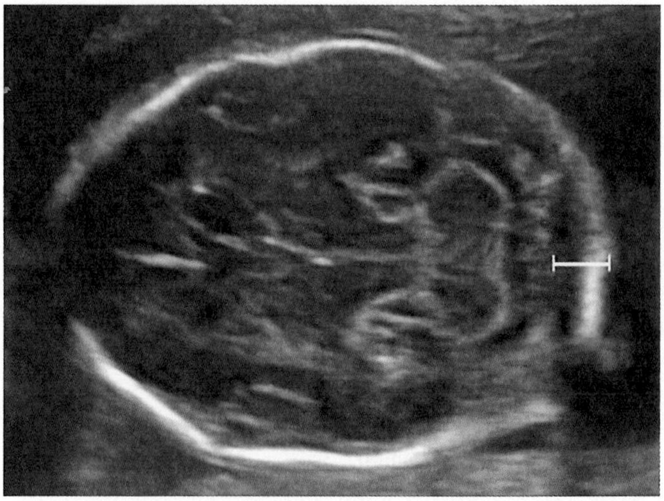

a. Increases to approximately 1:7

b. Increases to approximately 1:70

d. Increases to approximately 1:700

d. Risk is not modified because she already had low risk screening

14–21. Which of the following is not high on your differential of the following 19-week ultrasound finding?

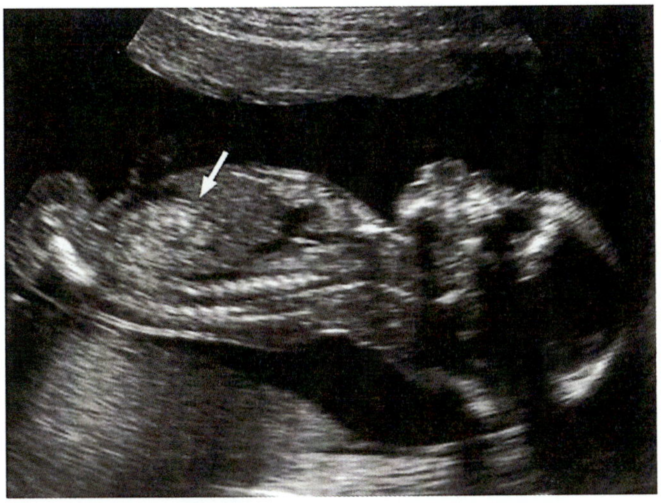

a. Trisomy 21
b. Cystic fibrosis
c. Toxoplasmosis infection
d. Prior intraamnionic hemorrhage

14–22. Which of the following skeletal findings during a 20-week ultrasound examination suggest an increased risk for trisomy 21 when seen in a patient with other risk factors?

a. Observed:expected femur ratio of $\leq$0.90
b. Observed:expected humerus ratio of $\leq$0.90
c. Femur length:abdominal circumference ratio of $\leq$0.90
d. Observed:expected biparietal diameter ratio of $\leq$0.90

14–23. During first-trimester screening with nuchal translucency, as shown here, what other findings can be used to modify aneuploidy risk?

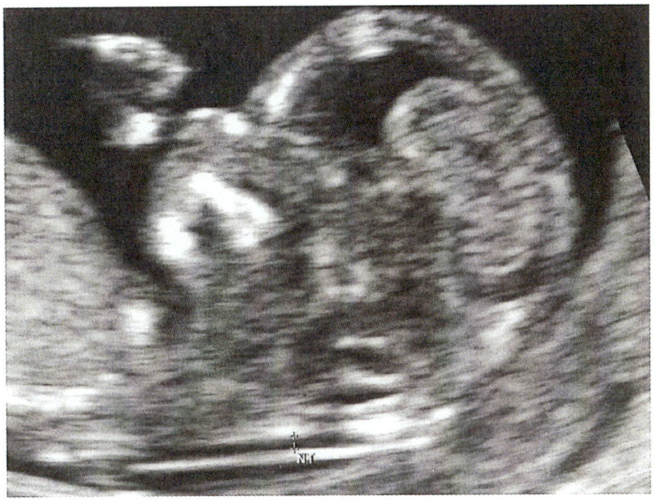

a. Absence of nasal bone
b. Presence of cystic hygroma
c. Early detection of many fetal anomalies
d. All of the above

14–24. Offering a commercially available pan-ethnic carrier screening panel to which of the following couples would be most beneficial?

a. A 33-year-old G0 with a history of hyperthyroidism presents with her 37-year-old husband. She identifies as multi-ethnic (Asian and African) and he identifies as Caucasian. No genetic disorders are uncovered on a pedigree.
b. A 36-year-old G0 with hypertension and her 34-year-old husband who both identify as being Asian. The husband's niece has just been diagnosed with cystic fibrosis and they report that her mutations have not been identified.
c. A 42-year-old G0 with diabetes and her 43-year-old husband who both identify as being of 100% Ashkenazi Jewish heritage. No genetic disorders identified in the family pedigrees of the couple. They are planning on pursuing donor frozen embryo transfer via in vitro fertilization.
d. All of the above

14–25. In their most recent recommendations, the American College of Obstetricians and Gynecologists recommend that which of the following be included in routine prenatal lab panels?

a. Cystic fibrosis

b. Spinal muscular atrophy

c. Both of the above

d. Neither of the above

14–26. Because of a recent diagnosis of cystic fibrosis in the daughter of her friend, a 26-year-old Caucasian G0 and her 27-year-old Ashkenazi Jewish husband are seen for preconception genetic counseling. After counseling they elect for the 23 mutation, pan-ethnic cystic fibrosis carrier screen. Her panel is negative for the mutations tested, but his shows that he carries the ΔF508 mutation. Based on this, what is the likelihood of them having a biological child with cystic fibrosis?

a. 1/8

b. 1/200

c. 1/400

d. 1/1600

14–27. Which of the following ethnicities is associated with the highest residual risk for spinal muscular atrophy after negative screening?

a. Asian

b. Caucasian

c. Multi-ethnic

d. African-American

14–28. What is the appropriate screening test for hemoglobinopathies in patients of African descent?

a. Sickle-prep

b. Peripheral blood smear

c. Hemoglobin electrophoresis

d. Complete blood count with differential

14–29. An Asian patient presents for prenatal care. Her intake complete blood count reveals microcytic anemia. What is the most appropriate next step in the evaluation of her anemia?

a. Iron studies

b. Peripheral blood smear

c. Hemoglobin electrophoresis

d. Alpha thalassemia molecular genetic testing

14–30. A 22-year-old Iranian primigravida at 9 weeks' gestation is noted to have anemia on her initial complete blood count. She reports that this was also noted a few months back at her annual exam, so her primary care physician had sent iron studies. She did not have iron deficiency on your review of her former lab studies. What is the next most appropriate step?

a. Intravenous iron infusion

b. Hemoglobin electrophoresis

c. Beta-globin chain gene sequencing

d. Parenteral vitamin B_{12} supplementation

14–31. Hexosaminidase A activity levels should be used in testing for Tay-Sachs disease in which of the following cases?

a. Chorionic villus sample of a pregnancy from parents who are both known to be Tay-Sachs carriers

b. Amnionic fluid sample of a pregnancy from parents who are both known to be Tay-Sachs carriers

c. Carrier testing for a male of sub-Saharan African descent whose wife is Ashkenazi Jewish and known to be a Tay-Sachs carrier

d. All of the above

14–32. In addition to cystic fibrosis and spinal muscular atrophy, the American College of Obstetricians and Gynecologists recommends that counseling and offering carrier screening for which of the following conditions be included in the care of Ashkenazi Jewish individuals?

a. Fanconi anemia, fragile X, and Tay-Sachs

b. Fragile X, Bloom syndrome, and Tay-Sachs

c. Canavan disease, familial dysautonomia, and Tay-Sachs

d. Niemann-Pick disease, phenylketonuria, and Tay-Sachs

14–33. A 26-year-old G1 presents at 12 weeks' gestation for nuchal translucency screening with the early fetal anatomical survey finding seen below. She was counseled on association with aneuploidy and is considering chorionic villus sampling or amniocentesis. Which of the following most accurately describes her invasive testing options?

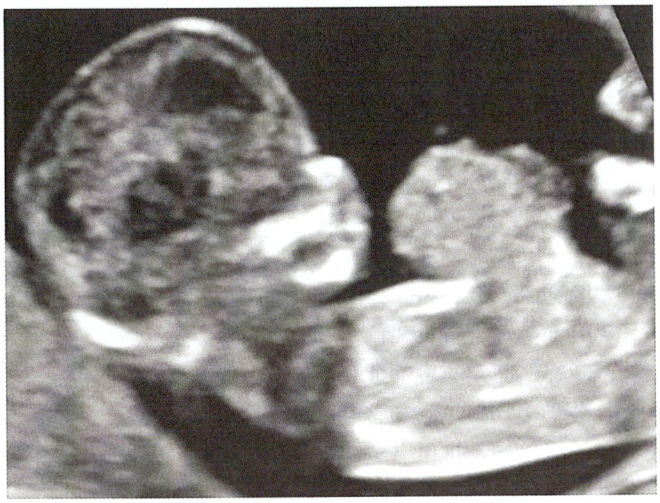

a. Procedure attributed loss rate is approximately 1 out of 400 for both CVS and amniocentesis

b. CVS can be performed earlier, but pregnancy loss after CVS is 2% compared to <1% after amniocentesis

c. CVS samples the placenta, so mosaicism that may be confined to the placenta is identified in up to 2%, whereas amniocentesis samples skin and other cells of fetal origin

d. All of the above

14–34. Compared to the baseline reported rate, the pregnancy loss rate is increased following amniocentesis in all except which of the following situations?

a. Twin gestation

b. Transplacental passage of needle

c. Maternal class 3 obesity (body mass index >40 kg/m^2)

d. All of the above

14–35. A 32-year-old multigravida is seen for suspected size/date discrepancy at 20 weeks' gestation, and ultrasound shows the following. Which modality provides the most rapid and complete assessment of etiology?

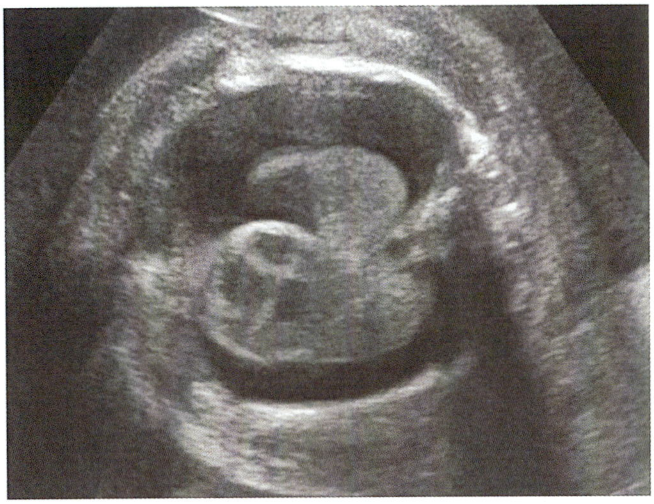

a. Amniocentesis

b. Magnetic resonance imaging

c. Percutaneous umbilical cord sampling

d. Detailed fetal anatomical survey and fetal echo

14–36. Compared to sampling a free loop of cord, fetal blood sampling performed at the placental insertion site is associated with which of the following?

a. Shorter procedure duration

b. Increased pregnancy loss rate

c. Increased procedure success rate

d. Decreased maternal blood contamination

14–37. As part of her recurrent pregnancy loss work-up, a 35-year-old G9P0 has been identified as having a balanced Robertsonian translocation involving chromosomes 14 and 21. She elects for in vitro fertilization to allow for preimplantation genetic screening. Which of the following is most appropriately included in their pre-procedure counseling?

a. Mosaicism is common in the cleavage state blastomere.

b. Aneuploidy screening or diagnostic testing is still recommended after preimplantation genetic screening.

c. Pregnancy rate after in vitro fertilization with preimplantation genetic screening is lower than in vitro fertilization without preimplantation genetic screening.

d. All of the above

CHAPTER 14 ANSWER KEY

Question number	Letter answer	Page cited	Header cited
14–1	**c**	p. 278	Historical Perspective
14–2	**b**	p. 278	Screening for Aneuploidy
14–3	**d**	p. 278	Screening for Aneuploidy
14–4	**d**	p. 279	Table 14-1 and Table 14-2
14–5	**a**	p. 279	Screening for Aneuploidy
14–6	**b**	p. 280 p. 285	Table 14-3 Cell-Free DNA Screening
14–7	**c**	p. 279	Statistical Considerations
14–8	**a**	p. 280	Table 14-4
14–9	**d**	p. 281	Traditional Aneuploidy Screening Tests
14–10	**c**	p. 281–282	Traditional Aneuploidy Screening Tests
14–11	**d**	p. 282	Unexplained Abnormalities of First-Trimester Analytes
14–12	**c**	p. 282–283	Second-Trimester Aneuploidy Screening
14–13	**c**	p. 283	Maternal Serum AFP Elevation: Neural-Tube Defect Screening
14–14	**d**	p. 283	Unexplained Abnormalities of Second-Trimester Analytes
14–15	**c**	p. 284	Low Maternal Serum Estriol Level
14–16	**d**	p. 284	Integrated and Sequential Screening
14–17	**a**	p. 285	Cell-Free DNA Screening
14–18	**b**	p. 285	Cell-Free DNA for Secondary Screening
14–19	**d**	p. 285	Cell-Free DNA Screening Limitations Comparison with Analyte-Based Screening
14–20	**b**	p. 287	Table 14-9
14–21	**c**	p. 288	Second Trimester Markers—"Soft Signs"
14–22	**a**	p. 288	Second Trimester Markers—"Soft Signs"
14–23	**d**	p. 281	First Trimester Aneuploidy Screening
14–24	**c**	p. 288	Carrier Screening for Genetic Disorders
14–25	**d**	p. 288	Carrier Screening for Genetic Disorders
14–26	**d**	p. 289	Table 14-11
14–27	**d**	p. 290	Spinal Muscular Atrophy
14–28	**c**	p. 290	Sickle Hemoglobinopathies
14–29	**a**	p. 290	Alpha Thalassemias
14–30	**b**	p. 290	Beta Thalassemias
14–31	**d**	p. 291	Tay-Sachs Disease
14–32	**c**	p. 291	Other Recessive Diseases in Ashkenazi Jewish Individuals
14–33	**d**	p. 294	Complications
14–34	**b**	p. 293	Complications
14–35	**c**	p. 294	Fetal Blood Sampling
14–36	**a**	p. 295	Complications
14–37	**d**	p. 296	Preimplantation Genetic Screening

CHAPTER 15

Fetal Disorders

15–1. Which of the following does not contribute to the low rate of alloimmunization in pregnancy?

a. Maternal-fetal ABO incompatibility

b. Administration of anti-D immune globulin

c. Low prevalence of incompatible red cell antigens

d. Consistent maternal immune response to the antigen

15–2. A 28-year-old G2P1 presents for prenatal care at 10 weeks' gestation. A type and screen is sent as part of her initial prenatal care labs, and it returns positive for anti-E antibodies at 1:8. What is the best first step in management?

a. Obtain paternal antigen testing

b. Repeat antibody titer in 4 weeks

c. Obtain paternal antibody testing

d. Obtain middle cerebral artery Doppler studies

15–3. For the patient in Question 15–2, paternal testing is not an option. The lab reports a critical titer of 1:16. What is the best next step in evaluation?

a. Repeat antibody titer in 4 weeks

b. Amniocentesis for fetal genotype

c. Amniocentesis for fetal phenotype

d. Serial middle cerebral artery Doppler studies starting at 16-18 weeks' gestation

15–4. For the patient in Question 15–2, at what antibody titer would you recommend initiation of screening for fetal anemia with middle cerebral artery Doppler studies?

a. 1:8

b. 1:16

c. 1:32

d. 1:64

15–5. A 36-year-old G3P2 at 28 weeks' gestation presents as a referral for sonographic abnormalities. On ultrasound fetal pleural effusions, skin edema, and polyhydramnios are noted, as shown below. Which of the following tests is indicated?

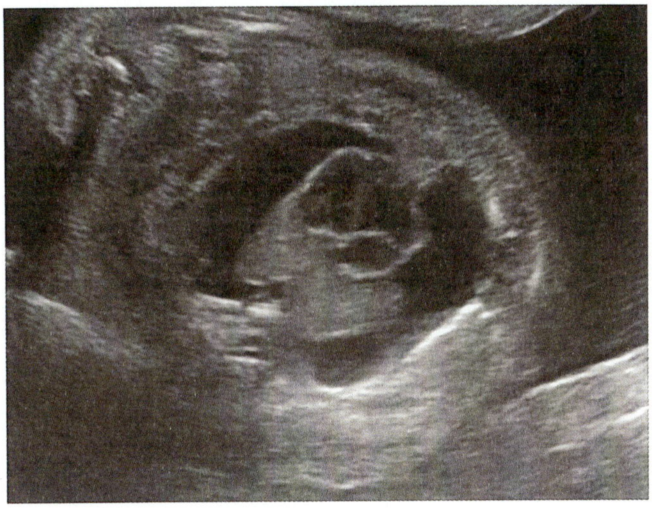

Used with permission from Dr. Jodi Dashe.

a. Middle cerebral artery Doppler studies

b. Maternal type and screen and syphilis testing

c. Amniocentesis for fetal chromosomal and infectious studies

d. All of the above

15–6. The patient in Question 15–5 is found to be O-negative with anti-D antibodies with a titer of 1:128. She denies a history of anti-D immune globulin administration in prior pregnancies. Fetal genotype from amniocentesis is pending. Using the reference below, which of the following results on middle cerebral artery Doppler studies at 28 weeks' gestation would prompt consideration of in utero transfusion?

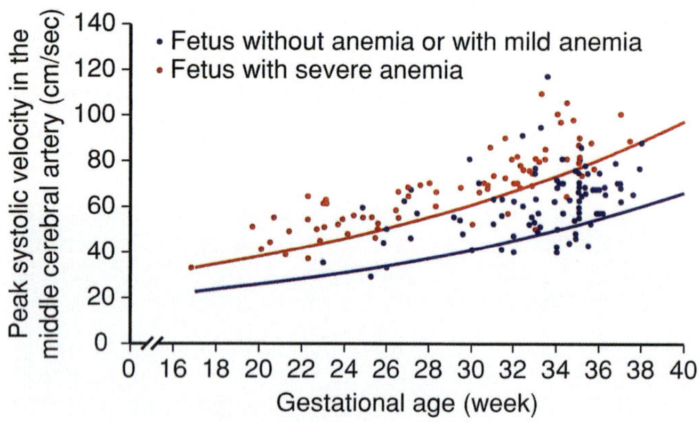

Reproduced with permission from Cunningham FG, Leveno KJ, Bloom SL, et al (eds): Fetal disorders. In William Obstetrics, 25th ed. New York, McGraw-Hill, 2018, Figure 15-1.

a. Peak systolic velocity of 22 cm/sec

b. Peak systolic velocity of 38 cm/sec

c. Peak systolic velocity of 45 cm/sec

d. Peak systolic velocity of 62 cm/sec

15–7. The patient in Question 15–5 has an abnormal middle cerebral artery peak systolic velocity and elects to proceed with fetal cord blood sampling and intrauterine transfusion. The estimated fetal weight is 1400 grams. Your pre-procedure counseling includes which of the following statements?

a. There is a 12% risk that the abnormal Doppler is a false-positive.

b. In her case, you expect the fetal hematocrit to be less than 15–20%, so you anticipate a transfusion volume of approximately 50 mL.

c. Once the transfusion is complete, she will undergo continued surveillance with weekly middle cerebral artery Doppler studies and repeat transfusion if the peak systolic velocity is greater than 1.5 multiples of the median.

d. All of the above

15–8. The patient described in Question 15–5 undergoes in utero transfusions at 29, 31, and 33 weeks' gestation with resolution of fetal hydrops following the first transfusion. She received a course of betamethasone for fetal lung maturity at 29 weeks' gestation. Middle cerebral artery peak systolic velocities rise to 1.8 multiples of the median at 35 weeks' gestation, as shown below. What is the recommended course of action?

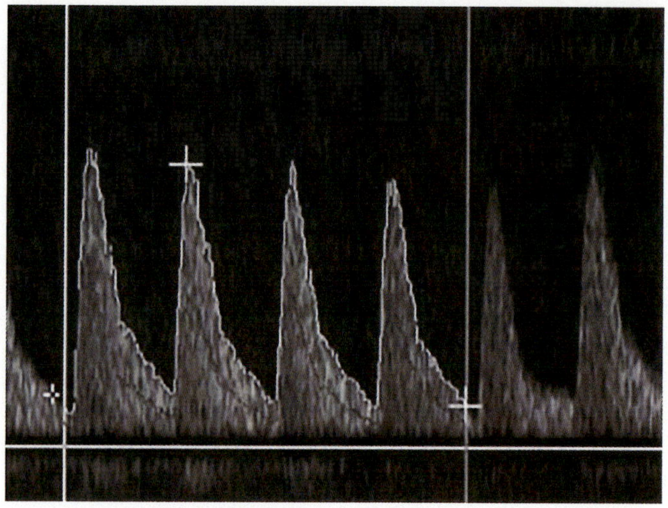

a. Repeat intrauterine transfusion

b. Expeditious delivery via induction of labor

c. Repeat middle cerebral artery Doppler studies in 24–48 hours

d. Administer a course of betamethasone followed by cesarean delivery

15–9. Which of the following immunoglobulin subtypes may contribute to fetal hemolytic anemia?

a. IgA

b. IgG

c. IgM

d. All of the above

15–10. What amount of fetal erythrocytes is required to sensitize a D-negative woman?

a. 10 mL

b. 0.1 mL

c. 1.0 mL

d. 0.01 mL

15–11. In regard to cell-free DNA testing and its utility in the management of fetal D genotyping in the United States, which of the following statements is currently false?

a. It is a cost-effective test.

b. It may decrease exposure to donor-related viral pathogens.

c. It decreases the number of women who require anti-D immune globulin by approximately 40%.

d. It is a reasonable alternative to amniocentesis for fetal genotype in the setting of maternal D sensitization.

15–12. According to the American College of Obstetricians and Gynecologists, at what titer of anti-Kell antibodies should surveillance for fetal anemia begin?

a. 1:8

b. 1:16

c. 1:32

d. Antibody titers are not appropriate for the monitoring of Kell-sensitized pregnancies.

15–13. A 26-year-old G2P1 is noted to have anti-Kell antibodies with a titer of 1:64 at her presentation for prenatal care. The father of the fetus is homozygous for the Kell antigen. At 20 weeks' gestation, middle cerebral artery Dopplers reveal a peak systolic velocity that is elevated to 1.6 multiples of the median with no evidence of fetal hydrops. When counseling her regarding the risks of intrauterine transfusions, which statement is most accurate?

a. The stillbirth risk is 15%.

b. The risk of fetal death is 2%.

c. The risk of emergent cesarean delivery is 1%.

d. The risk of preterm rupture of membranes is 5–10%.

15–14. What percent of alloimmunization occurs at the time of delivery?

a. 10%

b. 30%

c. 60%

d. 90%

15–15. A 23-year-old primigravida declines her indicated dose of anti-D immune globulin at 28 weeks' gestation. When questioned as the why, she reports she "does not like shots." During your counseling of the patient on the risks, you mention the increase in risk of alloimmunization associated with deferring the injection, which is approximately which of the following?

a. Four-fold

b. Five-fold

c. Ten-fold

d. Twenty-fold

15–16. The standard 300 μg dose of anti-D immune globulin covers what volume of fetal hemorrhage?

a. 10 mL of fetal whole blood

b. 30 mL of fetal whole blood

c. 10 mL of fetal red blood cells

d. 30 mL of fetal red blood cells

15–17. A 21-year-old G1 presents at 38 weeks' gestation with decreased fetal movement and is noted to have the fetal heart rate tracing shown below. An emergent cesarean delivery is done, and the neonate is noted to be depressed and pale. The Kleihauer-Betke test result is 2% and the maternal hematocrit is 35%. What is the best approximation of fetal hemorrhage?

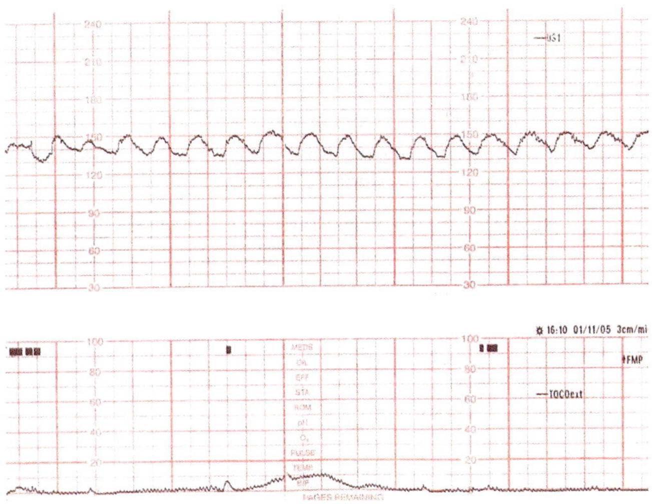

a. 50 mL fetal whole blood

b. 70 mL fetal whole blood

c. 90 mL fetal whole blood

d. 100 mL fetal whole blood

15–18. A 22-year-old primigravida delivers a term neonate without complications. Neonatal petechiae are noted, and platelet count at 4 hours of life is noted to be 12,000/μL. Maternal platelets trended downward during pregnancy reaching 89,000/μL at delivery. What is the most likely diagnosis?

a. Preeclampsia
b. Gestational thrombocytopenia
c. Idiopathic thrombocytopenic purpura
d. Neonatal alloimmune thrombocytopenia

15–19. The patient in Question 15–18 presents for counseling prior to pursuing future pregnancies. She has been tested and is HPA-1b homozygous with antibodies against the HPA-1a antigen. Which of the following statements most accurately reflects her risk of recurrence in future pregnancies with the same father?

a. 10%
b. 50%
c. 70–90%
d. 100%

15–20. The patient in Question 15–18 becomes pregnant again two years after her first delivery. What is the most appropriate treatment plan this pregnancy?

a. Serial fetal blood sampling starting at 20 weeks' gestation to follow platelet counts and initiate therapy when <50,000/μL.
b. IVIG 2 g/kg/week starting at 12 weeks' gestation, addition of corticosteroids at 32 weeks' gestation, and cesarean delivery at term.
c. IVIG 2 g/kg/week starting at 20 weeks' gestation, addition of corticosteroids at 32 weeks' gestation, and cesarean delivery at term.
d. IVIG 2 g/kg/week starting at 20 weeks' gestation, addition of corticosteroids at 32 weeks' gestation, and vaginal delivery at term.

15–21. A 32-year-old G2P1 at 38 weeks' gestation has a history of refractory idiopathic thrombocytopenic purpura, and despite treatment with steroids and a course of IVIG, her platelet count is 25,000/μL. She asks if a cesarean delivery would be best for her or the fetus. Which reply is most appropriate?

a. Fetal thrombocytopenia is rare, and vaginal delivery is recommended.
b. Fetal thrombocytopenia is common, and cesarean delivery is indicated to prevent fetal intracranial hemorrhage.
c. Fetal thrombocytopenia is common, and fetal blood sampling to guide determination of delivery method is recommended.
d. Fetal thrombocytopenia is common, but the available data suggests no increased risk of intracranial hemorrhage with vaginal delivery.

15–22. What was the most common cause of nonimmune hydrops in the large review done by Bellini in 2015?

a. Infectious
b. Lymphatic
c. Hematologic
d. Cardiovascular

15–23. A 34-year-old woman presents for routine fetal anatomy sonogram and has the findings shown below. What is the most likely cause of fetal hydrops diagnosed at 18 weeks' gestation?

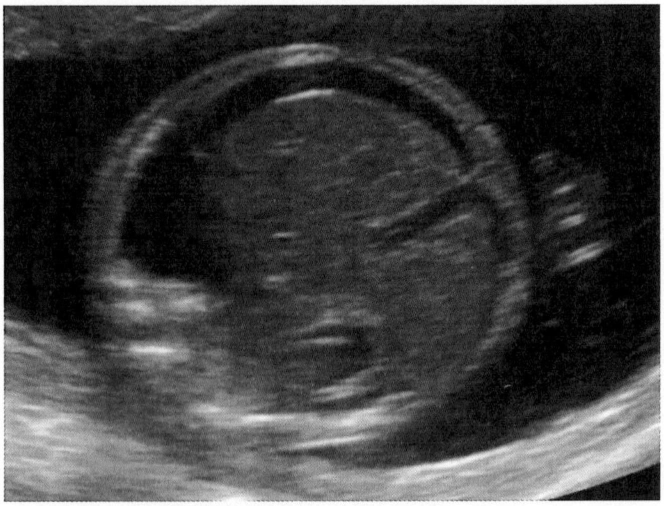

Used with permission from Dr. Jodi Dashe.

a. Infectious
b. Lymphatic
c. Chromosomal
d. Cardiovascular

15–24. A 42-year-old woman presents at 12 weeks' gestation with vaginal bleeding and transabdominal sonography reveals cystic hygromas, as show in the below images. She had "low-risk" cell-free DNA testing at 10 weeks' gestation for trisomy 13, 18, and 21 and was consistent with the absence of a Y chromosome. What is the most likely diagnosis?

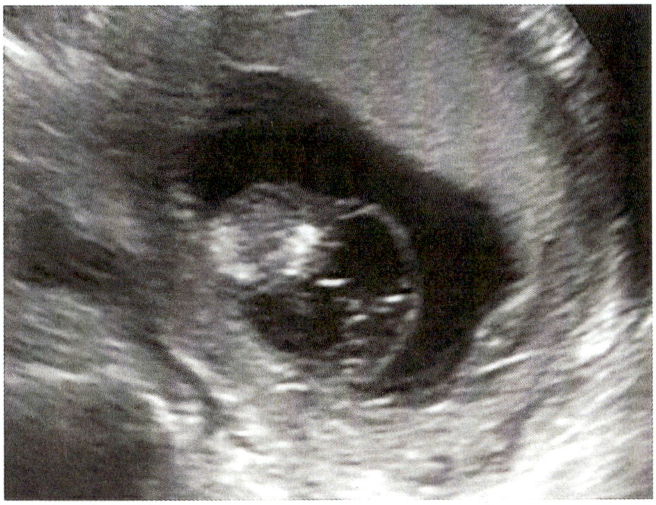

a. Trisomy 21
b. Trisomy 18
c. Turner syndrome
d. Noonan syndrome

15–25. A 19-year-old primigravida undergoes routine fetal anatomy sonogram at 19 weeks' gestation with the isolated finding as shown below. Which statement is correct?

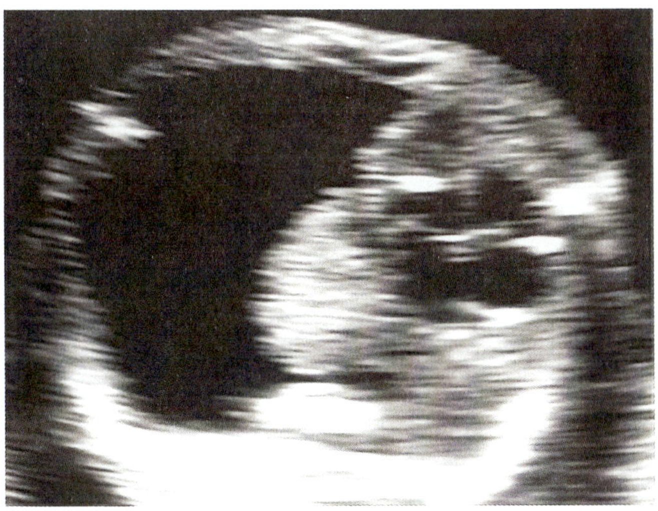

a. There is an indication for a fetal thoracentesis.
b. The risk of aneuploidy is significant, and diagnostic amniocentesis is recommended.
c. There is a significant risk of recurrence and progression to fetal hydrops following drainage of the pleural effusion.
d. All of the above statements are correct.

15–26. A 26-year-old G2P1 at 28 weeks' gestation presents with complaints of new-onset severe headache and generalized edema. Her pregnancy has been complicated by fetal cystic hygromas, diagnosis of trisomy 18, and progression to fetal hydrops. Her blood pressure is noted to be 170/102 mmHg, with 4+ proteinuria and an elevated serum creatinine. A fetal demise with severe polyhydramnios and placentomegaly is diagnosed. What is the most accurate diagnosis?

a. Mirror syndrome
b. Gestational hypertension
c. Preeclampsia with severe features
d. Disseminated intravascular coagulation

15–27. For the patient in Question 15–26, physical exam reveals significant leg swelling, left much greater than right. Doppler of her lower extremities reveals a new deep vein thrombosis in the left lower extremity. Her headache has worsened, and she has required multiple doses of intravenous anti-hypertensives. Fetal lie is noted to be transverse back up. What is the best next step in management?

a. Defer delivery and initiate full anticoagulation
b. Repeat cesarean delivery followed by initiation of full anticoagulation within 24 hours
c. Induction of labor with initiation of full anticoagulation immediately following delivery
d. Initiation of magnesium sulfate, intravenous anti-hypertensives as needed, and repeat cesarean delivery followed by initiation of full anticoagulation within 24 hours

15–28. Why does ABO incompatibility manifest in first-born neonates, despite the lack of prior maternal exposures?

a. Fetal red cells have more antigenic sites than adult cells.
b. Anti-A and anti-B antibodies can cross the placenta early in the first trimester.
c. Most group O women have previously been exposed to bacteria possessing A- or B-like antigens.
d. None of the above

15–29. What is the main reason that peak systolic velocity of the middle cerebral artery increases as fetal anemia worsens?

a. Fetal cardiac output increases
b. Fetal blood viscosity decreases
c. Preferential shunting of fetal blood to the brain
d. All of the above

15–30. The image shown below is a Kleihauer-Betke test, which is used to assess fetomaternal hemorrhage. Which of the following is not a limitation of this test?

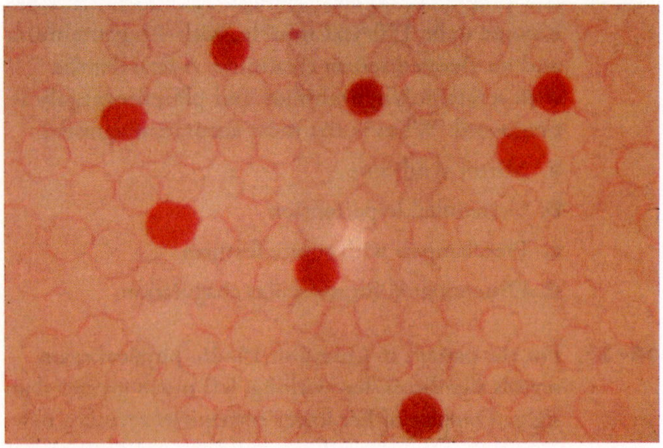

Reproduced with permission from Cunningham FG, Leveno KJ, Bloom SL, et al (eds): Fetal disorders. In William Obstetrics, 25th ed. New York, McGraw-Hill, 2018, Figure 15-3.

a. It is labor intensive.

b. It is only qualitative.

c. It is less accurate at term.

d. Interpretation is limited in the setting of maternal hemoglobinopathy.

15–31. Which of the following is not a treatable etiology of nonimmune hydrops?

a. Parvovirus

b. Chylothorax

c. α4-Thalassemia

d. Tachyarrhythmias

15–32. Red cells used for fetal transfusion should have which of the following characteristics?

a. Irradiated

b. Leukocyte enriched

c. Same ABO group as the mother

d. An approximate hematocrit of 50%

CHAPTER 15 ANSWER KEY

Question number	Letter answer	Page cited	Header cited
15–1	**d**	p. 301	Red Cell Alloimmunization
15–2	**a**	p. 303	Management of the Alloimmunized Pregnancy
15–3	**a**	p. 303	Management of the Alloimmunized Pregnancy
15–4	**c**	p. 301	Red Cell Alloimmunization
15–5	**d**	p. 309	Hydrops Fetalis
15–6	**d**	p. 304	Management of the Alloimmunized Pregnancy
15–7	**b**	p. 304	Management of the Alloimmunized Pregnancy
15–8	**b**	p. 304	Management of the Alloimmunized Pregnancy
15–9	**b**	p. 301	Red Cell Alloimmunization
15–10	**b**	p. 305	Prevention of Anti-D Alloimmunization
15–11	**a**	p. 303	Management of the Alloimmunized Pregnancy
15–12	**d**	p. 303	Red Cell Alloimmunization
15–13	**a**	p. 304	Management of the Alloimmunized Pregnancy
15–14	**d**	p. 305	Prevention of Anti-D Alloimmunization
15–15	**d**	p. 305	Prevention of Anti-D Alloimmunization
15–16	**b**	p. 305	Prevention of Anti-D Alloimmunization
15–17	**b**	p. 307	Hemorrhage Quantification
15–18	**d**	p. 308	Alloimmune Thrombocytopenia
15–19	**c**	p. 308	Alloimmune Thrombocytopenia
15–20	**c**	p. 308	Alloimmune Thrombocytopenia
15–21	**d**	p. 309	Immune Thrombocytopenia
15–22	**d**	p. 311	Nonimmune Hydrops
15–23	**c**	p. 310	Nonimmune Hydrops
15–24	**c**	p. 310	Nonimmune Hydrops
15–25	**d**	p. 311	Nonimmune Hydrops
15–26	**a**	p. 312	Mirror Syndrome
15–27	**d**	p. 312	Mirror Syndrome
15–28	**c**	p. 303	Red Cell Alloimmunization
15–29	**d**	p. 303	Management of the Alloimmunized Pregnancy
15–30	**b**	p. 307	Fetomaternal Hemorrhage
15–31	**c**	p. 309	Nonimmune Hydrops
15–32	**a**	p. 304	Management of the Alloimmunized Pregnancy

CHAPTER 16

Fetal Therapy

16–1. Fetuses with premature atrial contractions can later be found to have which of the following arrhythmias?

a. Atrial flutter

b. Atrial fibrillation

c. First-degree heart block

d. Supraventricular tachycardia

16–2. Sustained fetal tachyarrhythmias can lead to which of the following fetal complications?

a. Hydrops

b. Oligohydramnios

c. Fetal-growth restriction

d. All of the above

16–3. Which of the following agents are commonly administered to women to treat fetal tachyarrhythmias?

a. Sotalol

b. Digoxin

c. Flecainide

d. All of the above

16–4. The majority of cases of congenital adrenal hyperplasia are caused by which enzyme deficiency?

a. 21-Hydroxylase deficiency

b. 11β-Hydroxylase deficiency

c. 17α-Hydroxylase deficiency

d. 3β-Hydroxysteroid dehydrogenase deficiency

16–5. Before what gestational age does maternal treatment with dexamethasone need to commence to prevent virilization of a female fetus with congenital adrenal hyperplasia?

a. 6 weeks' gestation

b. 7 weeks' gestation

c. 9 weeks' gestation

d. 12 weeks' gestation

16–6. A 31-year-old woman presents with her husband for her screening ultrasound. At 19 weeks' gestation the fetal abnormality pictured below is found. You counsel her that as this mass expands, the fetus is at risk for which of the following?

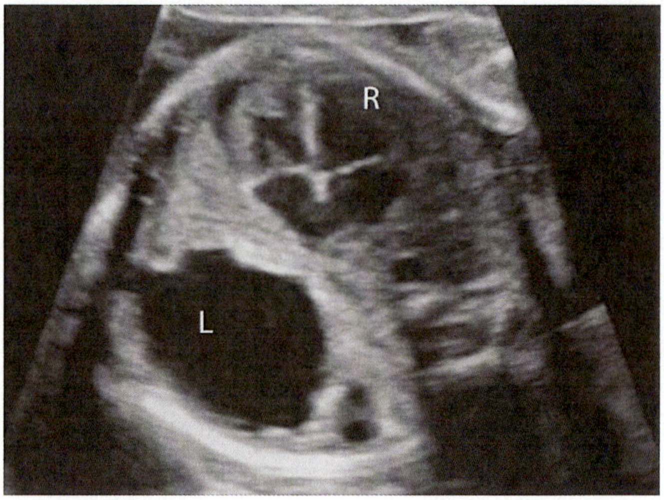

a. Fetal death

b. Hydrops fetalis

c. Depressed cardiac output

d. All of the above

16–7. For the patient in Question 16–6 you calculate a congenital cystic adenomatoid malformation volume ratio (CVR) of 1.4. What is the most appropriate next step in management based on this calculation?

a. Observation

b. Open fetal surgery

c. Medical therapy in pregnancy

d. Percutaneous thoraco-amnionic shunt placement

16–8. Which of the following fetal conditions cannot be treated with shunting?

a. Isolated pleural effusion

b. Lower urinary tract obstruction

c. Twin-twin transfusion syndrome

d. Congenital cystic adenomatoid malformation

16–9. The neural damage in myelomeningocele is the result of which of the following?

a. Hindbrain herniation

b. Trauma from a vaginal birth

c. Exposure to the amnionic fluid

d. Decreased fetal movement in utero

16–10. A 35-year-old woman's fetus is found to have the congenital anomaly pictured below. She inquires about fetal surgery. You counsel her that infants who underwent prenatal surgery in the Management of Myelomeningocele Study (MOMS) had which of the following outcomes compared with those that had postnatal surgery?

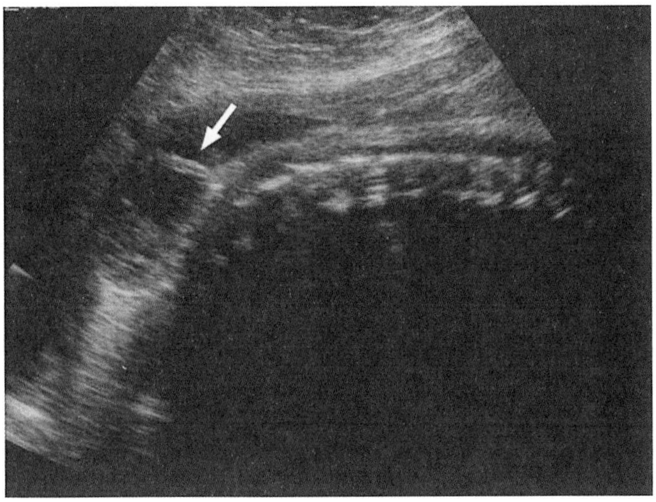

a. They experienced lower hindbrain herniation rates.

b. They were more likely to walk independently at 30 months.

c. They were less likely to require ventriculoperitoneal shunting by 1 year of age.

d. All of the above

16–11. The patient in Question 16–12 asks about the risks of fetal surgery. You counsel her that in the MOMS trial, all except which of the following morbidities occurred more frequently in the prenatal surgery group?

a. Preterm delivery

b. Placental abruption

c. Maternal hypertension

d. Maternal pulmonary edema

16–12. A 24-year-old presents for her rate of growth ultrasound at 28 weeks' gestation and the abnormality seen below is found. Hydrops fetalis can occur in these situations as a result of which of the following?

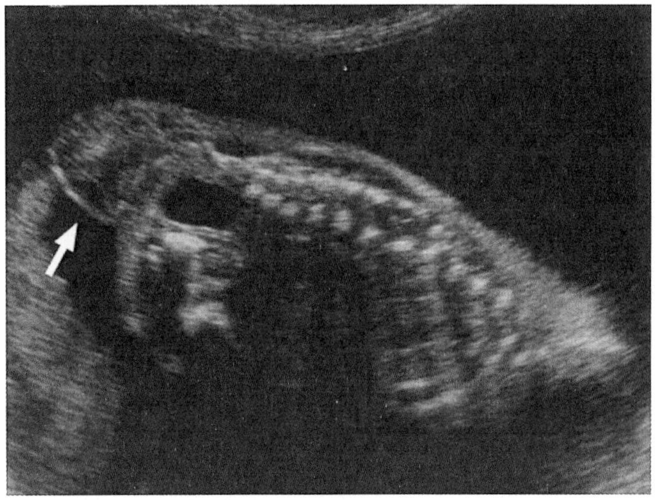

a. Lymphatic obstruction

b. Congestive heart failure

c. High-output heart failure

d. None of the above

16–13. In the United States, which of the following twin pregnancies would be a candidate for fetoscopic laser ablation therapy for twin-twin transfusion syndrome (TTTS)?

a. Dichorionic diamnionic twins at 19 weeks' gestation with stage II TTTS

b. Monochorionic diamnionic twins at 23 weeks' gestation with stage I TTTS

c. Monochorionic diamnionic twins at 15 weeks' gestation with stage IV TTTS

d. Monochorionic diamnionic twins at 21 weeks' gestation with stage III TTTS

16–14. A pair of monochorionic twins presents at 20 weeks' gestation. The sonographic findings displayed below are found. In addition, there is no growth discordance, umbilical Doppler studies are normal, and hydrops is not present. What would be the assigned Quintero stage?

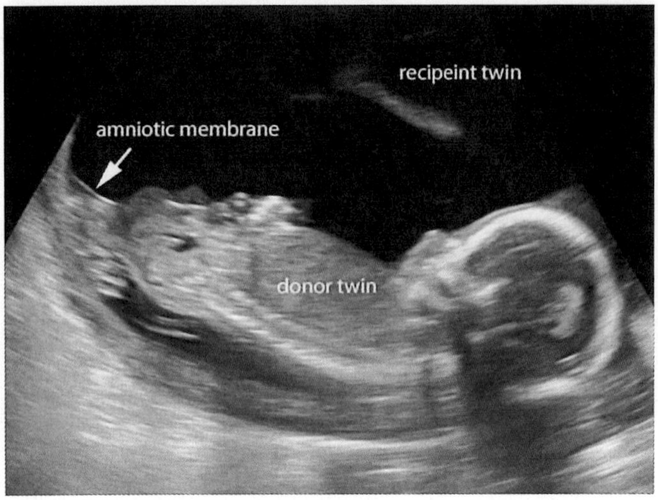

Used with permission from Dr. Ramen Chmait.

a. Stage I
b. Stage II
c. Stage III
d. Stage IV

16–15. Which of the following complications is least likely to occur with laser therapy for twin-twin transfusion syndrome?

a. Vascular laceration
b. Placental abruption
c. Grade III intraventricular hemorrhage
d. Preterm premature rupture of membranes

16–16. What is the main concern in the setting of an isolated congenital diaphragmatic hernia?

a. Liver herniation
b. Mediastinal shift
c. Bowel herniation
d. Low lung volumes

16–17. The increase in neonatal survival rates with congenital diaphragmatic hernias is due to which of the following advances?

a. In utero repair
b. Postnatal respiratory support
c. Ex-utero intrapartum treatment
d. Fetal endoscopic tracheal occlusion

16–18. Which of the following lung-to-head ratios predicts survival?

a. 0.5
b. 0.6
c. 1.1
d. 1.5

16–19. A 39-year-old woman is referred at 22 weeks' gestation with concern for fetal hydrops. A sonogram reveals the finding below. Work-up for this lesion consists of which of the following?

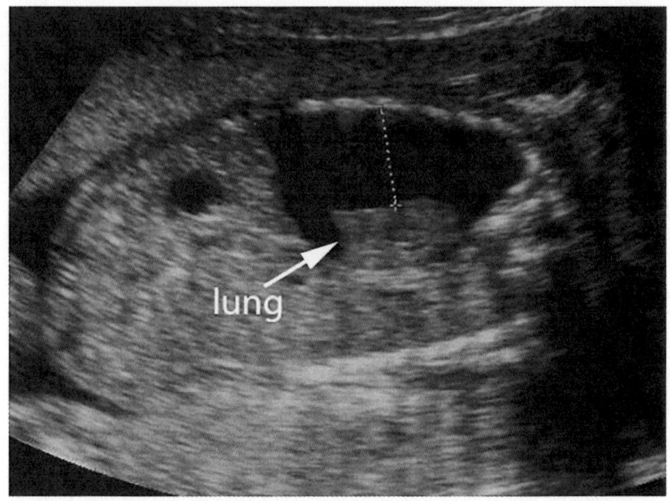

a. Fetal karyotype
b. Fetal echocardiogram
c. Maternal viral studies
d. All of the above

16–20. In the case in Question 16–19, what is the most likely etiology of the pleural effusion?

a. Trisomy 21
b. Fetal cardiac defect
c. Lymphatic obstruction
d. Fetal parvovirus infection

16–21. All except which of the following is not a sonographic finding of lower urinary tract obstruction?

a. Hydramnios
b. Dilated urethra
c. Dilated bladder
d. Bladder wall thickening

16–22. A patient presents for her screening ultrasound at 18 weeks' gestation, and the fetus had the sonographic finding shown below. Work-up for this abnormality does not include which of the following?

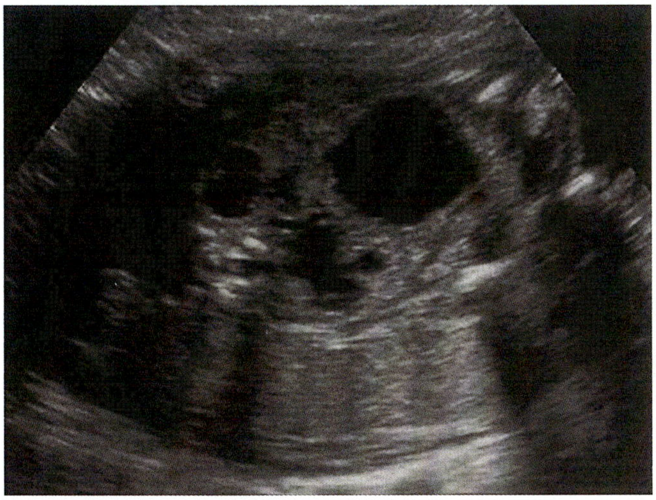

a. Vesicocentesis
b. Determination of gender
c. Amniocentesis for karyotype
d. Fetal magnetic resonance imaging

16–23. After determination that the fetus in Question 16–22 is a male with no other abnormalities, vesicocentesis is performed. All of the urinary indices are normal, and a vesicoamnionic shunt is placed. Which of the following is a goal of shunt placement?

a. Prevent skeletal deformities
b. Preservation of renal function
c. Prevent pulmonary hypoplasia
d. Prevent fetal-growth restriction

16–24. The finding of a female fetus in the setting of a lower urinary tract obstruction is associated with which of the following?

a. Increased risk of stillbirth
b. Increased likelihood of aneuploidy
c. Increased likelihood for complex malformations
d. Less likely to be candidates for vesicoamnionic shunts

16–25. All except which of the following would generally be considered contraindications to vesicoamnionic shunt placement in fetuses with bladder outlet obstruction?

a. Female sex
b. Aneuploidy
c. Presence of renal cysts
d. Urinary sodium of 80 mmol/L

16–26. All except which of the following urinary analytes are evaluated to predict renal prognosis in a fetus with bladder-outlet obstruction?

a. Sodium
b. Chloride
c. Potassium
d. β_2-Microglobulin

16–27. Which of the following is an indication for in utero fetal cardiac intervention?

a. Fetal atrial fibrillation
b. Critical aortic stenosis
c. Cardiac rhabdomyomas
d. Isolated pericardial effusion

16–28. The goal of fetal aortic valvuloplasty is which of the following?

a. Prevent fetal hydrops
b. Prevent development of mitral regurgitation
c. Prevent aortic valve replacement later in life
d. Preserve left ventricular function and prevent left hypoplastic heart syndrome

16–29. At delivery, ex-utero intrapartum treatment (EXIT) procedures may be indicated in the management of which of the following fetal conditions?

a. Large anterior encephalocele
b. Large sacrococcygeal teratoma
c. Hypoplastic left heart syndrome
d. Congenital high airway obstruction sequence

16–30. Which of the following is the goal of an ex-utero intrapartum treatment (EXIT) procedure?

a. Excision of a fetal tumor
b. Minimize maternal blood loss
c. Establishment of a fetal airway
d. Repair of a fetal myelomeningocele

16–31. Which of the following fetal conditions can cause hydrops fetalis?

a. Thyrotoxicosis
b. Sacrococcygeal teratoma
c. Congenital cystic adenomatoid malformation
d. All of the above

16–32. All except which of the following are examples of fetal conditions that may be amenable to medical therapy delivered transplacentally?

a. Fetal thyrotoxicosis
b. Sacrococcygeal teratoma
c. Supraventricular tachycardia
d. Congenital cystic adenomatoid malformation

CHAPTER 16 ANSWER KEY

Question number	Letter answer	Page cited	Header cited
16–1	**d**	p. 316	Premature Atrial Contractions
16–2	**a**	p. 316	Tachyarrhythmias
16–3	**d**	p. 316	Tachyarrhythmias
16–4	**a**	p. 317	Congenital Adrenal Hyperplasia
16–5	**c**	p. 317	Congenital Adrenal Hyperplasia
16–6	**d**	p. 318	Congenital Cystic Adenomatoid Malformation
16–7	**a**	p. 318	Congenital Cystic Adenomatoid Malformation
16–8	**c**	p. 319	Table 16-2
16–9	**c**	p. 319	Myelomeningocele Surgery
16–10	**d**	p. 319	Myelomeningocele Surgery
16–11	**c**	p. 320	Table 16-3
16–12	**c**	p. 321	Sacrococcygeal Teratoma
16–13	**d**	p. 321	Twin-Twin Transfusion Syndrome
16–14	**a**	p. 322	Twin-Twin Transfusion Syndrome
16–15	**a**	p. 322	Complications
16–16	**d**	p. 323	Congenital Diaphragmatic Hernia
16–17	**b**	p. 323	Congenital Diaphragmatic Hernia
16–18	**d**	p. 323	Lung-to-Head Ratio
16–19	**d**	p. 324	Thoracic Shunts
16–20	**c**	p. 324	Thoracic Shunts
16–21	**a**	p. 325	Urinary Shunts
16–22	**d**	p. 325	Urinary Shunts
16–23	**c**	p. 325	Urinary Shunts
16–24	**c**	p. 325	Urinary Shunts
16–25	**d**	p. 325	Urinary Shunts
16–26	**c**	p. 326	Table 16-4
16–27	**b**	p. 326	Fetal Intracardiac Catheter Procedures
16–28	**d**	p. 326	Fetal Intracardiac Catheter Procedures
16–29	**d**	p. 327	Ex-Utero Intrapartum Treatment
16–30	**c**	p. 327	Ex-Utero Intrapartum Treatment
16–31	**d**	p. 318 p. 318 p. 321	Fetal Thyrotoxicosis Congenital Cystic Adenomatoid Malformation Sacrococcygeal Teratoma
16–32	**b**	p. 315	Medical Therapy

CHAPTER 17

Fetal Assessment

17–1. What is a goal of antepartum fetal surveillance?

a. Predict timing of fetal death
b. Avoid unnecessary intervention
c. Improve positive predictive value of maternal kick counts
d. None of the above

17–2. Concerning antepartum testing, positive predictive values for true-positive abnormal test results approximate which of the following?

a. 5–10%
b. 10–40%
c. 40–60%
d. 60–80%

17–3. Which of the following statements concerning fetal movements is true?

a. Fetuses spend most of their time in behavioral states 2F and 3F after 36 weeks.
b. The average number of fetal movements increases weekly until 40 weeks' gestation.
c. General body movements become organized between 20 and 30 weeks' gestation.
d. Beyond 6 weeks' gestation, fetal movements are never absent for periods exceeding 13 minutes.

17–4. Which of the following findings have been attributed to studies in fetal movement?

a. Women are more likely to perceive fetal movements lasting more than 20 seconds.
b. Informal maternal perceptions of fetal movement are as valuable as formally recorded fetal movement.
c. Growth restricted fetuses were identified before birth more often when fetal movement count was used.
d. All of the above

17–5. Which of the following is true regarding fetal movements?

a. The lowest number of weekly fetal movements occurs at term.
b. The number of weekly fetal movements peaks at 32 weeks' gestation.
c. In a normal pregnancy there should be 10 counts in a 12-hour period.
d. Declining amnionic fluid volume and space account for decreased fetal movements at 30 weeks' gestation.

17–6. The type of breathing displayed below has been called which of the following?

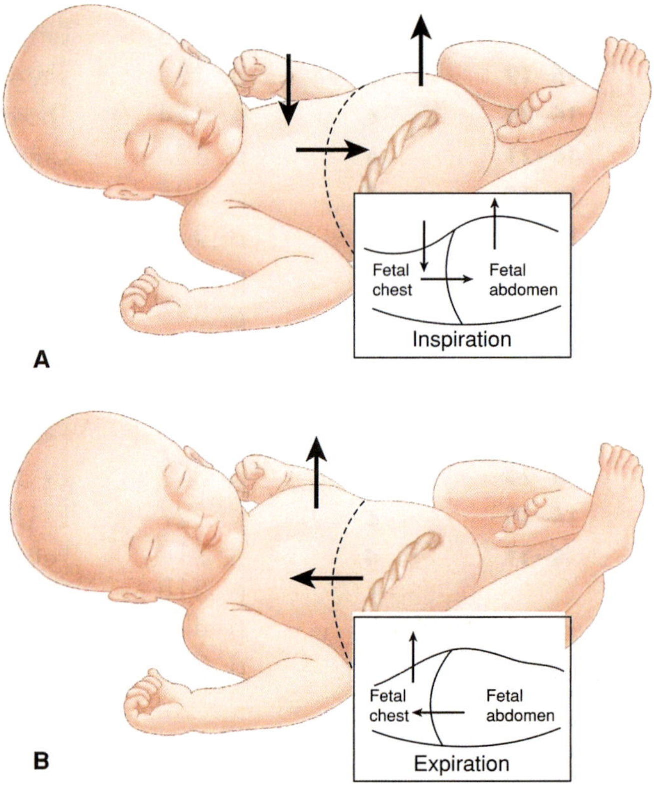

A

B

Reproduced with permission from Cunningham FG, Leveno KJ, Bloom SL, et al (eds): Fetal assessment. In Williams Obstetrics, 25th ed. New York, McGraw-Hill, 2018, Figure 17-3.

a. Paradoxical
b. Anatomical
c. Diaphragmatic
d. Late term fetal breathing

17–7. Which of the following statements are true concerning contraction stress tests?

a. Identifies uteroplacental insufficiency.

b. Average time to completion is 75 minutes.

c. Equivocal-suspicious tests should be repeated in 24 hours.

d. Variable decelerations are normal and do not require assessment.

17–8. A 36-year-old multiparous patient is undergoing a contraction stress test (CST). The nurse in the testing center calls and tells you the CST has adequate contractions, and late decelerations with every third contraction. How would this CST be interpreted?

a. Positive CST

b. Negative CST

c. Equivocal-suspicious CST

d. None of the above

17–9. Which of the following statements are true concerning nonstress tests?

a. They assess fetal condition rather than uteroplacental function.

b. It has a similar ability to predict fetal wellbeing as a contraction stress test.

c. The time to perform a nonstress test is much shorter than a contraction stress test.

d. All of the above

17–10. A 25-year-old primigravida with type 1 diabetes presents to labor and delivery at 28 weeks' gestation complaining of 3 days of nausea and vomiting and an inability to tolerate food. An arterial blood gas is performed showing a pH of 7.08. The fetal heart rate tracing on admission is shown below. Which of the following is the cause of the minimal variability and recurrent decelerations seen?

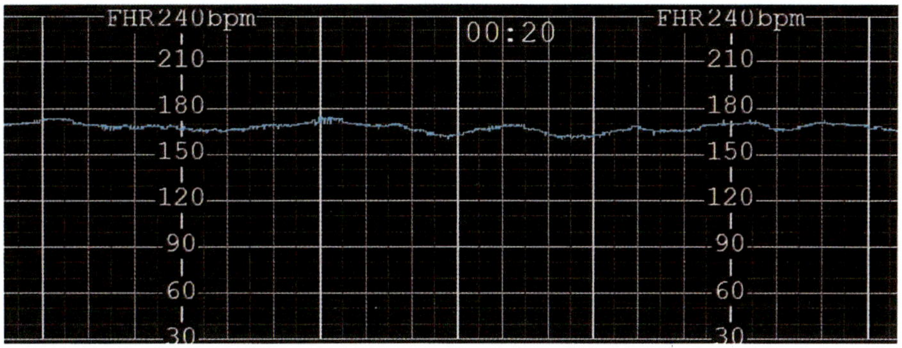

Used with permission from Dr. John Byrne.

a. Fetal sleep cycle

b. Maternal acidemia

c. Maternal blood glucose of 348 mg/dL

d. All of the above

17–11. A 34-year-old multigravida at 34 weeks' gestation presents to triage with complaints of decreased fetal movement. She undergoes a nonstress test as depicted below. Which statement is true regarding the nonstress test?

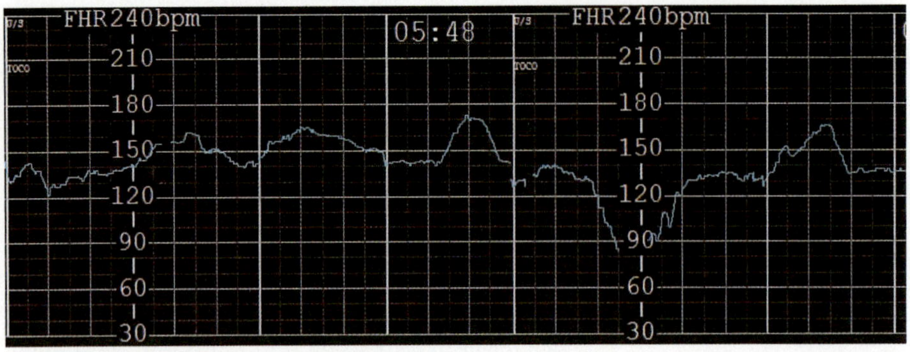

Used with permission from Dr. Molly Dubois.

a. It is a reactive nonstress test.

b. Fetal movement is not documented, so she cannot go home.

c. A full 40-minute test must be performed before she can go home.

d. The variable deceleration indicates she must undergo prolonged monitoring.

17–12. Which of the following statements regarding a nonstress test is not true?

a. They do not predict acute asphyxial events.

b. Vibroacoustic stimulation of the fetus is not allowed.

c. More than 20 minutes may be needed to account for fetal sleep cycles.

d. One acceleration is just as reliable as two in predicting healthy fetal status.

17–13. The components of a biophysical profile include all except which of the following?

a. Fetal tone

b. Fetal breathing

c. Contraction stress test

d. Amnionic fluid volume measurement

17–14. Which statement accurately reflects the image shown below?

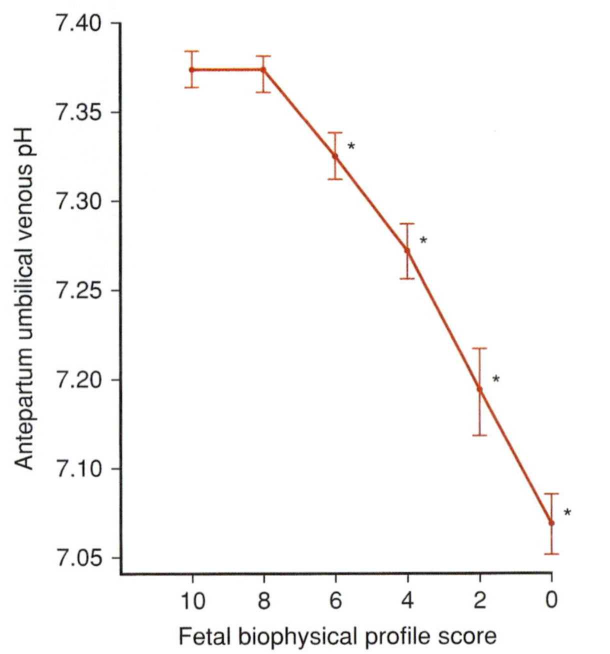

Reproduced with permission from Cunningham FG, Leveno KJ, Bloom SL, et al (eds): Fetal assessment. In Williams Obstetrics, 25th ed. New York, McGraw-Hill, 2018, Figure 17-9.

a. A score of 6/10 is indication to proceed with delivery.

b. A score of 0/10 is associated with almost certain asphyxia.

c. A score of 8/10 is associated with an umbilical venous pH ≤7.30.

d. A score of 4/10 is similar to 6/10 in regard to umbilical venous pH.

17–15. Which of the following statements is true regarding the modified biophysical profile?

a. It is associated with a false-positive rate of 1.5%.

b. It is associated with a false-negative rate of 0.8 per 1000.

c. The American College of Obstetricians and Gynecologists agrees that it is as good as any other fetal test of well-being.

d. All of the above

17–16. According to the American College of Obstetricians and Gynecologists, which of the following statements concerning amnionic fluid volume is true?

a. Best measurement to detect oligohydramnios is the deepest vertical pocket.

b. Decreased amnionic fluid volume usually represents decreased uteroplacental perfusion.

c. Use of the deepest vertical pocket to define oligohydramnios leads to fewer unnecessary interventions.

d. All of the above

17–17. When is umbilical artery velocimetry considered abnormal?

a. End-systolic flow is absent

b. Systolic-diastolic ratio is less than 2

c. Systolic-diastolic ratio is greater than 4

d. Systolic-diastolic ratio >95th percentile for given gestational age

17–18. Which of the following is true regarding the umbilical artery Doppler shown below?

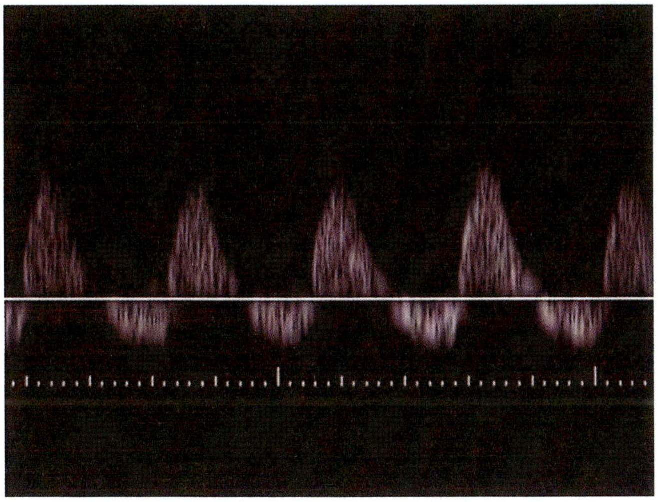

a. This is absent end-systolic flow.

b. This is reversed end-diastolic flow.

c. This finding is normal until 32 weeks' gestation.

d. This pattern indicates decreased resistance to umbilical artery blood flow.

17–19. Middle cerebral artery Doppler is useful in which of the following scenarios?

a. Fetal intrauterine growth restriction

b. Routine assessment of fetal well-being

c. Pregnancies complicated by alloimmunization

d. All of the above

17–20. Which of the following are true concerning Doppler of the ductus venosus?

a. Absent or reversed flow is a sign of multiorgan damage.

b. It can be used to prevent iatrogenic preterm delivery.

c. Correlates well with umbilical artery Doppler to predict fetal well-being.

d. It is a useful surveillance tool for fetuses with intrauterine growth restriction.

17–21. High resistance flow in the uterine artery between 22 and 24 weeks' gestation is correlated with which of the following?

a. Stillbirth

b. Abruption

c. Preeclampsia

d. All of the above

17–22. Concerning antenatal fetal testing, which of the following is true?

a. It is used to predict fetal wellness.

b. Each method is limited in some way.

c. Normal biological fetal variation makes interpretation challenging.

d. All of the above

17–23. A benefit from vibroacoustic stimulation is which of the following?

a. It increases the predictability of the nonstress test.

b. It makes a nonstress test feasible in the preterm infant.

c. It shortens the time necessary to perform a nonstress test.

d. None of the above

17–24. A 33-year-old with chronic hypertension at 36 weeks' gestation reports decreased fetal movement at her prenatal care appointment. Ultrasound shows a deepest vertical pocket of 4 cm. What is the next best step?

a. Nonstress test

b. Umbilical artery Doppler

c. Assessment of fetal growth

d. Prolonged monitoring on labor and delivery

17–25. The patient in Question 17–24 undergoes a nonstress test. A representation of the 20-minute tracing is shown below. What do you do next?

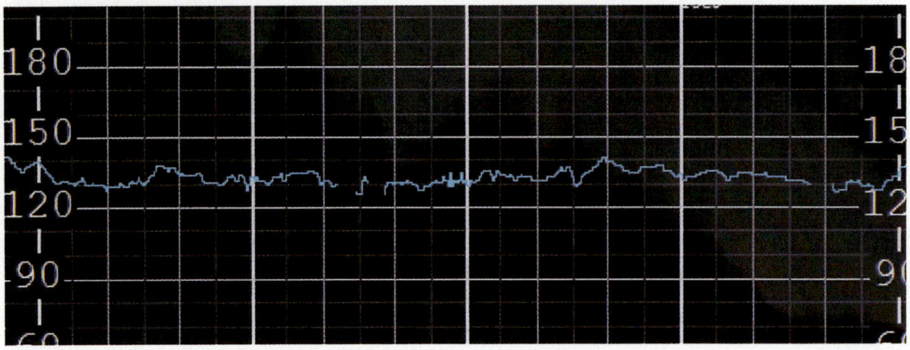

a. Send the patient to labor and delivery for delivery.

b. Leave the patient on the fetal monitor for 20 more minutes.

c. Send the patient to labor and deliver for cesarean delivery.

d. Send patient home and have her return the next day for repeat nonstress test.

17–26. The patient in Question 17–24 undergoes another 20 minutes of fetal heart rate monitoring and the remainder of the nonstress test (NST) is as shown below. What is your interpretation and plan?

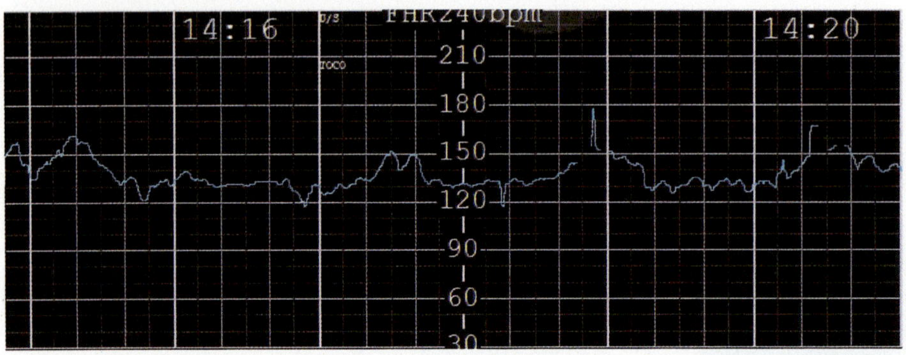

a. Reactive NST; return to clinic in 1 week

b. Reactive NST; proceed with biophysical profile

c. Nonreactive NST; use the vibroacoustic stimulator

d. Nonreactive NST; proceed with prolonged monitoring on labor and delivery

17–27. A 34-year-old at 35 weeks' gestation with gestational diabetes treated with insulin undergoes a biophysical profile (BPP). A score of 6/8 is obtained due to lack of fetal tone. What is your next best step?

a. Perform a nonstress test.

b. Send her to labor and delivery for delivery.

c. Send her to labor and delivery for a contraction stress test.

d. No further testing

17–28. A 30-year-old multigravida at 22 weeks' gestation has an anti-Kell titer of 1:64. What technique are you going to use to monitor this pregnancy?

a. Weekly nonstress test

b. Weekly biophysical profiles

c. Weekly middle cerebral artery Doppler

d. Nothing until she reports decreased fetal movement

17–29. Which fetal behavioral state is matched correctly?

a. Stage 1F—quiescent state

b. Stage 2F—vigorous body movements

c. Stage 3F—frequent gross body movements

d. Stage 4F—continuous eye movements only

17–30. Which of the following are methods to assess fetal movement?

a. Ultrasound

b. Tocodynamometer

c. Maternal perception

d. All of the above

17–31. Which of the following can affect fetal breathing?

a. Cervical exam

b. Amniocentesis

c. Maternal position

d. Fetal presentation

17–32. Fetal heart rate variability is influenced by all except which of the following?

a. Fetal sleep cycle

b. Maternal position

c. Maternal medication

d. Maternal cigarette smoking

CHAPTER 17 ANSWER KEY

Question number	Letter answer	Page cited	Header cited
17–1	**b**	331	Introduction
17–2	**b**	331	Introduction
17–3	**c**	331	Fetal Movement
17–4	**d**	332	Fetal Movement
17–5	**b**	332	Figure 17-2
17–6	**a**	333	Figure 17-3
17–7	**a**	334	Contraction Stress Test
17–8	**c**	334	Contraction Stress Test
17–9	**d**	335	Nonstress Test
17–10	**b**	336	Abnormal Nonstress Tests
17–11	**a**	335	Normal Nonstress Tests
17–12	**b**	335	Normal Nonstress Tests
17–13	**c**	337	Biophysical Profile
17–14	**b**	339	Figure 17-9
17–15	**d**	339	Modified Biophysical Profile
17–16	**d**	339	Amniotic Fluid Volume
17–17	**d**	339	Umbilical Artery Velocimetry
17–18	**b**	339	Umbilical Artery Velocimetry
17–19	**c**	340	Middle Cerebral Artery
17–20	**a**	340	Ductus Venosus
17–21	**d**	340	Uterine Artery
17–22	**d**	340	Antenatal Testing Summary
17–23	**c**	337	Acoustic Stimulation Tests
17–24	**a**	338	Modified Biophysical Profile
17–25	**b**	335	Normal Nonstress Tests
17–26	**a**	335	Normal Nonstress Tests
17–27	**a**	338	Table 17-3
17–28	**c**	340	Middle Cerebral Artery
17–29	**a**	331	Physiology
17–30	**d**	332	Clinical Application
17–31	**a**	333	Fetal Breathing
17–32	**b**	335	Fetal Heart Rate Acceleration

SECTION 6

EARLY PREGNANCY COMPLICATIONS

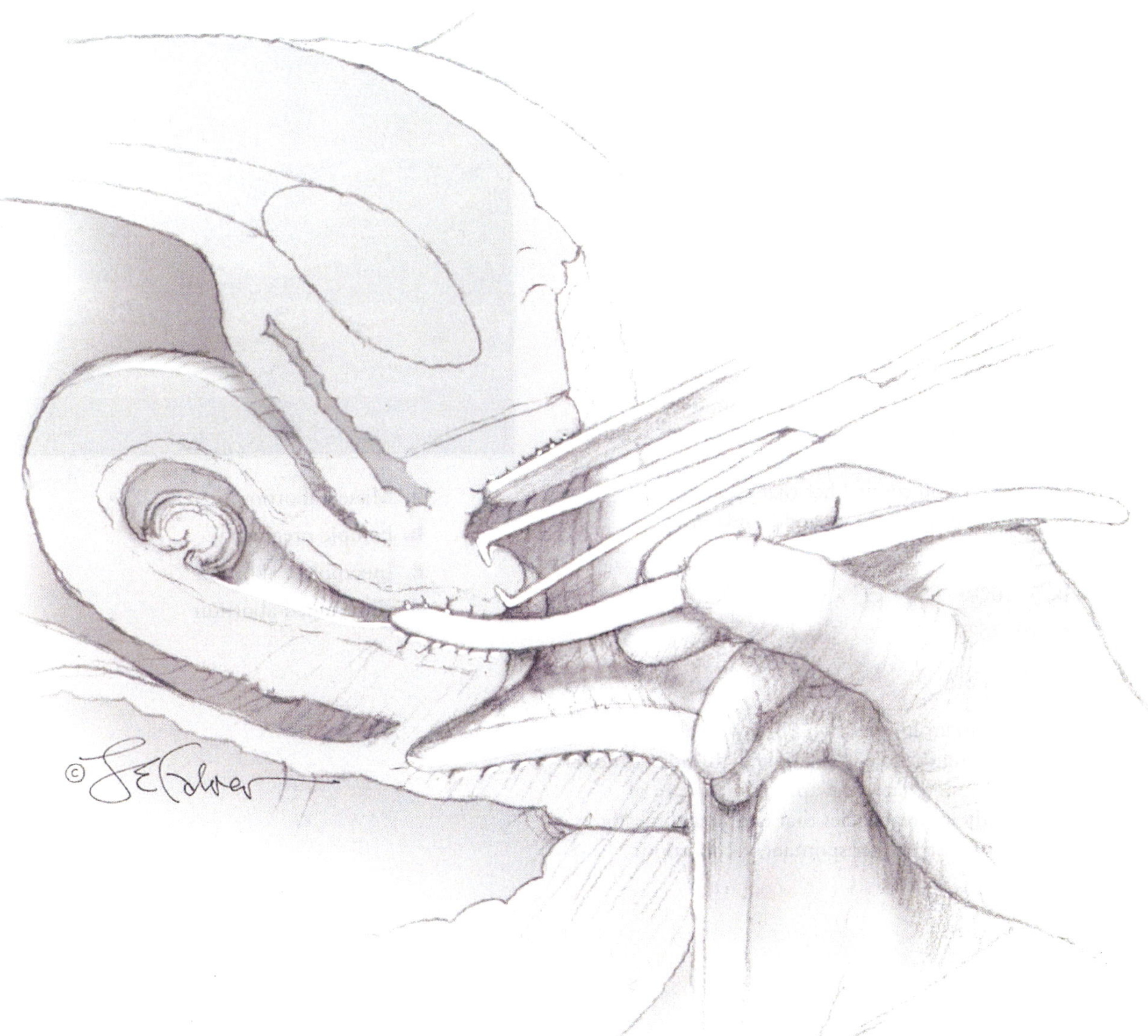

CHAPTER 18

Abortion

18–1. Which of the following sonogram findings is consistent with the American College of Obstetricians and Gynecologists definition of early pregnancy loss?

a. An anembryonic pregnancy

b. A crown-rump length of 7 mm with no cardiac motion

c. A fetus measuring 13 weeks' gestation with no cardiac motion

d. All of the above

18–2. What percent of spontaneous abortions occur within the first 12 weeks of gestation?

a. 60%

b. 70%

c. 80%

d. 90%

18–3. A 22-year-old G1P0 presents for a follow-up visit after receiving care for a spontaneous abortion at 8 weeks' gestation. She has many questions regarding the possible cause of her miscarriage, and the risk of recurrence. You counsel her that approximately what percentage of pregnancies end in miscarriage?

a. 3–5%

b. 5–10%

c. 10–25%

d. 40%

18–4. For the patient in Question 18–3, you also counsel her regarding the rate of aneuploidy in first-trimester miscarriages. What is the approximate rate of aneuploidy in pregnancies that end in a clinically apparent first trimester spontaneous abortion?

a. 10%

b. 20%

c. 33%

d. 50%

18–5. A patient presents for her first obstetrical visit at 8 weeks' gestation by last menstrual period with complaints of vaginal spotting; on exam the cervical os is closed without active bleeding. A sonogram is performed, as shown below, with no cardiac motion noted. What is the correct diagnosis?

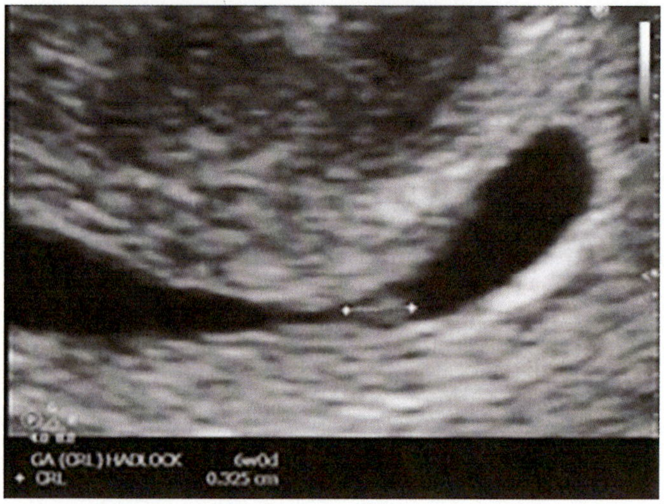

a. Missed abortion

b. Ectopic pregnancy

c. Incomplete abortion

d. Threatened abortion

18–6. The patient in Question 18–5 presents for repeat sonogram in 2 weeks, as shown below. She denies any complaints, and pelvic exam is unremarkable. No cardiac motion is noted. What is the correct diagnosis?

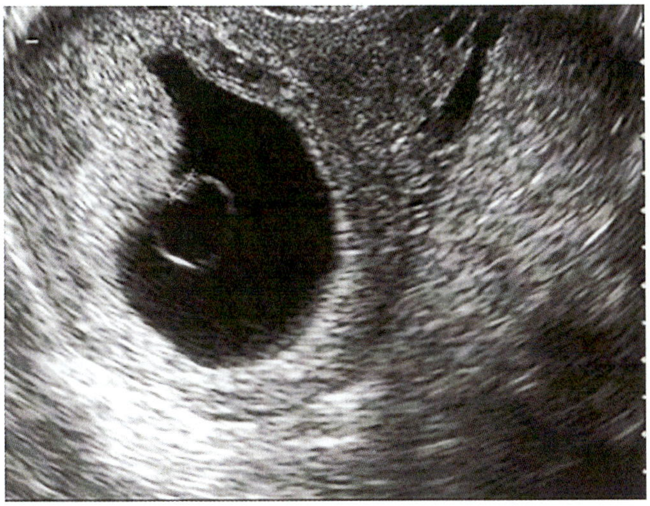

a. Missed abortion
b. Ectopic pregnancy
c. Incomplete abortion
d. Threatened abortion

18–7. Which of the following chromosomal abnormalities is most common in the setting of first-trimester spontaneous abortion?

a. Trisomy 18
b. Trisomy 21
c. Tetraploidy
d. Monosomy X (Turner syndrome)

18–8. A 40-year-old G5P1A3 at 7 weeks' gestation presents with a spontaneous abortion. Her medical history is remarkable for hypothyroidism with a TSH of 1.5 μIU/mL on levothyroxine, type 2 diabetes mellitus with a hemoglobin A_{1C} of 10% on metformin, and MTHFR heterozygous mutation. She underwent testing with another physician following her prior miscarriages, with normal maternal karyotype and negative antiphospholipid antibody syndrome testing. The products of conception are sent for karyotype, which is normal. Her 44-year-old husband is the father of all of her pregnancies. She requests use of prophylactic anticoagulation in future pregnancies to improve her pregnancy outcomes. Which of the following recommendations is most appropriate?

a. Initiation of insulin therapy
b. Increase dose of levothyroxine
c. Consider sperm donor given likely paternal factor
d. Begin heparin prophylaxis with missed menses next pregnancy

18–9. Consumption of which of the following legal substances in large quantities is most clearly associated with an increased risk of miscarriage?

a. Alcohol
b. Tobacco
c. Caffeine
d. Phthalates

18–10. A 20-year-old woman at 4–5 weeks' gestation by last menstrual period presents with vaginal spotting and cramping. On exam her cervical os is closed, and pelvic ultrasound image reveals no evidence of intrauterine pregnancy or adnexal masses (as shown below). Her progesterone level is 12 ng/mL, and β-hCG level is 456 mIU/mL. What is the correct diagnosis?

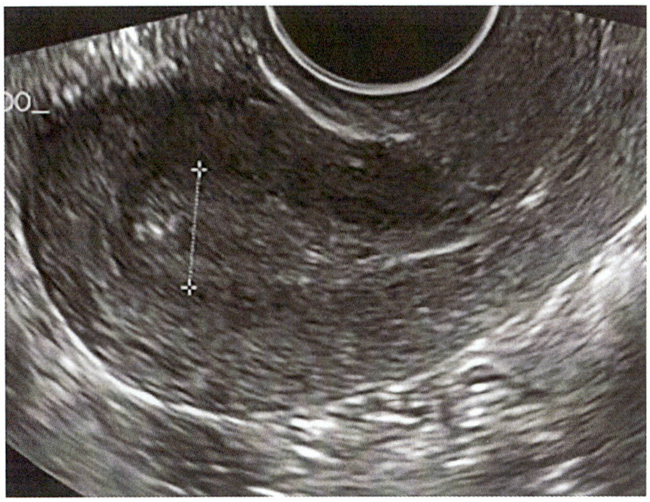

a. Missed abortion
b. Ectopic pregnancy
c. Threatened abortion
d. Pregnancy of unknown location

18–11. The patient in Question 18–10 presents for follow-up 48 hours later, she denies further bleeding or abdominal pain. Her β-hCG level is 796 mIU/mL. What is the most appropriate course of action?

a. Repeat pelvic sonogram
b. Administer methotrexate
c. Repeat β-hCG level in 48 hours
d. Administer supplemental progesterone

CHAPTER 18

18–12. The patient in Question 18–11 presents for follow-up with appropriately rising β-hCG levels and is eventually diagnosed with a threatened abortion. When counseling her regarding adverse outcomes related to threatened abortion, you inform her she may be at increased risk of which of the following?

a. Preterm birth
b. Placental previa
c. Placental abruption
d. All of the above

18–13. A 32-year-old G3P2 at 6 weeks' gestation by last menstrual period presents with vaginal spotting. A pelvic sonogram is done with the findings shown below. The gestational sac measures 22 mm × 20 mm × 31 mm. When counseling the patient regarding her management options, which is least appropriate?

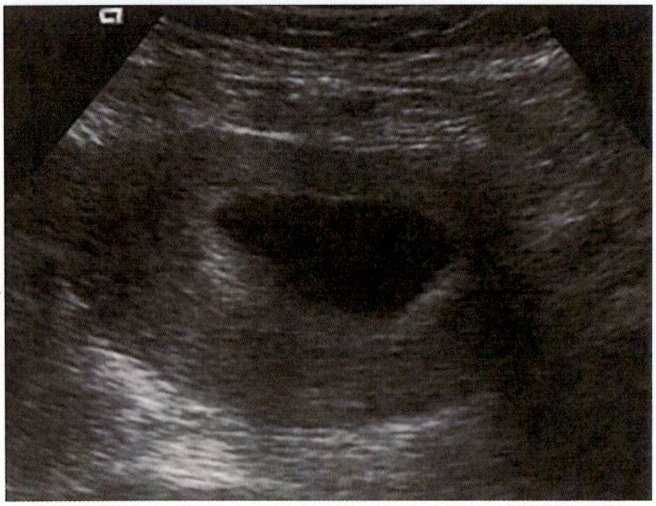

a. Expectant management
b. Administer misoprostol
c. Repeat sonogram in 2 weeks
d. Perform dilation and curettage

18–14. The patient in Question 18–13 elects for administration of misoprostol, 800 µg vaginally. When called for follow-up 48 hours later she reports some light spotting, but no bleeding or passage of tissue. She would like to avoid surgical dilation and curettage if possible. Which of the following regimens should be recommended?

a. Mifepristone 200 mg orally
b. Misoprostol 800 µg vaginally
c. Misoprostol 200 µg sublingual
d. Misoprostol 800 µg vaginally plus mifepristone 600 mg orally

18–15. A G1 at 17 weeks' gestation presents with complaint of leakage of fluid. On sterile speculum exam the cervix is closed and scant pooling of clear fluid is noted. Sonogram reveals anhydramnios as seen below. You counsel the patient on the high risk of delivery prior to viability with expectant management. Which statement is most correct regarding the risk of delivery with previable rupture of membranes?

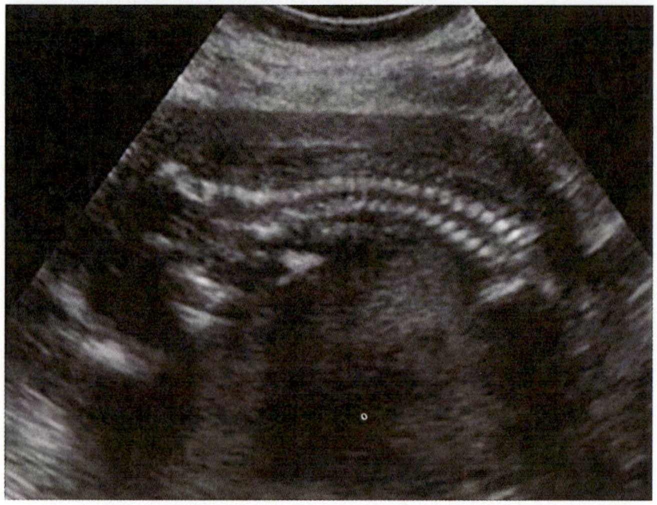

a. 10–20% within 1 week, 40–50% within 2–5 weeks
b. 20–30% within 1 week, 60–70% within 2–5 weeks
c. 40–50% within 1 week, 70–80% within 2–5 weeks
d. 60–70% within 1 week, 80–90% within 2–5 weeks

18–16. For the patient in Question 18–15, you counsel her that which of the following findings increases the risk of poor outcomes including pulmonary hypoplasia?

a. Anhydramnios
b. Short duration of latency
c. Gestational age at rupture
d. All of the above

18–17. A woman presents with her partner to the emergency department complaining of abdominal pain and fever. She has a temperature of 41°C, a blood pressure of 78/42 mmHg, no rebound or guarding, but exquisite cervical motion tenderness and generalized malaise. After asking her partner to leave the room, she discloses that she underwent an illegal abortion at approximately 8 weeks' gestation last night. You diagnose her with a septic abortion and begin broad-spectrum antibiotic therapy. Which pathogenic organism do you suspect given the severity of her illness?

a. *Escherichia coli*
b. *Mycoplasma hominis*
c. Group A streptococcus
d. Group B streptococcus

18–18. The patient in Question 18–17 improved with parenteral antibiotics and supportive care. Her blood type is noted to be A-negative. You explain the indication for a dose of anti-D immune globulin. You inform her that approximately what percentage of women undergoing induced abortion will become alloimmunized without immune globulin?

a. 1%
b. 2%
c. 4–5%
d. 8–10%

18–19. A 20-year-old G2P0A2 presents for follow-up after a spontaneous miscarriage at 7 weeks' gestation. She demands that you "do something" to prevent miscarriages in her future pregnancies. You offer evaluation for recurrent pregnancy loss, but provide reassurance that her likelihood of a successful next pregnancy is approximately what percent?

a. 74%
b. 82%
c. 86%
d. 92%

18–20. Which of the following is not a widely accepted cause of recurrent pregnancy loss?

a. Uterine structural abnormalities
b. Parental chromosomal abnormalities
c. Antiphospholipid antibody syndrome
d. Progesterone deficiency (luteal phase defect)

18–21. What percentage of recurrent pregnancy loss is due to parental chromosomal abnormalities?

a. 2–4%
b. 6–8%
c. 10%
d. 15%

18–22. Which of the following clinical scenarios is not an indication for antiphospholipid antibody testing?

a. History of three embryonic losses
b. History of fetal loss at 16 weeks' gestation
c. History of unexplained thromboembolism
d. History of severe preeclampsia requiring delivery at 38 weeks' gestation

18–23. A 38-year-old G1 undergoes a routine sonogram to survey fetal anatomy at 21 weeks' gestation. The cervical changes as shown below are found. She denies any complaints, including contractions. On sterile speculum exam she is noted to be dilated 1–2 cm with bulging membranes just past the level of the external os. She undergoes 24 hours of observation on labor and delivery without any change. What is the most likely diagnosis?

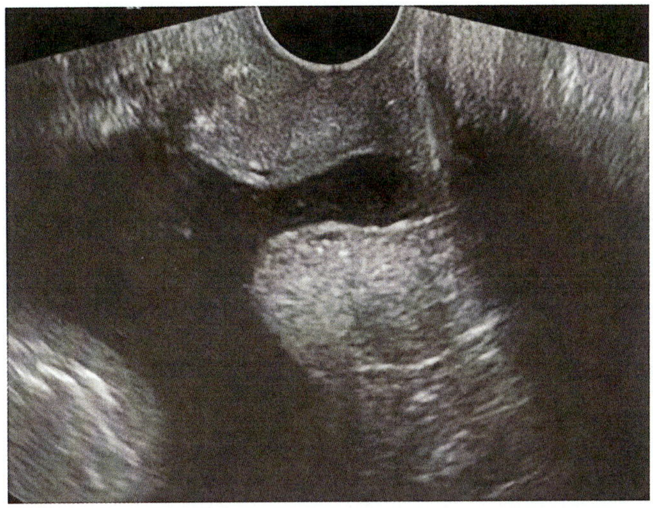

a. Inevitable abortion
b. Cervical insufficiency
c. Arrested preterm labor
d. None of the above

18–24. When counseling the patient in Question 18–23 regarding her management options, you offer her expectant management versus intervention. Which intervention is most appropriate?

a. Cerclage placement
b. Daily vaginal progesterone
c. 17-Hydroxyprogesterone acetate injections weekly
d. Expectant management with repeat cervical length in 1 week

18–25. The patient in Question 18–23 elects to proceed with cerclage placement. What is the most appropriate statement regarding her probable outcome?

a. There is a 20% risk of delivery prior to term.
b. There is a 33% risk of delivery prior to 35 weeks' gestation.
c. There is a 50% risk of delivery prior to 36 weeks' gestation.
d. There is at least a 50% risk of delivery prior to 28 weeks' gestation.

18–26. A 22-year-old G1 undergoes a routine sonogram to survey fetal anatomy at 20 weeks' gestation. The cervix is noted to appear short on transabdominal imaging and a transvaginal cervical length is performed, measuring 19 mm. According to the American College of Obstetricians and Gynecologists, what is the recommended therapy?

a. Cerclage placement
b. Daily vaginal progesterone
c. 17-Hydroxyprogesterone acetate injections weekly
d. Expectant management with repeat cervical length in 1 week

18–27. In a woman without history of prior cesarean delivery, at what gestational age is removal of a prophylactic transvaginal cerclage most reasonable?

a. 34 weeks' gestation
b. 37 weeks' gestation
c. 39 weeks' gestation
d. Defer until the onset of labor

18–28. Which of the following is an indication for transabdominal cerclage?

a. Twin gestation
b. History of cervical insufficiency
c. History of failed transvaginal cerclage
d. Prior preterm birth at 26 weeks' gestation

18–29. When counseling a patient regarding prophylactic cerclage placement, which of the following is a known risk?

a. Bleeding
b. Infection
c. Membrane rupture
d. All of the above

18–30. A 22-year-old primigravida is scheduled to undergo suction dilation and curettage for a missed abortion at 8 weeks' gestation. Prior to the procedure the decision is made to place hygroscopic dilators. A single Dilapan-S dilator is placed in the cervix, and a moist gauze is placed subsequently in the vaginal vault. How long will it take the dilator to reach its maximum diameter?

a. 1–2 hours
b. 2–4 hours
c. 4–6 hours
d. 6–12 hours

18–31. A 32-year-old multigravida is diagnosed with an embryonic demise at 7 weeks' gestation. When counseling her regarding options other than expectant management, you explain that as compared to suction curettage, which has an efficacy rate of 96–100%, medical abortion is associated with what risk of failure?

a. 2–17%
b. 4–9%
c. 5–26%
d. 10–20%

18–32. The patient in Question 18–31 elects to undergo dilation and curettage. Misoprostol is chosen for cervical ripening prior to the procedure. Which route of administration is thought to be least effective?

a. Oral
b. Vaginal
c. Sublingual
d. All are equivalent

18–33. Which regimen is recommended by the American College of Obstetricians and Gynecologists for prophylaxis for postabortive infection?

a. Ancef 2 g IV at time of the procedure
b. Clindamycin 900 mg IV at the time of the procedure
c. Doxycycline 100 mg BID × 14 days after the procedure
d. 100 mg doxycycline 1 hour prior and 200 mg doxycycline after the procedure

18–34. Which of the following is a relative contraindication to outpatient medical termination of pregnancy?

a. IUD in situ
b. Use of anticoagulation
c. Severe renal, liver, or cardiovascular disease
d. All of the above

18–35. A 22-year-old woman presents for elective termination of pregnancy at 7 weeks' gestation. After counseling she is prescribed mifepristone and misoprostol to complete outpatient medical abortion. She completes the dose of mifepristone in the office, but then calls back stating she has decided not to proceed with termination of pregnancy. You inform her of the risks of mifepristone exposure in pregnancy which include which of the following?

a. 28% risk of preterm birth
b. 5% risk of fetal malformations
c. 10–46% risk of pregnancy loss
d. None of the above

18–36. A 24-year-old woman with missed abortion at 6 weeks' gestation elects for outpatient medical treatment. You prescribe 800 μg of misoprostol to be taken up to 3 times 3 hours apart. What of the following are side effects of misoprostol?

a. Diarrhea

b. Vomiting

b. Fever and chills

c. All of the above

18–37. What is the risk of uterine rupture with medical termination of a second-trimester pregnancy in the setting of one prior cesarean delivery?

a. 0.2%

b. 0.4%

c. 0.6%

d. 0.8%

18–38. As compared to pregnancies that are continued, the maternal mortality rate with first-trimester termination of pregnancy is lower. What is the approximate mortality rate associated with induced abortion?

a. 1 per 100,000

b. 2 per 100,000

c. 5 per 100,000

d. 7 per 100,000

CHAPTER 18 ANSWER KEY

Question number	Letter answer	Page cited	Header cited
18–1	**a**	p. 347	Nomenclature
18–2	**c**	p. 347	First Trimester Spontaneous Abortion
18–3	**c**	p. 347	First Trimester Spontaneous Abortion
18–4	**d**	p. 347	First Trimester Spontaneous Abortion
18–5	**d**	p. 350	First Trimester Spontaneous Abortion
18–6	**a**	p. 350	First Trimester Spontaneous Abortion
18–7	**d**	p. 347	First Trimester Spontaneous Abortion
18–8	**a**	p. 347	First Trimester Spontaneous Abortion
18–9	**a**	p. 348	First Trimester Spontaneous Abortion
18–10	**d**	p. 348	First Trimester Spontaneous Abortion
18–11	**c**	p. 348	First Trimester Spontaneous Abortion
18–12	**d**	p. 349	First Trimester Spontaneous Abortion
18–13	**c**	p. 350	Frist Trimester Spontaneous Abortion
18–14	**b**	p. 351	First Trimester Spontaneous Abortion
18–15	**c**	p. 351	First Trimester Spontaneous Abortion
18–16	**d**	p. 351	First Trimester Spontaneous Abortion
18–17	**c**	p. 351	First Trimester Spontaneous Abortion
18–18	**c**	p. 351	First Trimester Spontaneous Abortion
18–19	**d**	p. 352	Recurrent Pregnancy Loss
18–20	**d**	p. 352	Recurrent Pregnancy Loss
18–21	**a**	p. 352	Recurrent Pregnancy Loss
18–22	**d**	p. 353	Recurrent Pregnancy Loss
18–23	**b**	p. 354	Midtrimester Abortion
18–24	**a**	p. 354	Midtrimester Abortion
18–25	**d**	p. 354	Midtrimester Abortion
18–26	**b**	p. 354	Midtrimester Abortion
18–27	**b**	p. 355	Midtrimester Abortion
18–28	**c**	p. 356	Midtrimester Abortion
18–29	**d**	p. 356	Midtrimester Abortion
18–30	**c**	p. 358	First Trimester Abortion Methods
18–31	**a**	p. 361	First Trimester Abortion Methods
18–32	**a**	p. 359	First Trimester Abortion Methods
18–33	**d**	p. 359	First Trimester Abortion Methods
18–34	**d**	p. 361	First Trimester Abortion Methods
18–35	**b**	p. 361	First Trimester Abortion Methods
18–36	**c**	p. 361	First Trimester Abortion Methods
18–37	**b**	p. 363	Second Trimester Abortion Methods
18–38	**a**	p. 364	Consequences of Elective Abortion

CHAPTER 19

Ectopic Pregnancy

19–1. What percentage of first-trimester pregnancies in the United States are ectopically located?

a. 0.1–0.5%

b. 0.2–1.0%

c. 0.5–1.5%

d. 1.0–2.0%

19–2. A 25-year-old nulligravida with Rh-negative blood type and a negative antibody screen is postoperative day 1 following salpingectomy for a 6-week ectopic pregnancy. What dose of IgG anti-D immunoglobulin is deemed sufficient prior to discharge?

a. 50 μg

b. 100 μg

c. 200 μg

d. 300 μg

19–3. Among women who become pregnant while using contraception, the relative number of ectopic pregnancies is increased with which of the following contraceptives?

a. Condoms

b. NuvaRing

c. Progestin-releasing intrauterine device

d. Estrogen-containing birth control pills

19–4. A 31-year-old G2P1 presents to the emergency room at 7 weeks by last menstrual period with pelvic pain. Her β-hCG level is 1234 mIU/mL, but no ultrasound is performed. When she returns to her obstetrician's office for follow-up 3 days later, her β-hCG is 1166 mIU/mL and ultrasound demonstrates a 5-cm complex left adnexal mass. A diagnostic laparoscopy is performed, and the surgical findings are shown in the image. What is the most likely diagnosis?

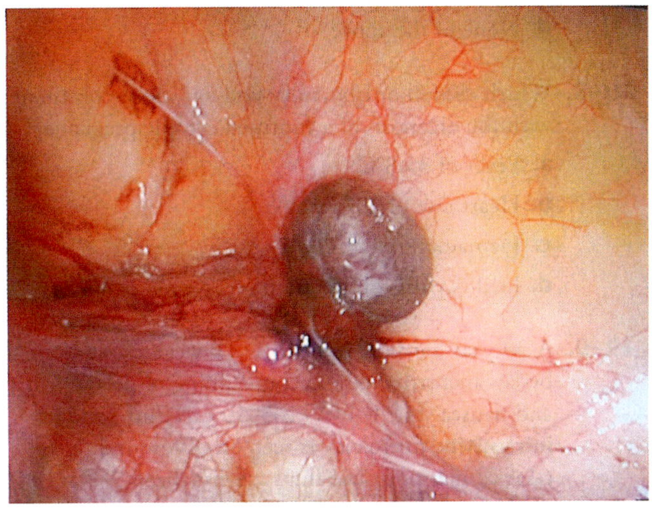

Used with permission from Dr. Eddie McCord.

a. Paratubal cyst

b. Serous cystadenoma

c. "Acute" ectopic pregnancy

d. "Chronic" ectopic pregnancy

19–5. In ectopic pregnancies, the absence of which tubal tissue layer facilitates rapid invasion of proliferating trophoblasts into the muscularis?

a. Serosa

b. Epithelium

c. Submucosa

d. Connective tissue

19–6. What is the classic triad of clinical symptoms of an ectopic pregnancy?

- **a.** Nausea, pain, and vaginal bleeding
- **b.** Delayed menstruation, pain, and vaginal bleeding
- **c.** Dizziness, delayed menstruation, and vaginal bleeding
- **d.** Shoulder pain, delayed menstruation, and vaginal bleeding

19–7. A 38-year-old G4P3 presents with a positive pregnancy test, vaginal bleeding, palpitations, and intense neck and shoulder pain, which is worse with inspiration. She is found to be tachycardic and hypotensive. Her ultrasound reveals a likely right ectopic pregnancy. What is the most likely cause of her neck and shoulder pain?

- **a.** A pulled back muscle
- **b.** Referred pain from her right fallopian tube
- **c.** Diaphragmatic irritation due to hemoperitoneum
- **d.** None of the above

19–8. Which clinical or laboratory finding is least consistent with the diagnosis of a ruptured ectopic pregnancy?

- **a.** Fever of 39.8°C
- **b.** Heart rate of 137 bpm
- **c.** Hematocrit of 21.2%
- **d.** Leukocytosis of 28,000 μL

19–9. A 30-year-old G2P1 presents at 6 weeks' gestation by last menstrual period complaining of pelvic pain and nausea. Her β-hCG is 3010 mIU/mL, and no intrauterine pregnancy is seen on ultrasound. No adnexal masses or free fluid are visualized. What is the best management strategy?

- **a.** No intervention
- **b.** Surgical therapy
- **c.** Methotrexate injection
- **d.** Expectant management with 48-hour follow-up

19–10. What is the discriminatory β-hCG level above which failure to visualize an intrauterine pregnancy likely indicates that a pregnancy either is not alive or is ectopically located?

- **a.** ≥100 mIU/mL
- **b.** ≥500 mIU/mL
- **c.** ≥1000 mIU/mL
- **d.** ≥1500 mIU/mL

19–11. A 21-year-old G1 presents at 6 weeks' gestation by last menstrual period complaining of pelvic pain. She is normotensive, her heart rate is 79 beats per minute, and there is mild right-sided abdominal discomfort on exam. Her β-hCG is 1345 mIU/mL, and her ultrasound findings are shown below. No adnexal masses or free fluid are seen. What is the best management strategy?

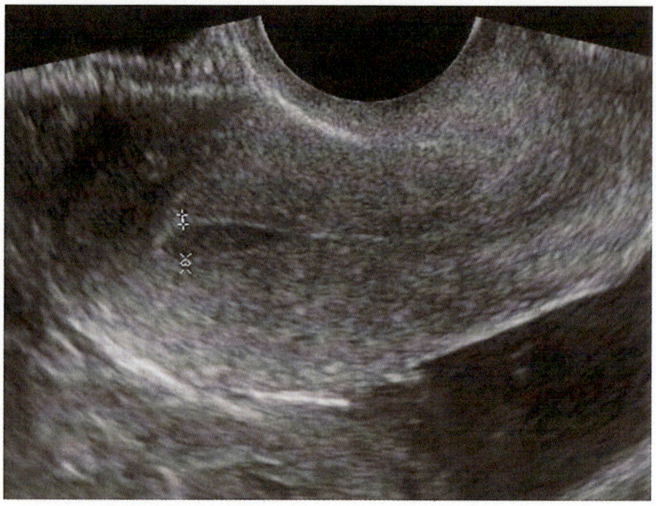

- **a.** Methotrexate
- **b.** Dilation and curettage
- **c.** Diagnostic laparoscopy
- **d.** Discharge home with follow-up β-hCG in 48 hours.

19–12. What is the minimum rise of β-hCG you expect in 48 hours from an early progressing intrauterine pregnancy?

- **a.** 12%
- **b.** 23%
- **c.** 53%
- **d.** 67%

19–13. What percentage of ectopic pregnancies demonstrate appropriately rising β-hCG levels?

- **a.** 15%
- **b.** 33%
- **c.** 42%
- **d.** 50%

19–14. A 27-year-old G3P2 was recently seen in the emergency room with vaginal bleeding and passed products of conception while undergoing evaluation. Her β-hCG at the time of presentation was 2500 mIU/mL. At her 7-day follow-up her β-hCG is again measured. What value is most consistent with a completed spontaneous abortion?

a. 500 mIU/mL

b. 1250 mIU/mL

c. 1750 mIU/mL

d. 2000 mIU/mL

19–15. What progesterone value threshold is most helpful to exclude ectopic pregnancy?

a. >10 ng/mL

b. >15 ng/mL

c. >20 ng/mL

d. >25 ng/mL

19–16. A 39-year-old G5P3 presents at 6 weeks' gestation with lower abdominal pain. A transvaginal ultrasound is performed for further evaluation. What findings would be expected on transvaginal ultrasound if her dates are correct and her pregnancy is viable?

a. Gestational sac only

b. Gestational sac and yolk sac

c. Gestational sac, yolk sac, and fetal pole with cardiac motion

d. Gestational sac, yolk sac, and fetal pole without cardiac motion

19–17. The sonographic finding pictured can be seen with which of the following condition(s)?

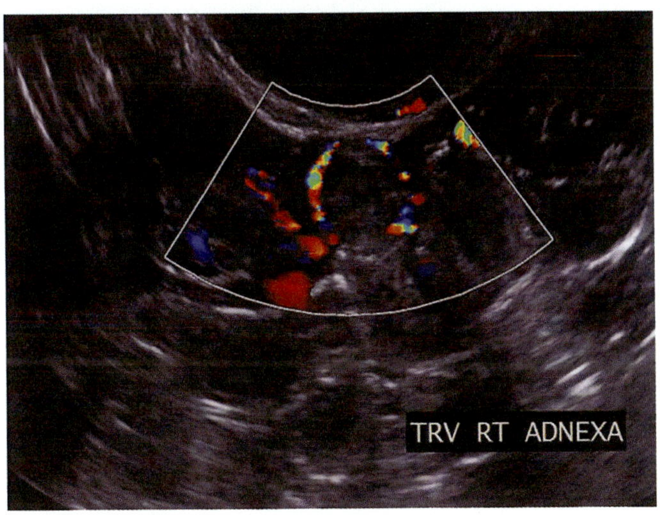

a. Ectopic pregnancy only

b. Corpus luteum cyst only

c. Corpus luteum cyst and ectopic pregnancy

d. None of the above

19–18. A 31-year-old G3P1 at 6 to 7 weeks' gestation by last menstrual period presents with severe abdominal pain, weakness, and dizziness. On sonographic evaluation, she is noted to have a complex left adnexal mass with free fluid in Morrison pouch. What is the minimum amount of accumulated hemoperitoneum which would be expected at the time of surgery?

a. 100–200 mL

b. 200–300 mL

c. 300–400 mL

d. 400–500 mL

19–19. What is the purpose of performing a dilation and curettage prior to administering methotrexate?

a. To confirm a secretory endometrium

b. To assess for endometrial decidualization

c. To confirm the absence of trophoblastic tissue

d. To avoid the heavy vaginal bleeding provoked by methotrexate

19–20. What is the cellular mechanism of action of methotrexate?

a. DNA intercalation

b. Inhibition of microtubule formation

c. Impedance of DNA and RNA synthesis

d. Alkylation of proteins, DNA, and RNA

19–21. What is the ectopic resolution rate following methotrexate administration?

a. 66%

b. 78%

c. 90%

d. 97%

19–22. A 35-year-old G4P2 presents at 7 to 8 weeks' gestation complaining of mild lower abdominal pain and spotting and is found to have a 3-cm left ectopic pregnancy. She has a history of severe persistent asthma and was treated for an asthma exacerbation 2 days ago. She also has a history of a prior ectopic pregnancy treated with salpingectomy, chronic hypertension for which she takes labetalol, and type 2 diabetes managed with insulin. What aspect of her history would preclude treatment with methotrexate?

a. Type 2 diabetes

b. Chronic hypertension

c. Severe persistent asthma with recent exacerbation

d. History of a prior ectopic pregnancy treated with salpingectomy

19–23. What is the single best predictor of successful treatment with single-dose methotrexate?

a. β-hCG
b. Progesterone level
c. Ectopic pregnancy size
d. Absence of fetal cardiac activity

19–24. A 23-year-old G1 is diagnosed with a right ectopic pregnancy and given a single dose of methotrexate. Her β-hCG is 3153 mIU/mL on day 1 following methotrexate administration, 3256 mIU/mL on day 4, and 2548 mIU/mL on day 7. What is the most appropriate course of action based on these values?

a. Diagnostic laparoscopy
b. Recheck β-hCG level in 1 week
c. Administer second dose of methotrexate
d. No further intervention or follow-up is required

19–25. What percentage of women treated with single-dose methotrexate therapy require an additional dose of medication for an inadequate clinical response?

a. 5–10%
b. 10–15%
c. 15–20%
d. 20–25%

19–26. You are evaluating a 26-year-old woman in the emergency room who presents with abdominal pain and is found to have a positive pregnancy test. Her heart rate is 105 beats per minute and her blood pressure is 82/50 mmHg. On ultrasound, you do not identify an intrauterine pregnancy, and a 3-cm left adnexal mass is identified with moderate complex fluid seen in the cul-de-sac. What is the best management for this patient?

a. Methotrexate
b. Dilation and curettage
c. Expectant management
d. Laparoscopic salpingectomy

19–27. Which of the following is not true regarding salpingostomy performed for an ectopic pregnancy?

a. Up to 15% have persistence of trophoblastic tissue
b. This is the procedure of choice for ruptured ectopic pregnancies
c. Mean resolution time to a negative β-hCG is 20 days following surgery
d. Subsequent pregnancy rates are comparable to those for ectopics managed by salpingectomy

19–28. In comparing medical versus surgical therapy, what is the clinical benefit of surgery compared to methotrexate?

a. Decreased risk of post-therapy depression
b. Improved pregnancy rates following surgery
c. Improved physical functioning immediately following therapy
d. All of the above

19–29. A 19-year-old G1 is diagnosed with a 2.3-cm right ectopic pregnancy. Her β-hCG is 1967 mIU/mL, her hematocrit is 37%, and she has a small amount of free fluid in her cul-de-sac. She strongly desires expectant management rather than immediate treatment. Which aspect of her history favors successful resolution with expectant management?

a. β-hCG < 2000 mIU/mL
b. Hematocrit above 35%
c. Free fluid in the cul-de-sac
d. Ectopic pregnancy size <3 cm

19–30. Which of the following is true regarding the condition depicted in the image?

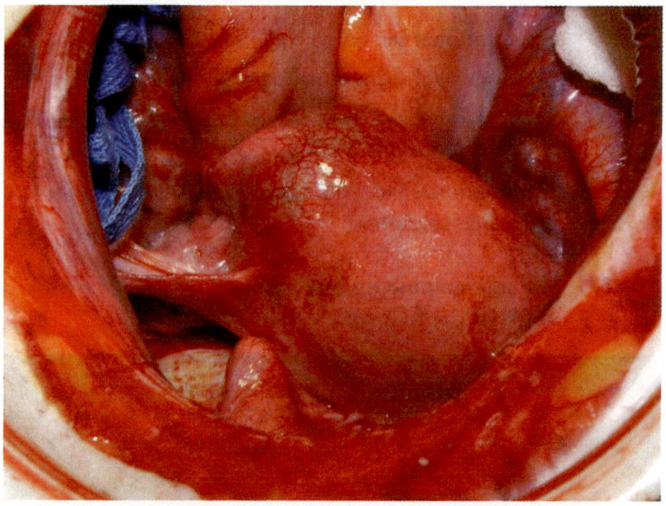

Reproduced with permission from Cunningham FG, Leveno KJ, Bloom SL, et al (eds): Ectopic pregnancy. In Williams Obstetrics, 25th ed. New York, McGraw-Hill, 2018, Figure 19-7.

a. Rupture usually occurs later at 8–16 weeks
b. Usually requires surgical treatment by means of a wedge resection
c. Hemorrhage can be more severe due to the proximity to uterine and ovarian arteries
d. All of the above

19–31. A 41-year-old G5P3 presents at 6–7 weeks' gestation by last menstrual period complaining of lower abdominal pain. She has a history of a tubal ligation 2 years ago during her third cesarean delivery. Her history is otherwise unremarkable. She undergoes transvaginal sonography with the image shown. What potential complication may result if she chooses to continue her pregnancy?

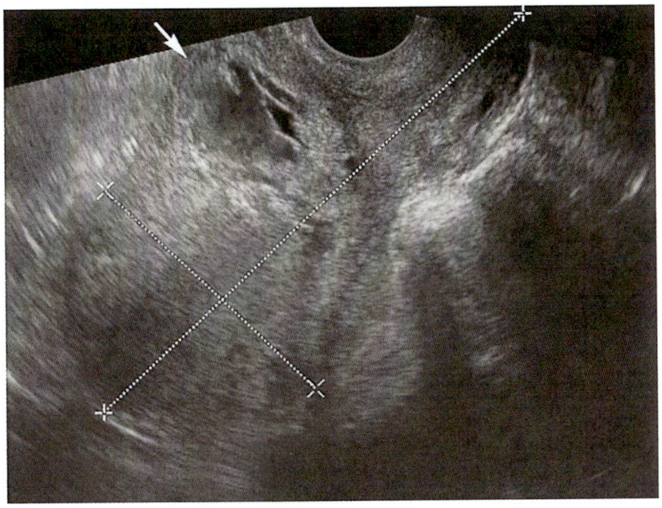

a. Placenta accreta
b. Placental abruption
c. Gestational diabetes
d. Premature rupture of membranes

19–32. What is the first-line treatment for a stable woman with the complication shown in the ultrasound image?

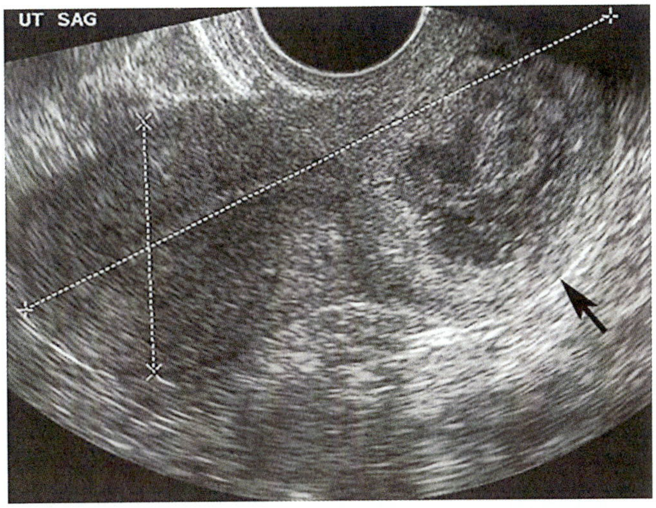

Reproduced with permission from Cunningham FG, Leveno KJ, Bloom SL, et al (eds): Ectopic pregnancy. In Williams Obstetrics, 25th ed. New York, McGraw-Hill, 2018, Figure 19-10.

a. Methotrexate
b. Expectant management
c. Exploratory laparotomy
d. Admission for serial pelvic exams

19–33. What adjunctive treatment can be employed to decrease or manage complications associated with a cervical ectopic pregnancy?

a. Uterine artery embolization
b. Foley catheter cervical tamponade
c. Fetal intracardiac potassium chloride injection
d. All of the above

CHAPTER 19 ANSWER KEY

Question number	Letter answer	Page cited	Header cited
19–1	**c**	p. 371	Introduction
19–2	**a**	p. 371	Classification
19–3	**c**	p. 372	Risks
19–4	**d**	p. 372	Evolution and Potential Outcomes
19–5	**c**	p. 372	Evolution and Potential Outcomes
19–6	**b**	p. 372	Clinical Manifestations
19–7	**c**	p. 372	Clinical Manifestations
19–8	**a**	p. 373	Clinical Manifestations
19–9	**d**	p. 373	Multimodality Diagnosis
19–10	**d**	p. 373	Multimodality Diagnosis
19–11	**d**	p. 373	Multimodality Diagnosis
19–12	**c**	p. 375	Multimodality Diagnosis
19–13	**b**	p. 375	Multimodality Diagnosis
19–14	**a**	p. 375	Multimodality Diagnosis
19–15	**d**	p. 375	Multimodality Diagnosis
19–16	**c**	p. 375	Multimodality Diagnosis
19–17	**c**	p. 375	Multimodality Diagnosis
19–18	**d**	p. 376	Multimodality Diagnosis
19–19	**c**	p. 376	Multimodality Diagnosis
19–20	**c**	p. 377	Medical Management
19–21	**c**	p. 377	Medical Management
19–22	**c**	p. 378	Medical Management
19–23	**a**	p. 378	Medical Management
19–24	**b**	p. 378	Medical Management
19–25	**c**	p. 378	Medical Management
19–26	**d**	p. 378	Medical Management
19–27	**b**	p. 379	Surgical Management
19–28	**a**	p. 379	Surgical Management
19–29	**d**	p. 380	Expectant Management
19–30	**d**	p. 380	Interstitial Pregnancy
19–31	**a**	p. 381	Cesarean Scar Pregnancy
19–32	**a**	p. 382	Cervical Pregnancy
19–33	**a**	p. 382	Cervical Pregnancy

CHAPTER 20

Gestational Trophoblastic Disease

20–1. As a group, gestational trophoblastic disease is typified by which of the following?

- **a.** Scant cytotrophoblast
- **b.** Perivillous fibrin deposition
- **c.** Villous mesenchymal hyperplasia
- **d.** Abnormal trophoblast proliferation

20–2. Measurement of which hormone is pivotal in the diagnosis, management, and surveillance of gestational trophoblastic disease?

- **a.** Estriol
- **b.** Alpha-fetoprotein
- **c.** Human chorionic gonadotropin
- **d.** All of the above

20–3. As illustrated by the microscopic differences seen here between (A) malignant invasive mole and (B) choriocarcinoma, hydatidiform moles as a group are differentiated histologically from other non-molar neoplasms by the presence of which of the following?

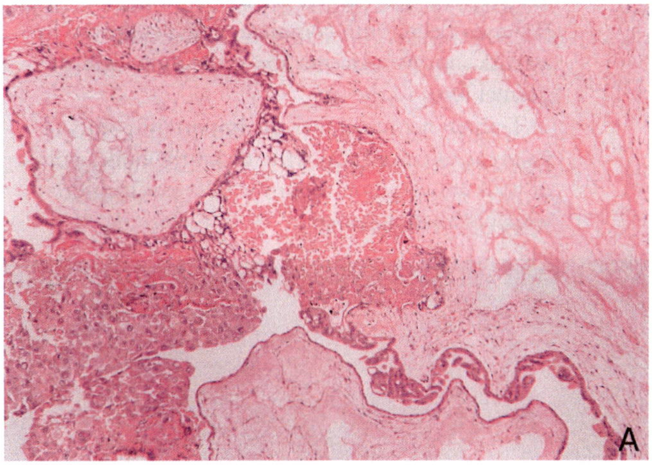

Used with permission from Dr. Ona Faye-Peterson.

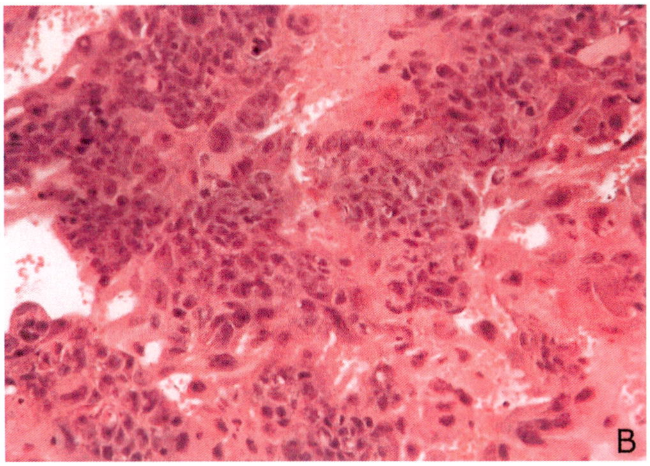

Reproduced with permission from Schorge JO: Gestational trophoblastic disease. In Hoffman BL, Schorge JO, Schaffer JI, et al (eds): Williams Gynecology, 2nd ed. New York, McGraw-Hill, 2012, Figure 37-8.

- **a.** Villi
- **b.** Nuclear atypia
- **c.** Marked angiogenesis
- **d.** p57 immunostaining

20–4. Gestational trophoblastic neoplasia includes all of the following except which one?

a. Invasive mole

b. Choriocarcinoma

c. Partial hydatidiform mole

d. Placental site trophoblastic tumor

20–5. Ms. Audi presents to you for a second opinion. She is 19 weeks' gestation and has a dichorionic diamnionic twin pregnancy. She tells you that her primary obstetrician told her that she was at very high risk for serious complications of pregnancy because something was wrong with one of her twins. You review the images of a magnetic resonance imaging study she had last week. A representative image is shown below with complete mole designated by asterisk, normal placenta above the mole, and the normal fetus to the left.

To help her remember the important points of your consultation, you write down the bullet points of your conversation. Your list does not include which of the following?

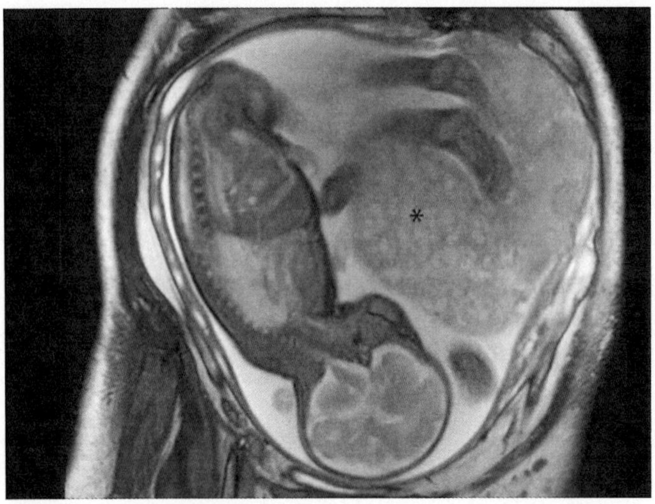

Used with permission from Dr. April Bleich.

a. Fewer than 50% of pregnancies like this reach term.

b. There is a high risk for needing preterm delivery due to preeclampsia or bleeding.

c. There is a 15–20% risk for developing gestational trophoblastic neoplasia, which is a malignancy.

d. Early termination of pregnancy reduces the subsequent risk for developing gestational trophoblastic neoplasia.

20–6. A 34-year-old multigravida presents for her first prenatal care visit. She is 9 weeks by her sure last menstrual period, and reports feeling much worse than she did in her last pregnancies. Which of the following sets of clinical data would increase your suspicion for molar pregnancy?

a. Pulse 54 bpm, TSH 4.0 U/ml, β-hCG 9,000 mIU/mL, uterus size = dates, and severe constipation

b. Pulse 84 bpm, TSH 2.0 U/ml, β-hCG 100,000 mIU/mL, uterus size $>$ dates, and profound fatigue

c. Pulse 60 bpm, TSH 0.09 U/mL, β-hCG 3000 mIU/mL, uterus size $<$ dates, and intermittent vaginal bleeding

d. Pulse 120 bpm, TSH 0.003 U/mL, β-hCG 310,000 mIU/mL, uterus size $>$ dates, and severe nausea and vomiting

20–7. The patient in Question 20–6 undergoes an ultrasound. Based on the ultrasound findings below, you suspect the genetic studies on the products of conception will show which of the following?

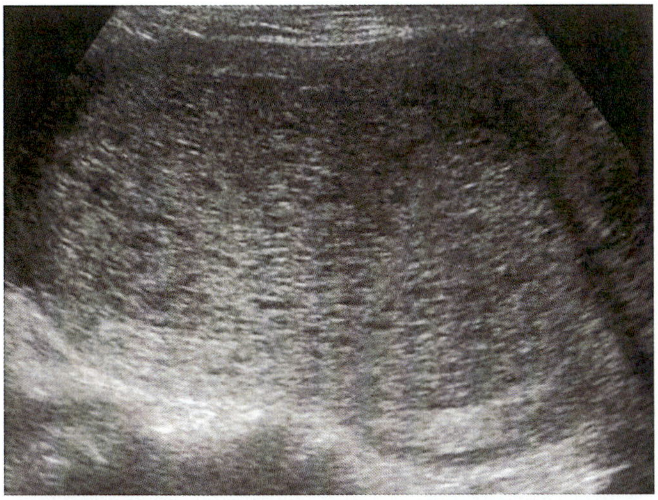

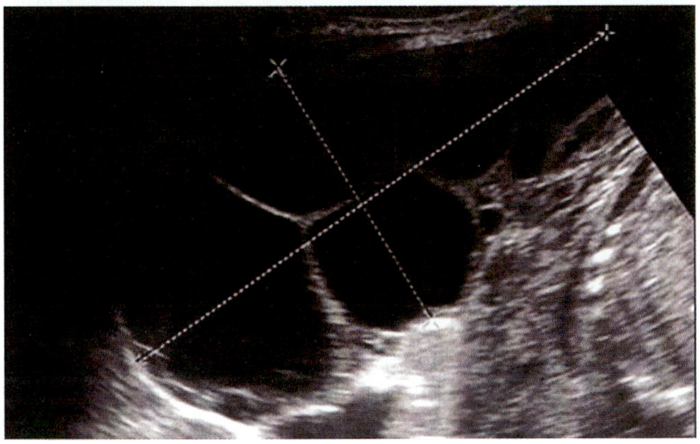

Used with permission from Dr. Jodi Dashe.

a. 46,XX
b. 47,XXY
c. 69,XXY
d. Any of the above could be seen

20–8. You explain the findings to the patient in Question 20–6. What do you recommend as the next step in management?

a. Schedule for hysterectomy
b. Schedule dilation and curettage
c. Schedule dilation and curettage, laparoscopic oophorectomy, and staging
d. Obtain pre-op labs and a chest radiograph, and review results prior to making definitive surgical plans

20–9. While consenting the patient in Question 20–6, you review which of the following risks associated with the planned procedure?

a. Hemorrhage requiring transfusion
b. Hemorrhage requiring hysterectomy
c. Respiratory distress, potentially requiring intensive care unit admission
d. All of the above

20–10. The patient in Question 20–6 does very well and goes home with no apparent complications. She returns to your office and you discuss the pathological diagnosis of complete hydatidiform mole. Which of the following explains the pathogenesis of a complete mole?

a. Androgenesis
b. Dispermic fertilization
c. Maternal chromosome inactivation
d. All of the above

20–11. You elucidate the recommended care plan for the patient in Question 20–6. Which of the following are important aspects in optimizing her care?

a. A copper intrauterine device is recommended for reliable birth control.
b. Serial β-hCG quantification is performed until undetectable and then monthly for 6 months.
c. Serial endometrial biopsies are recommended as surveillance for gestational trophoblastic neoplasia.
d. All of the above

20–12. The patient in Question 20–6 has a β-hCG level of 1500 mIU/mL at month 6 after 5 months of undetectable β-hCG levels. Which of the following factors does not increase the risk of this representing malignancy?

a. She did not do prophylactic chemotherapy.
b. She had a complete mole versus a partial mole.
c. Her theca-lutein cysts were 12 cm at diagnosis.
d. It took 4 months for her β-hCG to reach undetectable level after initial dilation and curettage.

20–13. Due to the increased β-hCG level, an ultrasound is ordered for the patient in Question 20–6. The results are shown below. How do you counsel her?

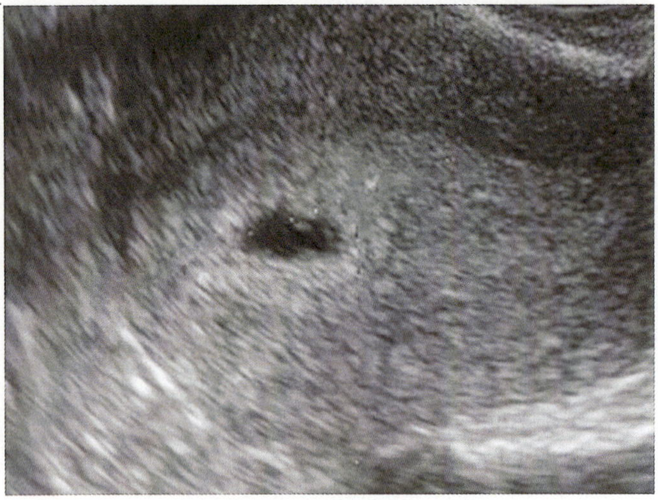

a. The risk of another mole is 0.9%.

b. If this is not a mole, live birth rate is equivalent to general population.

c. If this is not a mole, risk for congenital anomalies is not greater than baseline.

d. All of the above

20–14. As the patient in Question 20–6 progresses normally through a subsequent pregnancy, she is counseled that some alterations of routine care are recommended. Which of the following is not recommended because of her history of complete mole?

a. Recommendation for 6-week postpartum β-hCG level

b. Recommendation for pathological evaluation of placenta after delivery

c. Recommendation for amniocentesis due to increased risk for aneuploidy

d. All of the above are recommended

20–15. A primigravida who is 9 weeks by last menstrual period presents to the emergency room with vaginal bleeding. She is noted to have an open cervical os, and subsequently expels the products shown below. The patient is Rh negative. Does she need anti-D immune globulin prior to discharge?

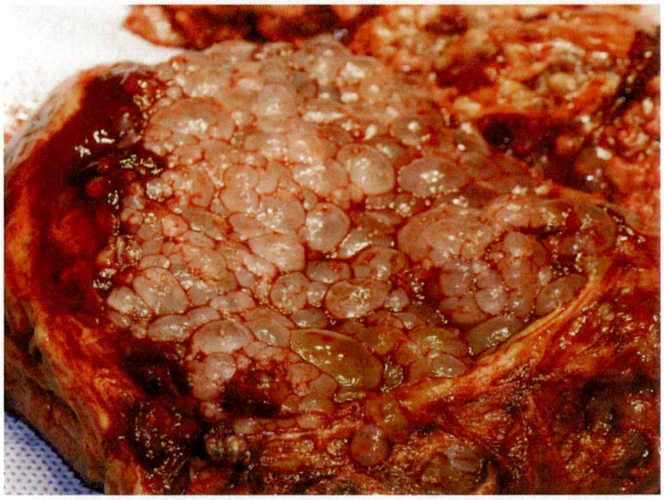

a. Yes, because there may be fetal tissue

b. Yes, because a dilation and curettage is necessary

c. No, because no fetal tissue is seen within the products

d. No, because the red cells cannot have the D-antigen

20–16. The process shown below can be confirmed pathologically by which of the following?

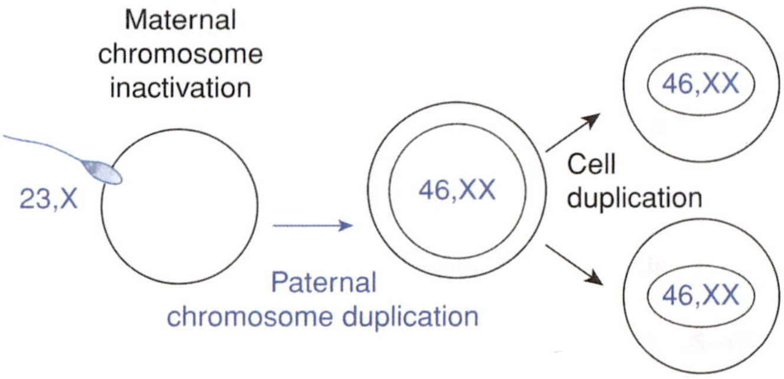

Reproduced with permission from Cunningham FG, Leveno KJ, Bloom SL, et al (eds): Gestational trophoblastic disease. In Williams Obstetrics, 25th ed. New York, McGraw-Hill, 2018, Figure 20-2a.

a. Co-existent presence of fetal tissue

b. Minimal trophoblastic proliferation

c. Absence of p57KIP2 immunostaining

d. Presence of p57KIP2 immunostaining

20–17. Which of the following are criteria for diagnosis of gestational trophoblastic neoplasia?

- **a.** Rise in β-hCG levels
- **b.** Plateau of β-hCG levels
- **c.** Persistence of β-hCG for 6 months or more
- **d.** All of the above

20–18. Gestational trophoblastic neoplasia may develop after which of the following?

- **a.** Evacuation of a partial mole
- **b.** Delivery of a normal term pregnancy
- **c.** Ectopic pregnancy in a fallopian tube
- **d.** All of the above

20–19. A patient is seen for a routine 6-week postpartum visit. She is still having daily vaginal bleeding, sometimes with clots. She had an uncomplicated term vaginal delivery and went home on postpartum day 2. Her bimanual and speculum examination are unremarkable. What is the first test you order?

- **a.** β-hCG
- **b.** Fibrinogen
- **c.** Bladder scan
- **d.** All of the above

20–20. According to the World Health Organization modified prognostic scoring system that was adapted by the International Federation of Gynecology and Obstetrics in 2009, which of the following is assessed and assigned a rating score during staging of gestational trophoblastic neoplasia?

- **a.** Parity
- **b.** Thyroid-stimulating hormone level
- **c.** Number of months from the antecedent pregnancy
- **d.** All of the above

20–21. Following dilation and curettage for a complete mole, Ms. Brown is being surveilled with serial β-hCG levels. For the past 3 weeks, the β-hCG levels have plateaued. Diagnostic evaluation reveals a metastatic lesion in her liver as shown in the image below. Given the extent of disease, what is her International Federation of Gynecology and Obstetrics stage?

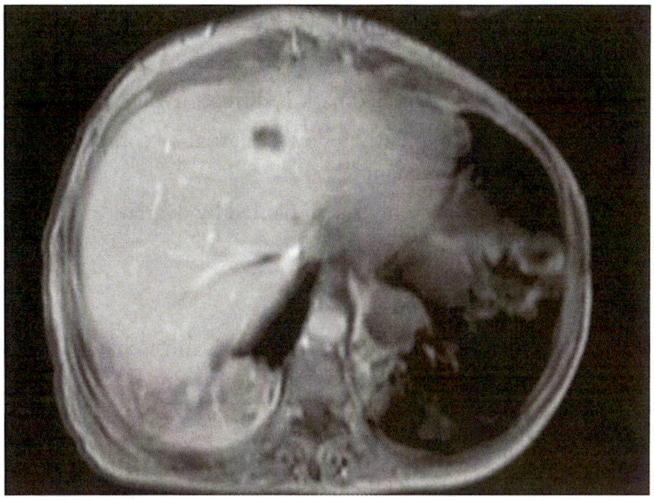

Used with permission from Dr. John Schorge.

- **a.** Stage I
- **b.** Stage II
- **c.** Stage III
- **d.** Stage IV

20–22. According to the World Health Organization modified prognostic scoring system that was adapted by the International Federation of Gynecology and Obstetrics, patients with scores at or above which of the following thresholds are assigned to the "high risk" gestational trophoblastic neoplasia group?

- **a.** ≥ 5
- **b.** ≥ 6
- **c.** ≥ 7
- **d.** ≥ 9

20–23. The most consistent finding with gestational trophoblastic neoplasia is which of the following?

- **a.** Seizures
- **b.** Uterine bleeding
- **c.** Hemorrhagic ascites
- **d.** Deep vein thrombosis

20–24. Which of the following features is most characteristic of an invasive mole?

a. Penetrates deeply into myometrium

b. Displays minimal trophoblastic growth

c. A hallmark is the association with distant metastases

d. Most frequently follows a term or preterm euploid pregnancy

20–25. Which of the following features is most characteristic of gestational choriocarcinoma?

a. Pathological hallmark is diffuse, hyperplastic villi

b. Most frequently follows a partial or complete molar pregnancy

c. Are commonly accompanied by ovarian theca-lutein cysts

d. All of the above

20–26. Which of the following features is most characteristic of placental site trophoblastic tumor?

a. A high proportion of free β-hCG is considered diagnostic

b. Is best treated by hysterectomy due to chemotherapy resistance

c. Arises from intermediate trophoblasts at the placental site

d. All of the above

20–27. Clinical features of epithelioid trophoblastic tumor are most similar to which other histological class of gestational trophoblastic neoplasia?

a. Invasive mole

b. Gestational choriocarcinoma

c. Complete hydatiform mole

d. Placental-site trophoblastic tumor

20–28. Metastatic spread of choriocarcinoma is most common via which of the following routes?

a. Lymphatic

b. Hematogenous

c. Cerebrospinal fluid

d. Peritoneal spread via fallopian tubes

20–29. Distant metastases from choriocarcinoma are most commonly found in which organ?

a. Lung

b. Liver

c. Brain

d. Spleen

20–30. A 42-year-old G3P3003 has been diagnosed with choriocarcinoma 6 months after her term vaginal delivery of a healthy female neonate. Her β-hCG was 1 million mIU/mL, and she had a single 2-cm metastasis identified in her liver. What is her stage per the International Federation of Gynecology and Obstetrics staging system?

a. Stage I

b. Stage II

c. Stage III

d. Stage IV

20–31. The patient in Question 20–30 is being seen for the first time since her diagnosis for a discussion of available treatments. She has had no intervention to date. What do you recommend?

a. She has low-risk disease; radical hysterectomy is curative

b. She has low-risk disease; single-agent chemotherapy is recommended as sole therapy

c. She has high-risk disease; combination chemotherapy is recommended as sole therapy

d. She has high-risk disease; combination chemotherapy is recommended as first-line therapy, but additional surgery or radiation may be indicated

20–32. Response to therapy by the patient in Question 20–30 will primarily be monitored with what method?

a. Serial β-hCG levels

b. Serial endometrial biopsies

c. Serial positron-emission tomographic scans

d. All of the above

20–33. The patient in Question 20–30 inquires as to the success rate of your recommended treatment plan for her disease. What percentage of women are cured?

a. Approximately 60% of women like her will be cured.

b. Approximately 70% of women like her will be cured.

c. Approximately 80% of women like her will be cured.

d. Approximately 90% of women like her will be cured.

CHAPTER 20 ANSWER KEY

Question number	Letter answer	Page cited	Header cited
20–1	d	p. 388	Gestational Trophoblastic Disease
20–2	c	p. 388	Gestational Trophoblastic Disease
20–3	a	p. 388	Gestational Trophoblastic Disease
20–4	c	p. 388	Gestational Trophoblastic Disease
20–5	d	p. 390	Twin Pregnancy
20–6	d	p. 390	Clinical Findings
20–7	a	p. 389	Pathogenesis
20–8	d	p. 392	Table 20-2
20–9	d	p. 393	Molar Pregnancy Termination
20–10	d	p. 389	Pathogenesis
20–11	b	p. 393	Postevacuation Surveillance
20–12	a	p. 392 p. 393	Molar Pregnancy Termination Postevacuation Surveillance
20–13	d	p. 389 p. 393	Epidemiology and Risk Factors Postevacuation Surveillance
20–14	c	p. 396	Subsequent Pregnancy
20–15	a	p. 393	Molar Pregnancy Termination
20–16	c	p. 390	Table 20-1
20–17	d	p. 394	Table 20-3
20–18	d	p. 393	Gestational Trophoblastic Neoplasia
20–19	a	p. 394	Diagnosis, Staging, and Prognostic Scoring
20–20	c	p. 394	Table 20-4
20–21	d	p. 394	Table 20-4
20–22	c	p. 394	Diagnosis, Staging, and Prognostic Scoring
20–23	b	p. 393	Clinical Findings
20–24	a	p. 394	Invasive Mole
20–25	c	p. 395	Gestational Choriocarcinoma
20–26	d	p. 395	Placental Site Trophoblastic Tumor
20–27	d	p. 395	Epithelioid Trophoblastic Tumor
20–28	b	p. 395	Choriocarcinoma
20–29	a	p. 395	Choriocarcinoma
20–30	d	p. 394	Table 20-4
20–31	d	p. 395	Treatment
20–32	a	p. 395	Treatment
20–33	d	p. 395	Treatment

SECTION 7

LABOR

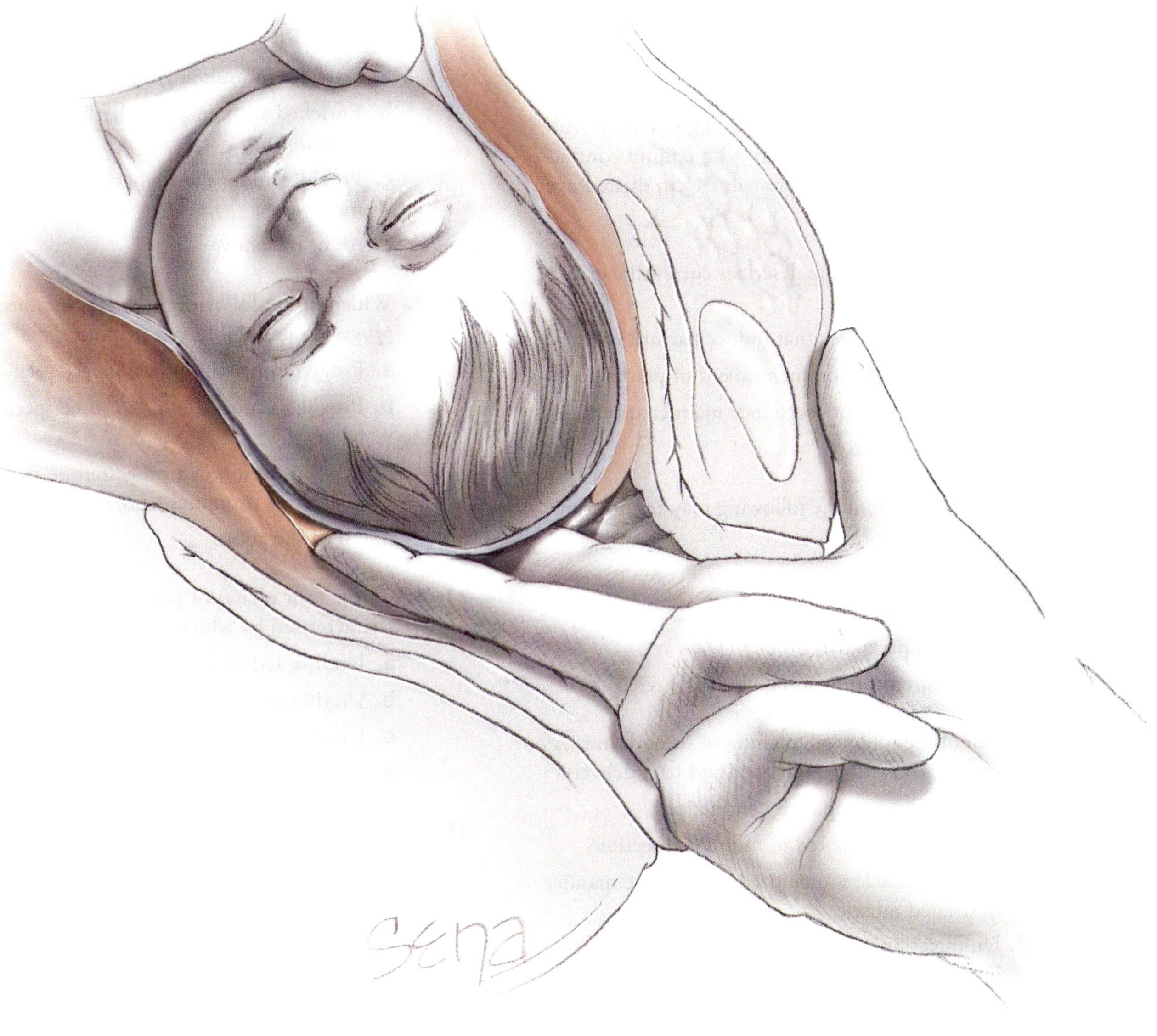

CHAPTER 21

Physiology of Labor

21–1. Which of the following patients are in labor?

a. A 23-year-old G1P0 at 38 weeks' gestation with painful contractions and a cervix that remains closed over 2 hours

b. A 33-year-old G2P1 at 38 weeks' gestation with nonpainful contractions and a cervix that changes to 3 cm dilated over 2 hours

c. A 33-year-old G2P1 at 38 weeks' gestation with one prior cesarean delivery with painful contractions and a cervix that remains closed over 2 hours

d. A 33-year-old G2P1 at 38 weeks' gestation with one prior cesarean delivery with painful contractions and a cervix that remains 1 cm dilated over 2 hours

21–2. Which of the following describes current theories of labor?

a. Synthesis of factors that induce parturition

b. Fetal source for commencement of parturition

c. Functional loss of pregnancy maintenance factors

d. All of the above

21–3. All except which of the following may result from abnormal parturition?

a. Dystocia

b. Preterm labor

c. Postterm pregnancy

d. Premature rupture of membranes

21–4. Which of the following qualities of smooth muscles is advantageous for contractions and fetal delivery?

a. Greater shortening with contractions

b. Forces are not exerted in multiple directions

c. Smooth muscle is organized in the same manner as striated muscle

d. Unidirectional force generation in the fundus and lower uterine segment

21–5. Which of the following is not a function of the cervix during pregnancy?

a. Preventing infection

b. Maintenance of competence

c. Extracellular changes for greater compliance

d. All of the above

21–6. Which of the following is a characteristic of the amnion?

a. Provides immunological acceptance

b. Enriched with enzymes that inactivate uterotonins

c. Provides all tensile strength to resist rupture of membranes

d. All of the above

21–7. Which of the following supports the theory that progesterone inhibits parturition?

a. Progesterone withdrawal precedes labor

b. Providing progesterone to some species delays labor

c. Administration of a progesterone-receptor antagonist promotes labor

d. All of the above

21–8. Of the four phases of parturition, phase 2 is characterized by which of the following?

a. Uterine activation, cervical ripening

b. Uterine quiescence, cervical softening

c. Uterine contraction, cervical dilatation

d. Uterine involution, cervical remodeling

21–9. Which phase of parturition corresponds to the clinical stages of labor?

a. Phase 1

b. Phase 2

c. Phase 3

d. Phase 4

21–10. Which of the following does not help achieve uterine quiescence?

a. Uterotonin degradation
b. Increased intracellular Ca^{2+}
c. Ion channel regulation of cell membrane potential
d. Activation of the uterine endoplasmic reticulum stress response

21–11. During which stage of labor is the fetus delivered?

a. Stage 1
b. Stage 2
c. Stage 3
d. Stage 4

21–12. Cervical softening in phase 1 of parturition results in part from which of the following?

a. Stromal atrophy
b. Increased stromal vascularity
c. Increased collagen monomer cross-linking
d. All of the above

21–13. Contraction-associated protein (CAP) within the uterine smooth muscle prepares it to contract during labor. CAP concentrations increase during phase 2 of parturition and include all except which of the following proteins?

a. Connexin 43
b. Oxytocin receptor
c. Progesterone A receptor
d. Prostaglandin F receptor

21–14. Compared to the uterine body, the cervix has a significantly lower percentage of which of the following?

a. Collagen
b. Proteoglycans
c. Smooth muscle
d. Glycosaminoglycans

21–15. A 23-year-old primigravida presents for induction of labor at 41 weeks' gestation. Her cervix is unfavorable with a Bishop score of 4. You proceed with cervical ripening using the agent depicted below. This medication belongs to which class of agents?

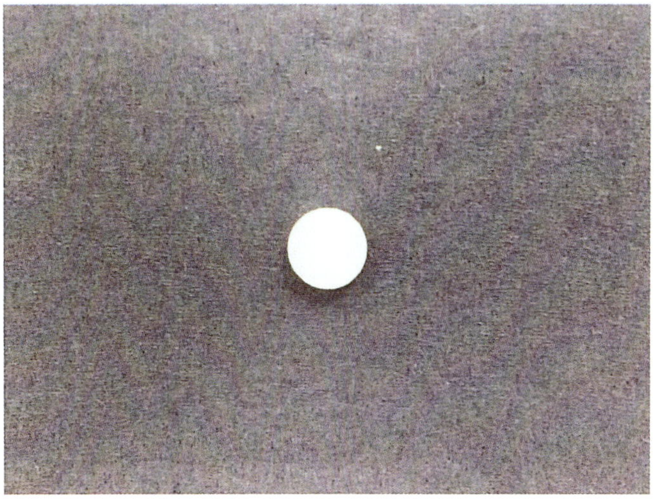

a. Oxytocin
b. Beta mimetics
c. Prostaglandins
d. Nonsteroidal inflammatory drugs

21–16. What is the primary source of corticotropin-releasing hormone in pregnancy?

a. Placental
b. Fetal adrenal
c. Fetal hypothalamus
d. Maternal hypothalamus

21–17. Which of the following are fetal contributors to the initiation of parturition?

a. Surfactant protein A
b. Corticotropin-releasing hormone
c. Senescent-associated secretory phenotype
d. All of the above

21–18. A fetus with a neural tube defect is shown below with the fetal orbits labeled O. Which of the following abnormalities of normal parturition has been associated with this anomaly?

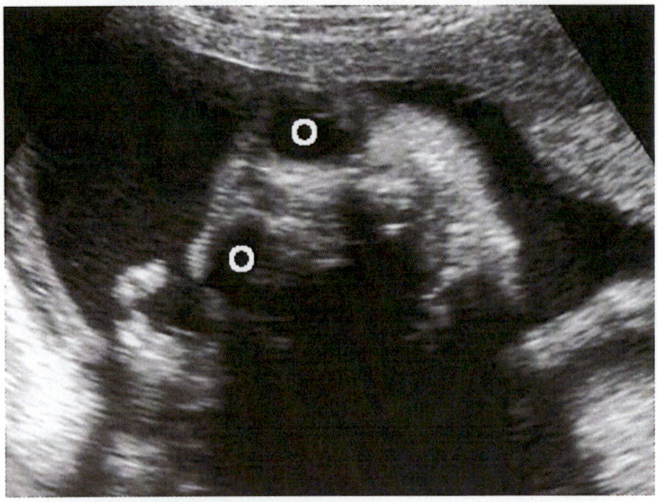

a. Preterm labor
b. Prolonged gestation
c. Uterine tachysystole
d. None of the above

21–19. Which of the following are plausible causes of uterine contraction pain?

a. Myometrial hypoxia
b. Uterine peritoneum stretch
c. Compression of nerve ganglia in the cervix
d. All of the above

21–20. A 30-year-old primigravida presents to your office at 39 weeks' gestation. She is exhausted and ready to be delivered but does not want to be induced. You suggest membrane stripping and inform her this will lead to a rise in which of the following prostaglandins?

a. I_2
b. E_2
c. H
d. F_{2a}

21–21. During cesarean delivery, the hysterotomy incision is ideally made in the lower uterine segment, shown here prior to bladder flap creation. Which of the following aids in development of this uterine segment during phase 3 of parturition?

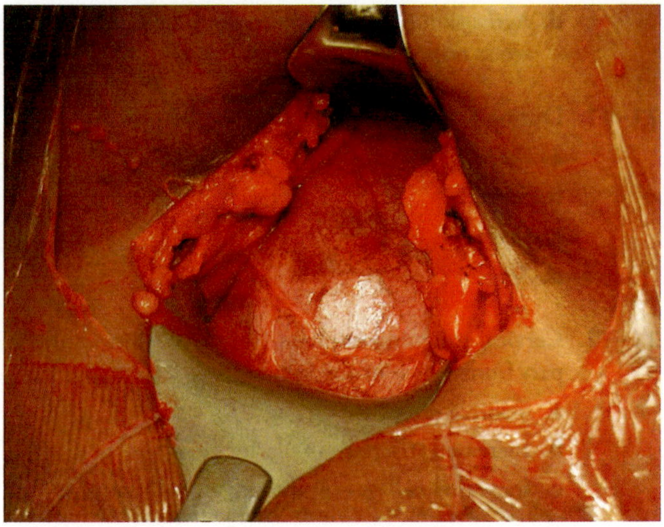

Used with permission from Dr. Sarah White.

a. Progressive thickening of the upper uterine segment with labor progression
b. Smooth muscle cell fibers of the fundus relax to their original length after each contraction
c. Smooth muscle cell fibers of the lower uterine segment relax to their original length after each contraction
d. All of the above

21–22. After the cervix is fully dilated, what is the most important force in fetal expulsion?

a. Uterine contractions
b. Intraabdominal pressure
c. Fetal head descending through the pelvis
d. None of the above

21–23. As a result of contraction forces, the cervix effaces and dilates by mechanisms that include all except which of the following?

a. Contraction forces create lateral pull against the cervix to open its canal.

b. Contraction forces are transferred directly through the presenting part to the cervix to dilate its canal.

c. Contraction forces pull smooth muscle fibers at the internal os up into the adjacent upper uterine segment to efface the cervix.

d. Contraction forces are translated into hydrostatic pressure within the amnionic sac, which presses against the cervix to dilate the cervical canal.

21–24. In which of the following women would you expect rapid descent of the fetal head?

a. A 23-year-old G1P0 at 40 weeks' gestation

b. A 23-year-old G3P2 at 40 weeks' gestation

c. A 33-year-old G1P0 at 28 weeks' gestation

d. A 33-year-old G1P0 at 37 weeks' gestation

21–25. Which of the following is the most important component of the pelvic floor?

a. Vaginal wall

b. Piriformis muscle

c. Coccygeus muscle

d. Levator ani muscle

21–26. What is the initial step that leads to placental separation following delivery of the infant?

a. Uterine contractions

b. Tension pulls it away from the implantation site

c. Formation of a hematoma behind the placenta with uterine involution

d. None of the above

21–27. In which mechanism of placental delivery does the placenta leave the body before the retroplacental hematoma?

a. Bandl mechanism

b. Duncan mechanism

c. Schultze mechanism

d. Chadwick mechanism

21–28. Which of the following is accurate regarding oxytocin?

a. Nanopeptide

b. Synthesized as a prohormone

c. Myometrial receptor numbers increase during phase 2

d. All of the above

21–29. Indomethacin, a nonsteroidal antiinflammatory drug (NSAID), has some tocolytic actions. As a group, NSAIDs target which enzyme in prostaglandin production?

a. Phospholipase A_2

b. Cyclooxygenase-1

c. Prostaglandin isomerase

d. Prostaglandin dehydrogenase

21–30. A 34-year-old G1P0 is undergoing induction of labor with misoprostol for cervical ripening. The nurse calls you for fetal heart rate decelerations, and you notice she is having prolonged contractions, as shown below. You administer terbutaline, a β_2 adrenergic receptor agonist, and initiate which of the following cellular responses to cause uterine relaxation?

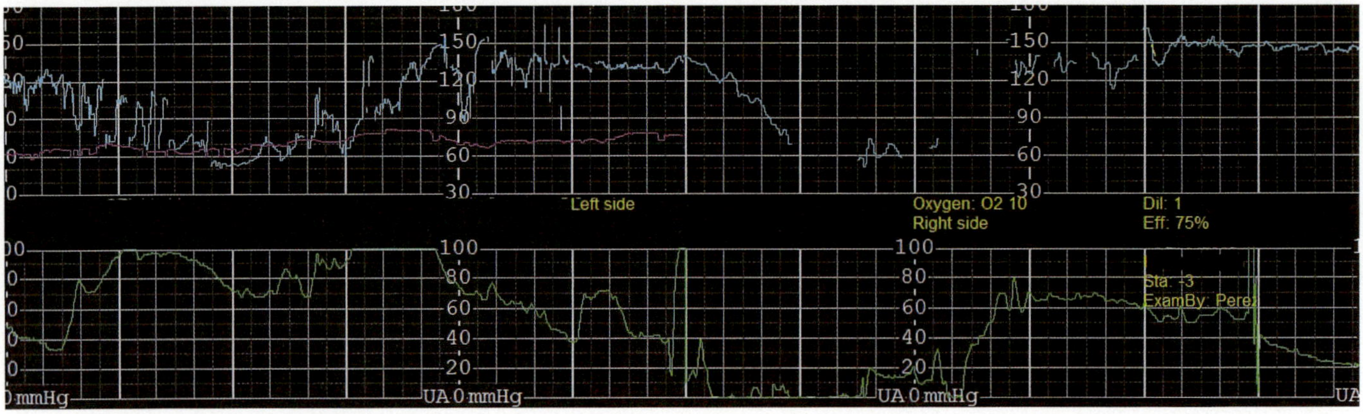

a. Increased intracellular Ca^{2+} levels

b. Increased extracellular Mg^{2+} levels

c. Increased cyclic adenosine monophosphate levels

d. Decreased cyclic guanosine monophosphate levels

21–31. A 34-year-old woman is scheduled to return for her postpartum visit 6 weeks after delivery. Given that you will discuss birth control options at that visit, what may be the optimal timing of that visit?

a. 6 weeks based on tradition

b. 4 weeks if she is breastfeeding

c. 6 weeks as long as she is breastfeeding

d. 4 weeks because ovulation returns 4–6 weeks after birth

21–32. Which of the following uterotonins plays a role in phase 3 of parturition?

a. Endothelin-1

b. Angiotensin II

c. Prostaglandins

d. All of the above

CHAPTER 21 ANSWER KEY

Question number	Letter answer	Page cited	Header cited
21–1	b	400	Introduction
21–2	d	400	Introduction
21–3	d	400	Introduction
21–4	a	401	Uterus
21–5	d	401	Uterus
21–6	c	401	Placenta
21–7	d	401	Sex Steroid Hormone Role
21–8	a	403	Figure 21-3
21–9	c	403	Figure 21-3
21–10	b	403	Myometrial Relaxation and Contraction
21–11	b	403	Figure 21-4
21–12	b	407	Cervical Softening
21–13	c	408	Myometrial Changes
21–14	c	409	Cervical Ripening
21–15	c	410	Induction of Cervical Ripening
21–16	a	410	Fetal Endocrine Cascade
21–17	d	411	Fetal Contributions to Labor
21–18	b	411	Fetal Anomalies and Delayed Parturition
21–19	d	412	Uterine Labor Contractions
21–20	d	412	Uterine Labor Contractions
21–21	a	412	Distinct Lower and Upper Uterine Segments
21–22	b	413	Ancillary Forces
21–23	c	413	Cervical Changes
21–24	b	414	Second Stage: Fetal Descent
21–25	d	414	Pelvic Floor Changes
21–26	b	415	Third Stage: Delivery of Placenta and Membranes
21–27	c	416	Third Stage: Delivery of Placenta and Membranes
21–28	d	416	Oxytocin
21–29	b	416	Prostaglandins
21–30	c	407	G-Protein–Coupled Receptors
21–31	d	417	Phase 4: The Puerperium
21–32	d	416	Uterotonins in Parturition Phase 3

CHAPTER 22

Normal Labor

22–1. What is the most common fetal lie?

a. Oblique

b. Unstable

c. Transverse

d. Longitudinal

22–2. When the fetus lies with the long axis transversely, what is the presenting part?

a. Knee

b. Head

c. Shoulder

d. Buttocks

22–3. What is the fetal attitude in the photo below?

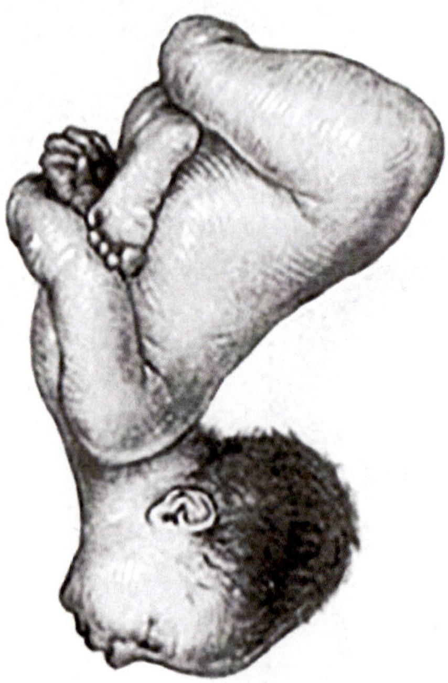

Reproduced with permission from Cunningham FG, Leveno KJ, Bloom SL, et al (eds): Normal labor. In Williams Obstetrics, 25th ed. New York, McGraw-Hill, 2018, Figure 22-1D.

a. Face

b. Brow

c. Vertex

d. Sinciput

22–4. In the photo below, the neck is only partly flexed and the anterior fontanel is presenting. What is the fetal attitude?

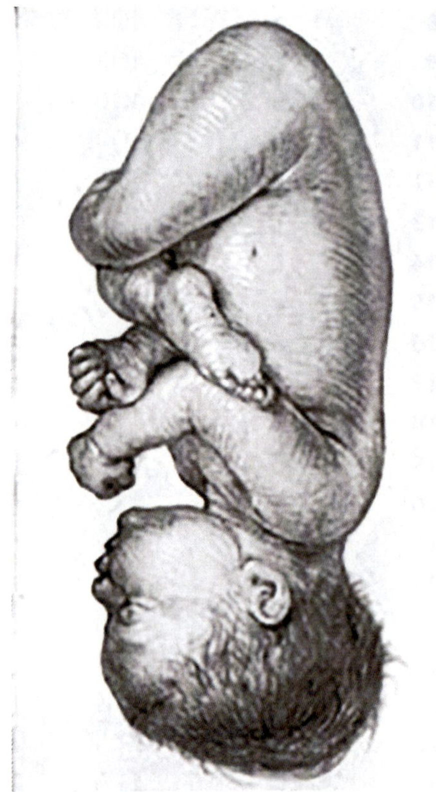

Reproduced with permission from Cunningham FG, Leveno KJ, Bloom SL, et al (eds): Normal labor. In Williams Obstetrics, 25th ed. New York, McGraw-Hill, 2018, Figure 22-1B.

a. Face

b. Brow

c. Occiput

d. Sinciput

22–5. What composes the cephalic pole?

a. Head

b. Head and upper extremities

c. Head, upper extremities, and trunk

d. Head, upper extremities, trunk, and lower extremities

22–6. Why is there a high incidence of breech among hydrocephalic fetuses?

- **a.** Increased intracranial pressure
- **b.** Podalic pole needs more room
- **c.** Cephalic pole needs more room
- **d.** Because the fetal head is small, it does not have the force to turn

22–7. What is the incidence of breech at term?

- **a.** 1%
- **b.** 3%
- **c.** 5%
- **d.** 10%

22–8. What is the fetal position in the drawing below?

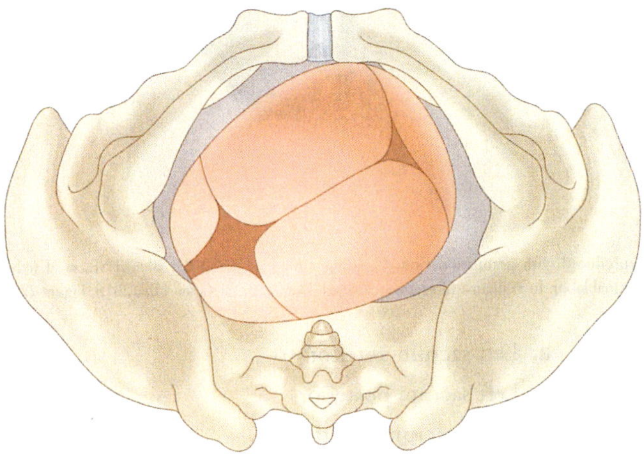

Reproduced with permission from Cunningham FG, Leveno KJ, Bloom SL, et al (eds): Normal labor. In Williams Obstetrics, 25th ed. New York, McGraw-Hill, 2018, Figure 22-2A.

- **a.** Left occiput anterior (LOA)
- **b.** Left occiput posterior (LOP)
- **c.** Right occiput anterior (ROA)
- **d.** Right occiput posterior (ROP)

22–9. What is the fetal position in the drawing below?

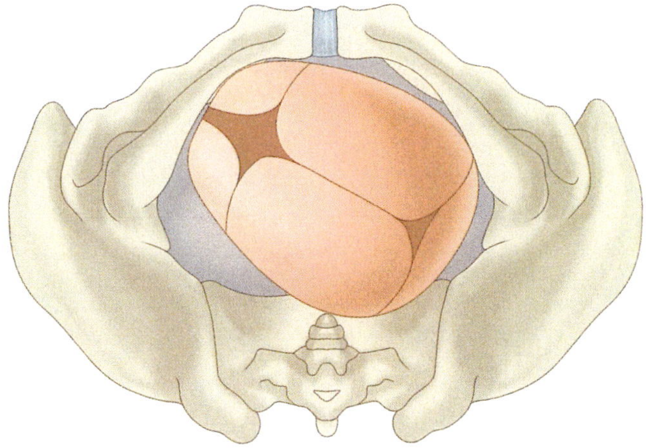

Reproduced with permission from Cunningham FG, Leveno KJ, Bloom SL, et al (eds): Normal labor. In Williams Obstetrics, 25th ed. New York, McGraw-Hill, 2018, Figure 22-2B.

- **a.** Left occiput anterior
- **b.** Left occiput posterior
- **c.** Right occiput anterior
- **d.** Right occiput posterior

22–10. What is the fetal position in the drawing below?

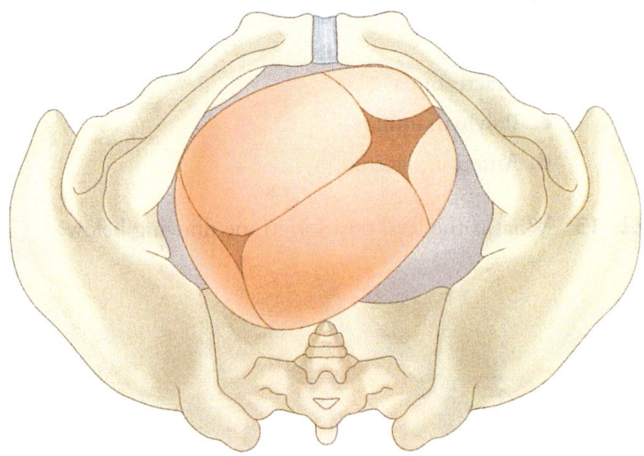

Reproduced with permission from Cunningham FG, Leveno KJ, Bloom SL, et al (eds): Normal labor. In Williams Obstetrics, 25th ed. New York, McGraw-Hill, 2018, Figure 22-3A.

- **a.** Left occiput anterior
- **b.** Left occiput posterior
- **c.** Right occiput anterior
- **d.** Right occiput posterior

SECTION 7

22–11. What is the fetal position in the drawing below?

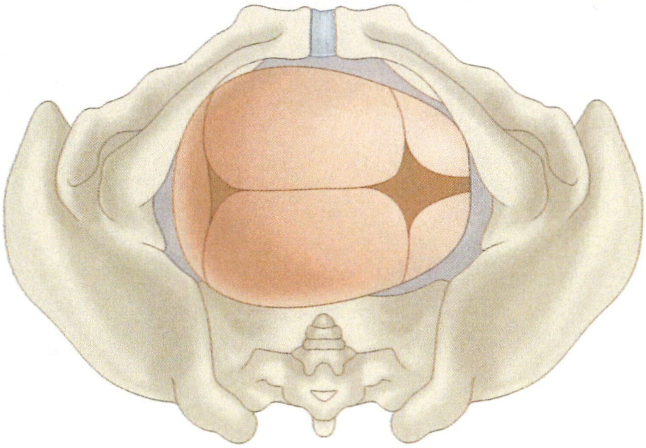

Reproduced with permission from Cunningham FG, Leveno KJ, Bloom SL, et al (eds): Normal labor. In Williams Obstetrics, 25th ed. New York, McGraw-Hill, 2018, Figure 22-3B.

a. Left occiput anterior
b. Right occiput anterior
c. Left occiput transverse
d. Right occiput transverse

22–12. Which of the following is least detrimental to the performance of Leopold maneuvers?

a. Obesity
b. Macrosomia
c. Polyhydramnios
d. Anterior placenta

22–13. What is the fetal position in the drawing below?

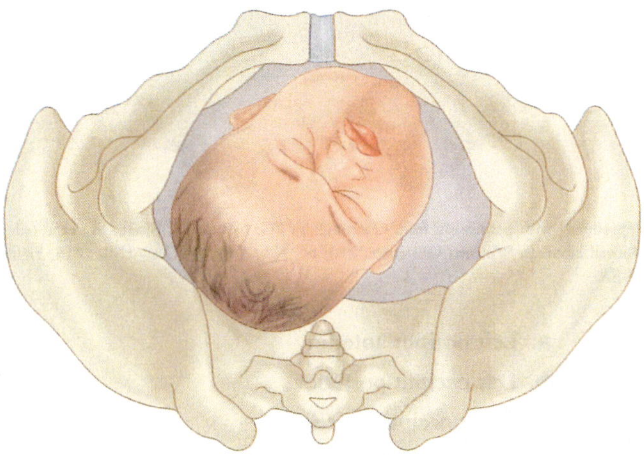

Reproduced with permission from Cunningham FG, Leveno KJ, Bloom SL, et al (eds): Normal labor. In Williams Obstetrics, 25th ed. New York, McGraw-Hill, 2018, Figure 22-5.

a. Left mento-anterior
b. Left mento-posterior
c. Right mento-anterior
d. Right mento-posterior

22–14. What is the fetal position in the drawing below?

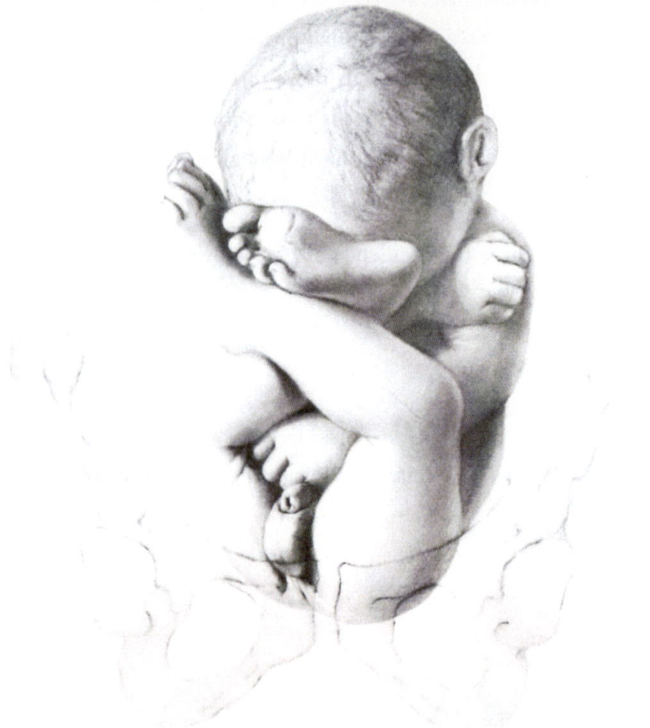

Reproduced with permission from Cunningham FG, Leveno KJ, Bloom SL, et al (eds): Normal labor. In Williams Obstetrics, 25th ed. New York, McGraw-Hill, 2018, Figure 22-6.

a. Left sacrum anterior
b. Left sacrum posterior
c. Right sacrum anterior
d. Right sacrum posterior

22–15. Which Leopold maneuver determines degree of fetal descent?

a. 1
b. 2
c. 3
d. 4

22–16. The term engagement refers to which of the following?

a. Top of the head passing through the pelvic inlet
b. Top of the head passing through the pelvic outlet
c. Biparietal diameter passing through the pelvic inlet
d. Biparietal diameter passing through the pelvic outlet

22–17. What is the term for lateral deflection of the sagittal suture toward the sacral promontory as depicted in the drawing below?

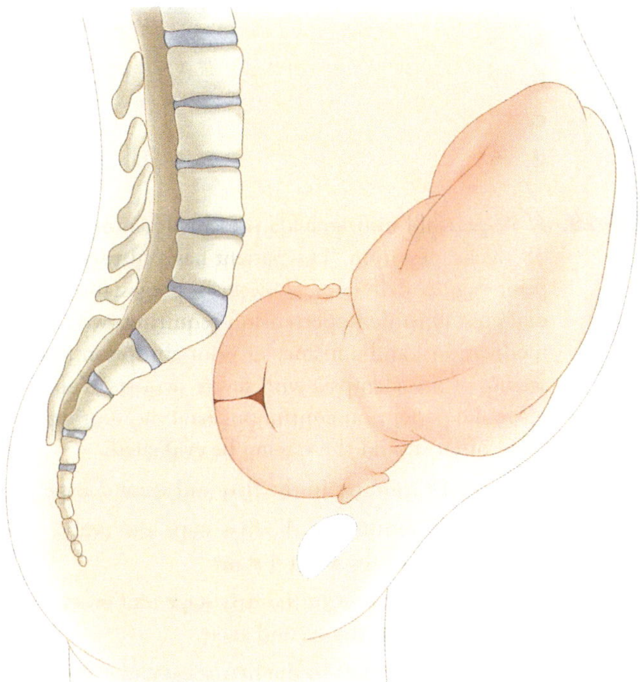

Reproduced with permission from Cunningham FG, Leveno KJ, Bloom SL, et al (eds): Normal labor. In Williams Obstetrics, 25th ed. New York, McGraw-Hill, 2018, Figure 22-12.

a. Normal asynclitism
b. Oblique asynclitism
c. Anterior asynclitism
d. Posterior asynclitism

22–18. Which of the following statements about the occiput posterior position is true?

a. They are more commonly seen in the setting of a posterior placenta.
b. Epidural anesthesia may predispose to incomplete rotation to the occiput anterior position.
c. The fetus is less likely to turn to the occiput anterior position if small for gestational age.
d. Extension of the fetal head improves the likelihood that it will turn from occiput posterior to occiput anterior.

22–19. Which of the following statements about the photo provided below is false?

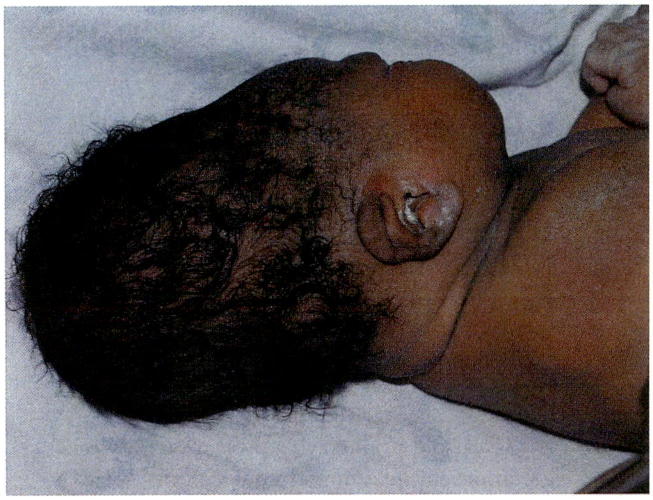

a. This is the product of rapid labor.
b. This can make it difficult to assess the sutures and fontanels.
c. Most of the time, these changes to the fetal head shape will resolve within a week of delivery.
d. These changes to the fetal head can facilitate a vaginal delivery in women with a contracted pelvis.

22–20. During which portion of labor does the cervix dilate very little but the connective tissue component change considerably?

a. Active phase
b. Acceleration phase
c. Dilational division
d. Preparatory division

22–21. Which of the following has been associated with prolonging labor?

a. Maternal fear
b. Maternal obesity
c. Epidural analgesia
d. All of the above

22–22. Which stage of labor is defined as the period of time from when the patient reaches complete cervical dilation through delivery of the fetus?

a. First stage
b. Second stage
c. Third stage
d. Fourth stage

22–23. Which of the following has not been associated with a prolonged second stage of labor?

a. Sedation

b. Macrosomia

c. Maternal obesity

d. Contracted maternal pelvis

22–24. What is the recommended nurse: patient ratio for a low-risk laboring patient?

a. 1:1

b. 1:2

c. 1:3

d. 2:1

22–25. A 25-year-old primigravida presents at 38 weeks' gestation complaining of contractions every 5–7 minutes. On exam, she is 1 cm dilated, 50% effaced, and the fetal head is at –1 station. Her membranes are intact and there is no vaginal bleeding seen. After 2 hours of observation, the fetal tracing is category I. The contractions have spaced out to every 15 minutes. The patient's cervix remains unchanged. Her vitals are within normal limits, and she has no medical problems. What is the best management plan for this patient?

a. Amniotomy induction

b. Continued monitoring

c. Oxytocin augmentation

d. Discharge home with labor precautions and instructions to follow up with her doctor

22–26. A 17-year-old primigravida at 38 weeks' gestation presents complaining of leakage of fluid. When performing nitrazine testing to assess for the presence of amniotic fluid in the vagina, which of the following would you expect to give you a false-negative result?

a. Blood

b. Semen

c. Scant fluid

d. Bacterial vaginosis

22–27. When the cervix becomes as thin as the adjacent lower uterine segment, what is the effacement?

a. 0%

b. 25%

c. 50%

d. 100%

22–28. A 28-year-old primigravida at term presents in labor. She is very uncomfortable. You go to examine the patient, and you note that the fetal head is visible at the introitus. What is the fetal station?

a. –5

b. –2

c. +2

d. +5

22–29. A 39-year-old multigravida presents for induction at 38 weeks' gestation. The patient has a history of two prior vaginal deliveries, cholestasis, pregestational diabetes, chronic hypertension requiring two medications, and a history of prior abruption in the setting of preeclampsia with severe features. You place the patient on continuous fetal monitoring. How often should the tracing be evaluated?

a. Every 15 minutes in the first and second stage.

b. Every 15 minutes in the first stage and every 5 minutes in the second stage.

c. Every 15 minutes in the first stage and every 30 minutes in the second stage.

d. Every 30 minutes in the first stage and every 15 minutes in the second stage.

22–30. A 30-year-old multigravida presents in active labor at term. She progresses from 4 cm to complete in 3 hours. She has the baby spontaneously 1 hour later. She has a third-degree laceration that is repaired. On postpartum day 1, she is found to have urinary retention. What is her risk factor for urinary retention?

a. Age

b. Rapid labor

c. Multiparity

d. Perineal laceration

22–31. A 22-year-old primigravida presents in active labor at 6 cm dilation. Her membranes are intact, the fetus is cephalic, and the fetal tracing is category I. Two hours later, she is still 4 cm dilated. Her contractions are every 7 minutes. What is the best next step in labor management?

a. Amniotomy

b. Continued observation

c. Amniotomy and oxytocin

d. Cesarean section for failure to progress

22–32. Should the patient in Question 22–31 achieve adequate uterine contractions, what is a reasonable minimum rate of cervical dilation?

a. 1 cm in 2 hours

b. 1–2 cm per hour

c. 2–3 cm per hour

d. 3–4 cm per hour

CHAPTER 22 ANSWER KEY

Question number	Letter answer	Page cited	Header cited
22-1	**d**	p. 422	Fetal Lie
22-2	**c**	p. 422	Fetal Presentation
22-3	**a**	p. 422	Figure 22-1
22-4	**d**	p. 422	Figure 22-1
22-5	**a**	p. 422	Cephalic Presentation
22-6	**c**	p. 422	Cephalic Presentation
22-7	**b**	p. 422	Breech Presentation
22-8	**a**	p. 423	Figure 22-2
22-9	**b**	p. 423	Figure 22-2
22-10	**d**	p. 424	Figure 22-3
22-11	**d**	p. 424	Figure 22-3
22-12	**b**	p. 424	Leopold Maneuvers
22-13	**a**	p. 425	Figure 22-5
22-14	**b**	p. 425	Figure 22-6
22-15	**d**	p. 426	Leopold Maneuvers
22-16	**c**	p. 427	Engagement
22-17	**c**	p. 429	Figure 22-12
22-18	**b**	p. 431	Occiput Posterior Presentation
22-19	**a**	p. 431	Figure 22-16
22-20	**d**	p. 432	First Stage of Labor
22-21	**d**	p. 433	Active Phase
22-22	**b**	p. 434	Second Stage of Labor
22-23	**c**	p. 434	Second Stage of Labor
22-24	**b**	p. 434	Table 22-2
22-25	**d**	p. 435	Identification of Labor
22-26	**c**	p. 435	Ruptured Membranes
22-27	**d**	p. 435	Cervical Assessment
22-28	**d**	p. 436	Cervical Assessment
22-29	**b**	p. 436	Intrapartum Fetal Monitoring
22-30	**d**	p. 438	Urinary Bladder Function
22-31	**a**	p. 439	Labor Management Protocols
22-32	**b**	p. 439	Labor Management Protocols

CHAPTER 23

Abnormal Labor

23–1. Which of the following may be responsible for dystocia in labor?

- **a.** Bony pelvis abnormalities
- **b.** Inadequate expulsive forces
- **c.** Soft tissue abnormalities of the reproductive tract
- **d.** All of the above

23–2. The majority of labor dystocia is due to which of the following?

- **a.** Asynclitism
- **b.** Fetal macrosomia
- **c.** Childhood rickets
- **d.** Premature rupture of membranes

23–3. Which of these factors influences the progress of labor?

- **a.** Prominent coccyx
- **b.** Pubic symphyseal separation
- **c.** Forward pressure by the leading fetal part
- **d.** Cervical dilation at the time of rupture of membranes

23–4. Since the 1960s, what significant advancement has been made in treating dysfunctional labor?

- **a.** Early artificial rupture of membranes
- **b.** Use of prostaglandins for cervical ripening
- **c.** Movement toward vacuum-assisted delivery in the setting of midpelvic arrest
- **d.** Realization that prolonged labor may lead to increased perinatal and maternal morbidity

23–5. Uterine contractions in normal labor are characterized by which of the following?

- **a.** Fundal dominance
- **b.** Contractions migrate from caudad to cephalad
- **c.** Pressure of an average spontaneous contraction is 15 mmHg
- **d.** Force of contractions is greatest at the lower uterine segment

23–6. Incoordinate uterine dysfunction refers to which of the following?

- **a.** The pressure gradient is distorted
- **b.** Basal uterine tone is appreciably elevated
- **c.** A more forceful contraction of the uterine midsegment than the fundus
- **d.** All of the above

23–7. The Montevideo group concluded that which of the following was the lowest contraction pressure necessary to cause cervical dilation?

- **a.** 15 mmHg
- **b.** 45 mmHg
- **c.** 60 mmHg
- **d.** 180 mmHg

23–8. When is the latent phase considered prolonged?

- **a.** 14 hours in nullipara
- **b.** 20 hours in mulitpara
- **c.** 10 hours in multipara
- **d.** None of the above

23–9. Which of the following is a protraction disorder?

- **a.** Prolonged active phase
- **b.** Protracted latent phase
- **c.** Prolonged deceleration phase
- **d.** Protracted active phase dilation

23–10. The World Health Organization has proposed a labor management partograph in which protraction is defined as ___ cm/hr cervical dilation for a minimum of ___ hours.

- **a.** 1, 3
- **b.** 2, 4
- **c.** 1, 4
- **d.** 2, 3

23–11. What are the Montevideo units in the tracing below?

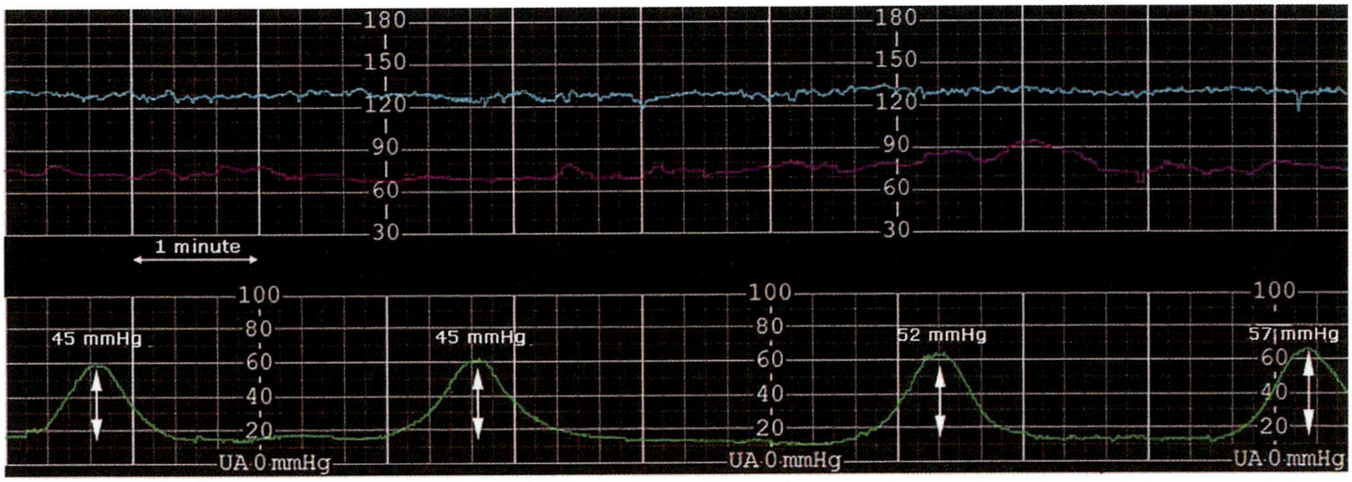

a. 50
b. 109
c. 142
d. 199

23–12. What is the threshold for adequate uterine contractions?

a. 180 Montevideo units
b. 200 Montevideo units
c. Contractions every 2 minutes
d. Five contractions in a 10-minute period

23–13. Which of the following statements comes from the Obstetric Care Consensus Committee of 2016?

a. The threshold for active labor is 4 cm.
b. A protraction disorder is an indication for a cesarean delivery.
c. A prolonged latent phase is not an indication for cesarean delivery.
d. Active phase arrest cannot be considered until the patient is 4 cm dilated and membranes are ruptured.

23–14. Which of the following statements is true comparing the Zhang versus Friedman curve?

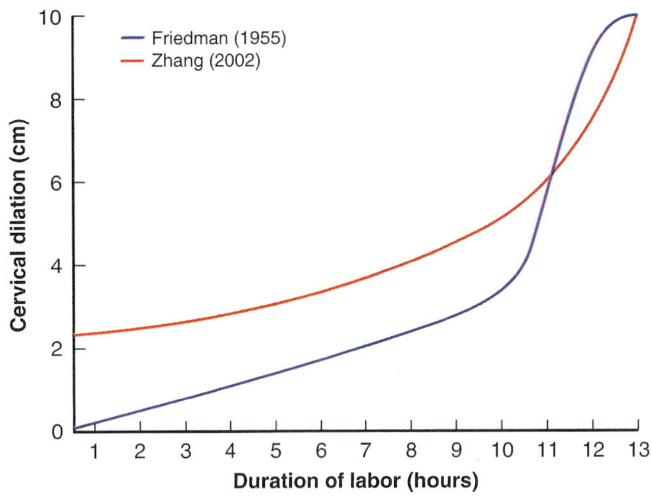

Reproduced with permission from Cunningham FG, Leveno KJ, Bloom SL, et al (eds): Abnormal labor. In Williams Obstetrics, 25th ed. New York, McGraw-Hill, 2018, Figure 23-3.

a. The Friedman curve begins to flatten at 3–4 cm.
b. In the Zhang curve the active phase of labor begins at 6 cm.
c. In the Friedman curve the active phase of labor begins at 6 cm.
d. All of the above

23–15. Which of the following accurately compares neuraxial and intravenous analgesia?

a. Time to delivery is lower with neuraxial analgesia.
b. Oxytocin augmentation was higher in the intravenous analgesia group.
c. Cesarean delivery rates are greater in the intravenous analgesia group.
d. None of the above

23–16. A 26-year-old multigravida at 40 weeks' gestation presents in labor at 6 cm. On repeat exam 4 hours later, she is still 6 cm. What other piece of information would you like to help determine your next step?

a. If she has any analgesia
b. The estimated fetal weight
c. If her membranes are ruptured
d. If her contractions are adequate

23–17. Regarding the patient in Question 23–16, you determine she has not had any analgesia, she is unruptured, and her contractions total 100 Montevideo units. What is the next best course of action?

a. Place neuraxial anesthesia
b. Augmentation with oxytocin
c. Provide intravenous analgesia
d. Proceed with cesarean delivery

23–18. Which of the following statements regarding the second stage of labor is false?

a. A prolonged first stage of labor correlates with a longer second stage.
b. No adverse maternal or neonatal outcomes are linked to delayed pushing.
c. The maximum length of time all women should spend in the second stage of labor is 4 hours.
d. Multiparous women should be allowed to push for 2 hours prior to diagnosing a second-stage labor arrest.

23–19. In laboring nulliparous women, fetal station above 0 at the time of admission is associated with which of the following?

a. A 25% cesarean rate
b. A 50% cesarean rate
c. An 86% cesarean rate
d. A higher cesarean rate than if the head is engaged

23–20. Which of the following statements is true concerning chorioamnionitis in labor?

a. Chorioamnionitis is associated with prolonged labor.
b. Chorioamnionitis in early labor is a consequence of dysfunctional labor.
c. Chorioamnionitis in the late stage of labor increases the risk for cesarean delivery.
d. All of the above

23–21. Which of the following is false regarding premature rupture of membranes at term?

a. Premature rupture of membranes complicates 8% of pregnancies.
b. Oxytocin induction leads to lower rates of chorioamnionitis.
c. Prophylactic antibiotics do not significantly lower the rates of chorioamnionitis.
d. The cesarean delivery rate is lower in women who are induced rather than managed expectantly.

23–22. Precipitous labor may result from which of the following?

a. Absence of painful sensations
b. Abnormally strong uterine contractions
c. Abnormally low resistance of the soft parts of the birth canal
d. All of the above

23–23. A 34-year-old multiparous woman presents in active labor at 38 weeks' gestation. She reports onset of contractions 1 hour ago and is 8 cm dilated on admission. She delivers an infant 1 hour later. What maternal risk is associated with precipitous labor?

a. Nerve injury
b. Uterine atony
c. Retained placenta
d. Bladder dysfunction

23–24. The infant delivered in Question 23–23 is at increased risk for which of the following?

a. Sepsis
b. Brachial plexus palsy
c. Meconium aspiration
d. Continuous positive airway pressure at birth

23–25. In obstetrics, which of the following defines a contracted pelvic inlet?

a. A transverse diameter <12 cm
b. An obstetric conjugate <10 cm
c. A diagonal conjugate <11.5 cm
d. An anteroposterior diameter <12 cm

23–26. Which of the following statements is true regarding contraction of the midpelvis?

a. It is less common than inlet contraction.
b. It causes transverse arrest of the fetal head.
c. It is suspected when the interspinous diameter is <11 cm.
d. It can be inferred when there are parallel vaginal sidewalls.

23–27. Which interischial tuberous diameter measurement serves as the threshold to define pelvic outlet contraction?

a. 7 cm

b. 8 cm

c. 9 cm

d. 10 cm

23–28. A 29-year-old primigravida presents for prenatal care at 10 weeks' gestation. She reports a history of a pelvic fracture 1 year ago. Which of the following is the most likely etiology of her fracture?

a. Fall

b. Assault

c. Gunshot wound

d. Automobile collision

23–29. The patient in Question 23–28 reports she was told she could never have a vaginal delivery. Which of the following is true?

a. Healing requires 8–12 weeks, so she can have a vaginal delivery.

b. If she has hardware in her pelvis she cannot have a vaginal delivery.

c. Hyperflexion of her hips during pushing may re-damage her pelvis.

d. If imaging shows any malalignment, she will have to undergo cesarean delivery.

23–30. The graphic below demonstrates the prevalence of cesarean deliveries after a failed forceps delivery attempt plotted against fetal birthweight. Which of the following is true regarding this data?

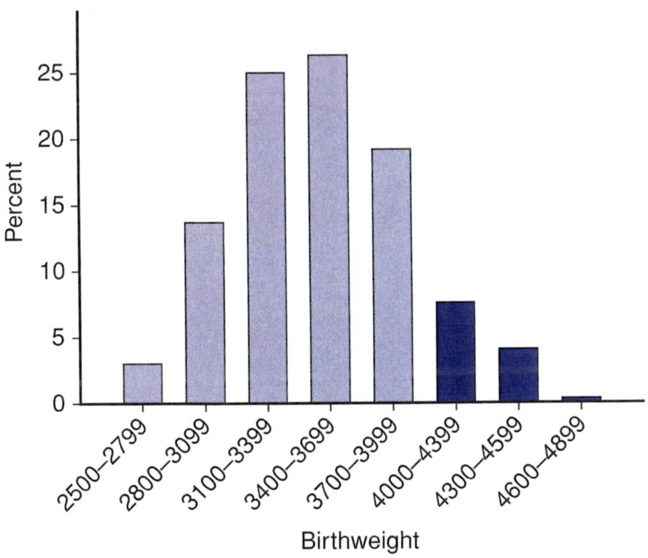

Reproduced with permission from Cunningham FG, Leveno KJ, Bloom SL, et al (eds): Abnormal labor. In Williams Obstetrics, 24th ed. New York, McGraw-Hill, 2014, Figure 23-5.

a. Most cesarean deliveries occurred in women with macrosomic infants.

b. Fetal size appears to be the significant contributor to failed forceps deliveries.

c. Malposition of the fetal head is a contributing factor to obstruction through the birth canal.

d. None of the above

23–31. Which of the following statements is true concerning face mentum posterior presentations?

a. Most will convert to mentum anterior.

b. Fetal macrosomia is the biggest risk factor.

c. Forceps should be applied when the station is +2.

d. A persistent mentum posterior presentation is never deliverable.

23–32. This image illustrates which fetal presentation?

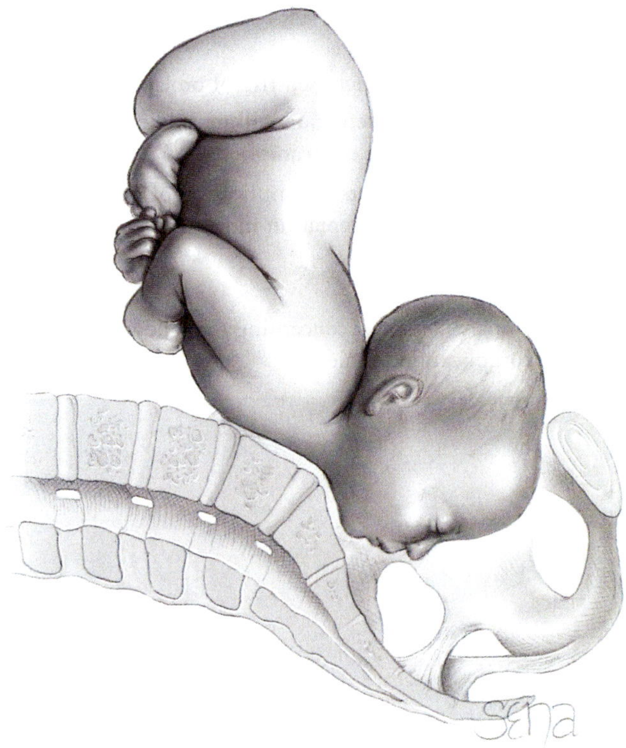

Reproduced with permission from Cunningham FG, Leveno KJ, Bloom SL, et al (eds): Abnormal labor. In Williams Obstetrics, 24th ed. New York, McGraw-Hill, 2014, Figure 23-6.

a. Face presentation

b. Brow presentation

c. Occiput presentation

d. Anteroposterior presentation

CHAPTER 23

23–33. Which statement below is accurate concerning the following presentation?

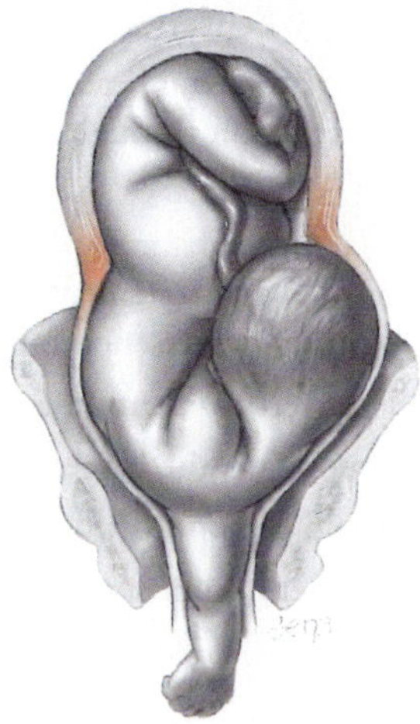

Reproduced with permission from Cunningham FG, Leveno KJ, Bloom SL, et al (eds): Abnormal labor. In Williams Obstetrics, 25th ed. New York, McGraw-Hill, 2018, Figure 23-10.

a. There is an increased risk of prolapsed cord.

b. This malpresentation will most likely be relieved with classical cesarean.

c. This represents a complication of persistent transverse presentation in labor.

d. All of the above

23–34. Which statement concerning the following labor complication is true?

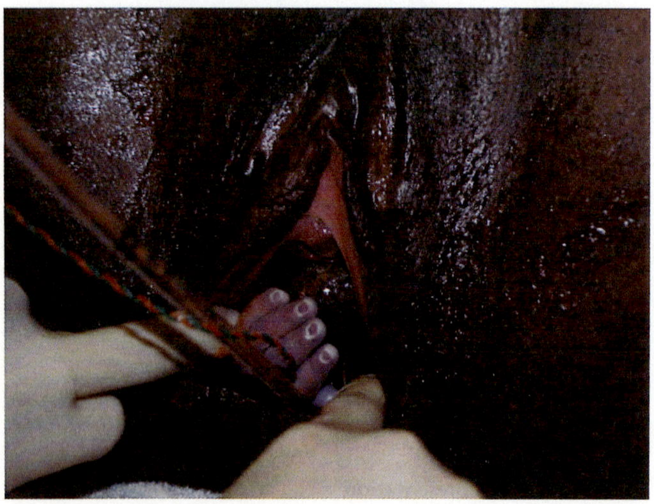

Used with permission from Dr. Elizabeth Mosier.

a. This is a composite presentation.

b. The forearm is frequently injured in this presentation.

c. In most cases the infant will deliver vaginally without difficulty.

d. The infant will sometimes withdraw its hand if "pinched" by the delivering obstetrician.

23–35. Which of the following are complications of labor dystocia?

a. Infection

b. Uterine rupture

c. Hysterotomy incision extensions

d. All of the above

23–36. A 24-year-old multigravida at 41 weeks' gestation with a body mass index of 38 kg/m^2 progresses through the first stage of labor and becomes complete at +2 station. She pushes for about 3 hours with neuraxial anesthesia. She delivers a 4200-gram infant with the assistance of forceps. The next day your patient reports lower extremity weakness with foot drop and pain. What is the most likely cause?

a. Obesity

b. Prolonged second stage

c. Forceps-assisted vaginal delivery

d. Complication of neuraxial anesthesia

CHAPTER 23 ANSWER KEY

Question number	Letter answer	Page cited	Header cited
23–1	d	442	Introduction
23–2	a	442	Descriptors
23–3	c	442	Mechanisms of Dystocia
23–4	d	442	Abnormalities of the Expulsive Forces
23–5	a	442	Types of Uterine Dysfunction
23–6	d	442	Types of Uterine Dysfunction
23–7	a	442	Types of Uterine Dysfunction
23–8	d	442	Labor Disorders
23–9	d	443	Table 23-2
23–10	c	443	Labor Disorders
23–11	c	443	Active-Phase Arrest
23–12	a	443	Active-Phase Arrest
23–13	c	444	Obstetric Care Consensus Committee
23–14	b	445	Background for the 6 cm rule
23–15	d	445	Table 23-5
23–16	d	444	Obstetric Care Consensus Committee
23–17	b	444	Obstetric Care Consensus Committee
23–18	c	447	Second Stage Descent Disorders Maternal Pushing Efforts
23–19	d	447	Fetal Station at Labor Onset
23–20	d	447	Risks for Uterine Dysfunction
23–21	d	448	Prematurely Ruptured Membranes at Term
23–22	d	448	Precipitous Labor and Delivery
23–23	b	448	Precipitous Labor and Delivery
23–24	b	448	Precipitous Labor and Delivery
23–25	a	448	Contracted Inlet
23–26	b	449	Contracted Midpelvis
23–27	b	449	Contracted Outlet
23–28	d	449	Pelvic Fractures
23–29	a	449	Pelvic Fractures
23–30	c	450	Fetal Body and Head Size
23–31	a	450	Face Presentation
23–32	a	450	Figure 23-6
23–33	d	453	Transverse Lie
23–34	c	454	Compound Presentation
23–35	d	454	Complications with Dystocia
23–36	b	455	Complications with Dystocia

CHAPTER 24

Intrapartum Assessment

24–1. Which portion of the fetal electrocardiogram is most reliably detected?

a. P wave

b. T wave

c. R-wave peaks

d. QRS complex

24–2. Which of the following is true regarding fetal heart monitoring through a fetal scalp electrode?

a. Heart rate is determined via time between R waves.

b. The maternal heart rate is also detected, but masked.

c. In the setting of an intrauterine fetal demise, the maternal heart rate will be recorded.

b. All of the above

24–3. Current fetal monitors can detect which of the following?

a. Maternal heart rate

b. Maternal pulse oximetry

c. Separate heart rates for a twin gestation

d. All of the above

24–4. Which of the following statements is true regarding the fetal heart rate pattern shown below?

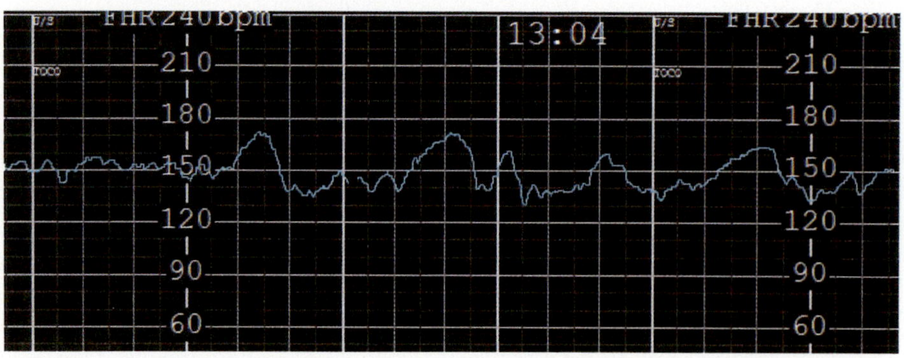

a. Does not require gel to obtain

b. Is not more difficult in obese women

c. Can be placed anywhere on the maternal abdomen

d. Uses ultrasound waves to detect the fetal heart rate

24–5. The NICHD Workshop standardized fetal heart rate interpretation in 2008. Which of the following factors makes interpreting fetal heart rate tracings difficult?

a. Paper speed at 3 cm/min

b. Interobserver agreement is low

c. Use of standardized terminology

d. Use of external monitors instead of internal monitors

24–6. Which of the following are descriptive characteristics of the fetal baseline heart rate?

a. Rate

b. Variability

c. Distinct patterns

d. All of the above

24–7. How is the fetal heart rate baseline determined?

a. Is determined over a 10-minute period

b. Increases with advancing gestational age

c. Is rounded to increments of 10 beats/minute

d. Minimum duration needed in a 10-minute period is 5 minutes

24–8. What fetal heart rates defines fetal bradycardia and fetal tachycardia, respectively?

a. <100 and >170

b. <110 and >170

c. <110 and >160

d. <120 and >160

24–9. A 24-year-old primigravida at 41 weeks' gestation is undergoing induction of labor. She is currently on intravenous oxytocin and reports abdominal pain that is not relieved by her epidural. The nurse calls you for the fetal heart rate pattern seen below. What is the likely etiology?

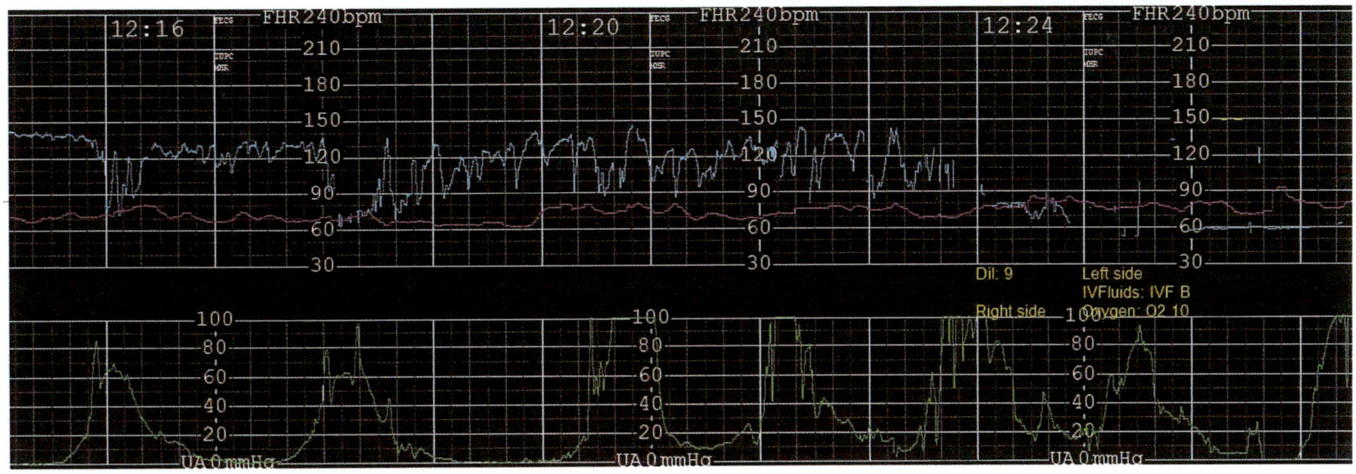

Used with permission from Dr. Travis Sims.

a. Fetal heart block

b. Rapid fetal descent

c. Placental abruption

d. Maternal hypothermia

24–10. What is the most common cause of fetal tachycardia?

a. Maternal pain

b. Chorioamnionitis

c. Maternal terbutaline

d. Fetal supraventricular tachycardia

24–11. What is the single most reliable sign of fetal compromise?

a. Decelerations

b. Fetal tachycardia

c. Change in baseline

d. Reduced variability

24–12. A 28-year-old primigravida is undergoing induction of labor. She experienced rupture of membranes 20 hours ago, and her cervical exam indicates she is 7 cm dilated. She receives intravenous butorphanol for pain. Which of the following is the etiology of the fetal heart rate variability seen below?

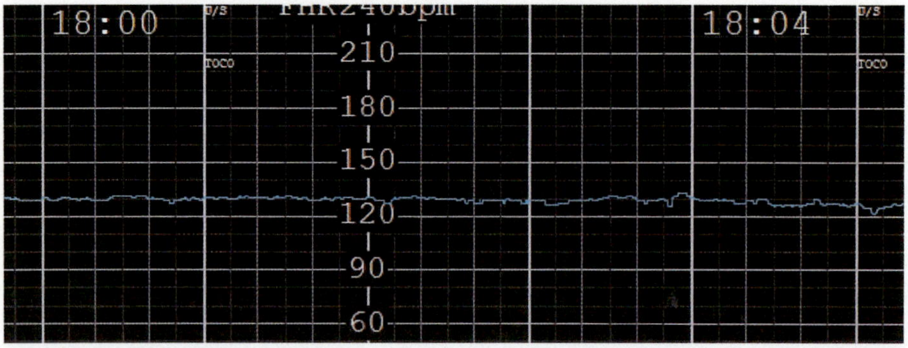

a. Active labor

b. Butorphanol

c. Oligohydramnios

d. Chorioamnionitis

24–13. Which of the following statements concerning fetal arrhythmias is true?

a. Are usually tachyarrhythmias

b. Are an indication for cesarean delivery

c. May hinder interpretation of the fetal heart rate tracings

d. All of the above

24–14. Sinusoidal fetal heart rate patterns are best described by which of the following statements?

a. Can be due to fetal sucking

b. Observed with mild fetal anemia

c. Frequency cycle of 2–5 cycles/minute

d. Baseline heart rate must be <120 beats/minute

24–15. Which of the following defines fetal heart rate decelerations as recurrent?

a. Occurring with ≥50% of contractions in a 10-minute period.

b. Occurring with ≥50% of contractions in a 20-minute period.

c. Occurring with >50% of contractions in a 10-minute period.

d. Occurring with >50% of contractions in a 20-minute period.

24–16. All except which of these statements is true regarding fetal heart rate accelerations?

a. Represent intact neurohormonal cardiovascular control mechanisms

b. Occur with fetal movement, scalp stimulation, and acoustic stimulation

c. Is considered prolonged if it is ≥2 minutes but <10 minutes in duration

d. At all gestational ages the peak is ≥15 beats per minute above the baseline

24–17. A deceleration that begins after the peak of the contraction and returns to baseline after the contraction ends is which of the following?

a. Late

b. Early

c. Variable

d. Prolonged

24–18. Which type of deceleration is pictured below?

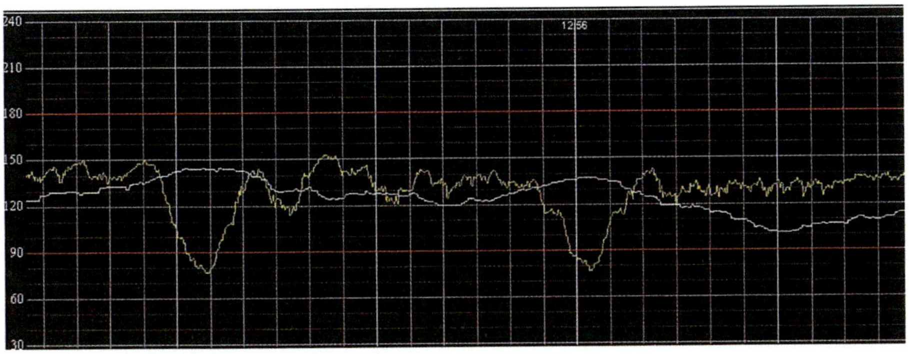

a. Late
b. Early
c. Variable
d. Prolonged

24–19. According to the American College of Obstetricians and Gynecologists, which of the following variable decelerations are abnormal?

a. Deep variables
b. Variables lasting >30 seconds
c. Variables with absent variability
d. Variables that take >30 seconds to reach their nadir

24–20. Which physiologic event results in initial compensatory rise in the fetal heart rate during a variable deceleration?

a. Acute increase in uterine tone
b. Occlusion of the umbilical vein
c. Occlusion of the umbilical artery
d. Occlusion of all umbilical vessels

24–21. A 25-year-old primigravida at 38 weeks' gestation is in the second stage of labor. Her fetal heart tracing is depicted below. Which of the following characteristics of the tracing increases her risk for fetal compromise?

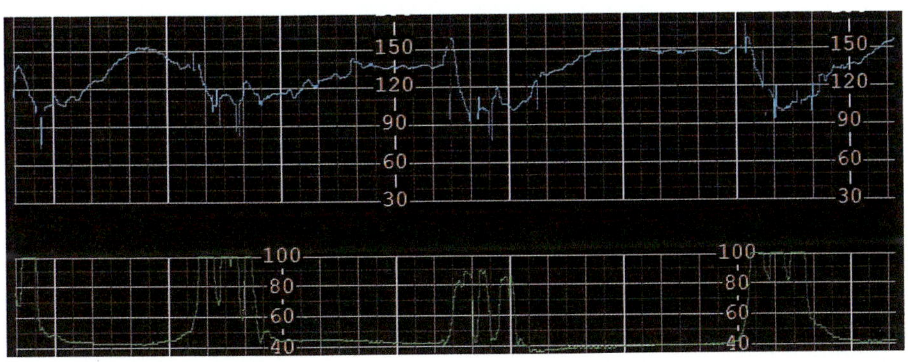

Used with permission from Dr. Noelle Zavala.

a. Normal baseline
b. Fetal tachycardia
c. Absent variability
d. All of the above

24–22. Which of the following statements is true regarding fetal heart rates in the second stage of labor?

a. Decelerations in the second stage of labor are ubiquitous.
b. If there is absent variability for longer than 4 minutes, acidemia can be predicted.
c. As the number of decelerations <30 beats per minute increases, the 5-minute Apgar score decreases.
d. All of the above

24–23. What effect do admission fetal monitoring programs have on low-risk women?

a. Improve neonatal outcomes
b. Decrease the number of interventions
c. Increase the number of cesarean deliveries
d. Decrease the number of operative deliveries

24–24. Which of the following is true for fetal scalp stimulation?

a. Accelerations predict a pH >7.2
b. Cannot be used in preterm infants
c. Lack of an acceleration predicts a pH <7.2
d. Cannot be used as a substitute for fetal scalp blood sampling

24–25. The use of fetal pulse oximetry has been shown to do which of the following?

a. Have no effect on the cesarean delivery rate
b. Increase the cesarean delivery rate for dystocia
c. Increase the cesarean delivery rate for nonreassuring status
d. Decrease the cesarean delivery rate for nonreassuring status

24–26. Why are the terms reassuring and nonreassuring imprecise and controversial?

a. Patterns change rapidly during labor.
b. The terms are subjective and without definition.
c. The terms reflect physiology rather than pathology.
d. All of the above

24–27. In 2008, the National Institute of Child Health and Human Development convened a conference and constructed a three-tiered system for fetal heart rate pattern classification. Which of the following accurately characterizes the different tiers?

a. Category I: absence of early decelerations and presence of normal baseline variability
b. Category II: presence of recurrent late decelerations and absent baseline variability
c. Category III: presence of recurrent variable decelerations and normal baseline variability
d. None of the above

24–28. Since the introduction of the new National Institute of Child Health and Human Development classification of fetal heart rate patterns, which of the following is true regarding its effect on perinatal and maternal morbidity?

a. Cesarean delivery rates have declined.
b. Identification of fetal acidosis is easier.
c. Neonatal morbidity rates have declined.
d. There is not a consensus on interpretation and management recommendations for fetal heart rate patterns.

24–29. Current guidelines from the American College of Obstetricians and Gynecologists recommend which of following regarding intrapartum neonatal suctioning in the presence of meconium?

a. Should be routinely performed in all infants
b. A credentialed team in neonatal resuscitation should be available
c. Routine intrapartum suctioning decreases the incidence of meconium aspiration syndrome
d. None of the above

24–30. In which of the following scenarios does the American College of Obstetricians and Gynecologists endorse amnioinfusion?

a. Meconium
b. Oligohydramnios
c. Variable decelerations
d. All of the above

24–31. The American College of Obstetricians and Gynecologists recommends collection of umbilical cord blood gases for which of the following conditions?

a. Low 5-minute Apgar score
b. Abnormal fetal heart rate tracing
c. Severe intrauterine growth restriction
d. All of the above

24–32. Which of the following statements are true concerning new uterine contraction terminology?

a. Hyperstimulation has been abandoned.
b. Tachysystole is defined as >5 contractions in 10 minutes averaged over 30 minutes.
c. Normal uterine activity is defined as ≤5 contractions in 10 minutes averaged over a 30-minute period.
d. All of the above

CHAPTER 24 ANSWER KEY

Question number	Letter answer	Page cited	Header cited
24–1	**c**	p. 458	Internal (Direct) Electronic Monitoring
24–2	**d**	p. 458	Internal (Direct) Electronic Monitoring
24–3	**d**	p. 459	Internal (Direct) Electronic Monitoring
24–4	**d**	p. 458	External (Indirect) Electronic Monitoring
24–5	**b**	p. 459	Fetal Heart Rate Patterns
24–6	**d**	p. 459	Baseline Fetal Heart Activity
24–7	**a**	p. 459	Baseline Fetal Heart Activity
24–8	**c**	p. 460	Table 24-1
24–9	**c**	p. 461	Baseline Fetal Heart Activity
24–10	**b**	p. 461	Baseline Fetal Heart Activity
24–11	**d**	p. 462	Baseline Fetal Heart Activity
24–12	**b**	p. 462	Baseline Fetal Heart Activity
24–13	**c**	p. 462	Baseline Fetal Heart Activity
24–14	**c**	p. 464	Baseline Fetal Heart Activity
24–15	**b**	p. 465	Periodic Fetal Heart Rate Changes
24–16	**d**	p. 465	Periodic Fetal Heart Rate Changes
24–17	**a**	p. 466	Periodic Fetal Heart Rate Changes
24–18	**c**	p. 466	Periodic Fetal Heart Rate Changes
24–19	**c**	p. 467	Periodic Fetal Heart Rate Changes
24–20	**b**	p. 467	Periodic Fetal Heart Rate Changes
24–21	**c**	p. 469	Fetal Heart Rate Patterns During Second-Stage Labor
24–22	**a**	p. 469	Fetal Heart Rate Patterns During Second-Stage Labor
24–23	**c**	p. 469	Admission Fetal Monitoring in Low-Risk Pregnancies
24–24	**a**	p. 470	Scalp Stimulation
24–25	**a**	p. 471	Fetal Pulse Oximetry
24–26	**d**	p. 472	Nonreassuring Fetal Status
24–27	**a**	p. 473	Table 24-2
24–28	**d**	p. 473	Diagnosis
24–29	**b**	p. 474	Meconium in Amnionic Fluid
24–30	**c**	p. 476	Management Options
24–31	**d**	p. 477	Fetal Heart Rate Patterns and Brain Injury
24–32	**d**	p. 480	Uterine Contraction Terminology

CHAPTER 25

Obstetrical Analgesia and Anesthesia

25–1. What percentage of maternal deaths in the United States are attributable to anesthesia?

a. 0.7%

b. 1.7%

c. 7.0%

d. 17%

25–2. A 25-year-old G2P1 is diagnosed with severe preeclampsia, with a platelet count of 40,000/μL, and requires a repeat cesarean delivery. You explain that the safest form of anesthesia is general endotracheal anesthesia. She states she has read in the recent media that anesthesia can be harmful to her fetus and requests more information. Which statement is true?

a. There is a significant lack of data to support the Food and Drug Administration's warning.

b. Most studies suggest that a single exposure of relatively short duration to general anesthesia has no effect on learning or behavior.

c. The Food and Drug Administration issued a warning that repeated or lengthy use of anesthesia during the third trimester may affect fetal brain development.

d. All of the above

25–3. Which statement regarding meperidine is true?

a. It readily crosses the placenta.

b. The neonatal half-life is 1–2 hours.

c. The metabolite normeperidine is not a respiratory depressant.

d. It is associated with higher Apgar scores in comparison to epidural analgesia.

25–4. You are called to evaluate an abnormal fetal heart rate tracing for a woman in labor. She recently received an intravenous medication for sedation and reports good pain relief. Ten minutes prior there was moderate variability and accelerations. The tracing is shown below. What is the most likely explanation for the below heart rate tracing?

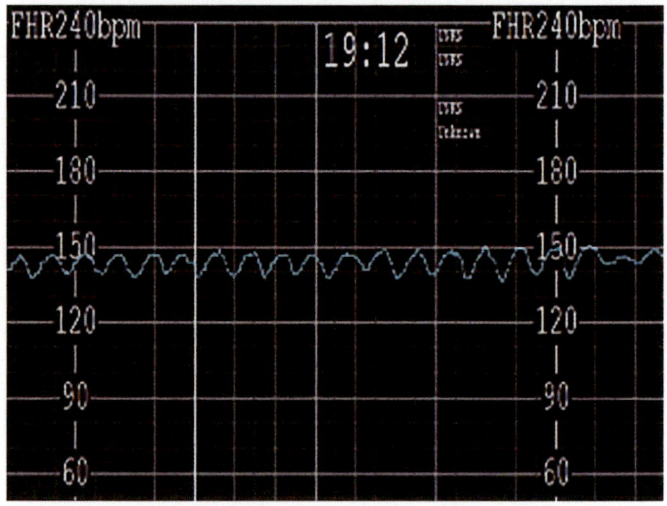

Used with permission from Dr. Ed Wells and Dr. F.G. Cunningham.

a. Fetal anemia

b. Fetal acidemia

c. Recent remifentanil administration

d. Recent butorphanol administration

25–5. A woman underwent a repeat cesarean delivery under spinal analgesia 2 hours ago and now complains of itching and some incisional discomfort. Which of the below medications will best address her complaints?

a. Fentanyl

b. Nalbuphine

c. Hydromorphone

d. Morphine sulfate

25–6. What is the primary and most important reason for administering an epidural test dose?

a. Rule out a high spinal
b. Rule out intravenous catheter placement
c. Ensure that anesthesia achieves a sufficient neurologic level
d. Give a bolus of narcotic to facilitate rapid pain relief

25–7. Which local anesthetic is associated with both neurotoxicity and cardiotoxicity at similar serum drug levels?

a. Lidocaine
b. Bupivacaine
c. Ropivacaine
d. 2-Chloroprocaine

25–8. A 22-year-old woman is undergoing labor induction. She has an epidural placed without complication and achieves excellent pain control. Two hours later she experiences acute-onset dizziness and tinnitus, and begins to demonstrate slurred speech. She then becomes hypotensive and unresponsive. Cardiopulmonary resuscitation is begun immediately and her airway is secured. The anesthesia provider notices that the epidural pump has been erroneously switched with her intravenous infusion line. What is the next best step of treatment after correcting this error?

a. Supportive care
b. Administer naloxone
c. Administer lipid emulsion
d. Place in left-lateral decubitus position

25–9. In the image shown below, which ligament is the needle passing through to reach the pudendal nerve?

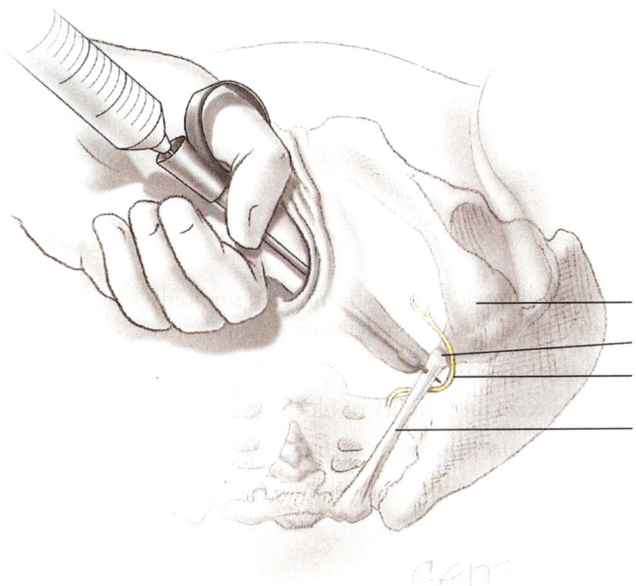

Reproduced with permission from Cunningham FG, Leveno KJ, Bloom SL, et al (eds): Obstetrical analgesia and anesthesia. In Williams Obstetrics, 25th ed. New York, McGraw-Hill, 2018, Figure 25-2.

a. Pudendal ligament
b. Sacroiliac ligament
c. Sacrospinous ligament
d. Sacrotuberous ligament

25–10. Which complication occurs with approximately 15% of paracervical blocks?

a. Infection
b. Hematoma
c. Fetal bradycardia
d. Intravascular injection

25–11. Which statement is true regarding spinal anesthesia in pregnancy as compared to nonpregnant individuals?

a. The subarachnoid space is larger in pregnant women.
b. A larger dose of anesthetic is required in pregnancy.
c. A dose of anesthetic achieves a lower blockade in pregnancy.
d. Associated hypotension may be more pronounced in pregnancy.

25–12. What level of blockade is desired with spinal anesthesia for cesarean delivery?

a. T4
b. T6
c. T8
d. T10

25–13. Which of the following is a benefit of adding opioids to spinal analgesia for cesarean delivery?

a. Opioids reduce shivering
b. Opioids increase the rapidity of blockade onset
c. Opioids minimize symptoms such as nausea and vomiting
d. All of the above

25–14. A 26-year-old G1 undergoing induction for severe preeclampsia undergoes epidural placement during labor. She receives a bolus of 1 liter crystalloid solution prior to epidural placement. Twenty minutes later the fetal heart rate tracing is as shown below, and maternal blood pressure is 92/54 mmHg. Prior to epidural placement, blood pressure range was 130–148/76–90 mmHg. Which intervention is most appropriate?

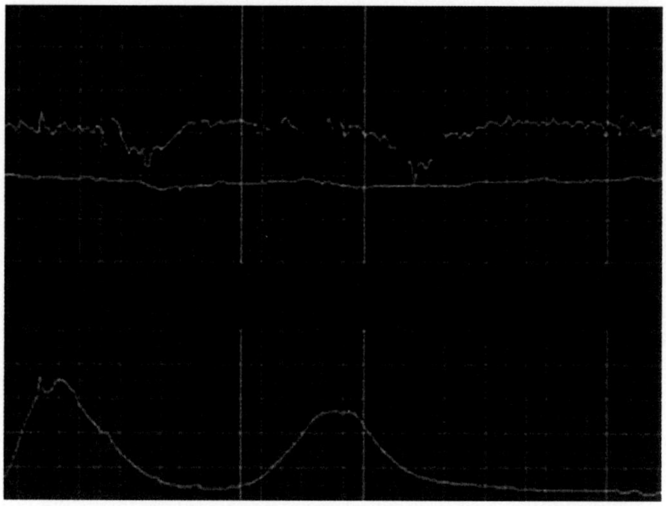

a. Administer IV ephedrine
b. Place supplemental oxygen
c. Emergent cesarean delivery
d. Bolus an additional 1 liter crystalloid

25–15. When used prophylactically in the obstetrical anesthesia setting, which vasopressor has been associated with fetal acidemia?

a. Ephedrine
b. Ergonovine
c. Phenylephrine
d. Methylergonovine

25–16. Which intervention is least effective for prevention of postdural puncture headache?

a. Use a small-gauge needle
b. Avoid multiple punctures
c. Use epidural analgesia when possible
d. Place patient in a flat supine position following puncture

25–17. Which of the below conditions is an absolute contraindication to neuraxial analgesia in labor?

a. Multiple sclerosis
b. Pulmonary hypertension
c. Cellulitis at the needle entry site
d. Received prophylactic unfractionated heparin 8 hours ago

25–18. Which structure is indicated by the arrow in the diagram below?

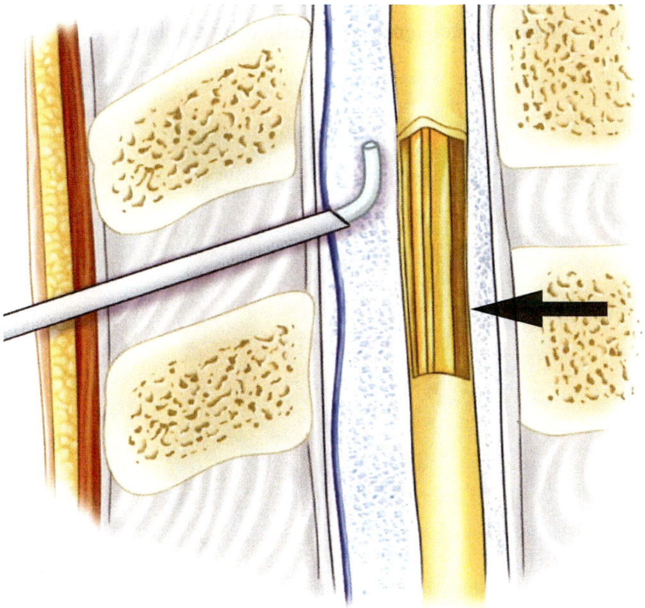

Reproduced with permission from Cunningham FG, Leveno KJ, Bloom SL, et al (eds): Obstetrical analgesia and anesthesia. In Williams Obstetrics, 25th ed. New York, McGraw-Hill, 2018, Figure 25-3.

a. Dura mater
b. Cauda equine
c. Ligamentum flavum
d. Vertebral venous plexus

25–19. Which of the following is the most common complication associated with epidural anesthesia?

a. Fever
b. Hypotension
c. Epidural hematoma
d. Ineffective analgesia

25–20. A 22-year-old primigravida is considering epidural analgesia during labor and inquires if undergoing epidural placement will affect her labor. Which of the following statements is most accurate?

a. Epidural use may prolong her labor
b. Epidural use may increase her need for oxytocin
c. Epidural use may increase her chance of operative delivery
d. All of the above

25–21. A 32-year-old G3P2 at 38 weeks' gestation with a history of a cesarean delivery and idiopathic thrombocytopenic purpura presents in early labor. She would like to undergo a repeat cesarean delivery. Her platelet count is 80,000/μL, which is stable from previous values. She desires to avoid general anesthesia if possible. What form of anesthesia is most reasonable to offer?

a. Spinal
b. Epidural
c. General anesthesia only
d. Combined spinal-epidural

25–22. Which step in patient preparation prior to intubation has most effectively reduced the maternal morbidity and mortality associated with general anesthesia for cesarean delivery?

a. Preoxygenation
b. Use of cricoid pressure
c. Antacid administration
d. Lateral uterine displacement

25–23. A 24-year-old woman presents at term with severe abdominal pain and fetal bradycardia. She is taken to the operating room to proceed with emergent cesarean delivery. Attempts at intubation after rapid sequence induction fail. Which of the following next steps is unacceptable?

a. Proceed with cesarean delivery
b. Establish adequate ventilation with laryngeal mask airway
c. Proceed with percutaneous or open cricothyrotomy
d. Allow the woman to awaken and use a different form of anesthesia

25–24. Which pulmonary lobe is most often involved in aspiration as a complication of general anesthesia?

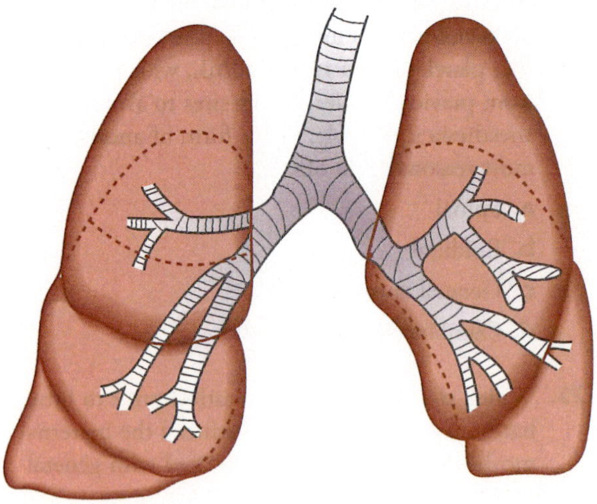

a. Left lower lobe
b. Right lower lobe
c. Right upper lobe
d. Right middle lobe

25–25. If a patient has emesis of gastric contents during induction of general anesthesia, which of the following steps is indicated to limit the complications of aspiration?

a. Saline lavage
b. Initiation of prophylactic antibiotics
c. Administration of corticosteroid therapy
d. Suctioning of inhaled fluid from pharynx and trachea

25–26. A patient requiring emergent cesarean delivery has a patchy epidural block and needs local infiltration of anesthesia to augment the blockade. In the image here, which nerve is identified by the letter X?

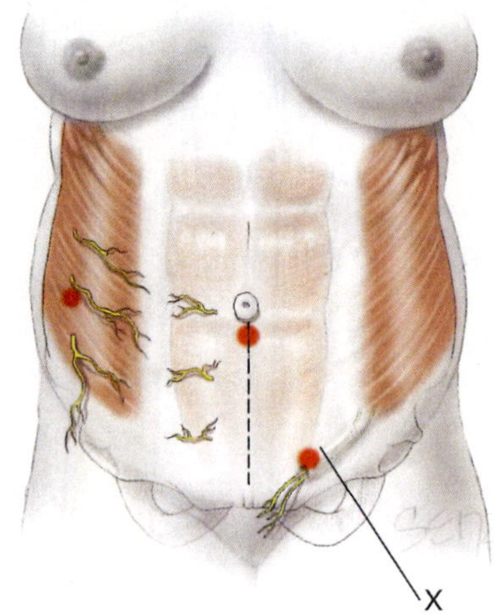

Reproduced with permission from Cunningham FG, Leveno KJ, Bloom SL, et al (eds): Obstetrical analgesia and anesthesia. In Williams Obstetrics, 25th ed. New York, McGraw-Hill, 2018, Figure 25-5.

a. Ischial nerve
b. Intercostal nerve
c. Ilioinguinal nerve
d. Hypogastric nerve

25–27. What is the rate of failed intubation for general anesthesia in pregnancy?

a. 1/100
b. 1/250
c. 1/400
d. 1/550

25–28. A patient with a known thrombophilia has just had a vaginal delivery under epidural anesthesia. She had discontinued her low-dose low-molecular-weight anticoagulant prior to induction of labor. When would it be safe to restart her anticoagulant postpartum?

a. Prior to removal of her epidural catheter
b. Directly following epidural catheter removal
c. At least 2 hours after epidural catheter removal
d. When her partial thromboplastin time is normal

25–29. A patient in early labor is sitting up for her epidural. An anesthetic test dose is given. The patient's heart rate and blood pressure rise immediately after administration of the test dose. What has most likely cause for this change in vital signs?

a. The test dose was given intravenously.

b. The patient experienced a contraction.

c. She is experiencing a high spinal blockade.

d. This is the normal response to a test dose.

25–30. Which nerve is primarily involved with the pain associated with perineal stretching?

a. Pudendal

b. Ilioinguinal

c. Genitofemoral

d. Frankenhäuser ganglion

25–31. What is the direct cause of most maternal deaths involving regional anesthesia?

a. Drug reaction

b. Cardiac arrhythmia

c. High spinal blockade

d. Central nervous system infection

25–32. Which of the below factors can influence the spread of anesthesia after continuous epidural catheter placement?

a. Maternal position

b. Dose of anesthetic

c. Location of catheter tip

d. All of the above

CHAPTER 25 ANSWER KEY

Question number	Letter answer	Page cited	Header cited
25–1	**a**	p. 485	Introduction
25–2	**d**	p. 486	Introduction
25–3	**a**	p. 488	Analgesia and Sedation During Labor
25–4	**d**	p. 488	Analgesia and Sedation During Labor
25–5	**b**	p. 488	Analgesia and Sedation During Labor
25–6	**b**	p. 489	Regional Anesthesia
25–7	**b**	p. 490	Regional Anesthesia
25–8	**c**	p. 490	Regional Anesthesia
25–9	**c**	p. 491	Regional Anesthesia
25–10	**c**	p. 490	Regional Anesthesia
25–11	**d**	p. 491	Neuraxial Analgesia
25–12	**a**	p. 491	Neuraxial Analgesia
25–13	**d**	p. 491	Neuraxial Analgesia
25–14	**a**	p. 492	Neuraxial Analgesia
25–15	**a**	p. 492	Neuraxial Analgesia
25–16	**d**	p. 492	Neuraxial Analgesia
25–17	**c**	p. 492	Neuraxial Analgesia
25–18	**a**	p. 493	Neuraxial Analgesia
25–19	**b**	p. 494	Neuraxial Analgesia
25–20	**d**	p. 495	Neuraxial Analgesia
25–21	**a**	p. 496	Neuraxial Analgesia
25–22	**c**	p. 498	General Anesthesia
25–23	**a**	p. 499	General Anesthesia
25–24	**b**	p. 499	General Anesthesia
25–25	**d**	p. 500	General Anesthesia
25–26	**c**	p. 497	Local Infiltration for Cesarean Delivery
25–27	**c**	p. 498	General Anesthesia
25–28	**c**	p. 496	Neuraxial Analgesia
25–29	**a**	p. 489	Regional Anesthesia
25–30	**a**	p. 490	Regional Anesthesia
25–31	**c**	p. 485	Introduction
25–32	**d**	p. 493	Neuraxial Analgesia

CHAPTER 26

Induction and Augmentation of Labor

26–1. A 19-year-old primigravida presents to the labor and delivery unit with the complaint of contractions following spontaneous rupture of membranes. Her initial cervical exam shows she is 2 cm dilated; 3 hours later she is 5 cm dilated. Over the next 4 hours there is no further cervical dilation, and oxytocin is started. The use of oxytocin in this setting would be described as which of the following?

a. Labor induction

b. Cervical ripening

c. Uterine maturation

d. Labor augmentation

26–2. Which of the following methods of uterine stimulation could not be employed in Question 26–1?

a. Oxytocin

b. Misoprostol

c. Dinoprostone

d. Extraamnionic saline infusion

26–3. Which of the following complications is increased in the setting of labor induction?

a. NICU admission

b. Postpartum hemorrhage

c. Amnionic fluid embolus

d. Umbilical artery pH <7.0

26–4. A 36-year-old G5P2 at 39 weeks' gestation presents for labor induction. Her previous largest infant weighed 3500 grams. She had a prior vertical cesarean section for a preterm breech presentation at 27 weeks' gestation, and has a history of herpes simplex type 1 infection. Which of the following is the correct first step in her evaluation for the appropriateness of labor induction?

a. Ultrasound for estimated fetal weight

b. Digital cervical exam to determine Bishop score

c. Speculum exam to look for herpes simplex lesions

d. None of the above

26–5. The results of an ultrasound for the patient in Question 26–4 are shown above. Which element in the patient's history is a contraindication to labor induction?

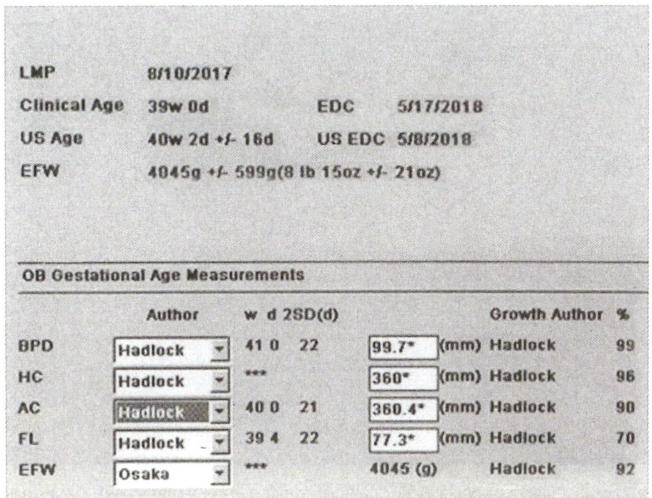

LMP 8/10/2017

Clinical Age 39w 0d EDC 5/17/2018

US Age 40w 2d +/- 16d US EDC 5/8/2018

EFW 4045g +/- 599g(8 lb 15oz +/- 21oz)

OB Gestational Age Measurements

	Author	w d	2SD(d)			Growth Author	%
BPD	Hadlock	41 0	22	99.7*	(mm)	Hadlock	99
HC	Hadlock	***		360*	(mm)	Hadlock	96
AC	Hadlock	40 0	21	360.4*	(mm)	Hadlock	90
FL	Hadlock	39 4	22	77.3*	(mm)	Hadlock	70
EFW	Osaka	***		4045 (g)		Hadlock	92

a. Grand multiparity

b. Prior vertical uterine incision

c. Suspicion of fetal macrosomia

d. Previous herpes simplex infection

26–6. A 27-year-old G2P1 had a prior low transverse cesarean section for breech presentation. Her gestational age is 37 weeks and her cervical exam shows she is dilated 3 cm, 50% effaced, and at –2 station with a cephalic presentation. Which of the following statements is most accurate in this scenario?

a. Labor induction is indicated because of concerns for cord prolapse.

b. Neonatal outcomes are equivalent at all gestational ages after 37 weeks.

c. Oxytocin is a safer option for labor induction compared to prostaglandin.

d. The risk for uterine rupture in not increased because of the location of the previous uterine incision.

26–7. The patient in Question 26–6 presents for amniotomy induction of labor 2 weeks later. Which of the following is more common with this labor induction method compared to awaiting spontaneous labor?

- **a.** Chorioamnionitis
- **b.** Shoulder dystocia
- **c.** Cervical laceration
- **d.** Placental abruption

26–8. What is the relative risk for the complication shown in the picture below when oxytocin is given to a patient with a history of prior uterine surgery?

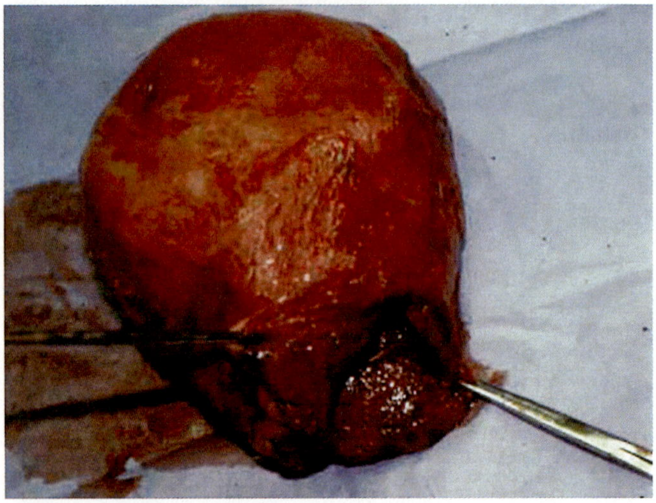

Reproduced with permission from Cunningham FG, Leveno KJ, Bloom SL, et al (eds): Obstetrical hemorrhage. In Williams Obstetrics, 25th ed. New York, McGraw-Hill, 2018, Figure 41-13.

- **a.** Twofold
- **b.** Threefold
- **c.** Tenfold
- **d.** Unchanged

26–9. What do the authors suggest contributed to the increase in postpartum hysterectomy between 1994 and 2007?

- **a.** Increased repeat cesarean sections
- **b.** Increased primary cesarean sections
- **c.** Increased frequency of labor inductions
- **d.** All of the above

26–10. A 27-year-old G1P0 with a body mass index of 29 kg/m^2 presents for labor induction. The estimated fetal weight is 4000 grams. Which factor portends a non-successful outcome?

- **a.** Nulliparity
- **b.** Younger age
- **c.** Body mass index <30 kg/m^2
- **d.** Estimated fetal weight <4000 grams

26–11. Which of the following is not used to calculate the Bishop score?

- **a.** Parity
- **b.** Effacement
- **c.** Fetal station
- **d.** Cervical dilation

26–12. The inclusion of this measurement into the Bishop score results in improved estimation of which of the following?

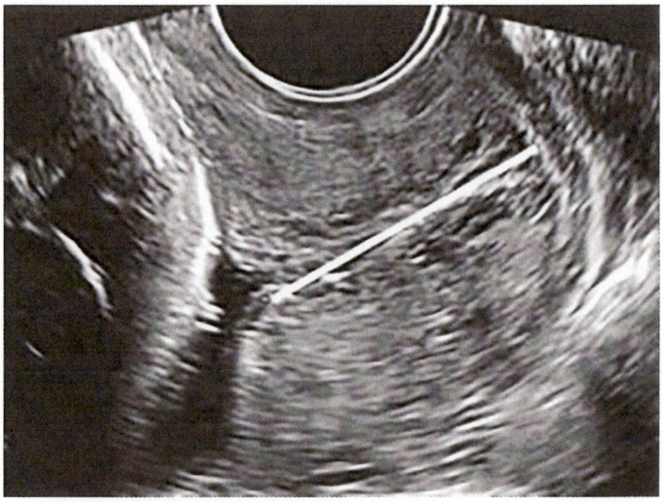

- **a.** Likelihood of cesarean section
- **b.** Prediction of successful vaginal delivery
- **c.** Estimation in length of stage 1 of labor
- **d.** None of the above

26–13. Dinoprostone, a synthetic analogue of prostaglandin E_2 used for cervical ripening and labor induction, is not available in which of the following formulations?

a. Gel

b. Intravenous

c. Vaginal suppository

d. Timed-release vaginal insert

26–14. Which of the following is a true statement with respect to the method of labor induction pictured below?

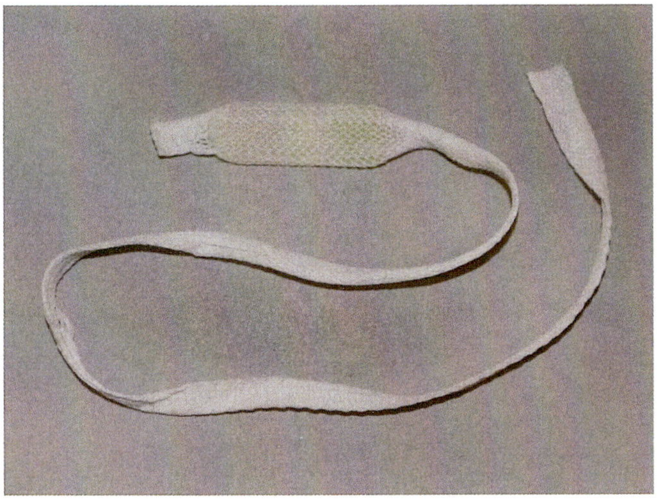

a. The tail facilitates removal from the vagina.

b. The insert is placed inside the dilated cervix.

c. Lubricant improves release of PGE_2 from the mesh sac.

d. It provides faster release of PGE_2 than gel formulation.

26–15. Following placement of the device shown in Question 26–14, a patient experiences uterine tachysystole with fetal heart rate abnormalities. Which is the appropriate response?

a. Remove insert

b. Intravenous fluid bolus

c. Subcutaneous terbutaline

d. Flush vagina with normal saline

26–16. A patient, G6P4A1, has a history of asthma and a hysteroscopic septum resection. The estimated weight of her fetus is 3800 grams. Which element of her history is a contraindication to labor induction using dinoprostone?

a. Parity

b. History of asthma

c. Previous uterine surgery

d. None of the above

26–17. A patient who underwent cervical ripening with a PGE_2 vaginal insert is ready for labor induction. What is the recommended period of time to wait after removing the insert?

a. 30 minutes

b. 2 hours

c. 6 hours

d. 12 hours

26–18. Misoprostol has FDA approval for use in what condition?

a. Menorrhagia

b. Medical abortion

c. Labor augmentation

d. Peptic ulcer prevention

26–19. With respect to efficacy of cervical ripening or labor induction, how does vaginally administered misoprostol compare to intracervical or intravaginal dinoprostone?

a. Increase in uterine tachysystole

b. No difference in rate of cesarean delivery

c. Increased rate of delivery within 24 hours

d. All of the above

26–20. A G2P1 at 41 weeks' gestation undergoes labor induction with oral misoprostol. Which of the following is a true statement?

a. Oral misoprostol is associated with higher Apgar scores than vaginal misoprostol.

b. The rate of cesarean delivery is reduced with oral misoprostol as compared to dinoprostone.

c. The success rate of vaginal delivery is higher with oral misoprostol as compared to oxytocin.

d. All of the above

26–21. Which of the following agents has the lowest clinical effectiveness for cervical ripening?

a. Misoprostol

b. Prostaglandin E_2

c. Isosorbide mononitrate

d. All have equivalent efficacy

26–22. Which of the following is not a benefit of mechanical techniques for preinduction cervical ripening?

a. Shorter length of stay

b. Decreased risk of tachysystole

c. Decreased rate of cesarean delivery

d. None of the above

26–23. Which of the following is increased when the technique shown below is used for cervical ripening compared to pharmacologic methods?

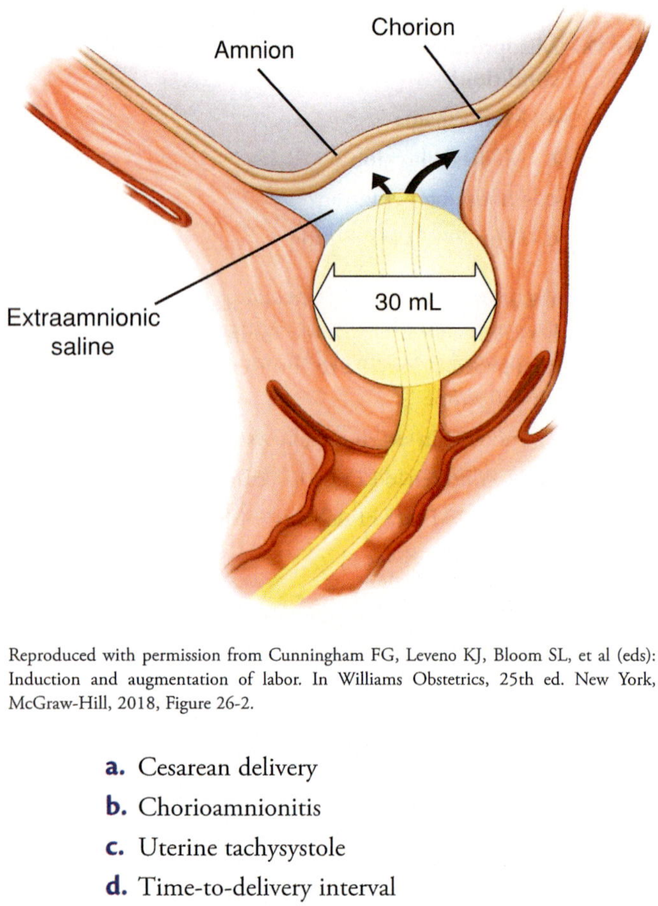

Reproduced with permission from Cunningham FG, Leveno KJ, Bloom SL, et al (eds): Induction and augmentation of labor. In Williams Obstetrics, 25th ed. New York, McGraw-Hill, 2018, Figure 26-2.

a. Cesarean delivery

b. Chorioamnionitis

c. Uterine tachysystole

d. Time-to-delivery interval

26–24. A 25-year-old primigravida presents to labor and delivery after spontaneous rupture of membranes at 37 weeks' gestation. She denies vaginal bleeding or regular contractions. What is the dose of oral misoprostol used to induce labor?

a. 25 mg

b. 100 mg

c. 100 mg

d. None of the above

26–25. Misoprostol fails to induce adequate contractions in the patient in Question 26–24, so oxytocin is started. The fetal heart rate tracing is shown below. What is the most appropriate response?

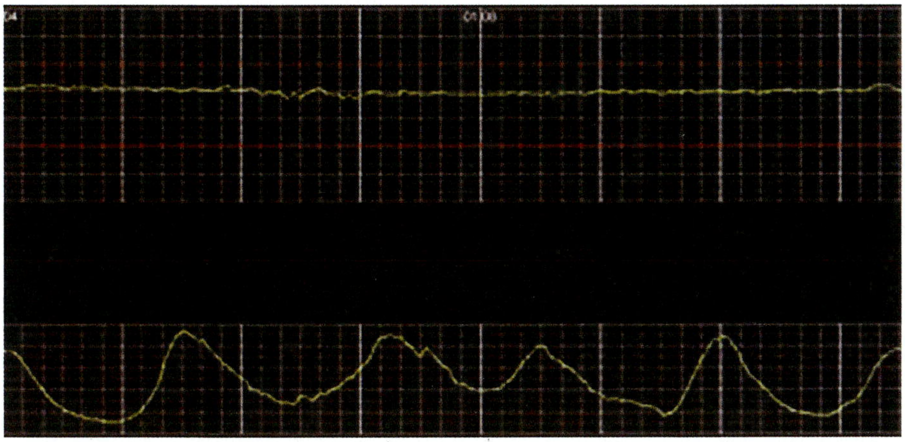

a. Do nothing
b. Stop oxytocin infusion
c. Perform cervical examination
d. Move the patient to the operating room for cesarean delivery

26–26. What is the half-life of oxytocin?

a. 30 seconds
b. 3 minutes
c. 30 minutes
d. 1 hour

26–27. A patient is undergoing labor augmentation. Her doctor ordered an oxytocin regimen that starts with an infusion rate of 6 mU/min and increases by 6 mU/min every 20 minutes. Which of the following is a benefit of this dosing regimen compared to one that uses 1 mU/min increments?

a. Reduced forceps delivery rate
b. Shorter mean admission-to-delivery time
c. Reduced rate of intrapartum chorioamnionitis
d. All of the above

26–28. In the previous scenario, what is the benefit of choosing a regimen that increases the infusion every 40 minutes instead of every 20 minutes?

a. Improved Apgar scores
b. Decreased neonatal sepsis
c. Reduced uterine tachysystole
d. Reduced cesarean delivery rate for dystocia

26–29. Oxytocin's similarity to arginine vasopressin accounts for which unwanted side effect?

a. Water intoxication
b. Hypertensive crisis
c. Uterine tachysystole
d. Amnionic fluid embolus

26–30. A patient in labor undergoes an amniotomy and oxytocin augmentation for arrest of the active phase of labor. Which of the following is true when compared to oxytocin administration alone?

a. The umbilical artery pH is decreased.
b. The time to delivery is slightly increased.
c. The rate of chorioamnionitis is increased.
d. There is a decreased rate of cesarean delivery.

26–31. Which of the following may help reduce the risk of cord prolapse during amniotomy?

a. Provide fundal pressure
b. Use a needle to puncture the membranes
c. Perform amniotomy during contraction
d. All of the above

26–32. Which of the following is a benefit of membrane stripping at term?

a. Shorter labor
b. Reduced active-phase labor arrest
c. Reduced incidence of postterm pregnancy
d. Reduced uterine tachysystole during labor

CHAPTER 26 ANSWER KEY

Question number	Letter answer	Page cited	Header cited
26–1	**d**	p. 503	Induction and Augmentation of Labor
26–2	**d**	p. 504	Techniques
26–3	**b**	p. 504	Risks
26–4	**d**	p. 504	Risks
26–5	**b**	p. 504	Risks
26–6	**c**	p. 504	Risks
26–7	**a**	p. 504	Risks
26–8	**b**	p. 504	Risks
26–9	**d**	p. 504	Risks
26–10	**a**	p. 504	Factors Affecting Induction Success
26–11	**a**	p. 505	Table 26-2
26–12	**d**	p. 506	Cervical "Favorability"
26–13	**b**	p. 506	Prostaglandin E_2
26–14	**a**	p. 507	Side Effects
26–15	**a**	p. 507	Side Effects
26–16	**d**	p. 507	Side Effects
26–17	**a**	p. 507	Administration
26–18	**d**	p. 507	Prostaglandin E_1
26–19	**d**	p. 507	Vaginal Administration
26–20	**d**	p. 507	Oral Administration
26–21	**c**	p. 507	Nitric Oxide Donors
26–22	**a**	p. 507	Mechanical Techniques
26–23	**b**	p. 508	Transcervical Catheter
26–24	**b**	p. 508	Prostaglandin E_1
26–25	**b**	p. 509	Intravenous Oxytocin Administration
26–26	**b**	p. 509	Intravenous Oxytocin Administration
26–27	**d**	p. 509	Oxytocin Regimes
26–28	**c**	p. 510	Interval between Incremental Dosing
26–29	**a**	p. 510	Risks versus Benefits
26–30	**c**	p. 511	Amniotomy for Induction and Augmentation
26–31	**d**	p. 511	Amniotomy for Induction and Augmentation
26–32	**c**	p. 512	Membrane Stripping for Labor Induction

SECTION 8

DELIVERY

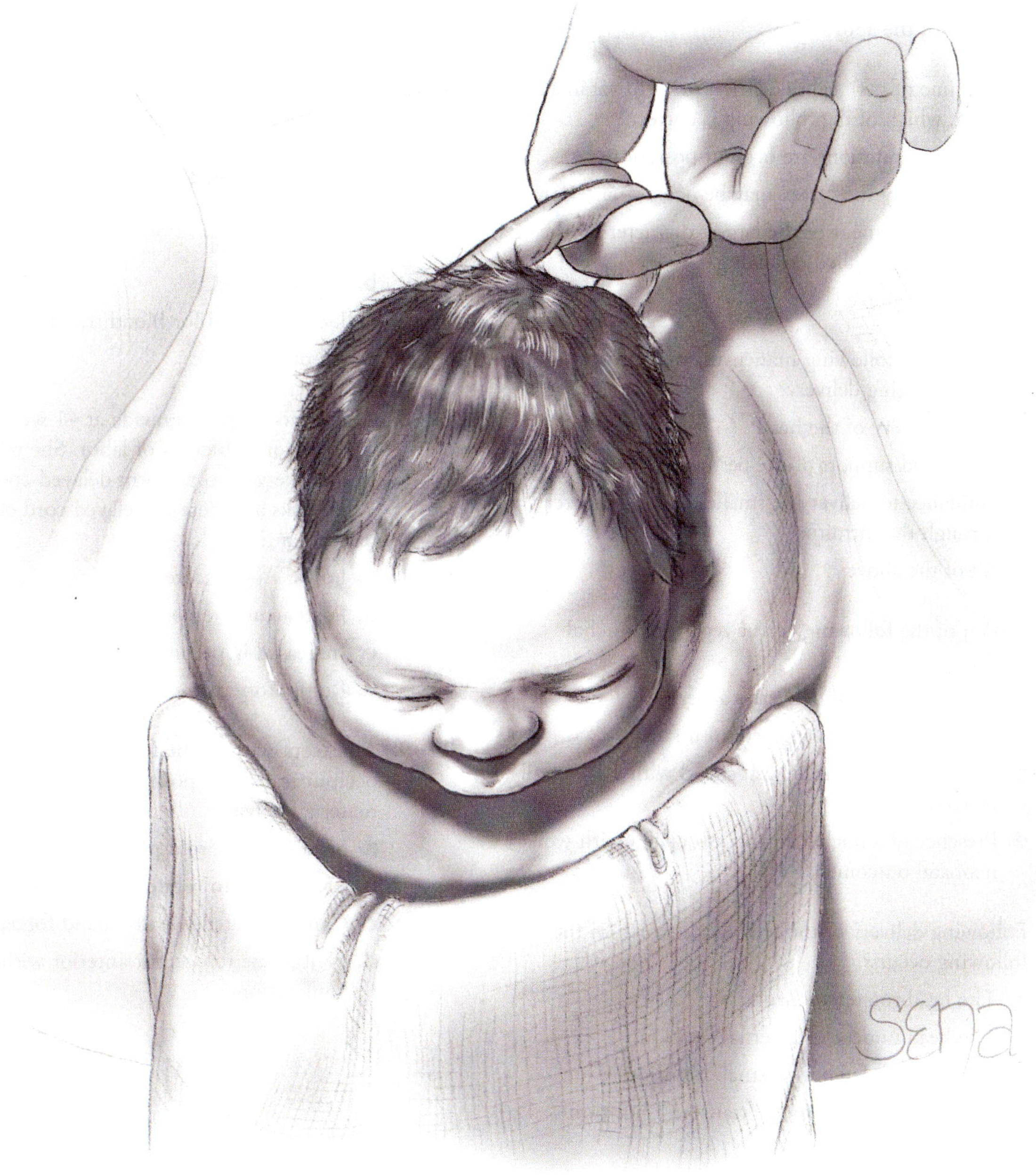

CHAPTER 27

Vaginal Delivery

27–1. The most common position for vaginal delivery is which of the following?

- **a.** Squatting
- **b.** Knee-chest
- **c.** Dorsal lithotomy
- **d.** None of the above

27–2. At the time of perineal distention prior to vaginal delivery, which of the following is correct?

- **a.** Most presentations are occiput posterior.
- **b.** Infrequently the vertex may be occiput anterior.
- **c.** The encirclement of the largest diameter by the vulvar ring is called crowning.
- **d.** All of the above

27–3. Which of the following maneuvers may protect the perineum during delivery?

- **a.** Slow delivery of the head
- **b.** One-hand support of the perineum
- **c.** Guidance to deliver the smallest head diameter through the introitus
- **d.** All of the above

27–4. Which of the following is true regarding nuchal cords?

- **a.** Found in 25% of deliveries at term
- **b.** Are more common in preterm infants
- **c.** Tight nuchal cords are associated with 10% of all deliveries
- **d.** Presence of a nuchal cord is associated with worse neonatal outcomes

27–5. Following delivery of the fetal head, which of the following occurs?

- **a.** The head rotates anterior
- **b.** The head undergoes internal rotation
- **c.** The head undergoes external extension
- **d.** The head rotates into the transverse position

27–6. All except which of the following statements regarding delivery of the fetal body are true?

- **a.** Usually delivers without delay after the shoulders.
- **b.** Hooking the axillae can be employed to hasten delivery of the body.
- **c.** Moderate outward traction on the head may be used to help delivery.
- **d.** Immediate nasopharyngeal suction should be performed after delivery.

27–7. What are the benefits of delayed cord clamping in preterm infants?

- **a.** Decrease IVH
- **b.** Decrease NEC
- **c.** Decrease need for blood transfusion
- **d.** All of the above

27–8. A 34-year-old primigravida at 41 weeks' gestation presents for induction of labor. She tells you she would like you to perform delayed cord clamping. What risks are there to delayed cord clamping in the term infant?

- **a.** Lower Apgar scores
- **b.** Postpartum hemorrhage
- **c.** Increased hyperbilirubinemia
- **d.** Respiratory distress syndrome from polycythemia

27–9. All except with of the following is true regarding occiput transverse position of the fetal head in the maternal pelvis?

- **a.** Seen with android pelvises
- **b.** Easiest way to rotate is manually
- **c.** Can be rotated with Kielland forceps
- **d.** Will rotate to occiput anterior with hypotonic contractions

27–10. Which of the following is true regarding persistent occiput posterior (OP) position in labor?

a. Seen more often in multiparous women

b. 2–10% of cephalic fetuses deliver in the OP position

c. Gynecoid pelvises predispose to persistent OP position

d. Epidural analgesia is not a risk for persistent OP position

27–11. For women who deliver vaginally with persistent occiput posterior (OP) position, which of the following is true?

a. Transabdominal ultrasound can aid in identifying the OP position.

b. There is increased blood loss compared to occiput anterior position.

c. There are more third- and fourth-degree lacerations compared to occiput anterior position.

d. All of the above

27–12. A 22-year-old primigravida has been pushing for 3 hours. The fetus is in persistent occiput posterior position with caput, and the fetal head is noted to protrude slightly through the introitus with each contraction. Which of the following features must be considered prior to attempted forceps delivery?

a. The head may not be engaged

b. At this station the pelvis is adequate

c. Diagnosed visually the station is +5

d. At this point low forceps may be applied without further evaluation

27–13. Which of the following defines shoulder dystocia?

a. Clinical perception of the delivering physician.

b. Maneuvers are needed to free the anterior shoulder.

c. Head to body delivery time is greater than 60 seconds.

d. All of the above

27–14. After a difficult delivery involving shoulder dystocia, the pediatrician tells you that the infant has suffered an injury. Which of the outcomes described below is most likely?

a. The mother had uterine atony.

b. The infant has a humeral fracture.

c. The infant has a clavicular fracture.

d. The infant exhibits a brachial plexus injury.

27–15. A 33-year-old multigravida is in clinic at 39 weeks' gestation and believes she has big baby. An ultrasound is performed, and the estimated fetal weight is 9 pounds. Which of the following is true?

a. Planned cesarean delivery may be offered.

b. Elective induction should be scheduled soon.

c. Shoulder dystocia may be accurately predicted.

d. Fetal macrosomia is a risk factor for shoulder dystocia.

27–16. The following illustration demonstrates which maneuver for reduction of shoulder dystocia?

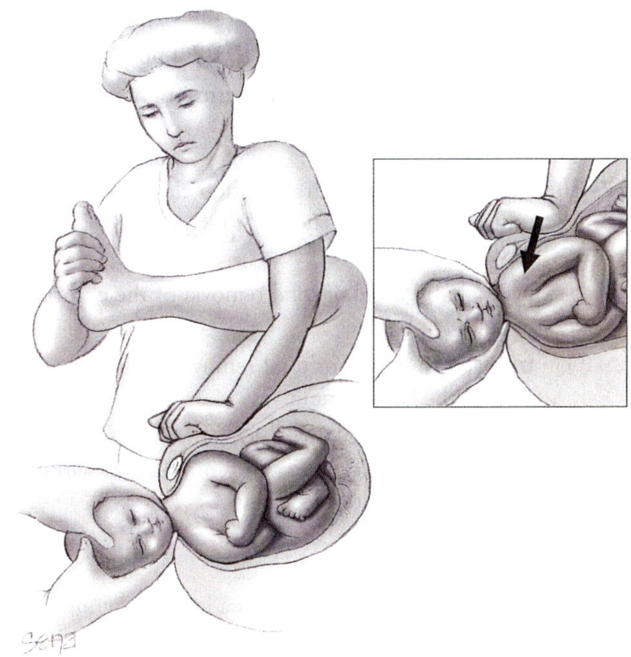

Reproduced with permission from Cunningham FG, Leveno KJ, Bloom SL, et al (eds): Vaginal delivery. In Williams Obstetrics, 25th ed. New York, McGraw-Hill, 2018, Figure 27-5.

a. Wood's screw

b. Rubin maneuver

c. McRoberts maneuver

d. Delivery of the posterior shoulder

27–17. The most common maneuver used to reduce a shoulder dystocia is which of the following?

a. Wood's screw

b. Rubin maneuver

c. Suprapubic pressure

d. McRoberts maneuver

27–18. Which of the following statistics concerning home birth is accurate?

a. 0.7% of deliveries in the United States are planned home births.

b. 0.2% of deliveries in the United States were unplanned home births.

c. In Norway 1.1% of unplanned home births ended in neonatal death.

d. All of the above

27–19. Which of the following is true concerning water birth?

a. Lower rates of anesthesia blocks

b. Increased rates of maternal infection

c. Risk for cord avulsion is 7/1000 births

d. Greater overall neonatal harm in low-risk populations

27–20. The World Health Organization classifies genital mutilation into four types. Which of the following descriptions is true?

a. Type I: Partial or total removal of the clitoris and/or prepuce

b. Type II: Partial or total removal of the clitoris and the labia minora

c. Type III: Partial or total removal of the labia minora and/or majora and infibulation without or without clitoridectomy

d. All of the above

27–21. When delivering a fetus with a lethal prognosis, you encounter shoulder dystocia. Which of the following maneuvers is least appropriate?

a. Cleidotomy

b. Cesarean delivery

c. Suprapubic pressure

d. McRoberts maneuver

27–22. A 35-year-old multigravida has just undergone a vaginal birth after cesarean delivery. Which of the following is a sign that the placenta is ready to be delivered?

a. Atonic fundus

b. Lengthening of the cord

c. Absence of vaginal bleeding

d. Fall of the uterus into the pelvis

27–23. Which of the following is true regarding oxytocin?

a. Side effect is hypotension

b. Mean half-life of 6–8 minutes

c. Onset of action is usually in 1 minute

d. Synthetic oxytocin is identical to that produced in the anterior pituitary

27–24. Approximately 2% of singleton births are accompanied by a delayed third stage. Possible reasons for this include which of the following?

a. Placenta adherens

b. Morbidly adherent placenta

c. Lower uterine segment contraction with a trapped placenta

d. All of the above

27–25. Which of the following descriptions of third-degree lacerations is accurate?

a. (1) <50% external anal sphincter tear

b. (2) 50% of external anal sphincter tear

c. (3a) >50% external anal sphincter tear

d. (3c) external anal sphincter plus internal anal sphincter tear

27–26. Risk factors for obstetrical anal sphincter injuries include which of the following?

a. Multiparity

b. Mediolateral episiotomy

c. Left occiput anterior position

d. None of the above

27–27. What is true concerning the illustrated perineal episiotomy below?

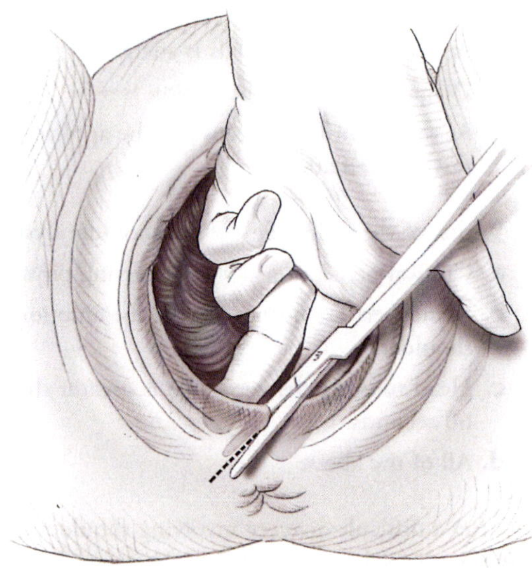

Reproduced with permission from Cunningham FG, Leveno KJ, Bloom SL, et al (eds): Vaginal delivery. In Williams Obstetrics, 25th ed. New York, McGraw-Hill, 2018, Figure 27-14.

a. Increased repair time

b. Increased dyspareunia

c. Increased rate of sphincter injury

d. All of the above

27–28. Indications for episiotomy include which of the following?

a. Breech delivery

b. Shoulder dystocia

c. Persistent occiput posterior position

d. All of the above

27–29. Which of the following is true regarding the repair of third-degree lacerations?

a. Antibiotics are not necessary.

b. The preferred suture is chromic.

c. The overlapping technique is only appropriate for type 3C lacerations.

d. The strength of the closure is derived from the striated muscle of the sphincter.

27–30. A 25-year-old G1P1 calls your office on postpartum day 6 complaining of increasing perineal pain for the last 24 hours. She underwent a successful forceps-assisted vaginal delivery complicated by a third-degree laceration. Which of the following is part of the differential diagnosis?

a. Wound infection

b. Urinary retention

c. Uterine involution

d. Excessive ambulation

27–31. After completion of a fourth-degree perineal laceration repair, you order which of the following medications?

a. Zosyn

b. Ampicillin

c. Dinoprostone

d. Second-generation cephalosporin

27–32. A 23-year-old G1P1 without medical problems has just undergone a spontaneous vaginal delivery. After delivery of the placenta, you note continued brisk bleeding. Exam suggests uterine atony. Which of the following is the next most appropriate medication?

a. Dinoprostone

b. Rectal misoprostol

c. Intravenous magnesium sulfate

d. Intramuscular methylergonovine

CHAPTER 27 ANSWER KEY

Question number	Letter answer	Page cited	Header cited
27–1	**b**	p. 516	Preparation for Delivery
27–2	**c**	p. 517	Delivery of the Head
27–3	**d**	p. 517	Delivery of the Head
27–4	**a**	p. 518	Delivery of the Shoulders
27–5	**d**	p. 518	Delivery of the Shoulders
27–6	**b**	p. 518	Delivery of the Shoulders
27–7	**d**	p. 519	Cord Clamping
27–8	**c**	p. 518	Cord Clamping
27–9	**d**	p. 519	Occiput Transverse Position
27–10	**b**	p. 519	Persistent Occiput Posterior Position
27–11	**d**	p. 519	Persistent Occiput Posterior Position
27–12	**a**	p. 520	Delivery
27–13	**d**	p. 520	Shoulder Dystocia
27–14	**d**	p. 520	Maternal and Neonatal Consequences
27–15	**d**	p. 520	Prediction and Prevention
27–16	**c**	p. 521	Figure 27-5
27–17	**c**	p. 521	Management
27–18	**d**	p. 524	Home Birth
27–19	**a**	p. 524	Water Birth
27–20	**d**	p. 525	Table 27-1
27–21	**b**	p. 525	Anomalous Fetuses
27–22	**b**	p. 526	Management of the Third Stage
27–23	**c**	p. 527	High-Dose Oxytocin
27–24	**d**	p. 527	Manual Removal of Placenta
27–25	**d**	p. 527	Birth Canal Lacerations
27–26	**d**	p. 529	Birth Canal Lacerations
27–27	**b**	p. 529	Episiotomy
27–28	**d**	p. 530	Indications
27–29	**c**	p. 532	Laceration and Episiotomy Repairs
27–30	**a**	p. 533	Perineal Laceration Care
27–31	**d**	p. 532	Laceration and Episiotomy Repairs
27–32	**d**	p. 527	Other Uterotonics

CHAPTER 28

Breech Presentation

28–1. Which of the following illustrations is labeled correctly?

a. Frank breech

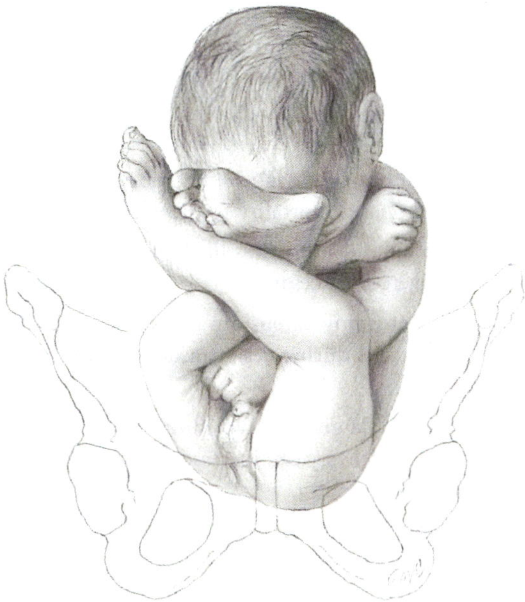

Reproduced with permission from Cunningham FG, Leveno KJ, Bloom SL, et al (eds): Breech delivery. In Williams Obstetrics, 25th ed. New York, McGraw-Hill, 2018, Figure 28-1.

b. Complete breech

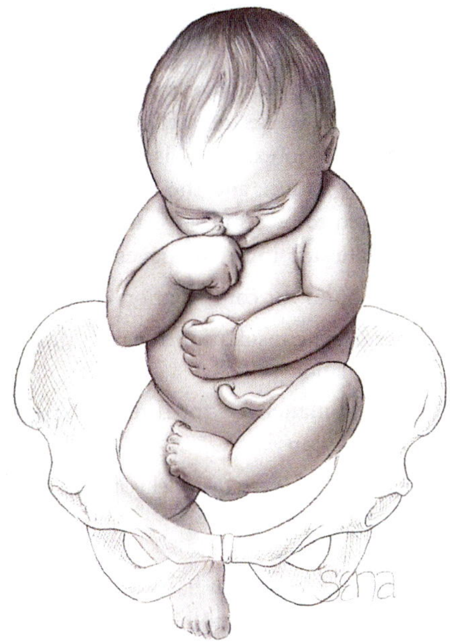

Reproduced with permission from Cunningham FG, Leveno KJ, Bloom SL, et al (eds): Breech delivery. In Williams Obstetrics, 25th ed. New York, McGraw-Hill, 2018, Figure 28-3.

c. Incomplete breech

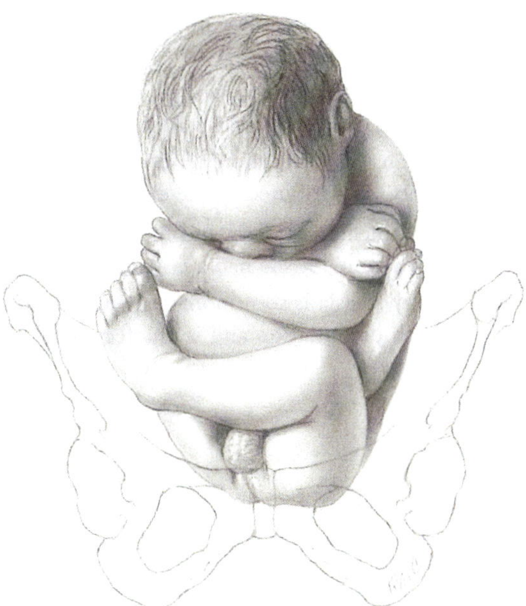

Reproduced with permission from Cunningham FG, Leveno KJ, Bloom SL, et al (eds): Breech delivery. In Williams Obstetrics, 25th ed. New York, McGraw-Hill, 2018, Figure 28-2.

d. None of the above

28–2. Among singleton pregnancies, breech presentation persists in what percentage at term?

a. 1–2%

b. 3–5%

c. 6–7%

d. 8–9%

28–3. Risk factors for breech presentation include which of the following?

a. Nulliparity

b. Prior breech fetus

c. Singleton gestation

d. None of the above

28–4. A 24-year-old primigravida presents to labor and delivery at 38 weeks' gestation. She is contracting regularly and on exam she is 4 cm dilated, 25% effaced, –3 station, and the fetal presenting part is suspected to be a foot. What is the next most appropriate step in her management?

a. Ultrasound for confirmation of fetal presentation

b. Anesthesia consultation for pain management during labor

c. Leopold maneuvers for further characterization of fetal position

d. Preparation for cesarean delivery due to non-cephalic presentation in labor

28–5. The Term Breech Trial has heavily influenced mode of delivery since its publication. Which of the following is a criticism of the study?

a. Mode of delivery was not randomized.

b. More than 10% of study participants had radiologic pelvimetry, which may have influenced management.

c. Many of the outcomes included in the "serious neonatal morbidity" composite did not portend long-term infant disability.

d. All of the above

28–6. Which of the following best characterizes the state of the literature regarding vaginal delivery of a term singleton breech?

a. Literature is mixed

b. Literature clearly shows trend to harm with planned vaginal delivery

c. Literature clearly shows no extra harm with planned vaginal delivery

d. None of the above

28–7. A 29-year-old multigravida is admitted to your antepartum service after premature rupture of membranes at 22 weeks' gestation. She is now 22 weeks 3 days and, after consultation with neonatology, she desires full resuscitation options at 23 weeks' gestation. Her fetus is breech. She understands that many factors are involved but inquires about which mode of delivery she should anticipate. Which of the following statements is most appropriate?

a. Cesarean would be considered after 23 weeks' gestation.

b. Cesarean would be recommended after 25 weeks' gestation.

c. Vaginal delivery would be recommended until 23 weeks' gestation.

d. All of the above

28–8. Which of the following is not true regarding maternal morbidity and mortality in breech delivery?

a. Maternal death is less likely if the breech fetus is delivered via cesarean.

b. Hysterotomy extensions can occur with the use of forceps during cesarean delivery of the breech fetus.

c. Anesthesia given to aid in uterine relaxation for vaginal delivery can increase the risk for postpartum hemorrhage.

d. Genital tract lacerations can occur with both vaginal and cesarean delivery of the breech fetus, and the risk of infection is increased.

28–9. A 28-year-old G3P2 presented in advanced labor with a fetus in frank breech presentation, and she delivered vaginally. Her 2-year-old is now undergoing therapy for hip dysplasia and Erb palsy. Which of the following is true regarding her daughter's condition?

a. Hip dysplasia is a known risk of vaginal breech delivery due to physical trauma.

b. Since it was not a shoulder dystocia, the Erb palsy cannot be attributed to the delivery.

c. Both the hip dysplasia and Erb palsy could have been avoided if she had a cesarean delivery.

d. Hip dysplasia is seen more frequently after breech presentation and is unaffected by mode of delivery.

28–10. When assessing candidacy for planned vaginal breech delivery, why are maternal pelvimetry and fetal ultrasound biometry correlation important?

a. The head is often larger than the breech.

b. The head of a breech fetus does not undergo molding during labor.

c. Ultrasound will help identify fetal anomalies that would alter candidacy.

d. All of the above

28–11. A 24-year-old multigravida at 39 weeks' gestation transfers care to you from her midwife due to breech presentation. She desires an unmedicated vaginal breech delivery. Which of the following in her history does not make her a good candidate for a vaginal breech delivery?

a. Diet-controlled gestational diabetes

b. A mid-pelvic interspinous distance of 11.9 cm

c. Ultrasound estimated fetal weight of 4200 grams

d. Desire to avoid anesthesia/analgesia during labor

28–12. What is the best indicator of pelvic adequacy for vaginal breech delivery?

a. Fetus in frank breech, right sacrum anterior position

b. Computed tomography scan of pelvic measurements

c. Steady cervical dilation and progressive descent of station with contractions

d. Clinical pelvimetry demonstrating inability to reach the sacral promontory

28–13. During a partial breech extraction, in the step pictured below, assisted delivery of the legs involves which of the following?

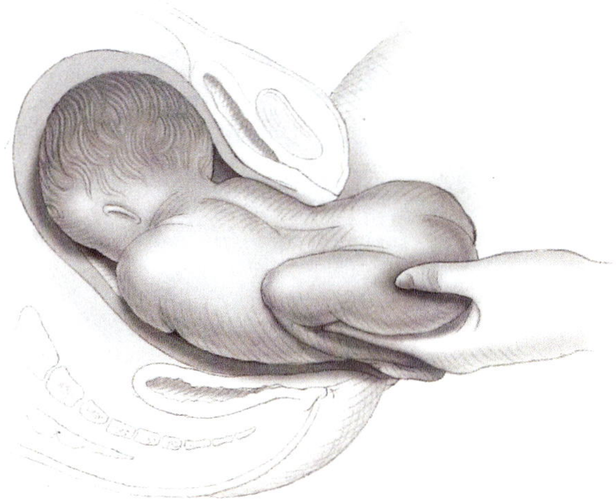

a. While holding the fetal buttock with one hand, the other hand sweeps up to find the fetal foot and downward traction results in delivery of the lower extremity.

b. While holding the fetal buttock with one hand, the other hand sweeps up to find the popliteal fossa and exerts pressure to adduct toward midline and sweep the leg downward.

c. While holding the fetal buttock with one hand, the other hand sweeps up to splint the femur with fingers parallel to the long axis and exerts pressure to abduct upward and laterally to sweep the leg away from midline.

d. None of the above

28–14. The image shown below demonstrates a fetus in which position?

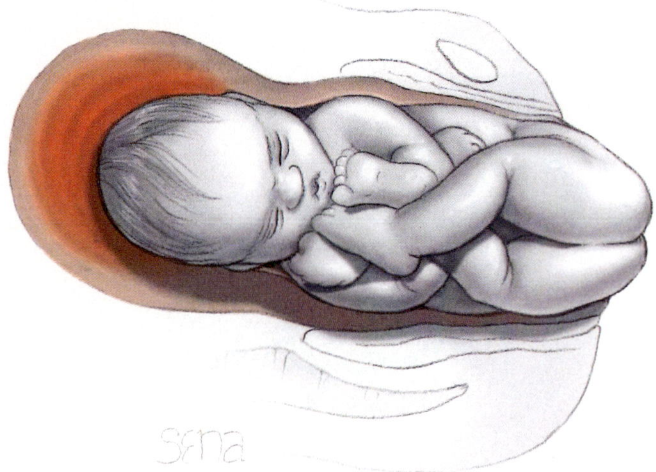

Reproduced with permission from Cunningham FG, Leveno KJ, Bloom SL, et al (eds): Breech delivery. In Williams Obstetrics, 25th ed. New York, McGraw-Hill, 2018, Figure 28-4.

a. Sacrum posterior

b. Left sacrum anterior

c. Right sacrum anterior

d. Left sacrum transverse

28–15. Which of the following statements is false regarding the tenets of partial breech extraction?

a. The breech is allowed to deliver spontaneously to the level of the umbilicus.

b. Following delivery of the legs, the fetal bony pelvis is grasped with both hands with fingers resting on the anterior superior iliac crests and thumbs on the sacrum.

c. After delivery of the fetal legs, steady, gentle, downward traction is employed until the lower halves of the scapulae are delivered with no effort to deliver shoulders and arms until one axilla is seen.

d. Once the breech has delivered to the level of the umbilicus, request cessation of maternal expulsive effort and patiently await spontaneous delivery of the shoulders with gentle support of the lower portion of the fetal body.

28–16. To resolve the complication shown in the image below, which of the following maneuvers should not be employed?

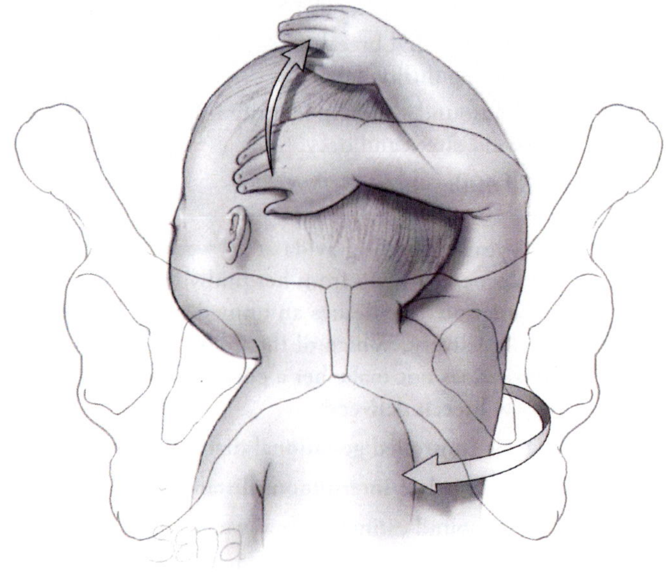

Reproduced with permission from Yeomans ER: Vaginal breech delivery. In Yeomans ER, Hoffman BL, Gilstrap LC III, et al (eds): Cunningham and Gilstrap's Operative Obstetrics, 3rd ed. New York, McGraw-Hill, 2017, Figure 31-13.

a. The fetus should be pulled downward to release the arm.

b. The fetus should be rotated 180 degrees clockwise in the case of the left arm.

c. The fetus should be rotated 180 degrees counterclockwise for the right arm.

d. The fetus is gently pushed upward back into the pelvis for second attempt at rotation if a primary maneuver is unsuccessful.

28–17. Which of the following correctly describes aspects of the Mariceau maneuver for delivery of the aftercoming head?

a. Suprapubic pressure is applied by an assistant to aid in keeping the head extended.

b. Two fingers of one hand grasp the shoulders of the back-down fetus from below while the other hand grasps both fetal feet, lifting up and over the maternal abdomen.

c. The index and middle finger of one hand are applied over the maxilla to flex the head while the fetal body rests on the palm of the same hand with legs straddling the forearm.

d. Once the suboccipital region of the fetal neck appears under the maternal symphysis, the fetal body is lowered below the plane of the maternal perineum to accomplish flexion and subsequent delivery of the head.

28–18. What is the utility of the maneuver demonstrated in the image below?

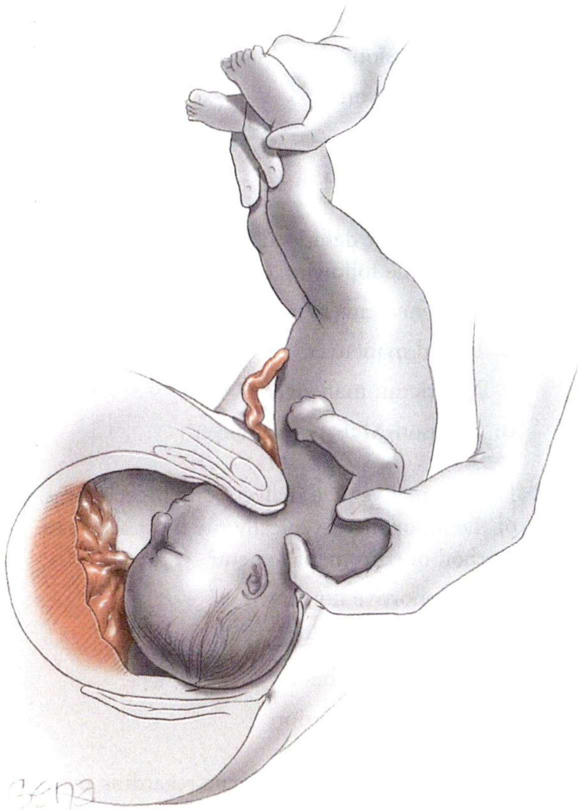

Reproduced with permission from Cunningham FG, Leveno KJ, Bloom SL, et al (eds): Breech delivery. In Williams Obstetrics, 25th ed. New York, McGraw-Hill, 2018, Figure 28-12.

- **a.** Safest maneuver for the delivery of the head of a preterm breech.
- **b.** Maneuver for delivery of the fetal head when the back is oriented posteriorly.
- **c.** Release of the aftercoming head in the setting of an incompletely dilated cervix.
- **d.** All of the above

28–19. Which of the following is true regarding the procedure being demonstrated in this image?

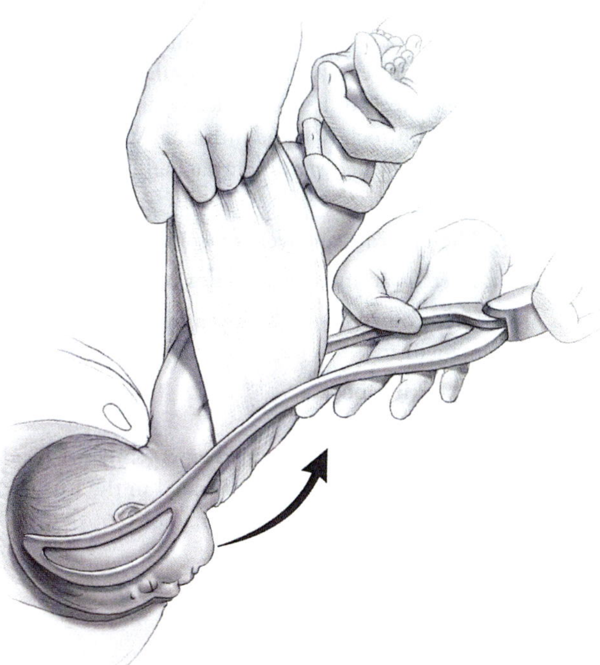

Reproduced with permission from Cunningham FG, Leveno KJ, Bloom SL, et al (eds): Breech delivery. In Williams Obstetrics, 25th ed. New York, McGraw-Hill, 2018, Figure 28-11c.

- **a.** The blades must be disarticulated prior to fetal head delivery.
- **b.** The blades are most easily placed with the provider elevated on a stool to achieve greater height.
- **c.** During application, the blade to be placed on the maternal left is held in the delivery provider's left hand with the provider's right hand protecting the maternal vaginal sidewall.
- **d.** The fetal body, wrapped in the towel, is allowed to rest on the shanks, and after the forceps are correctly placed, the forceps and fetal body are lowered to effect delivery of the head.

28–20. A 25-year-old G2P1001 at 30 weeks' gestation has been on the antepartum service for 2 weeks due to preterm rupture of membranes. Her most recent ultrasound showed an appropriately grown fetus in footling breech presentation with oligohydramnios. The nurse calls you because there are recurrent fetal heart rate decelerations to 70 beats per minute on her nonstress test. What is the initial verbal order you give to the nurse when you go to see the patient?

- **a.** Turn the patient on her left side
- **b.** Perform a sterile vaginal examination
- **c.** Start oxygen supplementation via facemask
- **d.** Obtain normal saline and an intrauterine pressure catheter so you can start an amnioinfusion.

28-21. The patient in Question 28–20 was determined to have two feet and a loop of umbilical cord at the vaginal introitus. Once in the operating room, general anesthesia is emergently induced and the fetal heart rate is 110 beats per minute. A repeat examination reveals that the scapulae of the fetus are past what feels to be a completely dilated cervix, and the fetal buttock is at the introitus. Which of the following is true regarding a vaginal breech delivery in this setting?

a. The Pinard maneuver is recommended.

b. There is an increased risk for head entrapment.

c. Uterotonics should be given during delivery maneuvers.

d. All of the above

28–22. Which maneuver, performed emergently for head entrapment, is being demonstrated in the image, and at what position are incisions made?

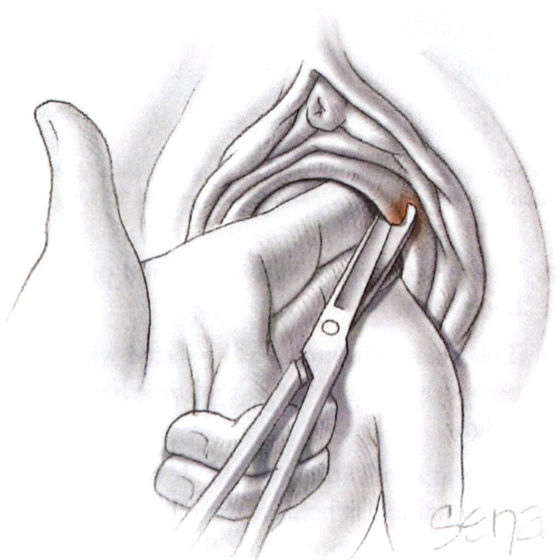

Reproduced with permission from Cunningham FG, Leveno KJ, Bloom SL, et al (eds): Breech delivery. In Williams Obstetrics, 25th ed. New York, McGraw-Hill, 2018, Figure 28-13.

a. Symphysiotomy at the symphyseal cartilage

b. Symphysiotomy at the symphyseal ligament

c. Dührssen incisions at 3:00, 9:00, and possibly 6:00

d. Dührssen incisions at 2:00, 10:00, and possibly 6:00

28–23. If the procedure performed in Question 28–23 is not successful, which of the following may aid in fetal delivery?

a. Piper forceps

b. Zavanelli maneuver

c. Suprapubic pressure

d. Subcutaneous nitroglycerine

28–24. What is the name of the process by which a frank breech fetus is manually converted to a footling breech presentation within the uterus during a cesarean or vaginal delivery?

a. Retroversion

b. Dextroflexion

c. Displacement

d. Decomposition

28–25. The maneuver described in Question 28–24 has which of the following eponyms?

a. Piper maneuver

b. Pinard maneuver

c. Mauriceau maneuver

d. Simpson-McLane maneuver

28–26. For planned vaginal delivery of a breech fetus, which of the following is typically the most adequate method of pain management?

a. A supportive doula

b. Pudendal anesthesia

c. Epidural anesthesia

d. Intravenous sedation

28–27. Which of the following is true regarding external cephalic version?

a. Overall success averages 80%

b. Success rate is lower with transverse lie than frank breech.

c. It is typically performed in women if breech persists at 36 weeks' gestation.

d. The American College of Obstetricians and Gynecologists recommends that version be offered and attempted whenever possible.

28–28. A 38-year-old multigravida is being seen for routine prenatal visit at 34 weeks' gestation. She had an ultrasound last week showing a fetus in breech presentation. She desires to avoid cesarean delivery and asks about external cephalic version. Which of the following statements is true?

a. Multiparity decreases the likelihood of a successful version.

b. External cephalic version is best offered at or after 36 weeks' gestation.

c. There is low chance for spontaneous vertex presentation at this gestational age.

d. Moxibustion is an alternative medicine technique that she could consider at this time.

28–29. Which of the following is an absolute contraindication to external cephalic version?

- **a.** Early labor
- **b.** Twin gestation
- **c.** Oligohydramnios
- **d.** Fetal-growth restriction

28–30. Which of the following is true regarding performance of external cephalic version?

- **a.** Immediate induction is indicated if version is successful.
- **b.** Anti-D immune globulin is administered to Rh-D negative women.
- **c.** Increased amnionic fluid is correlated with success, and amnioinfusion is routinely performed to increase version success.
- **d.** All of the above

28–31. External cephalic version success is improved with which of the following?

- **a.** Acute tocolysis
- **b.** Intravenous sedation
- **c.** Amnioinfusion to augment amnionic fluid volume
- **d.** All of the above

28–32. Internal podalic version is best characterized in which of the following?

- **a.** Manipulation within the uterus to yield a breech presentation, typically reserved for delivery of a second twin
- **b.** Manipulation within the uterus to yield a vertex presentation, typically reserved for the delivery of a second twin
- **c.** Manipulation within the uterus to yield a vertex presentation for a preterm breech fetus immediately after rupture of membranes
- **d.** None of the above

28–33. A patient presents for her postpartum visit after undergoing cesarean delivery at 40 weeks' gestation for breech presentation. No uterine anomaly was identified during the surgery. Is breech presentation more likely with her next pregnancy?

- **a.** Yes, with one prior breech presentation at term, recurrence is 6%.
- **b.** Yes, with one prior breech presentation at term, recurrence is 10%.
- **c.** Yes, with one prior breech presentation at term, recurrence is 28%.
- **d.** No, in the absence of a uterine anomaly, fetal presentation is random, and recurrence is not increased above baseline risk.

CHAPTER 28 ANSWER KEY

Question number	Letter answer	Page cited	Header cited
28–1	**a**	p. 539	Classification of Breech Presentations
28–2	**b**	p. 539	Introduction
28–3	**b**	p. 540	Risk Factors
28–4	**a**	p. 540	Examination
28–5	**c**	p. 541	Term Breech Fetus
28–6	**a**	p. 541	Term Breech Fetus
28–7	**d**	p. 541	Preterm Breech Fetus
28–8	**a**	p. 542	Delivery Complications
28–9	**d**	p. 542	Delivery Complications
28–10	**d**	p. 542	Imaging Techniques
28–11	**c**	p. 543	Table 28-1
28–12	**c**	p. 543	Vaginal Delivery Methods
28–13	**c**	p. 544	Partial Breech Extraction
28–14	**b**	p. 540	Examination
28–15	**d**	p. 545	Partial Breech Extraction
28–16	**a**	p. 546	Partial Breech Extraction
28–17	**c**	p. 546	Delivery of the Aftercoming Head
28–18	**b**	p. 547	Delivery of the Aftercoming Head
28–19	**c**	p. 547	Delivery of the Aftercoming Head
28–20	**b**	p. 548	Total Breech Extraction
28–21	**b**	p. 541 p. 548	Preterm Breech Fetus Head Entrapment
28–22	**d**	p. 548	Head Entrapment
28–23	**b**	p. 548	Head Entrapment
28–24	**d**	p. 549	Frank Breech
28–25	**b**	p. 549	Frank Breech
28–26	**c**	p. 543	Labor management
28–27	**d**	p. 549	External Cephalic Version
28–28	**d**	p. 550	External Cephalic Version
28–29	**b**	p. 550	External Cephalic Version
28–30	**b**	p. 550	External Cephalic Version
28–31	**a**	p. 550	External Cephalic Version
28–32	**a**	p. 549	External Cephalic Version
28–33	**b**	p. 540	Risk Factors

CHAPTER 29

Operative Vaginal Delivery

29–1. What is the ratio of vacuum-assisted to forceps-assisted vaginal deliveries?

a. 1:1

b. 2:1

c. 3:1

d. 4:1

29–2. All except which of the following are acceptable indications for operative vaginal delivery?

a. Aortic stenosis

b. Maternal exhaustion

c. Pelvic floor protection

d. 2nd stage labor $\geq$2 hours in a multipara with an epidural

29–3. A 31-year-old primigravida undergoing induction of labor reaches the 2nd stage of labor after 36 hours. Before beginning to push she says she is too tired and desires an operative vaginal delivery. Which of the following precludes her from having an elective operative vaginal delivery?

a. Head is at +1 station

b. Head is in occiput anterior position

c. Scalp is visible at the introitus without labial separation

d. All of the above

29–4. Which of the following is a prerequisite for vacuum extraction, but not a forceps-assisted vaginal delivery?

a. Epidural anesthesia

b. Minimum +2 station

c. Assistant to create suction

d. Minimum 34 weeks' gestation

29–5. Which of the following is true of high forceps?

a. No role in modern obstetrics

b. Indicated for fetal bradycardia

c. Forceps applied when the fetal head is engaged

d. Indicated for those with a prolonged second stage

29–6. Which of the following criteria must be met prior to performing an operative vaginal delivery?

a. Adequate anesthesia

b. Maternal bladder emptied

c. Known fetal head position

d. All of the above

29–7. A 32-year-old multigravida with an epidural in place has been pushing for 2 hours with poor descent. The fetal head is positioned left occiput posterior. Forceps delivery of this patient would be classified as which of the following?

a. Low

b. High

c. Outlet

d. Low outlet

29–8. Which of the following describes forceps that are applied to the fetal head with the scalp visible at the introitus without separation of the labia?

a. Low

b. Mid

c. High

d. Outlet

29–9. Maternal morbidity with forceps delivery is most closely predicted by which of the following?

a. Fetal station

b. Maternal parity

c. Fetal gestational age

d. Length of the second stage

29–10. In addition to operative vaginal delivery, which of the following is a risk factor for urinary retention?

a. Parity

b. Episiotomy

c. Labial swelling

d. Length of the second stage

29–11. Which of the following occurs more frequently with forceps-assisted vaginal delivery compared to vacuum-assisted vaginal deliveries?

a. Uterine atony
b. Urinary retention
c. Prolonged hospital stay
d. Vaginal wall lacerations

29–12. Which of the following interventions may reduce maternal perineal laceration during a forceps-assisted vaginal delivery?

a. Early disarticulation
b. Mediolateral episiotomy
c. Cessation of pushing during disarticulation
d. All of the above

29–13. The perinatal complication shown below is seen more frequently with which of the following delivery routes?

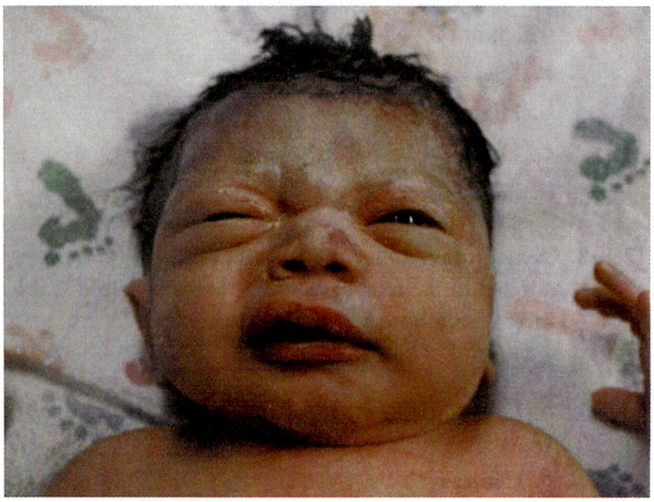

a. Forceps delivery
b. Cesarean delivery
c. Vacuum extraction
d. Spontaneous vaginal delivery

29–14. What is the mechanism for the injury pictured in Question 29–13?

a. Intracranial hemorrhage
b. Shoulder dystocia from a forceps delivery
c. Compression of the facial nerve by the forceps blade
d. None of the above

29–15. A subgaleal hemorrhage is seen more frequently with which of the following delivery routes?

a. Forceps delivery
b. Cesarean delivery
c. Vacuum extraction
d. Spontaneous vaginal delivery

29–16. A 32-year-old primigravida with an epidural has been pushing for 3 hours. Fetal position is occiput posterior, station is +2, and estimated fetal weight is 3400 grams. You consider an operative vaginal delivery for maternal exhaustion. Which of the following is associated with failure of an operative delivery?

a. Primigravida
b. Full maternal bladder
c. Occiput posterior position
d. Estimated fetal weight ≥3400 grams

29–17. The opening in this forceps blade mainly serves which of the following functions?

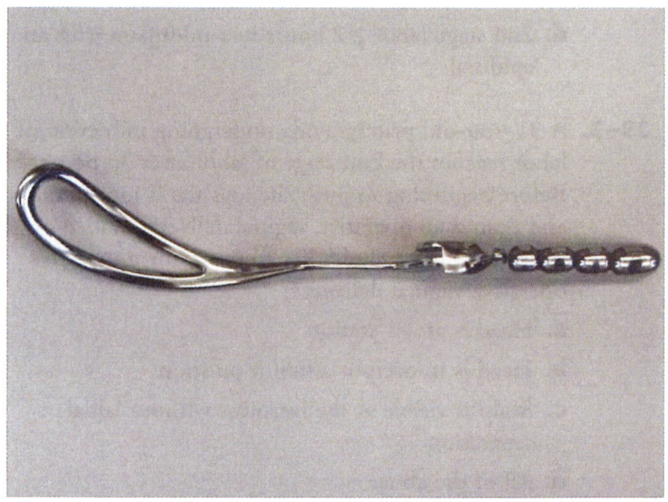

a. Protects the fetal ears
b. Allows blades to grip the fetal head firmly
c. Offers a smaller metal surface area against the fetal skull
d. Provides diminished traction forces against the maternal vaginal sidewall

29–18. During placement of a forceps blade, what is the purpose of having the right hand between the fetal head and the vaginal sidewall?

a. Protects the fetal ears
b. Identifies the ischial spines
c. Reduces maternal discomfort during placement
d. Guides the blade into position and protects the vaginal sidewall

29–19. In the setting of an occiput posterior position, correctly placed blades are equidistant from what landmark?

a. Fetal ears
b. Sagittal suture
c. Lambdoidal sutures
d. Midline of the face and brow

29–20. How is asynclitism resolved after placement of forceps?

a. It cannot be resolved
b. Removing and replacing the forceps
c. Pulling and/or pushing each branch along the long axis
d. Proceeding with downward traction, and it will spontaneously resolve

29–21. What forces are produced by a forceps-assisted vaginal delivery?

a. Friction
b. Traction
c. Compression
d. All of the above

29–22. Which of the following actions is necessary to rotate a fetus from an occiput posterior to an occiput anterior position?

a. Flexion of the fetal head
b. Disengaging the fetal head
c. Fundal pressure to allow easier access to the fetal head
d. All of the above

29–23. Which of the following pelvic types is generally associated with persistent occiput posterior position?

a. Android
b. Gynecoid
c. Anthropoid
d. Platypelloid

29–24. In attempting a rotation from occiput anterior to occiput posterior, which type of forceps is best employed?

a. Piper
b. Luikart
c. Kielland
d. Simpson

29–25. In all except which of the following presentations may forceps be used?

a. Mentum anterior
b. Occiput posterior
c. Mentum posterior
d. Occiput transverse

29–26. Which of the following is true concerning the vacuum device pictured below compared to a soft cup system?

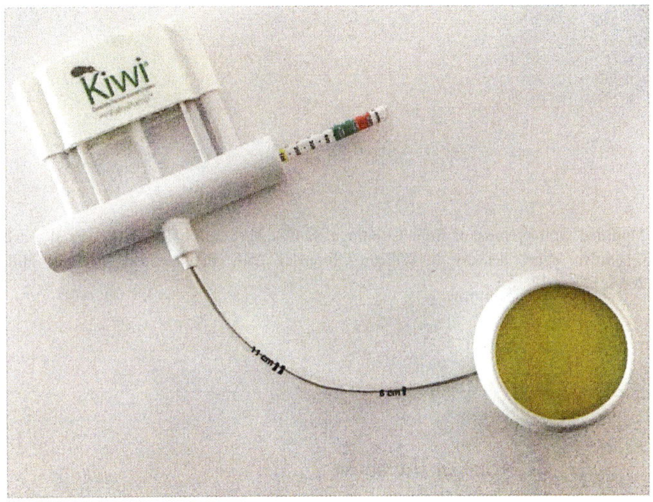

a. Allows easier placement
b. Allows more traction force
c. Higher scalp laceration rates
d. All of the above

SECTION 8

29–27. In the diagram below, which letter corresponds to the flexion point where the center of the cup should be placed?

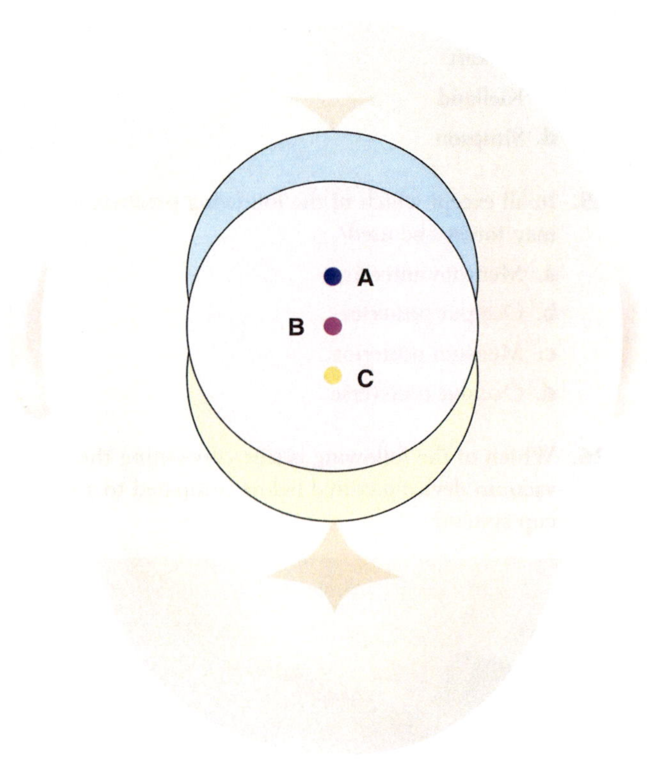

Modified with permission from Cunningham FG, Leveno KJ, Bloom SL, et al (eds): Operative vaginal delivery. In William Obstetrics, 24th ed. New York, McGraw-Hill, 2014, Figure 29-16.

- **a.** A
- **b.** B
- **c.** C
- **d.** None of the above

29–28. What is the purpose of placing the cup over the flexion point?

- **a.** Maximizes traction
- **b.** Minimizes cup detachment
- **c.** Delivers the smallest head diameter
- **d.** All of the above

29–29. Which of the following is the preferred total negative pressure generated prior to initiation of traction during vacuum extraction?

- **a.** 0.2 kg/cm^2
- **b.** 0.8 kg/cm^2
- **c.** 1.2 kg/cm^2
- **d.** 1.6 kg/cm^2

29–30. During a vacuum-assisted vaginal delivery, all except which of the following is the purpose of having the nondominant hand simultaneously on the cup and the fetal hand?

- **a.** Prevent a "pop-off"
- **b.** Gauge traction angle
- **c.** Detect cup separation
- **d.** Judge descent of the fetal head

29–31. In general, vacuum extraction would be contraindicated in all except which of the following clinical settings?

- **a.** 30-week fetus
- **b.** Fetal thrombocytopenia
- **c.** Inability to assess fetal station
- **d.** Occiput transverse presentation

29–32. Ideally, traction during vacuum extraction should be applied in which of the following manners?

- **a.** Continuously
- **b.** Intermittently and with contractions
- **c.** Intermittently and between contractions
- **d.** Intermittently with cycles of 20 seconds of traction followed by 1 minute of rest

CHAPTER 29 ANSWER KEY

Question number	Letter answer	Page cited	Header cited
29–1	**d**	p. 553	Introduction
29–2	**c**	p. 553	Indications
29–3	**a**	p. 553	Indications
29–4	**d**	p. 554	Classification and Prerequisites
29–5	**a**	p. 554	Classification and Prerequisites
29–6	**d**	p. 554	Table 29-1
29–7	**d**	p. 554	Table 29-1
29–8	**d**	p. 554	Table 29-1
29–9	**a**	p. 553	Classification and Prerequisites
29–10	**b**	p. 554	Classification and Prerequisites
29–11	**d**	p. 555	Lacerations
29–12	**d**	p. 555	Lacerations
29–13	**a**	p. 555	Acute Perinatal Injury
29–14	**c**	p. 556	Mechanisms of Acute Injury
29–15	**c**	p. 555	Acute Perinatal Injury
29–16	**c**	p. 556	Trial of Operative Vaginal Delivery
29–17	**b**	p. 557	Design
29–18	**d**	p. 557	Blade Application and Delivery
29–19	**d**	p. 558	Blade Application and Delivery
29–20	**c**	p. 558	Blade Application and Delivery
29–21	**d**	p. 560	Blade Application and Delivery
29–22	**a**	p. 561	Blade Application and Delivery
29–23	**c**	p. 561	Blade Application and Delivery
29–24	**a**	p. 561	Blade Application and Delivery
29–25	**c**	p. 562	Face Presentations
29–26	**d**	p. 562	Vacuum Extractor Design
29–27	**a**	p. 563	Technique
29–28	**d**	p. 563	Technique
29–29	**b**	p. 563	Technique
29–30	**a**	p. 564	Technique
29–31	**d**	p. 554	Table 29-1
29–32	**b**	p. 564	Technique

CHAPTER 30

Cesarean Delivery and Peripartum Hysterectomy

30–1. Of the following indications for primary cesarean delivery, which is least common?

- **a.** Fetal jeopardy
- **b.** Labor dystocia
- **c.** Placenta previa
- **d.** Malpresentation

30–2. Which of the following indications for primary cesarean delivery is most inappropriate?

- **a.** Malpresentation
- **b.** Prior cesarean delivery
- **c.** Unknown uterine scar type
- **d.** Early-onset severe preeclampsia

30–3. Which of the following is least likely to have contributed to the rising rate of primary cesarean delivery between 1970 and 2009?

- **a.** Abnormal placentation
- **b.** Electronic fetal monitoring
- **c.** Decrease in rates of vaginal birth after cesarean delivery
- **d.** Decrease in vaginal delivery rates for breech presentation

30–4. A 34-year-old primigravida at 39 weeks' gestation undergoes primary cesarean delivery on maternal request. Compared to a woman with a vaginal delivery, which of the following adverse neonatal outcomes is more likely to occur?

- **a.** Infection
- **b.** Birth trauma
- **c.** Respiratory distress syndrome
- **d.** Hypoxic ischemic encephalopathy

30–5. Which of the following maternal obstetrical complications is increased with cesarean delivery as compared to vaginal delivery?

- **a.** Infection
- **b.** Hemorrhage
- **c.** Thromboembolism
- **d.** All of the above

30–6. A 22-year-old G1 at 39 weeks' gestation with no prenatal care arrives on labor and delivery in active labor. When completing her delivery consents she declines all blood products due to religious beliefs. Which of the following interventions would be most helpful at this time?

- **a.** Minimize blood draws
- **b.** Erythropoietin administration
- **c.** Iron and folic acid administration
- **d.** Proactive administration of uterotonics if atony occurs

30–7. A 20-year-old primigravida presents at 40 weeks' gestation with elevated blood pressures and a headache. She is diagnosed with severe preeclampsia, and induction of labor is begun. After 28 hours she has made no cervical change and the decision is made to proceed with primary cesarean delivery. Which of the following interventions has been proven to decrease her risk of postoperative wound infection, in addition to 2 grams of cefazolin prior to skin incision?

- **a.** Shaving of surgical site
- **b.** Azithromycin 500 mg intravenous
- **c.** Preparation of the vagina with povidone-iodine
- **d.** All of the above

30–8. A 29-year-old woman at 40 weeks' gestation is scheduled to undergo primary cesarean delivery for malpresentation. She weighs 310 pounds, with a body mass index of 54 kg/m^2. She asks which type of skin incision is recommended, and you recommend a periumbilical vertical midline incision. Which of the following is true regarding a vertical midline as compared to transverse skin incision for this patient?

- **a.** Decreased risk of neuropathy
- **b.** Greater ease with wound care
- **c.** Decreased risk of subfascial hematoma
- **d.** All of the above

30–9. A 42-year-old G3P2 is scheduled to undergo a repeat cesarean delivery. She reports heavy menstrual bleeding outside of pregnancy and requests cesarean hysterectomy. You inform the patient this is not an indication for cesarean hysterectomy given the associated risks. You counsel her that cesarean hysterectomy increases her risk of which of the following?

a. Infection

b. Chronic pelvic pain

c. Urinary tract damage

d. None of the above

30–10. The patient in Question 30–9 is completing the consent for her repeat cesarean delivery. You discuss the risks of bowel, bladder, and ureteral injury. Which of the following most closely approximates the risk of ureteral injury at the time of cesarean delivery?

a. 1 in 500

b. 1 in 1000

c. 1 in 2000

d. 1 in 3000

30–11. A 25-year-old G2P1 at 39 weeks' gestation is undergoing trial of labor after a cesarean delivery in her previous pregnancy. She progresses to the second stage of labor, but after 3 hours of maternal effort a fetal bradycardia occurs for which an emergent cesarean delivery is performed. Which of the following circumstances increases her risk of unintentional cystotomy?

a. History of prior cesarean delivery

b. Need for emergent cesarean delivery

c. Cesarean delivery in the second stage of labor

d. All of the above

30–12. During the delivery in Question 30–11, an unintentional cystotomy occurs. It is noted to be present in the dome of the bladder, and good efflux is noted from bilateral ureteral orifices. Which suture is most appropriate for repair of the bladder mucosa and muscularis layers?

a. 3.0 vicryl

b. 1.0 chromic

c. 2.0 chromic

d. 4.0 monocryl

30–13. A 30-year-old G4P3 at 39 weeks' gestation undergoes repeat cesarean delivery, which is remarkable for extensive adhesive disease. Postoperatively she is noted to have minimal urine output, abdominal distention, and severe abdominal pain. Her vital signs are remarkable for mild tachycardia with blood pressure 118/78 mmHg, and her hematocrit is noted to be stable from the preoperative value of 32%. Her Foley is replaced and she receives multiple boluses of crystalloid without improvement in urine output. What is the next best step in management?

a. Transfusion

b. Lasix administration

c. Intravenous pyelography

d. Abdominal computed tomography with cystography

30–14. A 30-year-old G3P3 presents to the emergency department on postoperative day 4 complaining of 24 hours of severe abdominal pain and intractable nausea and vomiting. Her oral temperature is 39 °C; she is tachycardic with a heart rate of 140 bpm and appears pale and diaphoretic. What is the best next step in management?

a. Intravenous antibiotics

b. Exploratory laparotomy

c. Placement of nasogastric tube, bowel rest

d. None of the above

30–15. Which of the following is a risk factor for urinary retention after cesarean delivery?

a. Hemorrhage

b. Prior cesarean delivery

c. Postoperative narcotic analgesia

d. All of the above

30–16. A 21-year-old primigravida at 41 weeks' gestation is undergoing labor induction for oligohydramnios. She progresses to the second stage of labor, but the fetal head does not descend below 0 station despite 3 hours of pushing efforts. Cesarean delivery is undertaken, but extraction is difficult and requires upward pressure from the vagina. A radiograph of the newborn head is shown here and reveals a depressed skull fracture (*white arrow*). Approximately what percentage of cesarean deliveries is complicated by some type of fetal injury?

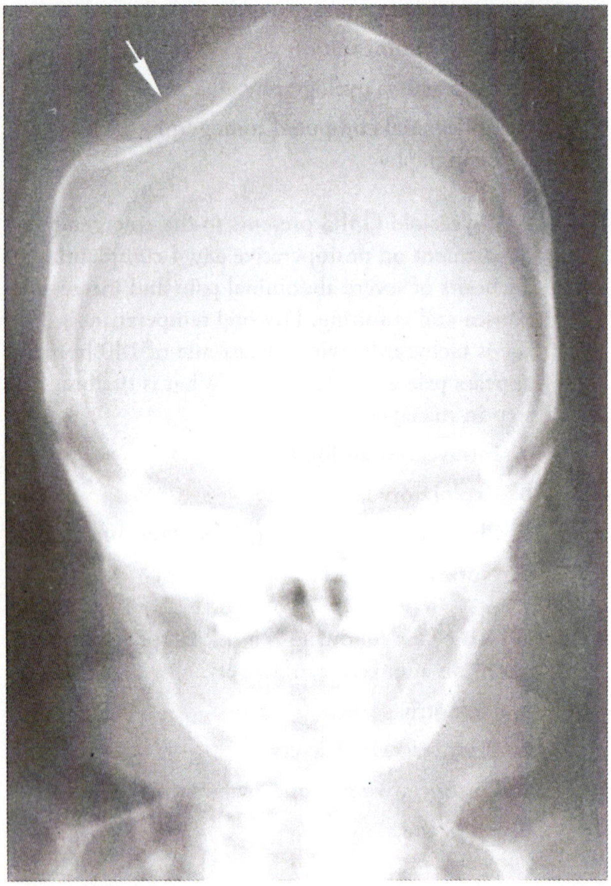

Reproduced with permission from Cunningham FG, Leveno KJ, Bloom SL, et al (eds): Diseases and injuries of the term newborn. In Williams Obstetrics, 24th ed. New York, McGraw-Hill, 2014, Figure 33-1.

a. 0.1%
b. 0.5%
c. 1.0%
d. 2.0%

30–17. Although not recommended by the American College of Obstetricians and Gynecologists, elective cesarean delivery on maternal request should only be considered as an option when which of the following criteria have been met?

a. Permanent sterilization will be performed
b. There is concern for inadequate pain control in labor
c. The pregnancy has reached at least 39 completed weeks
d. The patient has a history of fetal injury in a prior delivery

30–18. Which of the following preoperative interventions is no longer recommended to decrease maternal risk at the time of cesarean delivery?

a. Antacid administration
b. Foley catheter placement
c. Shaving of pubic hair with a razor
d. Administration of antibiotics prior to skin incision

30–19. Recommendations for antibiotic prophylaxis at cesarean delivery for women with a significant penicillin allergy include a single dose of which of the following agents?

a. Levofloxacin
b. Clindamycin
c. Gentamicin plus clindamycin
d. Vancomycin plus piperacillin-tazobactam

30–20. To reduce postoperative morbidity, the American College of Obstetricians and Gynecologists recommends antibiotic prophylaxis be given within how many minutes prior to skin incision?

a. 10 minutes
b. 30 minutes
c. 60 minutes
d. 90 minutes

30–21. When creating a Pfannenstiel skin incision, which vessels should be anticipated halfway between the skin and fascia, several centimeters from the midline?

a. Inferior epigastrics
b. External pudendals
c. Superficial epigastrics
d. Superficial circumflex iliacs

30–22. Compared with a vertical midline incision, a Pfannenstiel incision offers which of the following benefits?

a. Less postoperative pain
b. Improved cosmetic result
c. Less risk of incisional hernia
d. All of the above

30–23. When performing dissection through a Pfannenstiel incision, the two fascial layers are incised as illustrated in this image. The first layer encountered, which is incised in this image, is the aponeurosis of what muscle?

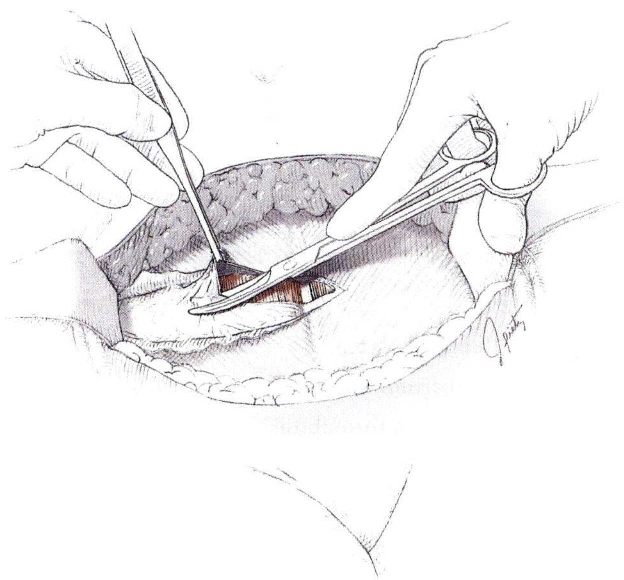

Reproduced with permission from Word L, Hoffman BL: Surgeries for benign gynecologic conditions. In Hoffman BL, Schorge JO, Schaffer JI, et al (eds) Williams Gynecology, 2nd ed. New York, McGraw-Hill, 2012, Figure 41-2.1.

a. Transversalis
b. Internal oblique
c. External oblique
d. Transversus abdominis

30–24. Which of the following benefits are seen with low transverse uterine incisions in comparison to classical incisions?

a. Ease of closure
b. Less likely to rupture in subsequent pregnancies
c. Lower risk of incisional adhesions to bowel or omentum
d. All of the above

30–25. Failure to recognize dextrorotation of the uterus prior to hysterotomy increases the risk of damage to which structure?

a. Left ureter
b. Right ureter
c. Left uterine artery
d. Right uterine artery

30–26. Extension of the hysterotomy may be accomplished with two different methods, as shown below. Compared with blunt extension, the use of bandage scissors for sharp extension has been associated with an increase in which of the following?

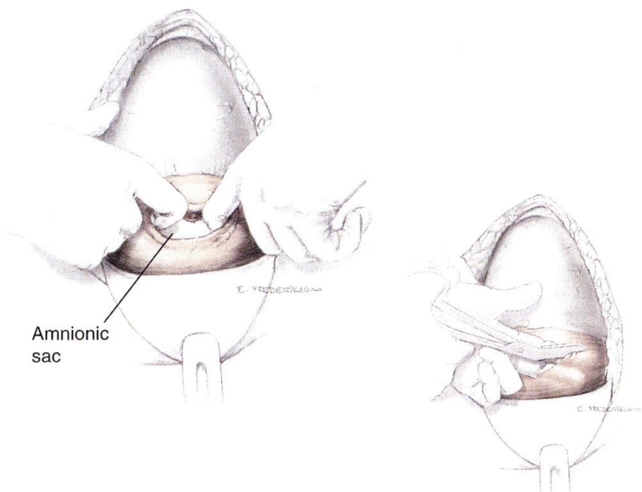

Reproduced with permission from Cunningham FG, Leveno KJ, Bloom SL, et al (eds): Cesarean delivery and peripartum hysterectomy. In Williams Obstetrics, 25th ed. New York, McGraw-Hill, 2018, Figure 30-5.

a. Blood loss
b. Operative time
c. Unintended extensions
d. All of the above

30–27. During cesarean delivery a hysterotomy is made in the lower uterine segment, as shown here. In which of the following settings should the incision be made relatively higher on the uterus to avoid uterine vessel laceration or unintended entry into the vagina?

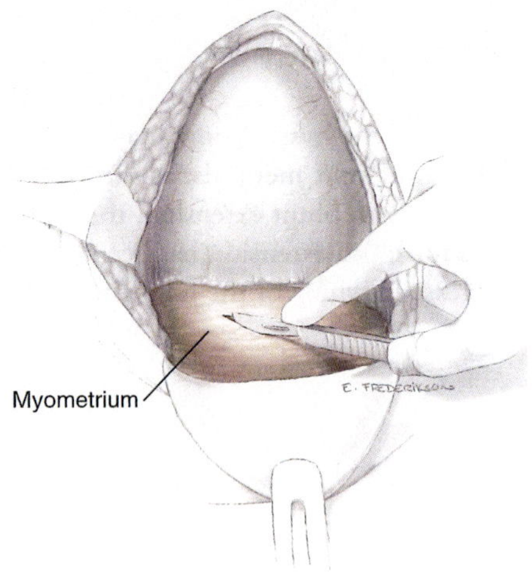

Reproduced with permission from Cunningham FG, Leveno KJ, Bloom SL, et al (eds): Cesarean delivery and peripartum hysterectomy. In Williams Obstetrics, 25th ed. New York, McGraw-Hill, 2018, Figure 30-4.

- **a.** Maternal anemia
- **b.** Fetal malpresentation
- **c.** A completely dilated cervix
- **d.** Cesarean performed prior to onset of labor

30–28. Compared with manual extraction, spontaneous delivery of the placenta with fundal massage, as shown below, has been shown to reduce the risk of which complication?

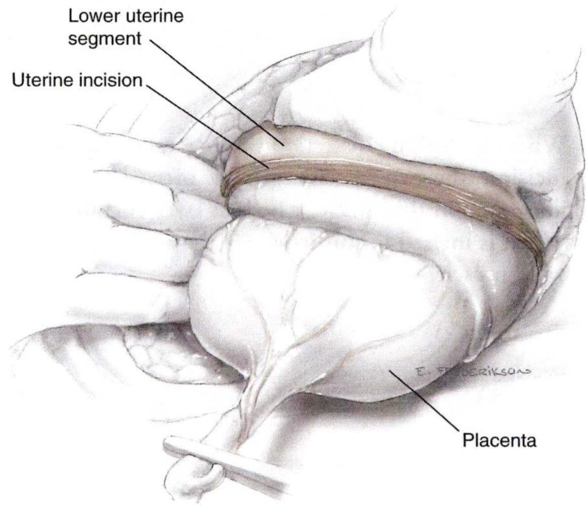

Reproduced with permission from Cunningham FG, Leveno KJ, Bloom SL, et al (eds): Cesarean delivery and peripartum hysterectomy. In Williams Obstetrics, 25th ed. New York, McGraw-Hill, 2018, Figure 30-9.

- **a.** Retained placenta
- **b.** Postpartum infection
- **c.** Deep-vein thrombosis
- **d.** Amniotic fluid embolism

30–29. Which of the following is a disadvantage of uterine exteriorization for repair of the hysterotomy, as show below?

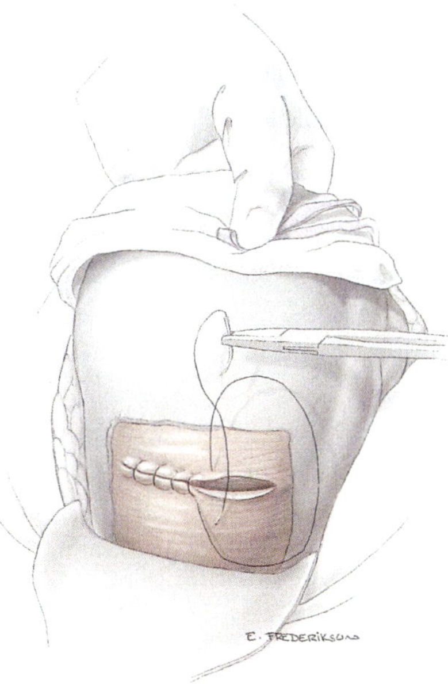

Reproduced with permission from Cunningham FG, Leveno KJ, Bloom SL, et al (eds): Cesarean delivery and peripartum hysterectomy. In Williams Obstetrics, 25th ed. New York, McGraw-Hill, 2018, Figure 30-10.

a. Increased blood loss
b. Increased febrile morbidity
c. Increased nausea and vomiting
d. Increased postoperative infection

30–30. Which of the following interventions is most likely to decrease adhesion formation at the time of cesarean delivery?

a. Achieving hemostasis
b. Closure of the peritoneum
c. Placement of an adhesion barrier at the hysterotomy
d. All of the above

30–31. What is a potential advantage of closure of the parietal peritoneum prior to closure of the fascia at the time of cesarean delivery?

a. Shorter operative time
b. Less adhesion formation
c. Decreased postoperative pain
d. Avoidance of distended bowel at the time of fascial closure

30–32. Which of the following is a theoretical benefit of using a monofilament suture such as polydioxanone (PDS) to close the fascial layer, as opposed to a braided suture such as polyglactin (vicryl)?

a. Decreased risk of infection
b. Lower half-life tensile strength
c. Decreased risk of knot slippage
d. All of the above

30–33. Which of the following is a potential indication for a classical hysterotomy, as shown below?

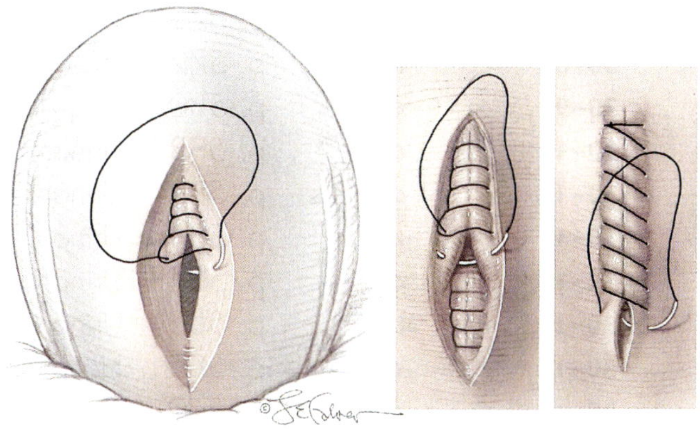

Reproduced with permission from Cunningham FG, Leveno KJ, Bloom SL, et al (eds): Cesarean delivery and peripartum hysterectomy. In Williams Obstetrics, 25th ed. New York, McGraw-Hill, 2018, Figure 30-12.

a. Maternal morbid obesity
b. Densely adherent bladder
c. Back-down transverse fetal lie
d. All of the above

30–34. A 33-year-old G3P2 with two prior cesarean deliveries presents at 35 weeks' gestation with active vaginal bleeding and fetal heart rate decelerations. She is taken for emergent repeat cesarean delivery and is found to have a placenta previa with accreta that requires cesarean hysterectomy. Compared with patients who have this procedure planned, this woman is at increased risk for which of the following complications?

a. Bladder injury
b. Ureteral injury
c. Blood transfusion
d. All of the above

30–35. Women who have normal blood volume expansion in pregnancy and a hematocrit of at least 30% will usually tolerate blood loss up to what volume without hemodynamic compromise?

a. 2000 mL
b. 3000 mL
c. 4000 mL
d. 5000 mL

CHAPTER 30 ANSWER KEY

Question number	Letter answer	Page cited	Header cited
30–1	c	p. 567	Cesarean Delivery in the United States
30–2	d	p. 568	Cesarean Delivery in the United States
30–3	a	p. 568	Cesarean Delivery in the United States
30–4	c	p. 569	Cesarean Delivery Risks
30–5	d	p. 568	Cesarean Delivery Risks
30–6	d	p. 569	Cesarean Delivery Risks
30–7	b	p. 571	Patient Preparation
30–8	d	p. 572	Cesarean Delivery Technique
30–9	c	p. 580	Peripartum Hysterectomy
30–10	d	p. 583	Urinary Tract or Bowel Injury
30–11	d	p. 583	Urinary Tract or Bowel Injury
30–12	a	p. 584	Urinary Tract or Bowel Injury
30–13	d	p. 584	Urinary Tract or Bowel Injury
30–14	b	p. 585	Urinary Tract or Bowel Injury
30–15	c	p. 585	Hospital Care until Discharge
30–16	c	p. 569	Cesarean Delivery Risks
30–17	c	p. 569	Cesarean Delivery Risks
30–18	c	p. 570	Patient Preparation
30–19	c	p. 571	Patient Preparation
30–20	c	p. 571	Patient Preparation
30–21	c	p. 572	Cesarean Delivery Technique
30–22	d	p. 571	Cesarean Delivery Technique
30–23	c	p. 572	Cesarean Delivery Technique
30–24	d	p. 573	Cesarean Delivery Technique
30–25	c	p. 573	Cesarean Delivery Technique
30–26	d	p. 575	Cesarean Delivery Technique
30–27	c	p. 574	Cesarean Delivery Technique
30–28	b	p. 576	Cesarean Delivery Technique
30–29	c	p. 577	Cesarean Delivery Technique
30–30	a	p. 578	Cesarean Delivery Technique
30–31	d	p. 578	Cesarean Delivery Technique
30–32	a	p. 578	Cesarean Delivery Technique
30–33	d	p. 578	Cesarean Delivery Technique
30–34	d	p. 582	Peripartum Hysterectomy
30–35	a	p. 585	Postoperative Care

CHAPTER 31

Prior Cesarean Delivery

31–1. Which of the following factors favors a successful trial of labor in a woman with a prior cesarean delivery?

- **a.** White race
- **b.** Single mother
- **c.** Increased maternal age
- **d.** Short interdelivery interval

31–2. What is the estimated relative risk of uterine rupture in women undergoing trial of labor after cesarean delivery compared to those choosing elective repeat cesarean delivery?

- **a.** 5
- **b.** 10
- **c.** 15
- **d.** 20

31–3. Which maternal complication is not increased in women undergoing trial of labor after cesarean delivery compared to those electing repeat cesarean delivery?

- **a.** Transfusion
- **b.** Hysterectomy
- **c.** Uterine infection
- **d.** Uterine dehiscence

31–4. You are taking care of a 25-year-old G2P1 at 36 weeks' gestation who underwent emergent primary cesarean delivery for suspected fetal distress in her first pregnancy. Her uterine incision closure from the time of surgery is pictured. If she chooses a trial of labor for this pregnancy, what is her absolute risk of uterine rupture?

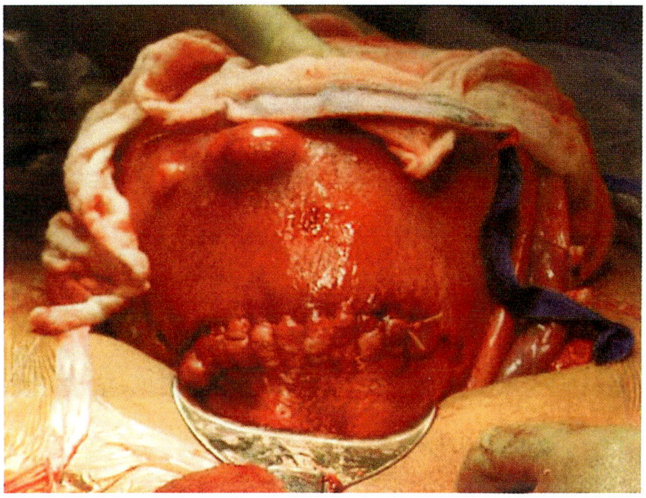

- **a.** 3/1000
- **b.** 7/1000
- **c.** 13/1000
- **d.** 19/1000

31–5. Which of the following neonatal morbidities are increased with trial of labor after cesarean delivery compared to elective repeat cesarean delivery?

- **a.** Respiratory distress syndrome
- **b.** Hypoxic ischemic encephalopathy
- **c.** Transient tachypnea of the newborn
- **d.** All of the above

31–6. You are caring for a 26-year old G2P1 who presents at 39 weeks' gestation in active labor. She has a history of prior cesarean delivery for breech presentation in her last pregnancy. This pregnancy has otherwise been uncomplicated. What is her approximate chance of a successful trial of labor?

a. 30%

b. 55%

c. 75%

d. 95%

31–7. What is the chance of uterine rupture based on the scar type shown in the photograph?

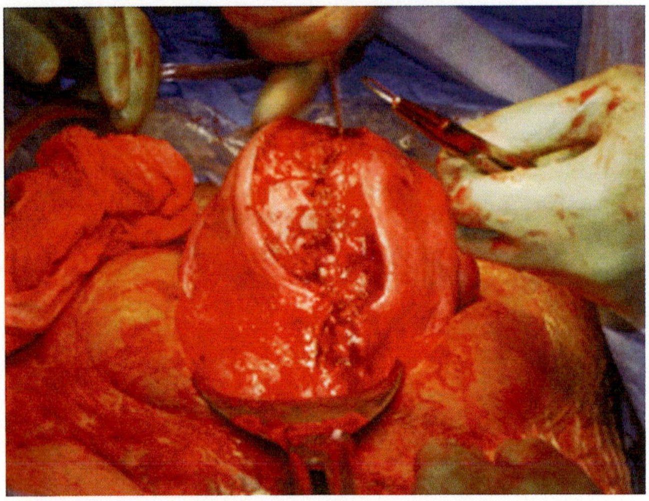

a. 0.2–0.9%

b. 1–7%

c. 2–6%

d. 2–9%

31–8. The majority of women delivering via cesarean delivery prior to 26 weeks' gestation require what type of uterine incision?

a. Classical incision

b. Pfannenstiel incision

c. Low-vertical incision

d. Low-transverse incision

31–9. You are performing a primary low-transverse cesarean delivery on a term patient for failure to progress. Which of the following operative techniques may decrease her risk of uterine rupture in a subsequent pregnancy?

a. Locking stitches

b. Double-layer closure

c. Placement of Floseal over the hysterotomy

d. None of the above

31–10. You see a patient at 34 weeks' gestation. She had a primary low-transverse cesarean delivery for failure to progress 18 months ago. On ultrasound, the lower uterine segment thickness measures 2.6 mm. How should you counsel the patient based on the sonographic findings?

a. This finding has no prognostic significance.

b. This finding is associated with a low risk of uterine rupture.

c. This finding is associated with a high risk of uterine rupture.

d. This finding is associated with an intermediate risk of uterine rupture.

31–11. A 30-year-old G2P1 presents for her confirmation of pregnancy visit. She underwent cesarean delivery during her last pregnancy 1 year ago for malpresentation. Her ultrasound results are shown below. What is the most appropriate counseling based on the findings?

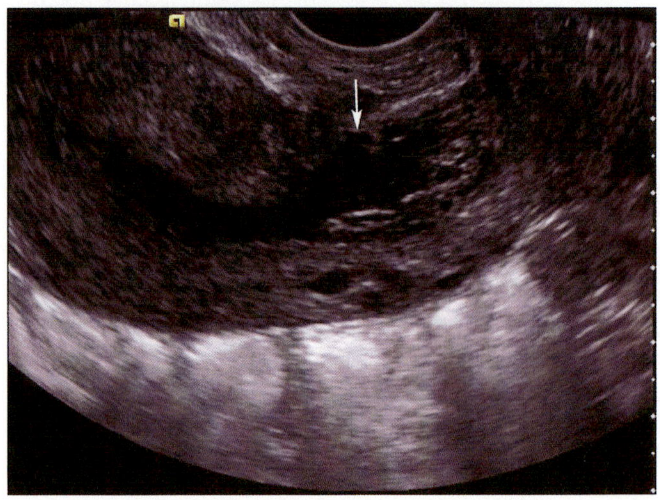

a. Her risk of uterine rupture is negligible.

b. Her risk of uterine rupture is decreased because of the ultrasound findings.

c. Her risk of uterine rupture is unchanged because of the ultrasound findings.

d. Her risk of uterine rupture is further increased because of the ultrasound findings.

31–12. Which risk factor confers the highest risk of uterine rupture in a subsequent pregnancy?

a. Interdelivery interval <6 months

b. Prior upper segment uterine rupture

c. Maternal body mass index >30 kg/m^2

d. Smallest myometrial thickness <2.0 mm

31–13. What is the approximate chance of successful vaginal birth after cesarean delivery in a patient with a body mass index exceeding 40 kg/m^2?

a. 50%
b. 60%
c. 70%
d. 80%

31–14. Which of the following is true regarding a woman who attempts a trial of labor with a 32-week preterm gestation?

a. The chance of uterine rupture is lower than with a term gestation.
b. The chance of successful vaginal delivery is higher than with a term gestation.
c. There is an increased risk of perinatal morbidity and mortality compared to a term gestation.
d. All of the above

31–15. Which of the following does not support performing an elective repeat cesarean delivery at 39 weeks' gestation without confirmation of fetal lung maturity by amniocentesis?

a. Fetal heart sounds have been documented for 30 weeks by Doppler ultrasound.
b. A positive serum or urine β-hCG test result has been documented for ≥36 weeks.
c. Sonographic measurements taken before 20 weeks' gestation support a gestational age ≥39 weeks.
d. All of the above

31–16. Which of the following statements is true regarding elective repeat cesarean deliveries based on the figure that is shown?

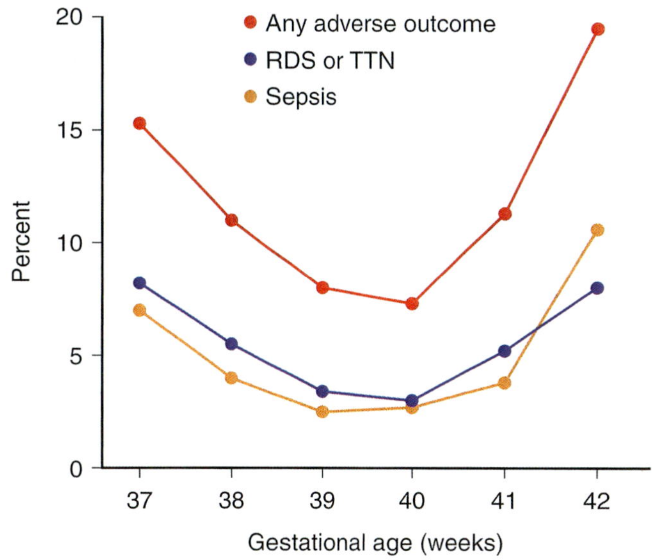

Reproduced with permission from Cunningham FG, Leveno KJ, Bloom SL, et al (eds): Prior cesarean delivery. In Williams Obstetrics, 25th ed. New York, McGraw-Hill, 2018, Figure 31-4.

a. Neonatal respiratory morbidity is lowest at 40 weeks' gestation.
b. The risk of any adverse neonatal outcome is highest at 37 weeks' gestation.
c. There is no increased neonatal morbidity with elective cesarean delivery at 38 weeks' gestation.
d. None of the above

31–17. Which of the following induction agents or methods confers the highest risk of uterine rupture in a woman with a prior cesarean delivery?

a. Oxytocin
b. Prostaglandin E_1
c. Prostaglandin $F_{2\alpha}$
d. Transcervical foley catheter

31–18. What is the most likely sign or symptom of a uterine scar rupture in a laboring woman with a history of a prior cesarean delivery?

a. Pain
b. Bleeding
c. Decreased fetal movement
d. Fetal heart rate decelerations

31–19. Which of the following has been demonstrated in women with a labor epidural who have an increased risk of uterine rupture?

a. Adequate pain relief is never achieved
b. More frequent epidural dosing is required
c. Successful epidural placement is more difficult
d. None of the above

31–20. What percentage of successful vaginal births after cesarean delivery were completed via operative assistance with either vacuum or forceps?

a. 5%
b. 15%
c. 25%
d. 35%

31–21. Which of the following statements is true regarding uterine scar exploration following successful vaginal birth after previous cesarean delivery?

a. Routine scar examination is recommended.
b. The chance of identifying a defect is <0.1%.
c. Any identified defect requires immediate exploratory laparotomy.
d. The need for exploratory laparotomy is determined by the extent of the defect and the presence of active bleeding.

31–22. You are augmenting a term patient who is attempting a vaginal birth after cesarean delivery. She is 6 cm dilated, 90% effaced, and –1 station and was comfortable with her epidural anesthesia when you checked her 10 minutes ago. You notice the heart rate tracing abnormalities that are pictured. You recheck the patient, but can no longer feel the fetal head. The maternal heart rate is 85 beats per minute, blood pressure 84/46 mmHg, and respirations 18 breaths per minute. What is the best intervention based on the findings?

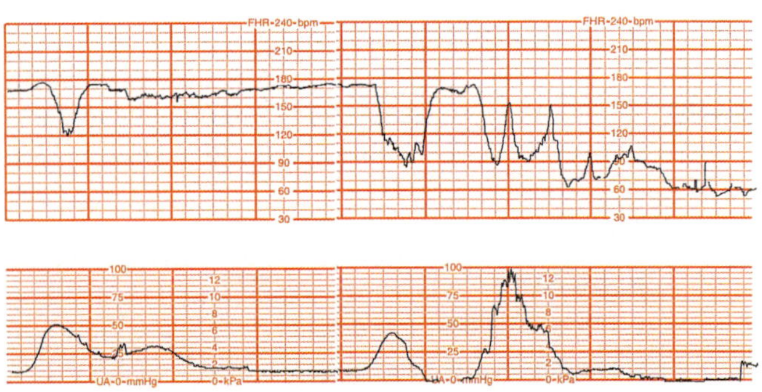

Reproduced with permission from Cunningham FG, Leveno KJ, Bloom SL, et al (eds): Prior cesarean delivery. In Williams Obstetrics, 25th ed. New York, McGraw-Hill, 2018, Figure 31-5.

a. Administer ephedrine
b. Reposition the patient
c. Attempt forceps placement
d. Proceed with emergent cesarean delivery

31–23. Uterine scar rupture can mimic which of the following obstetric emergencies?

a. Placental abruption
b. Pulmonary embolus
c. Amniotic fluid embolus
d. All of the above

31–24. Which of the following findings is not helpful to diagnose a uterine rupture during labor?

a. Fetal distress
b. Uterine tenderness
c. A firmly contracted uterus
d. Decreased resting tone based on an intrauterine pressure catheter reading

31–25. As you are caring for a laboring patient at term who is attempting a vaginal birth after having a previous cesarean delivery, you observe sudden and prolonged fetal bradycardia based on a fetal scalp electrode monitor. You proceed with an emergent cesarean delivery with the intraabdominal findings pictured. The fetus has been extruded into the abdominal cavity. What are the chances of fetal survival in this situation?

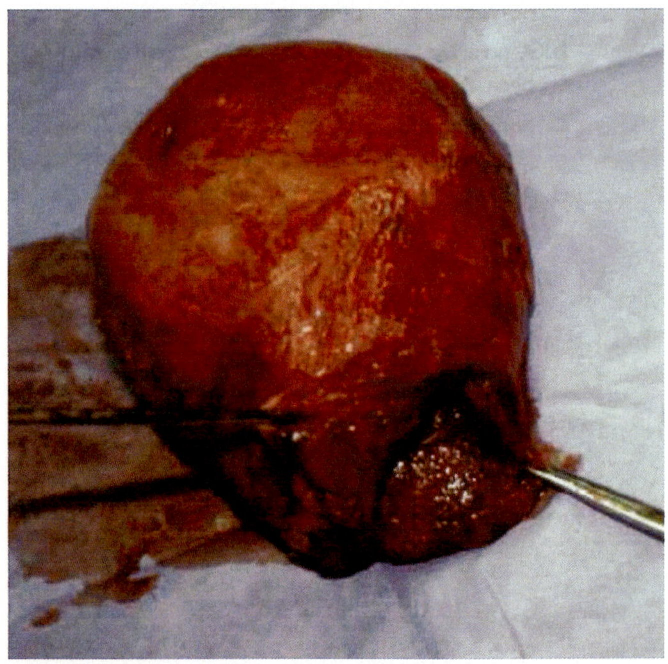

Reproduced with permission from Cunningham FG, Leveno KJ, Bloom SL, et al (eds): Obstetrical hemorrhage. In Williams Obstetrics, 25th ed. New York, McGraw-Hill, 2018, Figure 41-13.

a. 5–15%
b. 10–25%
c. 25–50%
d. 50–75%

31–26. According to published studies, what is the critical time threshold from decision to delivery to avoid long-term neurological impairments in the infant?

a. Less than 9 minutes
b. Less than 18 minutes
c. Less than 31 minutes
d. Less than 45 minutes

31–27. In a developed country, what are the risks of maternal and neonatal mortality, respectively, if a uterine rupture does occur during labor?

a. 0.2% and 5%
b. 0.5% and 7%
c. 0.2% and 7%
d. 0.5% and 5%

31–28. Which of the following statements is true based on the figure that is shown?

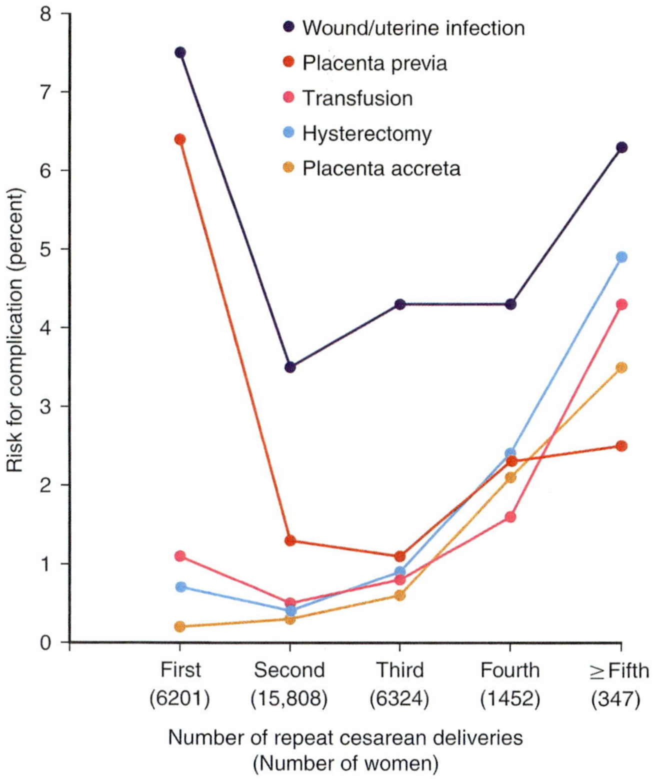

Reproduced with permission from Cunningham FG, Leveno KJ, Bloom SL, et al (eds): Prior cesarean delivery. In Williams Obstetrics, 25th ed. New York, McGraw-Hill, 2018, Figure 31-6.

a. Placenta previa complicates approximately 6% of first repeat cesarean deliveries.
b. The risk of wound infection is halved with the second repeat cesarean delivery.
c. The risk of placenta accreta continues to increase as the number of repeat cesarean deliveries increases.
d. All of the above

31–29. In a conservative approach to trial of labor following cesarean delivery, which of the following would not be considered cautionary before pursuing a labor induction in a patient with a history of cesarean delivery?

a. High station
b. A Bishop score of 10
c. Unknown incision type
d. Closed cervix at 41 weeks

31–30. When should discussion of the risks and benefits of a trial of labor following cesarean delivery ideally begin?

a. Preconceptionally
b. At the first prenatal visit
c. Prior to the start of the second trimester
d. After the patient presents to labor and delivery with contractions

31–31. Which of the following led to the decrease in rates of trial of labor after cesarean delivery after 1996?

a. Reports of maternal mortality from uterine rupture
b. Reports of perinatal mortality from uterine rupture
c. American College of Obstetricians and Gynecologists recommended that a physician be immediately available
d. All of the above

31–32. Which of the following is associated with the highest vaginal birth after cesarean delivery rate?

a. Prior vaginal delivery
b. Normal body mass index
c. Estimated fetal weight <4000 grams
d. Prior cesarean delivery for a nonrecurring indication

CHAPTER 31 ANSWER KEY

Question number	Letter answer	Page cited	Header cited
31–1	**a**	p. 592	Influencing Factors
31–2	**d**	p. 593	Maternal Risks
31–3	**b**	p. 594	Table 31-2
31–4	**b**	p. 593	Maternal Risks
31–5	**b**	p. 593	Fetal and Neonatal Risks
31–6	**c**	p. 594	Candidates for Trial of Labor
31–7	**d**	p. 594	Table 31-3
31–8	**a**	p. 595	Prior Uterine Incision
31–9	**d**	p. 595	Prior Uterine Incision
31–10	**b**	p. 595	Prior Uterine Incision
31–11	**c**	p. 595	Prior Uterine Incision
31–12	**b**	p. 596	Candidates for Trial of Labor
31–13	**b**	p. 595	Prior Uterine Incision
31–14	**d**	p. 595	Prior Uterine Incision
31–15	**d**	p. 597	Labor and Delivery Considerations
31–16	**a**	p. 597	Labor and Delivery Considerations
31–17	**b**	p. 597	Cervical Ripening and Labor Stimulation
31–18	**d**	p. 598	Epidural Anesthesia
31–19	**b**	p. 598	Epidural Anesthesia
31–20	**c**	p. 598	Epidural Anesthesia
31–21	**d**	p. 598	Uterine Scar Exploration
31–22	**d**	p. 598	Uterine Scar Exploration
31–23	**d**	p. 598	Uterine Scar Rupture
31–24	**d**	p. 598	Uterine Scar Rupture
31–25	**c**	p. 599	Decision-to-Delivery Time
31–26	**b**	p. 599	Decision-to-Delivery Time
31–27	**a**	p. 599	Decision-to-Delivery Time
31–28	**d**	p. 599	Multiple Repeat Cesarean Deliveries
31–29	**b**	p. 600	Conservative Guidelines to Approach a TOLAC
31–30	**a**	p. 600	Vaginal Birth After Cesarean—2017
31–31	**d**	p. 591	100 Years of Controversy
31–32	**d**	p. 596	Candidates for Trial of Labor

SECTION 9

THE NEWBORN

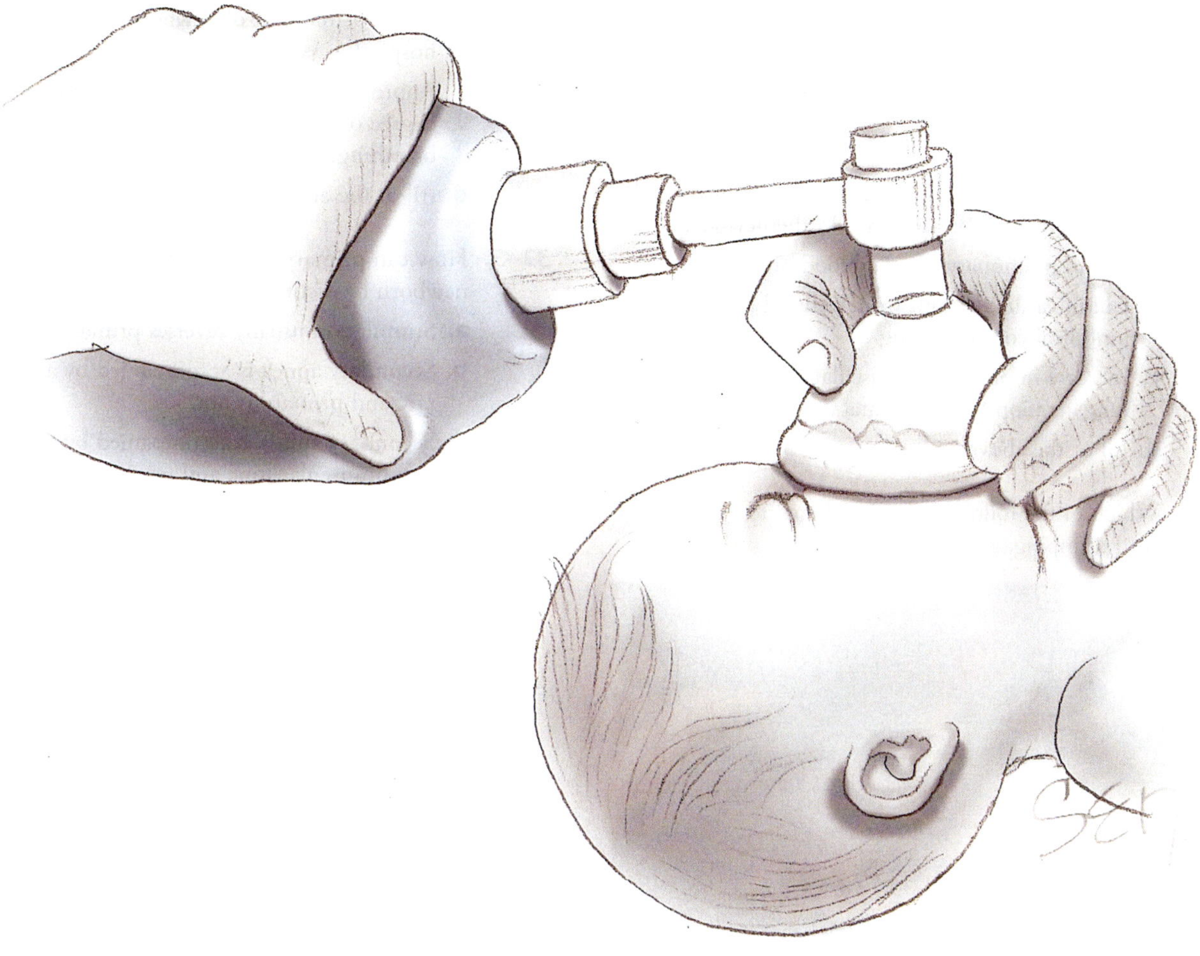

CHAPTER 32

The Newborn Infant

32–1. After delivery, clearance of the amnionic fluid that fills the fetal lungs occurs via which of the following mechanisms?

a. Physical compression of the fetal thorax

b. Absorption of fluid into the neonatal pulmonary circulation

c. Absorption of fluid into the neonatal pulmonary lymphatic system

d. All of the above

32–2. Which of the following postnatal changes promotes closure of the ductus arteriosus in the newborn?

a. Fall in pulmonary arterial blood pressure

b. Fall in cardiac output from reduced preload after umbilical cord clamping

c. Increase in pulmonary vascular compression after lung aeration from neonatal inspiration

d. All of the above

32–3. Which of the following is not a benefit of delayed cord clamping, as pictured below?

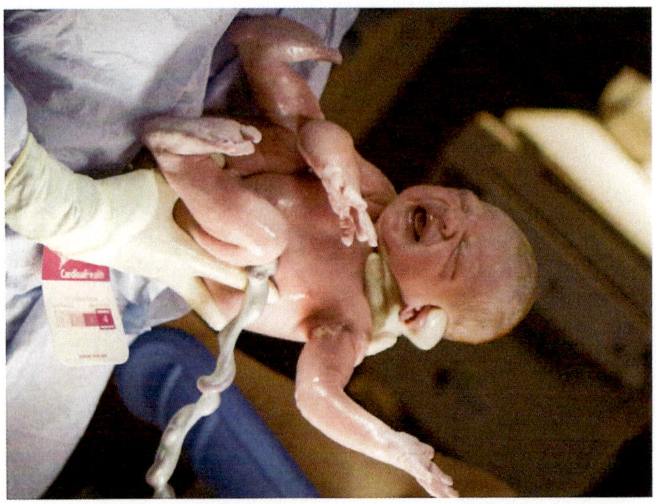

a. Increased iron stores

b. Reduced risk of neonatal bradycardia

c. Reduced hyperbilirubinemia and need for phototherapy

d. Reduced necrotizing enterocolitis in preterm neonates

32–4. Which of the following is true regarding neonatal resuscitation?

a. Approximately 1% of newborns need extensive resuscitation after delivery.

b. Newborns delivered at home face risk of death that is 5-fold that of newborns delivered in the hospital.

c. Approximately 30% of newborns require some degree of active resuscitation to stimulate breathing.

d. All of the above

32–5. How can primary and secondary apnea in the newborn be distinguished from each other?

a. Stimulation usually reverses primary apnea.

b. Secondary apnea is accompanied by a fall in heart rate and primary is not.

c. Secondary apnea is accompanied by loss of neuromuscular tone and primary is not.

d. All of the above

32–6. A 26-year-old multigravida presents in spontaneous labor at 39 weeks 3 days. She had spontaneous rupture of membranes with clear amnionic fluid and delivered spontaneously with a category I fetal heart rate tracing. The neonate was vigorous and crying immediately after delivery. What is the next best step in the management of this newborn?

a. Bulb suctioning of oropharyngeal secretions

b. Cord clamping and transfer to the radiant warmer

c. Placement on maternal abdomen for drying and evaluation of tone, heart rate, and respiratory effort

d. Hold infant in fully supported prone position and deliver 3 gentle back thumps to aid in initial secretion clearance.

32–7. Although initially vigorous and crying, the newborn in Question 32–6 became apneic with a heart rate that was 90 beats per minute at 50 seconds of life. The following is most appropriately initiated?

a. Secretions are suctioned

b. Positive pressure ventilation is administered

c. Newborn is stimulated, and head placed in the sniffing position

d. All of the above

32–8. The newborn in Question 32–6 was given positive pressure ventilation. Nonetheless, the newborn's heart rate at 80 seconds of life is 86 beats per minute. What is the next most appropriate step?

a. Chest compressions
b. Placement of an endotracheal tube
c. Placement of an umbilical vein catheter
d. Mask adjustment and airway repositioning

32–9. A preterm neonate born at 29 weeks' gestation is undergoing resuscitation and requires endotracheal ventilation. Which of the following is most correct regarding endotracheal tube– assisted ventilation of this newborn?

a. Positive pressure ventilation is delivered at a rate of 30 breaths per minute.
b. Opening pressure of 30–40 cm H_2O, greater than that for a term neonate, is typical.
c. Methods of confirming tracheal intubation include detection of end-tidal CO_2, increasing fetal heart rate, and visualization of symmetric chest wall motion.
d. All of the above

32–10. When chest compressions are indicated for newborn resuscitation, which of the following best describes the technique?

a. Compressions are delivered at a 2:1 ratio with ventilation
b. Two hands encircle the chest of the neonate with two thumbs used to deliver compressions
c. Compression depth is approximately one half of the anterior-posterior diameter of the neonate's chest
d. All of the above

32–11. Which site in the image below depicts the correct location of fingers for chest compressions in the neonate?

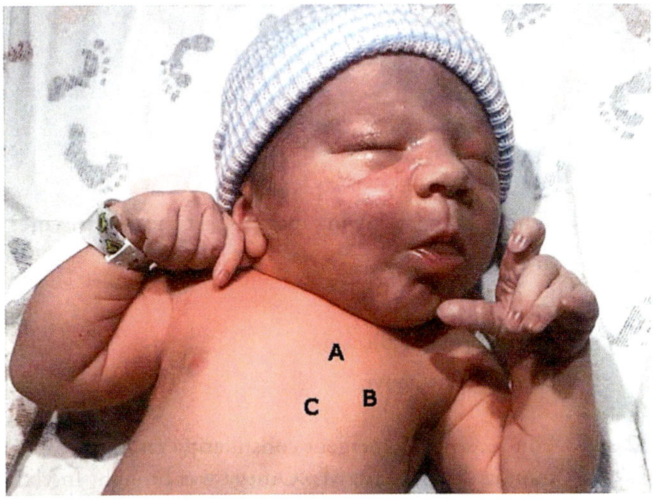

Used with permission from Dr. David Nelson.

a. A
b. B
c. C
d. None of the above

32–12. If the neonate's heart rate remains less than or equal to 60 beats per minute after adequate ventilation and chest compressions, which of the following is a recommended pharmacological intervention?

a. Epinephrine delivered via endotracheal tube at 0.05–0.1 mg/kg
b. Epinephrine delivered intravenously at 0.05–0.1 mg/kg
c. Ephedrine delivered via endotracheal tube at 0.05–0.1 mg/kg
d. Ephedrine delivered intravenously at 0.01–0.03 mg/kg

32–13. Which of the following statements are true regarding Apgar scores?

a. Apgar score assesses 5 characteristics and either 0 or 2 points are awarded.
b. Apgar score effectively assesses newborn health and effectiveness of resuscitation.
c. Five-minute Apgar score is predictive of neonatal survival in term but not preterm neonates.
d. In term neonates, Apgar score <7 at 5 minutes can be used to correlate a hypoxic event as a cause of cerebral palsy.

32–14. A term newborn has a heart rate of 128 beats per minute, is pink except for her feet and hands, is crying spontaneously and loudly, and is kicking both legs. What is her Apgar score?

a. 7

b. 8

c. 9

d. 10

32–15. Which of the following may impact the Apgar score?

a. Prematurity

b. Fetal malformation

c. Maternal medications

d. All of the above

32–16. You receive an emergent consultation from the trauma department. Ms. Omega was brought in via emergency medical transport after a motor vehicle collision. She has a tourniquet around her left upper arm proximal to an apparent traumatic amputation at the elbow. Another individual from the accident is awake and alert and states that Ms. Omega is 39 weeks pregnant and was on the way to the hospital for labor. You quickly perform an exam and note that the fetal head is at the perineum. Delivery is accomplished easily and on initial survey the neonate is pale with no respiratory effort or response to stimulation, and has a pulse of 80 beats per minute. An umbilical cord blood gas is obtained. Which of the following is most likely given the history?

a. Base deficit is 14 mEq/L

b. Umbilical artery pH is 7.19

c. One-minute Apgar score is 3

d. Respiratory acidemia is present

32–17. How do normal umbilical cord blood gas results differ between umbilical venous and umbilical arterial samples?

a. HCO_3^- is higher in a venous sample

b. The pCO_2 is lower in a venous sample

c. The pH is higher in an arterial sample

d. The base excess is lower in an arterial sample

32–18. A 27-year-old primigravida at 33 weeks' gestation has been on the antepartum unit for 6 days for preterm rupture of membranes. An image from her admission ultrasound is shown below. You get a stat page from the nurse informing you the patient is being wheeled over emergently with cord prolapse. Emergent cesarean delivery is performed with delivery approximately 24 minutes from the prolapse. Umbilical artery cord blood gas results are: pH 6.95, pCO_2 90 mmHg, HCO_3^- 18 mEq/L, and base deficit 8 mEq/L. One-minute Apgar score is 3 and five-minute Apgar score is 8. After the case you find her family to review the events. Which of the following is an appropriate statement?

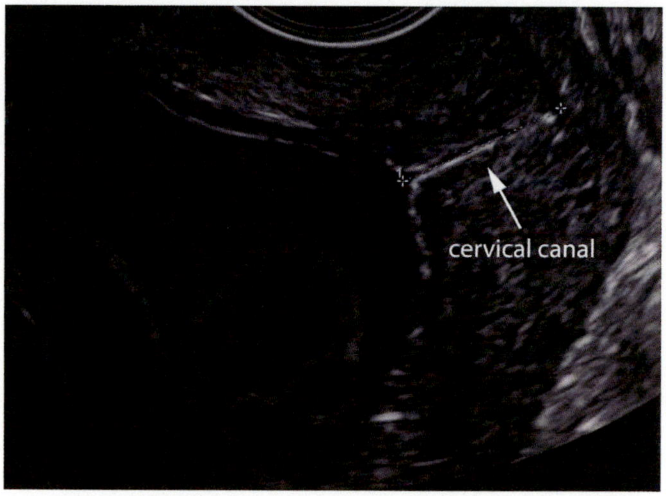

a. Findings are consistent with a metabolic acidosis

b. Findings suggest that the low pH was related to an acute event

c. Findings suggest high likelihood of a hypoxic-ischemic encephalopathy

d. All of the above

32–19. A 23-year-old primigravida at 38 weeks' gestation presents to labor and delivery after a witnessed seizure at home. Her initial blood pressure is 130/80 mmHg, and pulse is 140 beats per minute. The fetal heart rate tracing shows a heart rate of 100 beats per minute, absent variability, and late decelerations. She is having frequent contractions, and exam shows she is 3 cm dilated. She is taken back for emergent cesarean delivery, and bloody fluid is noted upon uterine entry. Placental findings are depicted below. Umbilical artery blood gas pH is 6.9 and base deficit is 14 mEq/L. Five-minute Apgar score is 2. Which of the following statements is evidence-based?

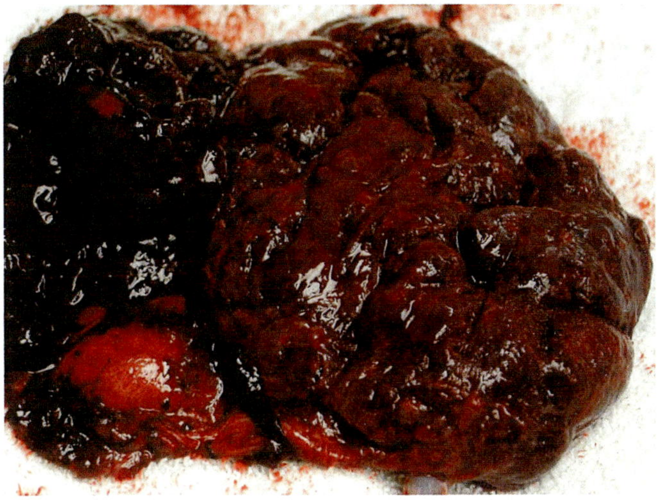

Used with permission from Dr. Anne Ambia.

a. Speed of resolution of the acidemia after birth is associated with outcome.

b. There is a high likelihood of multiorgan dysfunction in this neonate.

c. These initial findings are poorly predictive of subsequent neurological impairment.

d. All of the above are evidence-based statements related to the details of this case.

32–20. Ms. Cox was treated for *Neisseria gonorrhoeae* 3 weeks prior to presentation for a term vaginal delivery. She reports several episodes of unprotected intercourse since then, and does not feel confident that her partner sought treatment as recommended. Which of the following is the most appropriate initial intervention for her neonate?

a. Test for gonococcal and chlamydial infection

b. Single dose ceftriaxone 100 mg/kg intramuscular injection

c. Single application of 1% silver nitrate solution to both eyes

d. Single application of 0.5% erythromycin ointment to both eyes

32–21. Ms. Smith presents for her 6-week postpartum visit. She is doing well, and is excited to show you her newborn daughter, who is doing well overall. She has noticed some eye drainage the last few days, and you observe the findings depicted below. Which of the following statements is true?

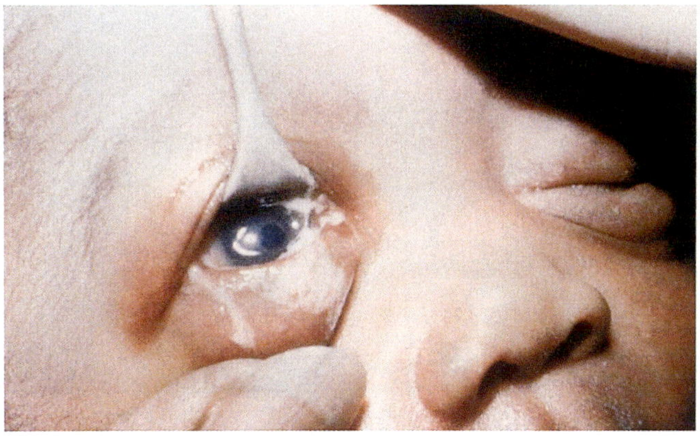

Reproduced with permission from Levsky ME, DeFlorio P: Ophthalmologic complications. In Knoop KJ, Stack LB, Storrow AB, et l (eds): The Atlas of Emergency Medicine, 3rd ed. New York, McGraw-Hill, 2010, Figure 2-1.

a. Prophylactic topical eye treatments given to the neonate do not reliably reduce the incidence of chlamydial conjunctivitis.

b. 12–25% of neonates delivered vaginally of mothers with chlamydia will develop conjunctivitis, but this manifests within 3 weeks of delivery.

c. Some form of conjunctivitis affects 1–12% of all neonates, but gonococcal and chlamydial infections are among the least common.

d. All of the above

32–22. During her prenatal care, Ms. Oliver is noted to be positive for both hepatitis B surface antigen and hepatitis B e antigen. Which of the following is the most appropriate evaluation and management of her term newborn?

a. Neonatal hepatitis B viral load to guide subsequent management

b. Administration of hepatitis B immune globulin as passive immunization after delivery

c. Administration of hepatitis B immune globulin after delivery and administration of the first dose of the hepatitis B vaccine series prior to discharge

d. Administration of hepatitis B immune globulin if mother is planning lactation, and administration of the first dose of the hepatitis B vaccine series prior to discharge

32–23. Why is the infant below receiving an injection of vitamin K within 1 hour of birth?

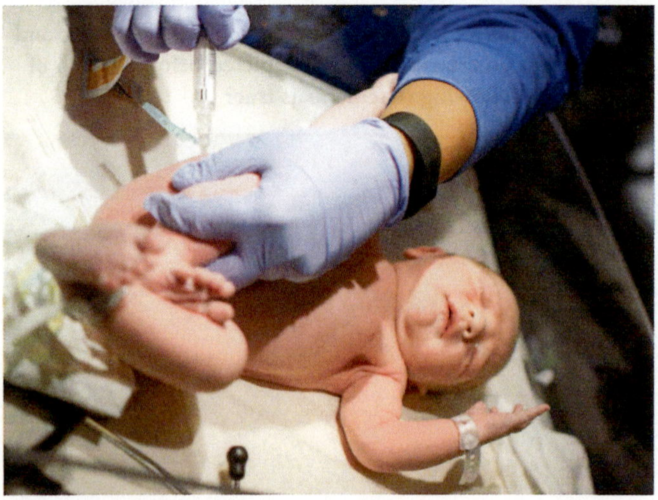

a. To enhance newborn bone development

b. To prevent vitamin K–dependent hemorrhagic disease of the newborn

c. To reduce the incidence of necrotizing enterocolitis in premature infants

d. To augment the lower vitamin K levels noted in breast milk compared to commercially produced infant formula

32–24 Which of the following is the most accurate statement regarding newborn screening?

a. Newborn screening panels are consistent across the United States.

b. The United States federal government mandates newborn screening.

c. The American Academy of Pediatrics dictates the content of the newborn screening panel.

d. None of the above

32–25. During her first trimester, Ms. Harris traveled to a country that is known to be an endemic area for Zika virus. Subsequently her serological testing was positive. Ultrasound surveillance of the fetus has been performed, including the 32-week assessment of fetal head biometrics shown here. Which of the following is not included in the recommended neonatal evaluation?

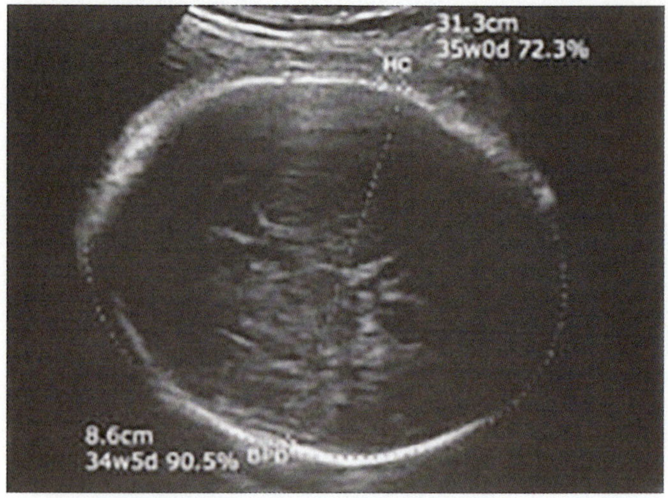

a. Newborn neurological assessment

b. Neonatal Zika virus laboratory testing

c. Neonatal magnetic resonance imaging

d. Standard newborn hearing screen prior to discharge

32–26. Ms. Blake comes to see you on postpartum day 5 for a blood pressure check. She had a spontaneous vaginal delivery at term complicated by preeclampsia and chorioamnionitis. The neonate never had a fever and has been feeding, voiding, and stooling well since discharge. Ms. Blake shows you the umbilical cord stump, which is depicted below. What is the appropriate response to her concern?

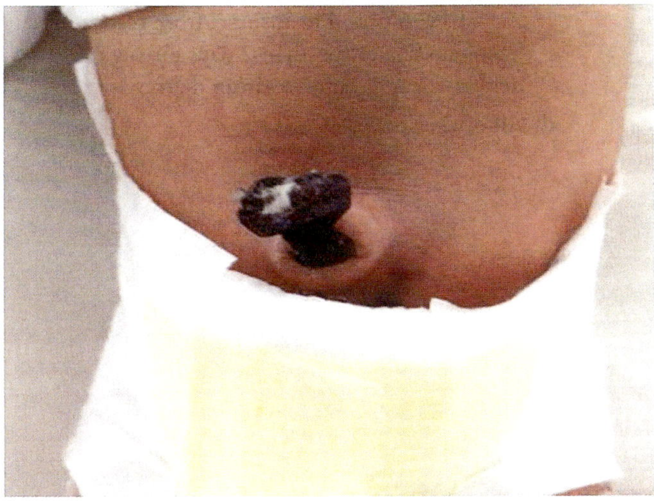

Used with permission from Kelly Yanes.

a. Provide reassurance of the normal finding with no new recommendations.

b. Recommend covering the stump with petroleum jelly and a gauze pad to hasten cord separation.

c. Recommend she proceed to the emergency room due to concern for necrosis and need for resection.

d. Recommend she proceed to her pediatrician's office due to concern for omphalitis with need for antibiotics.

32–27. A 31-year-old primigravida undergoes a spontaneous vaginal delivery at 40 weeks' gestation, delivering a female infant weighing 7 lb 9 oz. They are both discharged home on postpartum day 2. She has been home for 2 days and calls your office worried that the baby weighs 7 lb today. What is the most appropriate response?

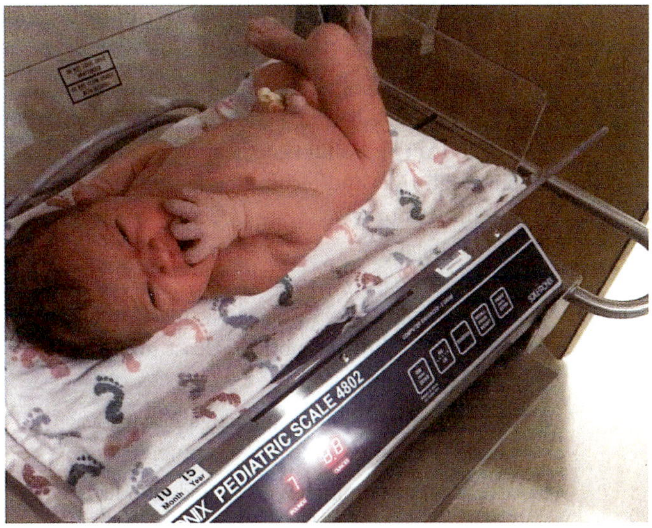

Used with permission from Dr. David Nelson.

a. If any further weight loss occurs, supplement breastfeeding with formula until her weight stabilizes.

b. Recommend converting to a high calorie commercial formula and schedule a weight check with the pediatrician in 3 days.

c. This amount of weight loss is within expectations. Observe wet diapers and continue breastfeeding with expectation to regain birthweight by 10 days.

d. None of the above

32–28. The American College of Obstetricians and Gynecologists recommend exclusive breastfeeding for how long?

a. 1 month

b. 3 months

c. 6 months

d. 12 months

32–29. Passage of meconium in the delivery room is associated with which of the following?

a. Necrotizing enterocolitis

b. Gastrointestinal tract patency

c. Fetal distress and lower Apgar score

d. Increased risk for Hirschsprung disease

32–30. Ms. Lewis is pregnant with a male fetus. She asks you about circumcision. Which of the following is not true?

a. Newborn male circumcision rate is estimated to be approximately 55% in the latest Centers for Disease Control report.

b. Circumcision lowers the incidence of human papilloma virus related penile cancer in males and cervical cancer in their partners.

c. In their 2012 policy statement, the American Academy of Pediatrics Task Force on Circumcision concluded that health benefits of male circumcision outweigh risks and recommended the procedure for all newborns.

d. All of the above

32–31. You are teaching a new intern about male circumcision. Which of the following points is least important in safe surgical technique?

a. Never use injectable local analgesia with a vasoactive compound such as epinephrine.

b. The Mogen technique is associated with less apparent discomfort for the newborn.

c. Newborn circumcision is an elective procedure to be performed only on healthy neonates with no family history of a bleeding disorder.

d. Careful inspection of the external genitalia is imperative to rule out any congenital disorders that are contraindications to routine circumcision.

32–32. Which of the following is true regarding hospital stay after delivery?

a. Early discharge is associated with increased neonatal mortality.

b. Early discharge is associated with increased neonatal readmission rates for dehydration and jaundice.

c. The Newborns' and Mothers' Health Protection Act of 1996 prohibits insurers from restricting hospital stays to less than 2 days for vaginal delivery or 4 days for cesarean delivery.

d. All of the above

CHAPTER 32 ANSWER KEY

Question number	Letter answer	Page cited	Header cited
32–1	**d**	p. 607	Transition to Air Breathing
32–2	**a**	p. 607	Transition to Air Breathing
32–3	**c**	p. 607	Transition to Air Breathing Umbilical Cord Clamping
32–4	**a**	p. 607	Newborn Resuscitation
32–5	**a**	p. 608	Newborn Resuscitation
32–6	**c**	p. 608	Resuscitation Protocol
32–7	**d**	p. 609	Figure 32-2
32–8	**d**	p. 610	Table 32-1
32–9	**c**	p. 608	Alternative Airway
32–10	**b**	p. 609	Chest Compressions
32–11	**c**	p. 609	Chest Compressions
32–12	**a**	p. 610	Epinephrine
32–13	**b**	p. 610	Apgar Score
32–14	**c**	p. 610	Apgar Score
32–15	**d**	p. 611	Apgar Score
32–16	**a**	p. 611	Fetal Acid–Base Physiology
32–17	**b**	p. 612	Table 32-3
32–18	**b**	p. 612 p. 613	Figure 32-4 Respiratory Acidemia
32–19	**c**	p. 612	Clinical Significance of Acidemia
32–20	**a**	p. 613	Eye Infection Prophylaxis
32–21	**a**	p. 613	Eye Infection Prophylaxis
32–22	**c**	p. 614	Hepatitis B Immunization
32–23	**b**	p. 614	Vitamin K
32–24	**d**	p. 614	Newborn Screening
32–25	**c**	p. 614	Zika Virus
32–26	**a**	p. 615	Care of Skin and Umbilical Cord
32–27	**c**	p. 615	Feeding and Weight Loss
32–28	**c**	p. 615	Feeding and Weight Loss
32–29	**b**	p. 615	Stools and Urine
32–30	**c**	p. 615	Male Circumcision
32–31	**d**	p. 616	Male Circumcision
32–32	**d**	p. 616	Rooming In and Hospital Discharge

CHAPTER 33

Diseases and Injuries of the Term Newborn

33–1. Which of the following is the most common reason for respiratory distress in term infants?

- **a.** Severe asphyxia
- **b.** Infection/sepsis
- **c.** Meconium aspiration
- **d.** Elective cesarean delivery

33–2. What is the incidence of meconium-stained amnionic fluid in term laboring women?

- **a.** 1–2%
- **b.** 10–20%
- **c.** 30–50%
- **d.** 60–70%

33–3. Which of the following is effective at reducing meconium aspiration syndrome?

- **a.** Amnioinfusion
- **b.** Oropharyngeal suctioning
- **c.** Cesarean delivery to avoid fetal heart tracing abnormalities
- **d.** None of the above

33–4. Which of the following has been used for the treatment of meconium aspiration syndrome?

- **a.** Intubation
- **b.** Inhaled corticosteroids
- **c.** Extracorporeal membrane oxygenation
- **d.** All of the above

33–5. In order to be diagnosed with neonatal encephalopathy, a neonate must be born at a minimum of what gestational age?

- **a.** 24 weeks' gestation
- **b.** 28 weeks' gestation
- **c.** 32 weeks' gestation
- **d.** 35 weeks' gestation

33–6. Which of the following forms of cerebral palsy can result from acute peripartum ischemia?

- **a.** Ataxia
- **b.** Hemiplegia
- **c.** Spastic diplegia
- **d.** Spastic quadriplegia

33–7. Which of the following is not consistent with an acute peripartum or intrapartum event leading to hypoxic ischemic encephalopathy?

- **a.** Umbilical artery pH <7
- **b.** Multisystem organ injury
- **c.** Apgar of >7 at 5 and 10 minutes
- **d.** Sentinel hypoxic or ischemic event immediately before or during delivery

33–8. Which of the following is the best imaging modality for visualizing the neonatal brain in cases of suspected hypoxic-ischemic encephalopathy?

- **a.** Cranial ultrasound
- **b.** Computed tomography
- **c.** Magnetic resonance imaging
- **d.** All listed modalities are equally good

33–9. All except which of the following are considered sentinel events when assessing for hypoxic-ischemic encephalopathy?

- **a.** Nuchal cord
- **b.** Uterine rupture
- **c.** Amnionic fluid embolus
- **d.** Severe placental abruption

33–10. Which of the following is not a risk factor for neonatal acidosis?

- **a.** Chorioamnionitis
- **b.** Regional anesthesia
- **c.** Advanced maternal age
- **d.** Emergency cesarean delivery

33–11. What is the prevalence of cerebral palsy in the United States?

a. 1/1000 children
b. 2/1000 children
c. 10/1000 children
d. 50/1000 children

33–12. What is the single most important risk factor for cerebral palsy?

a. Hydramnios
b. Preterm birth
c. Maternal obesity
d. Chorioamnionitis

33–13. What fetal heart abnormality predicts cerebral palsy and should thus prompt emergent intervention if present?

a. Tachysystole
b. Variable decelerations
c. Minimal beat-to-beat variability
d. No specific fetal heart rate pattern predicts cerebral palsy

33–14. You are seeing a patient and her husband after the delivery of their first child. The patient had preeclampsia with severe features and a placental abruption for which you performed an emergency cesarean delivery. The couple is very concerned about their infant. You want them to be counseled thoroughly by the neonatologists, but they are anxious for any information you can give them on their baby's outcome. You know that the 10-minute Apgar score was 2. Based on that, what is the risk of cerebral palsy?

a. 1%
b. 5%
c. 10%
d. 25%

33–15. What is the threshold for clinically significant cord gas acidemia?

a. pH <7.2
b. pH <7.1
c. pH <7.0
d. pH <6.9

33–16. Which of the following statements about neuroimaging studies for neonatal encephalopathy and cerebral palsy is true?

a. They can precisely time injuries.
b. Findings are not dependent on gestational age.
c. Magnetic resonance imaging findings correlate with severity of disability.
d. Sonographic studies and computed tomography scans are generally normal on the first day of life.

33–17. Which of the following is a major predictor of seizure disorders?

a. Neonatal seizures
b. Fetal malformations
c. Family history of seizure disorder
d. All of the above

33–18. Which of the following is not seen in neonatal abstinence syndrome?

a. Seizures
b. Irritability
c. Hypotonia
d. Poor suck reflex

33–19. Which of the following is a known complication of delayed cord clamping?

a. Plethora
b. Petechiae
c. Neonatal anemia
d. Hyperbilirubinemia

33–20. When do serum bilirubin levels peak in newborns?

a. Day of life 1
b. Day of life 2
c. Day of life 3–4
d. Day of life 7–10

33–21. The infant pictured below is being treated for neonatal hyperbilirubinemia. What is first-line treatment?

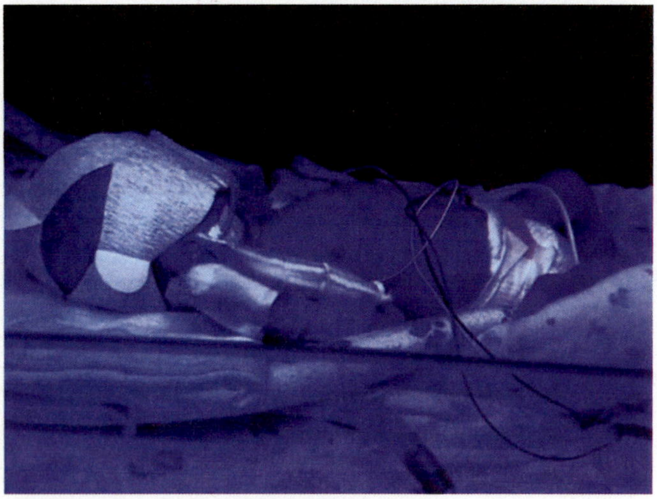

Used with permission from Dr. Stephanie Chang.

a. Dialysis
b. Phototherapy
c. Exchange transfusion
d. Glucose-6-phosphate replacement

33–22. Which of the following is not a vitamin K–dependent clotting factor?

a. Factor V
b. Factor VI
c. Factor VII
d. Factor XIII

33–23. What is the American College of Obstetricians and Gynecologists' recommended dose of vitamin K for routine prophylaxis against hemorrhagic disease of the newborn?

a. 2.0 mg orally
b. 0.5–1.0 mg orally
c. 2.0 mg intramuscularly
d. 0.5–1.0 mg intramuscularly

33–24. A 26-year-old primigravida presents in labor at term. The patient has a history of systemic lupus erythematosus for which she takes prednisone. After an uncomplicated vaginal birth, the neonate is noted to have mild thrombocytopenia for the first 2 days of life. What is the most likely cause?

a. Preeclampsia
b. Antiplatelet IgG
c. Undiagnosed parvovirus B19
d. Prednisone crossing the placenta

33–25. Which of the following carries the highest incidence of major birth trauma?

a. Failed forceps delivery
b. Failed vacuum delivery
c. Successful forceps delivery
d. Cesarean delivery in the setting of labor

33–26. A 27-year-old G1P1 had a spontaneous vaginal delivery at 26 weeks' gestation. The baby was diagnosed with an intracranial hemorrhage. What is the most likely etiology of this bleed?

a. Trauma
b. Hypoxia/ischemia
c. Thrombocytopenia
d. Arteriovenous malformation

33–27. Which of the following types of neonatal intracranial hemorrhage is common and almost always benign?

a. Subdural
b. Intracerebellar
c. Intraventricular
d. Primary subarachnoid

33–28. Present at birth and gone within hours or days, the schematic below depicts which of the following?

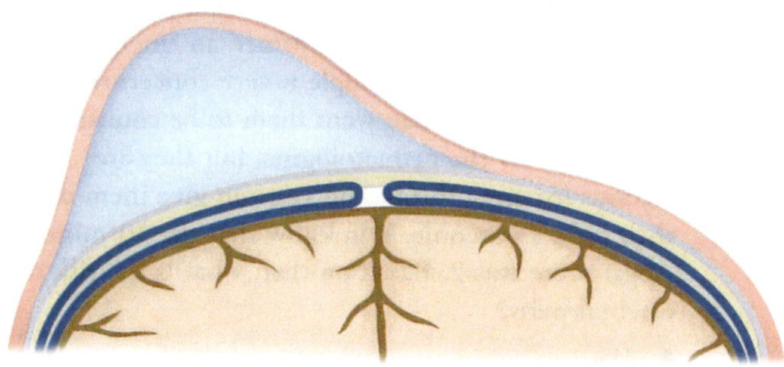

Reproduced with permission from Cunningham FG, Leveno KJ, Bloom SL, et al (eds): Diseases and injuries of the term newborn. In William Obstetrics, 25th ed. New York, McGraw-Hill, 2018, Figure 33-2.

a. Preparietal bleed
b. Cephalohematoma
c. Caput succedaneum
d. Subgaleal hemorrhage

33–29. With mortality rates of 12–18% from blood loss, the schematic below depicts which of the following?

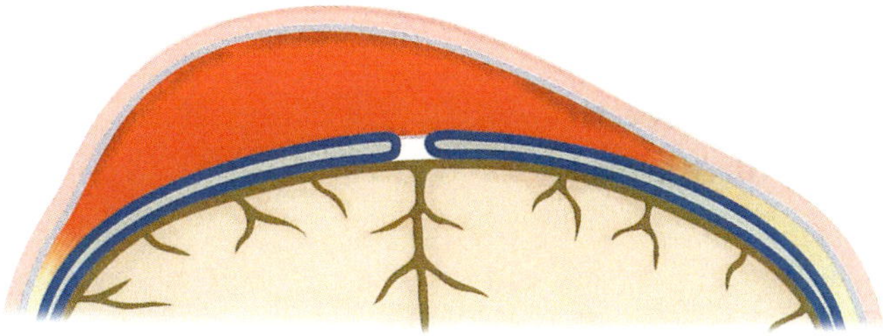

Reproduced with permission from Cunningham FG, Leveno KJ, Bloom SL, et al (eds): Diseases and injuries of the term newborn. In William Obstetrics, 25th ed. New York, McGraw-Hill, 2018, Figure 33-2.

a. Preparietal bleed
b. Cephalohematoma
c. Caput succedaneum
d. Subgaleal hemorrhage

33–30. The result of shearing forces, the schematic below depicts which of the following?

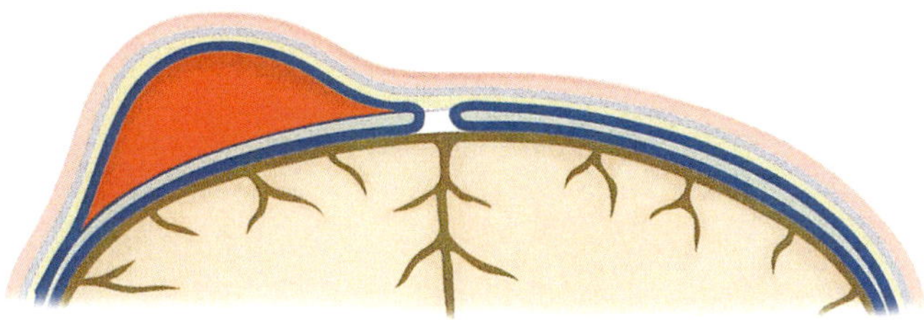

Reproduced with permission from Cunningham FG, Leveno KJ, Bloom SL, et al (eds): Diseases and injuries of the term newborn. In William Obstetrics, 25th ed. New York, McGraw-Hill, 2018, Figure 33-2.

a. Preparietal bleed
b. Cephalohematoma
c. Caput succedaneum
d. Subgaleal hemorrhage

33–31. A 17-year-old G1P1 presented at term in labor. She progressed to complete dilation. After pushing for 3 hours, she was taken for a cesarean delivery for failure to descend. The head was wedged deep in the pelvis. An assistant had to provide a vaginal hand to dislodge the head. After birth, a radiograph of the neonate's head was performed and is shown below. What is the diagnosis?

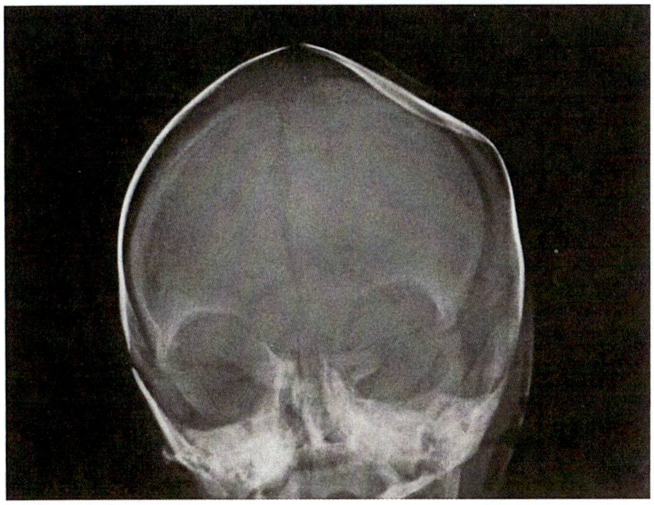

Reproduced with permission from Cunningham FG, Leveno KJ, Bloom SL, et al (eds): Diseases and injuries of the term newborn. In William Obstetrics, 25th ed. New York, McGraw-Hill, 2018, Figure 33-3.

a. Linear fracture
b. Craniosynostosis
c. Occipital osteodiastasis
d. Depressed skull fracture

33–32. A 24-year-old G1P1 gave birth to a term infant. The infant weighed 9 pounds at birth. The pediatrician noted that the newborn's left arm was held straight and internally rotated, the elbow was extended, and the wrist and fingers were flexed. The fingers did move freely. What nerve root is affected?

a. C_4
b. $C_{5\text{-}6}$
c. C_8-T_1
d. None of the above

33–33. A 22-year-old G1P1 presented at term in active labor. She had an uncomplicated vaginal delivery. A picture of her newborn is provided below. What nerve was injured?

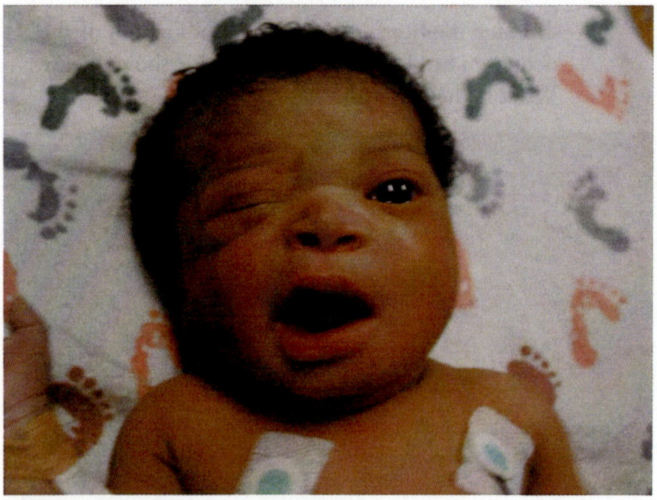

Used with permission from Dr. Barbara Hoffman.

a. Facial
b. Optic
c. Vagus
d. Trigeminal

33–34. Which of the following neonatal long-bone fractures is the most common?

a. Femoral
b. Humeral
c. Clavicular
d. Mandibular

CHAPTER 33 ANSWER KEY

Question number	Letter answer	Page cited	Header cited
33–1	**b**	p. 619	Respiratory Distress Syndrome
33–2	**b**	p. 620	Meconium Aspiration Syndrome
33–3	**d**	p. 620	Prevention
33–4	**d**	p. 620	Treatment
33–5	**d**	p. 621	Neonatal Encephalopathy
33–6	**d**	p. 621	Neonatal Encephalopathy
33–7	**c**	p. 621	Table 33-1
33–8	**c**	p. 622	Criteria for Hypoxic-Ischemic Encephalopathy
33–9	**a**	p. 622	Criteria for Hypoxic-Ischemic Encephalopathy
33–10	**b**	p. 622	Criteria for Hypoxic-Ischemic Encephalopathy
33–11	**b**	p. 622	Cerebral Palsy
33–12	**b**	p. 623	Incidence and Epidemiological Correlates
33–13	**d**	p. 623	Intrapartum Fetal Heart Rate Monitoring
33–14	**c**	p. 624	Apgar Scores
33–15	**c**	p. 624	Umbilical Cord Blood Gas Studies
33–16	**d**	p. 624	Neuroimaging in Neonatal Period
33–17	**d**	p. 625	Intellectual Disability and Seizure Disorders
33–18	**c**	p. 625	Neonatal Abstinence Syndrome
33–19	**d**	p. 625	Anemia
33–20	**c**	p. 626	Hyperbilirubinemia
33–21	**b**	p. 626	Prevention and Treatment
33–22	**b**	p. 626	Hemorrhagic Disease of the Newborn
33–23	**d**	p. 626	Hemorrhagic Disease of the Newborn
33–24	**b**	p. 627	Immune Thrombocytopenia
33–25	**b**	p. 627	Table 33-4
33–26	**b**	p. 628	Intracranial Hemorrhage
33–27	**d**	p. 628	Table 33-5
33–28	**c**	p. 629	Figure 33-2
33–29	**d**	p. 629	Figure 33-2
33–30	**b**	p. 629	Figure 33-2
33–31	**d**	p. 629	Skull Fractures
33–32	**b**	p. 630	Brachial Plexopathy
33–33	**a**	p. 630	Figure 33-4
33–34	**c**	p. 630	Fractures

CHAPTER 34

The Preterm Newborn

34–1. Compared to term infants, neonates born prematurely have higher associated rates of which of the following?

a. Sleep apnea
b. Developmental delay
c. Congenital malformations
d. All of the above

34–2. What is a reason for the decrease in preterm birth from 12% in 2007 to 10% in 2014?

a. Liberalized use of cerclage
b. Decrease in teen birth rate
c. Universal cervical length screening
d. Use of 17-alpha hydroxyprogesterone caproate

34–3. Respiratory distress syndrome contributes to which of the following comorbidities?

a. Neurological damage
b. Pulmonary hypertension
c. Necrotizing enterocolitis
d. All of the above

34–4. What is the mechanism of action by which surfactant prevents respiratory distress syndrome in neonatal lungs?

a. Clears fluid from the lungs
b. Dilates the pulmonary vasculature
c. Lowers surface tension in the alveoli
d. Aids in maturation of the terminal bronchioles

34–5. Respiratory distress syndrome can develop in the term infant as surfactant can be inactivated by which of the following substances?

a. Blood
b. Vernix
c. Meconium
d. All of the above

34–6. What is the etiology of the diffuse reticulogranular infiltrate seen on the chest radiograph below?

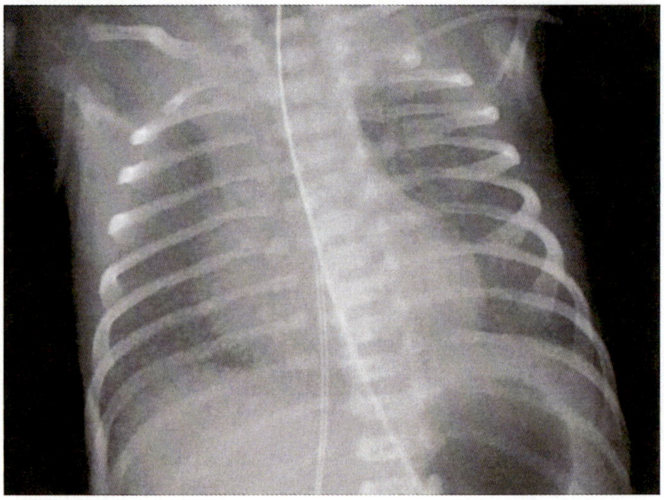

Used with permission from Dr. Becky Ennis.

a. Persistent fetal circulation
b. Bronchopulmonary dysplasia
c. Respiratory distress syndrome
d. Transient tachypnea of the newborn

34–7. A 32-year-old primigravida delivers a neonate at 31 weeks' gestation due to preeclampsia with severe features. She received a course of antenatal corticosteroids prior to delivery, but in the delivery room the neonate receives the intervention pictured below. The neonate likely displayed all except which of the following clinical signs?

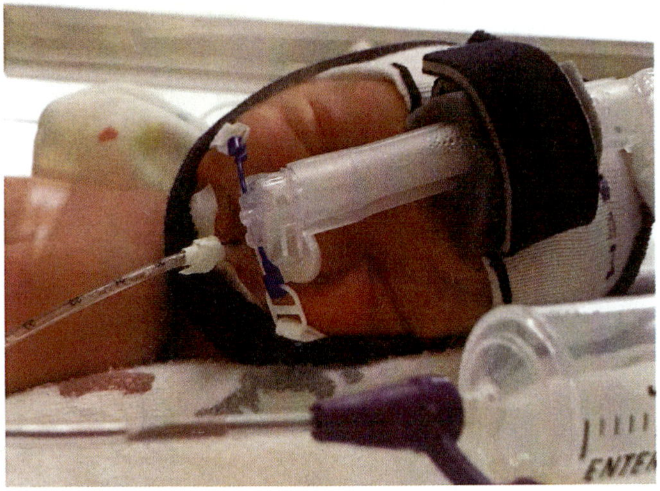

a. Tachypnea
b. Arrhythmia
c. Hypotension
d. Hypertension

34–8. The neonate in Question 34–7 continued to show a respiratory acidosis despite continuous positive airway pressure (CPAP). According to the American Academy of Pediatrics, what is the next best course of action?

a. Intubation
b. Nitric oxide
c. Glucocorticoids
d. Surfactant administration

34–9. Respiratory distress syndrome can be caused by which of the following?

a. Infection
b. Heart failure
c. Meconium aspiration
d. All of the above

34–10. A 37-year-old multigravida presents for a 6-week postpartum visit after delivering her son prematurely at 28 weeks' gestation. She informs you that he developed severe respiratory distress syndrome and was on a mechanical ventilator for many weeks. She is worried he will develop bronchopulmonary dysplasia (BPD). Which of the following medications have not been shown to prevent BPD?

a. Caffeine
b. Vitamin A
c. Glucocorticoids
d. Inhaled nitric oxide

34–11. Surfactant has been shown to reduce the rates of which of the following complications?

a. Intubation
b. Pneumothorax
c. Childhood asthma
d. Necrotizing enterocolitis

34–12. In which of the following scenarios are you least likely to give prophylactic surfactant?

a. A 33-week infant who did not receive antenatal corticosteroids.
b. A 27-week infant who received a course of "rescue steroids" prior to delivery.
c. A 37-week infant with respiratory distress syndrome requiring intubation.
d. A 26-week infant who received antenatal corticosteroids and continuous positive airway pressure in the delivery room.

34–13. The American College of Obstetricians and Gynecologists considers women candidates for antenatal corticosteroid therapy if they are at risk for preterm delivery at what gestational ages?

a. 22–34 weeks
b. 23–34 weeks
c. 24–32 weeks
d. 23–36 weeks

34–14. Antenatal corticosteroids have been shown to reduce which of the following complications of prematurity?

a. Respiratory distress syndrome and intraventricular hemorrhage
b. Bronchopulmonary dysplasia and intraventricular hemorrhage
c. Respiratory distress syndrome and necrotizing enterocolitis
d. Bronchopulmonary dysplasia and necrotizing enterocolitis

34–15. At what gestational age does the concentration of lecithin relative to sphingomyelin rise?

a. 23 weeks
b. 29 weeks
c. 30 weeks
d. 34 weeks

34–16. Which of the following are methods to assess fetal lung maturity?

a. Foam stability test
b. Lamellar body count
c. Fluorescence polarization test
d. All of the above

34–17. Which of the following methods to assess fetal lung maturity is considered the gold standard?

a. Foam stability test
b. Lamellar body count
c. Lecithin-sphingomyelin ratio
d. All of the above

34–18. A 26-year-old primigravida presents for her prenatal visit at 36 weeks' gestation and inquires about scheduling an induction of labor. At her first visit she was unsure of her last menstrual period, and she was dated by a 22-week ultrasound. At what gestational age does the American College of Obstetricians and Gynecologists (ACOG) recommend delivery?

a. 39 weeks
b. 41 weeks
c. 39 weeks after amniocentesis documenting fetal lung maturity
d. 41 weeks after amniocentesis documenting fetal lung maturity

34–19. A 29-year-old primigravida underwent a cesarean delivery of a female infant at 32 weeks' gestation secondary to preeclampsia with severe features and fetal-growth restriction. The infant weighed 1498 grams at birth. Which of the characteristics of this infant, pictured below, is not a risk factor for the development of necrotizing enterocolitis?

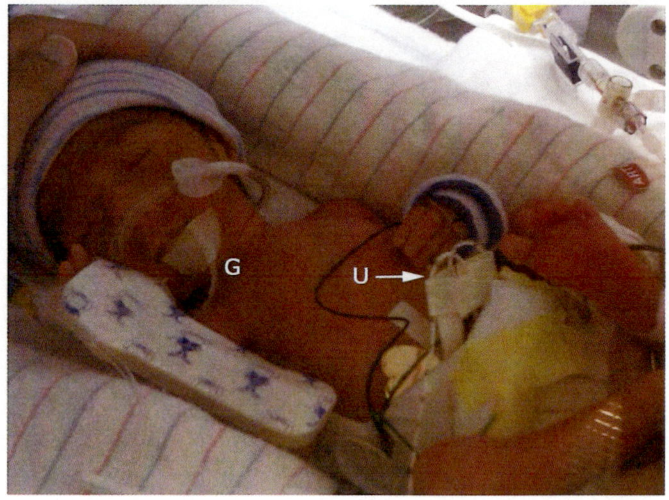

a. Female gender
b. Very low birthweight
c. Umbilical catheterization (U)
d. Supplementation of cow milk formula (G)

34–20. The neonate in Question 34–19 develops abdominal distention, fever, and intolerance of nasogastric feeds. An abdominal radiograph is performed and shown below. What is thought to be the pathophysiology of this condition?

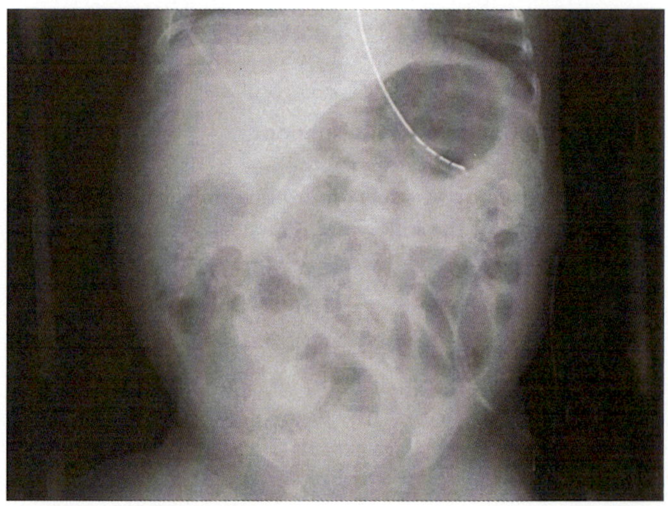

Used with permission from Dr. Natalie Frost.

a. Intestinal immaturity
b. Exposure to enteral feeds
c. Highly immunoreactive intestinal mucosa
d. All of the above

34–21. How does hyperoxemia lead to retinopathy of prematurity?

a. Causes centripetal vascularization of retina

b. Causes hemorrhage from retinal vessels and subsequent aberrant neovascularization

c. Causes severe retinal vasoconstriction, vessel obliteration, and subsequent aberrant neovascularization

d. Causes dilation of the retinal vessels, increase in angiogenic factors, and subsequent aberrant neovascularization

34–22. The infant pictured below was born at 34 weeks' gestation by cesarean delivery due to preeclampsia with severe features. The infant's birthweight was 1928 grams. Even at this gestational age, low birthweight is a risk factor for which of the following complications of prematurity?

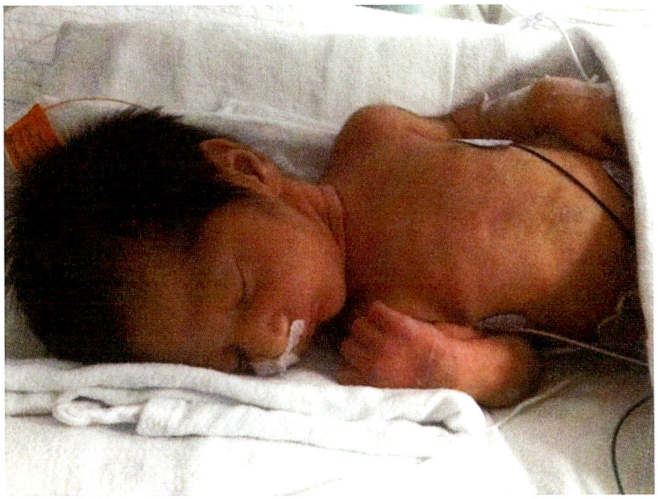

a. Necrotizing enterocolitis

b. Retinopathy of prematurity

c. Intraventricular hemorrhage

d. Respiratory distress syndrome

34–23. All except which of the following are cerebral lesions seen in the preterm infant?

a. Cerebellar hemorrhage

b. Middle cerebral artery stroke

c. Cystic periventricular leukomalacia

d. Periventricular hemorrhagic infarction

34–24. Which of the following is seen more typically in a term infant rather than a preterm infant?

a. Subdural hemorrhage

b. Cerebellar hemorrhage

c. Subarachnoid hemorrhage

d. Intraventricular hemorrhage

34–25. Which of the following is the preferred initial modality for identifying brain abnormalities in the newborn?

a. Sonography

b. Computed tomography

c. Magnetic resonance imaging

d. Positron emission tomography

34–26. Which of the following contributes to the increased risk of intraventricular hemorrhage in preterm infants?

a. Venous stasis and congestion

b. Impaired vascular autoregulation

c. Poor vessel support by the subependymal germinal matrix

d. All of the above

34–27. A 34-year-old multigravida presents for her postpartum visit and informs you her infant, born at 25 weeks' gestation, has a bleed in its brain. She reports she was told the bleeding has extended into the tissue. What grade intraventricular hemorrhage does her infant have?

a. Grade I

b. Grade II

c. Grade III

d. Grade IV

34–28. Which of the following medications has been shown to reduce neurodevelopmental impairment in the preterm infant?

a. Vitamin E

b. Indomethacin

c. Phenobarbital

d. Magnesium sulfate

34–29. Which of the following women are candidates for a course of antenatal corticosteroids according to the American College of Obstetricians and Gynecologists?

a. 26 weeks' gestation dilated to 3 cm contracting every 2 minutes

c. 23 weeks' gestation dilated to 2 cm contracting every 5 minutes

c. 33 weeks' gestation dilated to 3 cm who received a course of steroids 21 days ago on presentation for preterm premature rupture of membranes

d. All of the above

34–30. All except which of the following are risk factors for development of cerebral palsy?

a. Ischemia

b. Chorioamnionitis

c. Operative vaginal delivery

d. Intraventricular hemorrhage

34–31. Which of the following types of cerebral palsy is the least common?

a. Diplegia

b. Hemiplegia

c. Spastic quadriplegia

d. Choreoathetoid types

34–32. Which of the following statements about periventricular leukomalacia are true?

a. It is associated with cerebral palsy

b. Damage is irreversible because brain tissue does not regenerate

c. Due to lack of gliosis the areas appear as echolucent cysts on imaging

d. All of the above

34–33. All except which of the following substances have been shown to be toxic to brain tissue?

a. Calcium

b. Glutamate

c. Magnesium

d. Tumor necrosis factor

CHAPTER 34 ANSWER KEY

Question number	Letter answer	Page cited	Header cited
34–1	c	p. 636	Introduction
34–2	b	p. 636	Introduction
34–3	d	p. 636	Respiratory Distress Syndrome
34–4	c	p. 637	Etiopathogenesis
34–5	c	p. 637	Etiopathogenesis
34–6	c	p. 637	Clinical Course
34–7	c	p. 637	Treatment
34–8	d	p. 637	Treatment
34–9	d	p. 637	Clinical Course
34–10	d	p. 637	Treatment
34–11	b	p. 638	Surfactant Prophylaxis and Rescue
34–12	d	p. 638	Surfactant Prophylaxis and Rescue
34–13	b	p. 638	Prevention
34–14	a	p. 638	Prevention
34–15	d	p. 638	Prevention
34–16	d	p. 638	Prevention
34–17	c	p. 638	Prevention
34–18	b	p. 638	Prevention
34–19	a	p. 639	Necrotizing Enterocolitis
34–20	d	p. 639	Necrotizing Enterocolitis
34–21	c	p. 639	Retinopathy of Prematurity
34–22	a	p. 639	Necrotizing Enterocolitis
34–23	b	p. 639	Brain Disorders
34–24	a	p. 639	Intracranial Hemorrhage
34–25	a	p. 639	Brain Disorders
34–26	d	p. 639	Periventricular-Intraventricular Hemorrhage
34–27	d	p. 640	Periventricular-Intraventricular Hemorrhage
34–28	d	p. 640	Periventricular-Intraventricular Hemorrhage
34–29	d	p. 641	Periventricular-Intraventricular Hemorrhage
34–30	c	p. 641	Risks
34–31	d	p. 641	Cerebral Palsy
34–32	d	p. 640	Periventricular Leukomalacia
34–33	c	p. 641	Risks

CHAPTER 35

Stillbirth

35–1. When a standardized evaluation including autopsy, placental pathology, and testing of maternal and fetal tissues such as karyotype is conducted, in what percent of stillbirths can a probable or possible cause be identified?

a. 34%

b. 58%

c. 76%

d. 90%

35–2. Which of the following requirements must be met for reporting a fetal death in all U.S. states?

a. Weight >350 grams

b. Weight >500 grams

c. Gestational age >20 weeks

d. None of the above—the requirements vary by state

35–3. What was the most common cause of stillbirth in the Stillbirth Collaborative Research Network Study?

a. Undetermined

b. Fetal malformations

c. Placental abnormalities

d. Obstetrical complications

35–4. Which of the following is considered a risk factor for stillbirth?

a. Obesity

b. Nulliparity

c. Advanced maternal age

d. All of the above

35–5. Which of the following maternal risk factors carries the highest risk of stillbirth?

a. Prior stillbirth

b. Chronic hypertension

c. Cholestasis of pregnancy

d. Systemic lupus erythematosus

35–6. A 28-year-old primigravida with uncomplicated prenatal care presents to the labor unit at 38 weeks' gestation with contractions and decreased fetal movement. A diagnosis of fetal demise is made. Which of the following is true regarding establishing a cause of stillbirth?

a. May aid maternal coping

b. Allows accurate counseling regarding recurrence risk

c. May prompt therapy or intervention to prevent a similar outcome in a future pregnancy

d. All of the above

35–7. The patient in Question 35–6 declines autopsy but remains undecided regarding chromosomal analysis. Gross examination of the fetus reveals no obvious abnormalities or dysmorphology. How should the patient be counseled?

a. Chromosomal analysis is not indicated.

b. The risk of a chromosomal abnormality is up to 5%.

c. The risk of a chromosomal abnormality is up to 14%.

d. The risk of a chromosomal abnormality is up to 25%.

35–8. Recently, chromosomal microarray became the recommended method for chromosomal analysis in the setting of stillbirth. Which of the below statements regarding the benefit of chromosomal microarray compared to traditional karyotype is correct?

a. Chromosomal microarray provides quicker results

b. Chromosomal microarray results are more accurate

c. Chromosomal microarray results are more easily interpreted

d. Chromosomal microarray does not require dividing cells

35–9. A 25-year-old primigravida presents at 37 weeks' gestation with decreased fetal movement and is diagnosed with a fetal demise. On ultrasound amnionic fluid appears normal. She undergoes induction of labor without complications and delivers a stillborn infant that appears normal on examination. Examination of the placenta demonstrates no obvious abnormalities. Which of the maternal serum tests below is not indicated?

- **a.** Glucose level
- **b.** Kleihauer-Betke
- **c.** Type and screen
- **d.** Factor V Leiden testing

35–10. When a patient declines autopsy following stillbirth, which of the following tests may be useful, in addition to a fetogram such as the one shown below?

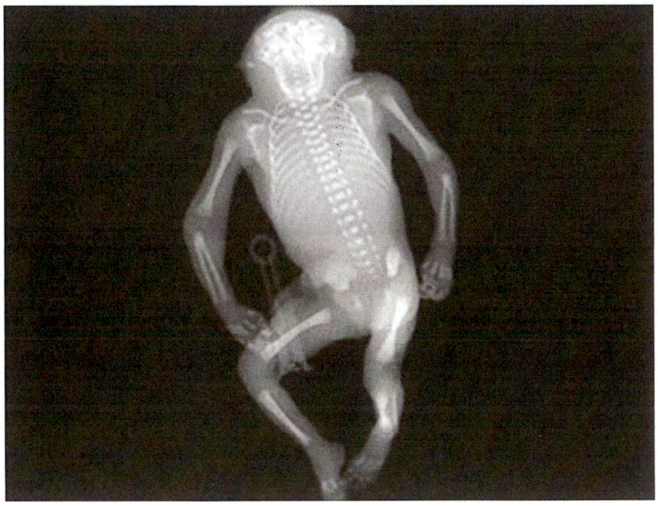

- **a.** Photography
- **b.** Bacterial cultures
- **c.** Magnetic resonance imaging
- **d.** All of the above

35–11. After delivery of a stillborn infant, a woman is unsure whether to pursue autopsy. Which counseling is most correct regarding the utility of autopsy?

- **a.** It rarely alters the presumed cause of death.
- **b.** It rarely alters future pregnancy management.
- **c.** It provides new information in approximately 25% of cases.
- **d.** It provides new information in approximately 75% of cases.

35–12. How often do autopsy results change the recurrence risk estimates and parental counseling following stillbirth?

- **a.** 5–10% of cases
- **b.** 10–20% of cases
- **c.** 25–50% of cases
- **d.** 50–75% of cases

35–13. A 35-year-old primigravida presents with fetal demise at 30 weeks' gestation. Which of the following may be associated with poor coping and greater risk of postpartum depression?

- **a.** Lack of keepsake items or photos
- **b.** Having her infant taken away due to need for testing
- **c.** Prolonged interval between diagnosis and induction
- **d.** All of the above

35–14. A 38-year-old G4P3 at 36 weeks' gestation by last menstrual period consistent with a first-trimester sonogram presents with a fetal demise. Her pregnancy was complicated by poorly controlled insulin-dependent type 2 diabetes mellitus, and a body mass index of 36 kg/m^2. She undergoes uncomplicated vaginal delivery of a 2000-gram infant without any visible abnormalities; placental pathology demonstrates a placenta which is small for gestational age with extensive perivillous thrombin deposition and maternal floor infarction, as shown in the image below. Of the factors possibly contributing to the patient's fetal demise, which is modifiable?

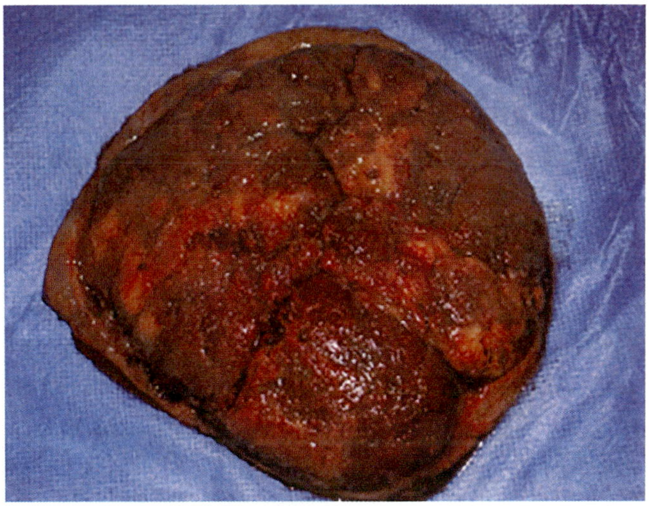

Used with permission from Dr. Ed Wells.

- **a.** Diabetes mellitus
- **b.** Placental insufficiency
- **c.** Fetal growth restriction
- **d.** None of the above

35–15. Which of the following recommendations could be made to the patient in Question 35–14 to decrease her future risk of recurrent stillbirth?

- **a.** Maternal karyotype
- **b.** Thrombophilia testing
- **c.** Preconception weight loss
- **d.** None of the above

35–16. For the patient in Question 35–14, which of the following interventions would be most appropriate in her future pregnancies?

- **a.** Full anticoagulation
- **b.** Prophylactic anticoagulation
- **c.** Delivery at 36 weeks' gestation
- **d.** Serial sonograms for growth in the third trimester

35–17. Which statement is not true regarding biophysical profiles in the setting of prior stillbirth?

- **a.** They increase the iatrogenic preterm birth rate.
- **b.** They are proven to decrease the risk of recurrent stillbirth.
- **c.** They are recommended by the American College of Obstetricians and Gynecologists after 32 weeks' gestation.
- **d.** All of the above

35–18. In the United States, which of the following gestational ages has the lowest associated fetal mortality rate per 1000 births?

- **a.** 20 weeks
- **b.** 30 weeks
- **c.** 39 weeks
- **d.** 42 weeks

35–19. In the United States, the definition of fetal death includes which of the following characteristics?

- **a.** No signs of life apparent at birth
- **b.** Induced terminations are included
- **c.** All pregnancies greater than 14 weeks' gestation
- **d.** None of the above

35–20. A 41-year-old G6P5 presents for fetal sonographic evaluation at 19 weeks' gestation. The following image is obtained, which demonstrates an absent calvarium (an arrow indicates the chin and asterisks mark the eyes). Her medical history is significant for poorly controlled hypertension and diabetes. Her obstetrical history is significant for having a previous child with Down syndrome and a major cardiac defect. Which of the following conditions likely contributed to this particular fetal anomaly?

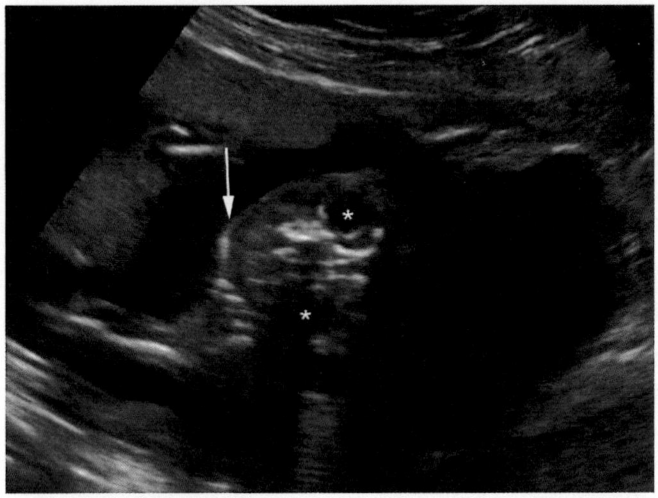

- **a.** Diabetes mellitus
- **b.** Advanced maternal age
- **c.** History of aneuploidy in a prior pregnancy
- **d.** History of anomalous infant in a prior pregnancy

35–21. The ient in Question 35–5 presents at 35 weeks' ge on for a prenatal care visit and is found to h a stillbirth. Induction is undertaken, and she vers the infant pictured below. Based on the llbirth Collaborative Research Writing Group's ategories, how would this stillbirth be classified with regard to the underlying cause?

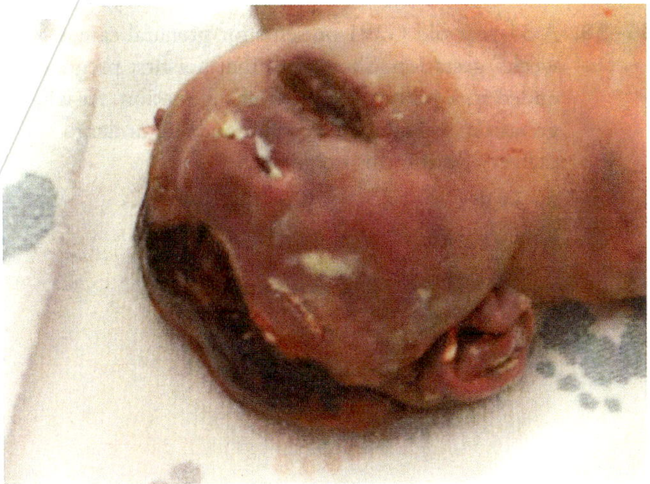

Used with permission from Dr. Tiffany Woodus.

a. Possible
b. Definite
c. Probable
d. Unknown

35–22. A 40-year-old G6P5 presents at 36 weeks' gestation with complaints of contractions and vaginal bleeding. Her prenatal care was routine other than administration of anti-D immune globulin at 28 weeks' gestation. On admission her blood pressure is 166/98 mmHg and proteinuria is found on urinalysis. Her cervix is 8 cm dilated and there is active vaginal bleeding. No fetal heart tones can be found, and a stillbirth is confirmed by sonographic examination. At delivery the placenta is noted to have the following appearance. What is the most common associated risk factor for this condition?

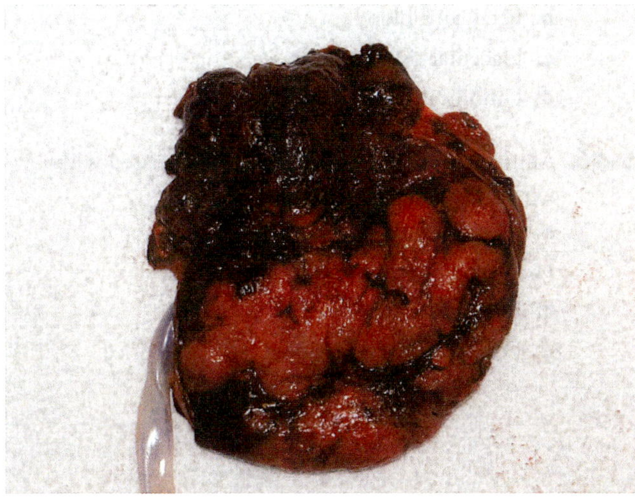

a. Hypertension
b. Hypothyroidism
c. Grand multiparity
d. Advanced maternal age

35–23. For the patient in Question 35–21, what additional testing is recommended?

a. Autopsy
b. Placental pathology
c. Chromosomal microarray
d. All of the above

35–24. For the patient in Question 35–21, which additional maternal blood test would be most useful in this clinical situation?

a. Kleihauer-Betke test

b. Thrombophilia testing

c. Lupus anticoagulant testing

d. Serum glucose measurement

35–25. Which specimen is most desirable for chromosomal microarray analysis of the stillborn infant?

a. Amnionic fluid

b. Fetal cord blood

c. Placental tissue sample

d. Umbilical cord segment

35–26. Almost half of all fetal deaths are associated with what pregnancy complication?

a. Preeclampsia

b. Oligohydramnios

c. Fetal malformations

d. Fetal growth restriction

35–27. At what gestational age should antenata[illegible]ting begin in women with a history of prior s[illegible]irth?

a. 28 weeks

b. 32 weeks

c. 34 weeks

d. 38 weeks

35–28. A 34-year-old G2P1 presents for prenatal care at [illegible] weeks' gestation. She reveals that her first pregnanc[illegible] ended in a stillbirth at 36 weeks' gestation. At what gestational age do you recommend she undergo delivery during this pregnancy?

a. 34 weeks

b. 36 weeks

c. 38 weeks

d. 39 weeks

CHAPTER 35 ANSWER KEY

Question number	Letter answer	Page cited	Header cited
35–1	**c**	p. 645	Causes of Fetal Death
35–2	**d**	p. 645	Definition of Fetal Mortality
35–3	**d**	p. 646	Causes of Fetal Death
35–4	**d**	p. 646	Risk Factors
35–5	**d**	p. 647	Risk Factors
35–6	**d**	p. 647	Evaluation of the Stillborn Fetus
35–7	**b**	p. 647	Evaluation of the Stillborn Fetus
35–8	**d**	p. 647	Evaluation of the Stillborn Fetus
35–9	**d**	p. 648	Evaluation of the Stillborn Fetus
35–10	**d**	p. 648	Evaluation of the Stillborn Fetus
35–11	**c**	p. 648	Evaluation of the Stillborn Fetus
35–12	**c**	p. 648	Evaluation of the Stillborn Fetus
35–13	**d**	p. 648	Psychological Aspects
35–14	**a**	p. 648	Prior Stillbirth
35–15	**c**	p. 648	Prior Stillbirth
35–16	**d**	p. 648	Prior Stillbirth
35–17	**b**	p. 649	Prior Stillbirth
35–18	**b**	p. 645	Figure 35-2
35–19	**a**	p. 645	Definition of Fetal Mortality
35–20	**a**	p. 646	Risk Factors
35–21	**c**	p. 646	Causes of Fetal Death
35–22	**a**	p. 646	Causes of Fetal Death
35–23	**d**	p. 646	Evaluation of the Stillborn Fetus
35–24	**a**	p. 646	Evaluation of the Stillborn Fetus
35–25	**b**	p. 647	Evaluation of the Stillborn Fetus
35–26	**d**	p. 648	Prior Stillbirth
35–27	**b**	p. 649	Prior Stillbirth
35–28	**d**	p. 648	Prior stillbirth

SECTION 10

THE PUERPERIUM

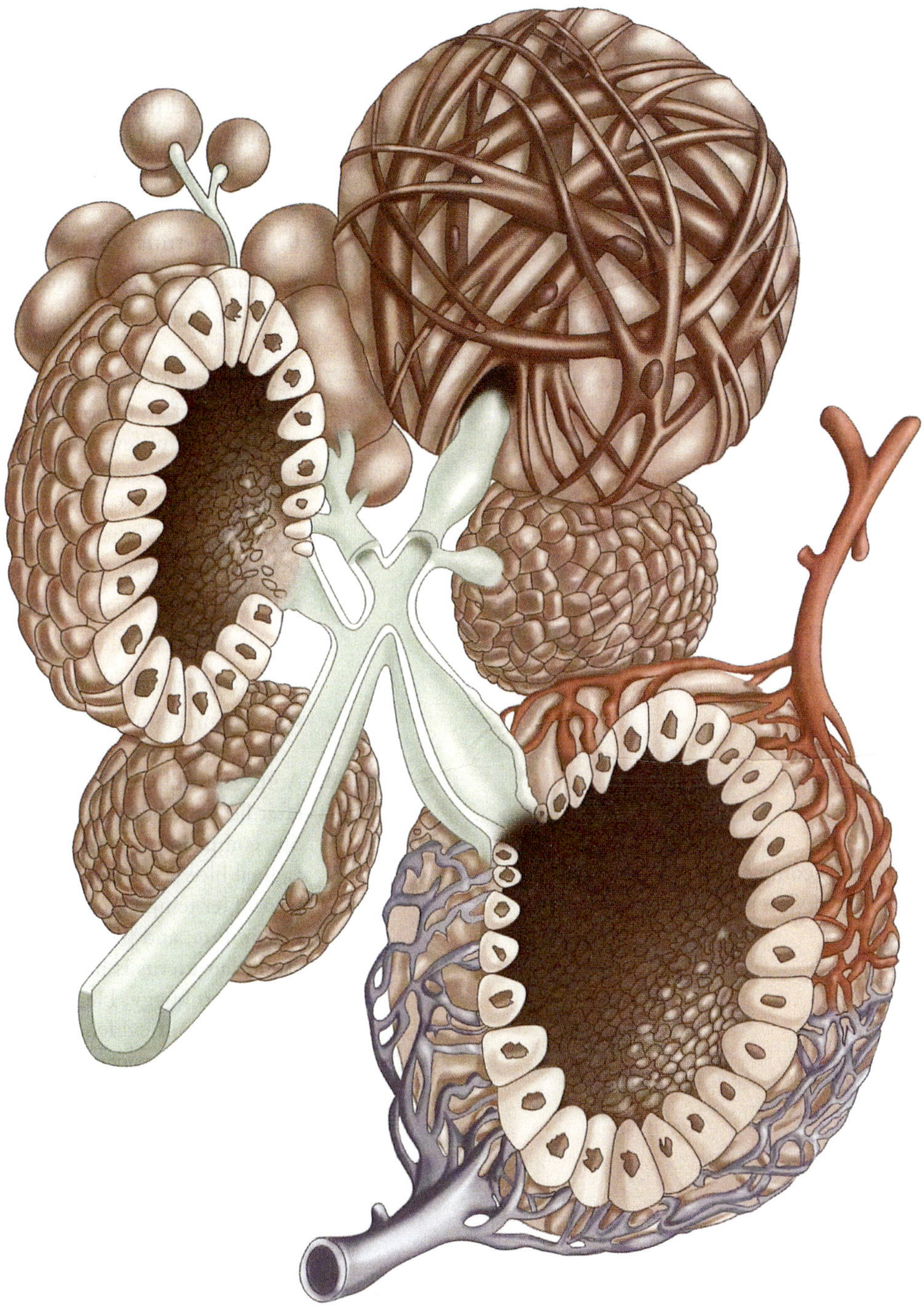

CHAPTER 36

The Puerperium

36–1. What duration of time is encompassed in the puerperium?

a. 2–4 weeks
b. 4–6 weeks
c. 6–8 weeks
d. 10–12 weeks

36–2. What are myrtiform caruncles?

a. Vaginal rugae
b. Scarred tags of hymenal tissue
c. A sexually transmitted infection
d. Microscopic tears in the vaginal epithelium

36–3. At what point in the puerperium does the endocervical canal reform?

a. 1 week postpartum
b. 2 weeks postpartum
c. 3 weeks postpartum
d. 4 weeks postpartum

36–4. What percentage of women experience regression of high-grade dysplasia following delivery?

a. 10%
b. 33%
c. 35%
d. 50%

36–5. How long does complete uterine involution take following delivery?

a. 1 week
b. 2 weeks
c. 3 weeks
d. 4 weeks

36–6. A 26-year-old G3P3 is postpartum day 1 following an uncomplicated vaginal delivery. She reports sharp, intermittent lower abdominal pain, which is more severe than in her prior deliveries. Her heart rate is 84 beats per minute, blood pressure 110/60 mmHg, and her temperature 99.3 °F. Her abdomen is soft on exam and there is no uterine tenderness. A scant amount of lochia is appreciated on bimanual exam. What is the most likely diagnosis?

a. Afterpains
b. Endometritis
c. Bladder flap hematoma
d. Septic pelvic thrombophlebitis

36–7. A 20-year-old G1P1 presents to the emergency room 10 days after an uncomplicated vaginal delivery complaining of fever, nausea/vomiting, abdominal pain, and increased vaginal discharge. On arrival, she is febrile to 38.6 °C and she has fundal tenderness on exam. Which of the following tests would be least helpful for further evaluation?

a. A complete blood count
b. A basic metabolic profile
c. A transvaginal ultrasound
d. A Gram stain of her vaginal discharge

36–8. A 40-year-old G2P2 presents to your office 2 weeks after her scheduled cesarean delivery for follow-up. She complains of intermittent episodes of heavy vaginal bleeding, occurring as recently as the day prior. Her temperature is 99.6°F, heart rate 98 beats per minute, and blood pressure 120/80 mmHg. On exam, her uterus is noted to be enlarged to 20 weeks in size and boggy. Her incision appears well approximated without evidence of infection. The most appropriate management includes which of the following?

a. A complete blood count
b. Methergine administration
c. Empiric antibiotic treatment
d. All of the above

36–9. Secondary postpartum hemorrhage is defined as uterine hemorrhage occurring during what timeframe after delivery?

a. 24 hours to 6 weeks

b. 48 hours to 6 weeks

c. 24 hours to 12 weeks

d. 48 hours to 12 weeks

36–10. What are common features of the urinary bladder in the postpartum period?

a. Increased capacity

b. Incomplete emptying

c. Insensitivity to intravesical pressures

d. All of the above

36–11. A 24-year-old G1P1 complains of abdominal pain and subjective fever 1 day following an uncomplicated vaginal delivery. Which of the following physical exam signs or laboratory values would be most helpful to make a diagnosis of endometritis in this postpartum patient?

a. Fundal tenderness

b. An absolute neutrophilia

c. White blood cell count of 25,000/μL

d. All of the above

36–12. After delivery, how long do cardiovascular parameters including cardiac output, heart rate, and blood pressure take to return to nonpregnant levels?

a. 48 hours

b. 72 hours

c. 7 days

d. 10 days

36–13. You counsel your puerperal patient that most women first approach their prepregnancy weight by which time interval following delivery?

a. 3 months

b. 6 months

c. 9 months

d. 12 months

36–14. Your patient is postoperative day 2 following a primary cesarean delivery for failure to progress. She is frustrated because she is only getting small drops of thick yellow liquid from her breasts. How long would you tell her to expect colostrum production before beginning her conversion to a more mature milk?

a. 2 to 5 days

b. 2 to 10 days

c. 5 to 14 days

d. 5 to 21 days

36–15. What vitamin is virtually absent in human breast milk?

a. Vitamin C

b. Vitamin A

c. Vitamin K

d. All vitamins are equally represented in breast milk

36–16. Which hormone is most responsible for milk expression during lactation?

a. Prolactin

b. Oxytocin

c. Dopamine

d. Progesterone

36–17. How would you advise a patient who is exclusively breastfeeding 4 weeks after delivery and develops nipple fissures?

a. Wash the area with mild soap and water daily.

b. Apply a steroid cream and use a nipple shield temporarily.

c. Continue exclusive breastfeeding without interruption.

d. Do not allow infant to feed on the affected side and empty the breast regularly with a pump.

36–18. All except which of the following conditions are contraindications to breastfeeding?

a. Infant with galactosemia

b. Maternal hepatitis B infection

c. Human immunodeficiency virus infection

d. Maternal active and untreated tuberculosis

36–19. A 21-year-old G1P1 presents to your office 4 days following an uncomplicated vaginal delivery complaining of breast pain and difficulty with breastfeeding. Her temperature is 37.8°C, heart rate 102 beats per minute, and respiratory rate 22 breaths per minute. The appearance of her breasts is similar to that pictured in the image. No erythema or fluctuance is appreciated on exam. What should you recommend to the patient?

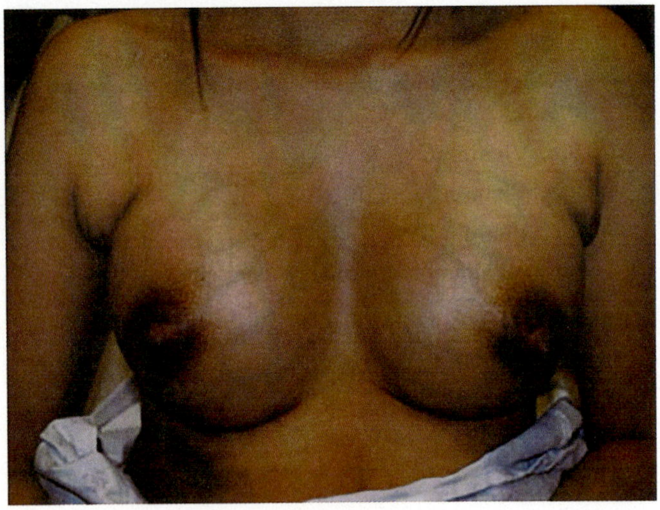

a. Initiation of dicloxacillin

b. Admission to the hospital

c. Stop breastfeeding immediately and use a breast binder

d. Oral analgesics, cool packs, and frequent feeding or pumping

36–20. Your patient presents 5 days postpartum with an axillary mass. She noted it during pregnancy although reports it was much smaller. Yesterday, she noticed that the mass became larger and more tender. Her face is shielded and a sagittal photograph of her breast, axilla, and arm is show below. She denies fever and has no additional complaints. Management of the patient should primarily include which of the following?

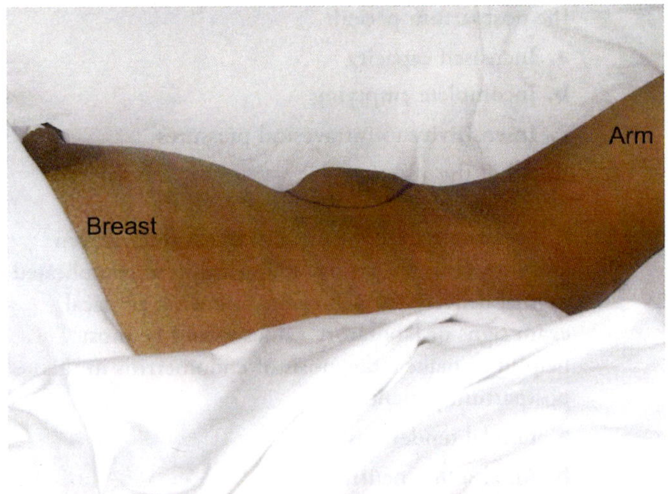

a. Needle aspiration

b. Observation and reassurance

c. Axillary lymph node excision

d. Antibiotic therapy with gram-positive coverage

36–21. A 34-year-old G3P3 with a history of migraine headaches calls your office 1 week following an uncomplicated vaginal delivery complaining of severe headaches. She did receive epidural anesthesia during her labor course, but review of her chart confirms that the epidural placement was easy and uncomplicated. The patient reports that the headaches began a few days following delivery and are associated with nausea, but no vomiting, and are minimally improved with either rest or over-the-counter analgesics. What is the most likely trigger of this patient's postpartum headaches?

a. Dural puncture

b. Estrogen withdrawal

c. Progesterone withdrawal

d. Intracerebral hemorrhage

36–22. Your patient had a 4-hour second stage of labor and vaginal delivery without laceration. As her epidural analgesia subsides, she complains of perineal pain. Her temperature is a 37.0°C, pulse 84 beats per minute, and blood pressure 120/68 mmHg. Her first void yielded 300 mL of urine. Management of the patient should primarily include which of the following?

a. Perineal cool pack
b. Surgical evacuation
c. Diagnostic needle aspiration
d. Broad-spectrum intravenous antibiotic therapy

36–23. A 19-year-old G1P1 complains of worsening vulvar pain in the recovery room 6 hours following a vaginal delivery. The delivery was complicated by a prolonged second stage and a third degree laceration. On further evaluation, her temperature is 37.2°C, heart rate 130 beats per minute, blood pressure 86/52 mmHg, and respiratory rate 28 breaths per minute. She appears pale and mildly diaphoretic. Examination of the perineum reveals the findings shown in the photo below. What is the next best course of action?

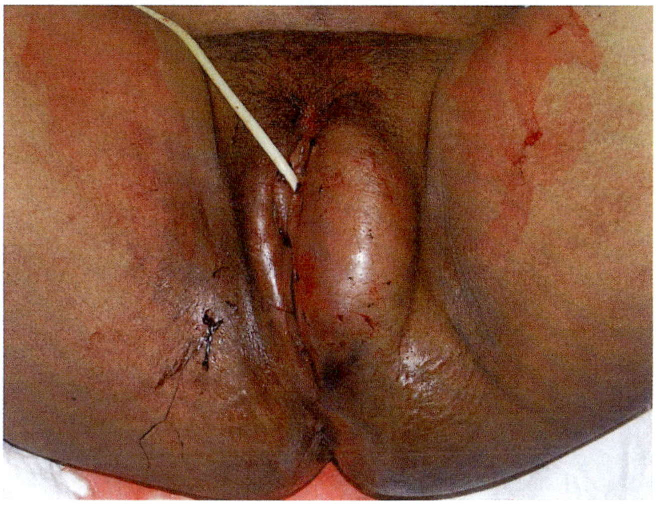

a. Urgent surgical evacuation
b. Place a vaginal pack and Foley catheter
c. Check a complete blood count and observe closely
d. Start intravenous antibiotics with gram-negative coverage

36–24. A 29-year-old G2P2 with an 18-hour labor course is unable to void 5 hours following a vaginal delivery. What is the best management option?

a. A single in-and-out catheterization
b. Place a Foley catheter for 24 hours
c. Continue close observation without intervention
d. Encourage increased fluid intake since the bladder is likely empty following delivery

36–25. Which of the following is true regarding the postpartum blues?

a. May be affected by body image concerns
b. Usually lasts for no more than 10 days after delivery
c. Effective treatment involves recognition and reassurance
d. All of the above

36–26. A 30-year-old G1P1 complains of difficulty with ambulation on postpartum day 1 following a labor and delivery course, which lasted 24 hours and included 3 hours of pushing in stirrups. You perform an exam and note bilateral foot drop on exam. Injury to what nerve is the most likely cause of the patient's ambulation difficulty?

a. Femoral nerve
b. Ilioinguinal nerve
c. Common peroneal nerve
d. Lateral femoral cutaneous nerve

36–27. Which of the following is true regarding the condition shown in the pelvic radiograph?

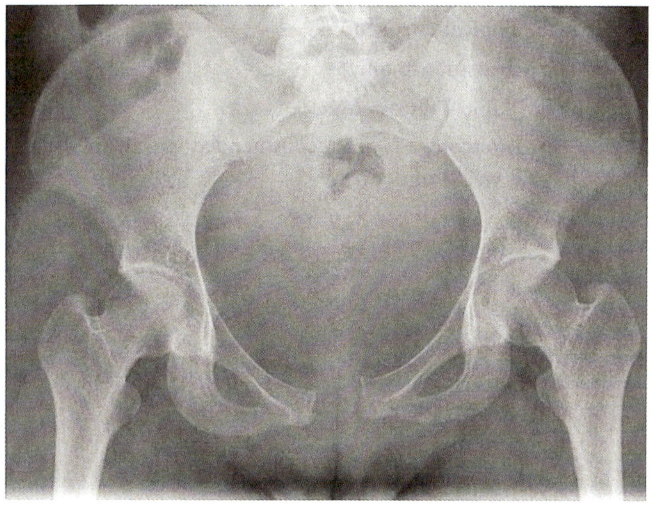

Reproduced with permission from Cunningham FG, Leveno KJ, Bloom SL, et al (eds): The Puerperium. In Williams Obstetrics, 25th ed. New York, McGraw-Hill, 2018, Figure 36-7.

a. Symphyseal separation >1.5 cm is diagnostic.
b. Surgery is usually necessary for separation >3 cm.
c. Treatment is generally conservative and consists of rest and placement of a pelvic binder.
d. All of the above

36–28. What is the mean time to ovulation resumption in a postpartum woman who elects not to breastfeed?

a. 4 weeks
b. 5 weeks
c. 6 weeks
d. 7 weeks

36–29. Your patient presents for her 6-week follow-up visit after having a primary cesarean delivery for breech presentation. She is trying to breastfeed exclusively but reports issues with milk supply. What contraceptive option would you not recommend for this patient?

a. Progestin-only pills

b. Estrogen-progestin patch

c. Depot medroxyprogesterone

d. A levonorgestrel intrauterine device

36–30. Following an uncomplicated vaginal delivery, when can women be advised to resume coitus based on desire and comfort?

a. 1 week postpartum

b. 2 weeks postpartum

c. 3 weeks postpartum

d. 4 weeks postpartum

36–31. What treatment can be offered to the postpartum woman who is exclusively breastfeeding and complains of vaginal dryness during intercourse 7 weeks following delivery?

a. Topical estrogen

b. Reassurance only

c. Topical testosterone

d. Intercourse is not recommended within the first 8 weeks of delivery.

36–32. Approximately what percentage of postpartum women require readmission to the hospital within 8 weeks of delivery?

a. <1%

b. 3%

c. 7%

d. 10%

36–33. A 29-year-old G1P1 presents for a follow-up visit 4 weeks postpartum following an uncomplicated spontaneous vaginal delivery. She is overall doing well and has returned to most of her usual activities. However, she complains of low energy levels despite the fact that her baby is sleeping for long intervals at night. What should you offer her?

a. Reassurance only

b. Psychiatry referral

c. Check her thyroid hormone levels

d. All of the above

CHAPTER 36 ANSWER KEY

Question number	Letter answer	Page cited	Header cited
36–1	b	p. 652	Introduction
36–2	b	p. 652	Birth Canal
36–3	a	p. 653	Uterus
36–4	d	p. 653	Uterus
36–5	d	p. 653	Uterus
36–6	a	p. 654	Afterpains
36–7	d	p. 654	Lochia
36–8	d	p. 654	Subinvolution
36–9	c	p. 654	Late Postpartum Hemorrhage
36–10	d	p. 655	Urinary Tract
36–11	a	p. 655	Hematological and Coagulation Changes
36–12	d	p. 655	Pregnancy Induced Hypervolemia
36–13	b	p. 656	Postpartum Diuresis
36–14	c	p. 656	Breast Anatomy and Secretory Products
36–15	c	p. 656	Breast Anatomy and Secretory Products
36–16	b	p. 656	Endocrinology of Lactation
36–17	d	p. 658	Care of Breasts
36–18	b	p. 658	Contraindications to Breastfeeding
36–19	d	p. 659	Breast Engorgement
36–20	b	p. 659	Other Issues with Lactation
36–21	b	p. 660	Hospital Care
36–22	a	p. 660	Perineal Care
36–23	a	p. 660	Perineal Care
36–24	b	p. 660	Bladder Function
36–25	d	p. 661	Pain, Mood and Cognition
36–26	c	p. 661	Neuromusculoskeletal Problems
36–27	c	p. 661	Musculoskeletal Injuries
36–28	d	p. 662	Contraception
36–29	b	p. 663	Contraception
36–30	b	p. 663	Coitus
36–31	a	p. 663	Coitus
36–32	b	p. 663	Late Maternal Morbidity
36–33	a	p. 663	Follow-up Care

CHAPTER 37

Puerperal Complications

37–1. What percentage of non-breastfeeding women develop fever from breast engorgement postpartum?

a. 15%
b. 25%
c. 35%
d. 55%

37–2. What is the most common etiology of persistent fevers after childbirth?

a. Atelectasis
b. Pyelonephritis
c. Breast engorgement
d. Genital tract infections

37–3. What physiological process in the postpartum period causes urinary tract infections to be uncommon?

a. Diuresis
b. Passage of lochia
c. Uterine involution
d. Immunosuppression

37–4. Which of the following is the single most significant risk factor for development of an uterine infection?

a. Route of delivery
b. Use of internal monitors
c. Artificial rupture of membranes
d. Group B streptococcus colonization

37–5. A 35-year-old multigravida at 39 weeks' gestation undergoes an induction for elevated blood pressures at term. After 24 hours, placement of internal monitors, and 10 cervical exams, the patient undergoes a cesarean delivery for failure to progress. Which of the following is not a risk factor for her developing an uterine infection?

a. Multiparity
b. Prolonged labor
c. Cesarean delivery
d. Placement of internal monitors

37–6. What organism has been implicated in late-onset, indolent metritis?

a. *Proteus*
b. *Klebsiella*
c. *Chlamydia*
d. *Peptostreptococcus*

37–7. What is the most important criterion for the diagnosis of postpartum metritis?

a. Fever
b. Leukocytosis
c. Foul-smelling lochia
d. Parametrial tenderness

37–8. A 20-year-old G1P1 underwent a cesarean delivery for failure to progress. Just prior to surgery, the patient was diagnosed with metritis and started on broad-spectrum antibiotics, which were continued postpartum. The patient continues to have fever on postoperative day 5. She does not appear septic. She is frustrated that she can't go home. Which of the following is the least likely diagnosis?

a. Infected hematoma
b. Parametrial phlegmon
c. Septic pelvic thrombophlebitis
d. Antimicrobial-resistant bacteria

37–9. What is the difference in treatment for metritis in cases of vaginal delivery versus cesarean section?

a. Dosing of antibiotics
b. Coverage of anaerobes
c. Duration of treatment
d. Route of administration of antibiotics

37–10. Which of the following regimens is the gold standard for treatment of a pelvic infection following a cesarean delivery?

a. Meropenem
b. Vancomycin
c. Clindamycin and aztreonam
d. Clindamycin and gentamicin

37–11. A 22-year-old primigravida at term is diagnosed with failure to progress, and the plan is made for cesarean delivery. The patient has no medical problems other than a body mass index of 50 kg/m^2. She also denies any allergies. The anesthesiologist asks if you would like routine perioperative antimicrobial prophylaxis. Which antibiotic do you ask for to further reduce her chance of a postoperative infection?

a. 3 grams instead of 2 grams of cefazolin

b. Vancomycin instead of the routine cefazolin

c. Routine 2 grams of cefazolin prior to skin incision

d. Ampicillin, gentamicin, and clindamycin for 24 hours after the surgery

37–12. Which of the following has not been shown to lower the risk for infection after cesarean delivery?

a. Spontaneous separation of the placenta

b. Chlorhexidine-alcohol skin preparation

c. Single-dose antibiotics prior to skin incision

d. Surgeons changing gloves after delivery of the placenta

37–13. In more than 90% of women, metritis responds to treatment with antibiotics within what period of time?

a. 12–24 hours

b. 24–36 hours

c. 48–72 hours

d. 72–96 hours

37–14. Which of the following is an evidence-based statement about the use of vacuum-assisted wound closure devices in obstetrics?

a. It prevents wound infection.

b. It is superior to standard dressings.

c. Provider time is decreased substantially.

d. It is significantly more cost effective than standard dressings.

37–15. A 30-year-old G2P2 presents on postoperative day 6 to the emergency room complaining of drainage from her cesarean incision. The cesarean delivery was for failure to progress after a long induction. The patient is currently afebrile. Her body mass index is 47 kg/m^2. The patient reports that she sat down yesterday and felt a pop. Shortly thereafter, she noticed pink/light brown drainage coming from her incision. She endorses chills and skin irritation around the incision. Lochia has been normal. On your exam, her skin is erythematous near the incision. There is serosanguinous drainage from the wound. Although the patient has good pain tolerance, why do you elect to take her to the operating room to evaluate the incision?

a. You plan to proceed with hysterectomy.

b. You want to open the wound, debride necrotic tissue, and then close it back up using en bloc closure.

c. You want to place a negative-pressure wound therapy system and that can only be done in the operating room.

d. You are concerned that the fascia may not be intact and if so, the fascia needs to be closed in the operating room.

37–16. Which of the following statements about necrotizing fasciitis is false?

a. It is common with low mortality rates.

b. Three risk factors are diabetes, obesity, and hypertension.

c. Surgical debridement of infected tissue should leave wide margins of healthy bleeding tissue.

d. Early diagnosis, surgical debridement, antimicrobials, and intensive care are paramount to successful treatment.

37–17. Which of the following statements about an ovarian abscess in the puerperium is true?

a. Rupture is rare

b. Usually affects both ovaries

c. Women present 4–6 weeks after delivery

d. It is thought to be caused by bacterial invasion of the ovary through a rent in the capsule.

37–18. Which of the following is frequently the first sign/symptom of peritonitis in a postpartum woman?

- **a.** Diarrhea
- **b.** Skin erythema
- **c.** Adynamic ileus
- **d.** Abdominal rigidity

37–19. Which of the following statements about the phlegmon illustrated in the figure below is true?

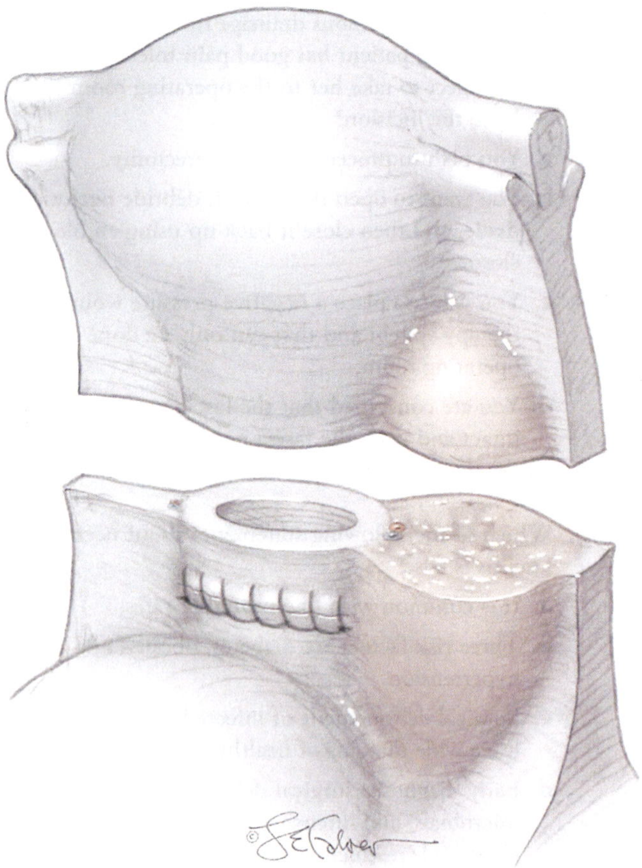

Reproduced with permission from Cunningham FG, Leveno KJ, Bloom SL, et al (eds): Puerperal complications. In Williams Obstetrics, 25th ed. New York, McGraw-Hill, 2018, Figure 37-3.

- **a.** This is usually a bilateral process.
- **b.** Rarely is this limited to the parametrium.
- **c.** Typically fever resolves in 5–7 days with broad-spectrum antibiotics.
- **d.** The most common route of extension is posteriorly into the rectovaginal septum.

37–20. Which of the following is least likely to occur during surgery for uterine incisional necrosis?

- **a.** Transfusion
- **b.** Hysterectomy
- **c.** Surgical debridement
- **d.** Bilateral salpingo-oophorectomy

37–21. What is the overall incidence of septic pelvic thrombophlebitis?

- **a.** 1/100
- **b.** 1/200
- **c.** 1/2000–1/3000
- **d.** 1/20,000–1/30,000

37–22. A 19-year-old primigravida undergoes a cesarean delivery for failure to progress. Her course is complicated by chorioamnionitis for which she receives broad-spectrum antibiotics. On postoperative day 5, the patient is still having fevers. She feels well and is becoming annoyed that she can not go home. Her incision is healing nicely with no erythema or drainage. On computed tomography imaging, the patient is noted to have a clot that extends to the ovarian vein. An image is provided below. What is the next step in your management?

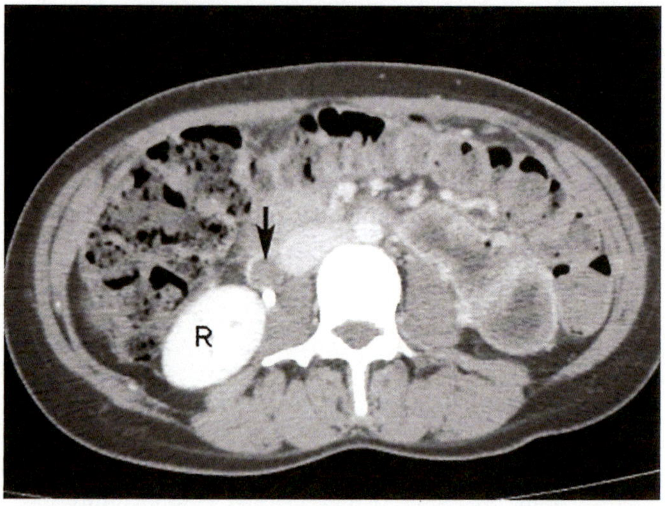

Reproduced with permission from Worley KC: Postoperative complications. In Yeomans ER, Hoffman BL, Gilstrap LC III, et al (eds). Cunningham and Gilstrap's Operative Obstetrics, 3rd ed. New York, McGraw Hill Education, 2017.

- **a.** Therapeutic heparin
- **b.** Continuation of antibiotic therapy
- **c.** Consult interventional radiology about removing the clot and/or placing a filter.
- **d.** Stop all medications and discharge home, so she can walk, reducing further clot risk.

37–23. Which of the following is a risk factor for episiotomy dehiscence?

- **a.** Smoking
- **b.** Infection
- **c.** Genital warts
- **d.** All of the above

37–24. A 22-year-old G1P1 presents 6 days after a vaginal delivery. Her course was complicated by chorioamnionitis and a second-degree perineal laceration. The patient is complaining of pain and drainage from her vagina. On exam, her laceration repair is open and draining purulent material. Which of the following would not be a step in your management?

- **a.** Intravenous antibiotics
- **b.** Debridement of necrotic tissue
- **c.** Establishment of adequate analgesia prior to debridement
- **d.** Intravenous antibiotics, debridement of necrotic tissue in the operating room, and then immediate closure of the laceration

37–25. What is the case-fatality rate of toxic shock syndrome?

- **a.** 1–2%
- **b.** 5–6%
- **c.** 10–15%
- **d.** 20–25%

37–26. A 20-year-old G1P1 presents 3 days postpartum after a vaginal delivery for fever, headache, nausea/vomiting, and lower abdominal pain. The patient's boyfriend reports that she got sick very quickly and is "not making sense when she talks." On exam, the patient has severe abdominal pain and foul-smelling lochia. She is hypotensive and tachycardic. She appears extremely ill. Which of the following is the most likely diagnosis?

- **a.** Listeriosis
- **b.** Pyelonephritis
- **c.** Gastroenteritis
- **d.** Toxic shock syndrome

37–27. Which of the following is the best treatment for toxic shock syndrome?

- **a.** Supportive care
- **b.** Supportive care and antibiotics
- **c.** Supportive care, antibiotics, and wound debridement if necessary
- **d.** There is no necessary treatment as it will resolve on its own over time

37–28. What is the incidence of mastitis?

- **a.** 1%
- **b.** 3%
- **c.** 10%
- **d.** 15%

37–29. When is mastitis most likely to occur?

- **a.** Postpartum day 1
- **b.** Postpartum day 5
- **c.** 3–4 weeks postpartum
- **d.** 6–9 months postpartum

37–30. What percentage of women with mastitis develop an abscess?

- **a.** 1%
- **b.** 3%
- **c.** 10%
- **d.** 15%

37–31. Which of the following is not expected in cases of mastitis?

- **a.** Fever
- **b.** Chills
- **c.** Breast firmness
- **d.** Symptoms in both breasts

37–32. A 32-year-old G4P2 presents 3 weeks after undergoing a cesarean delivery for breech presentation. She has been exclusively breastfeeding and feeling well. She now complains of a 2-day history of fever, chills, and breast pain. She finds it difficult to feed the infant on the affected side. On exam, the breast is warm, red, and tender. You expect mastitis at the least, are not sure if there is an abscess. You obtain an ultrasound and the image is shown below. What is the best management plan?

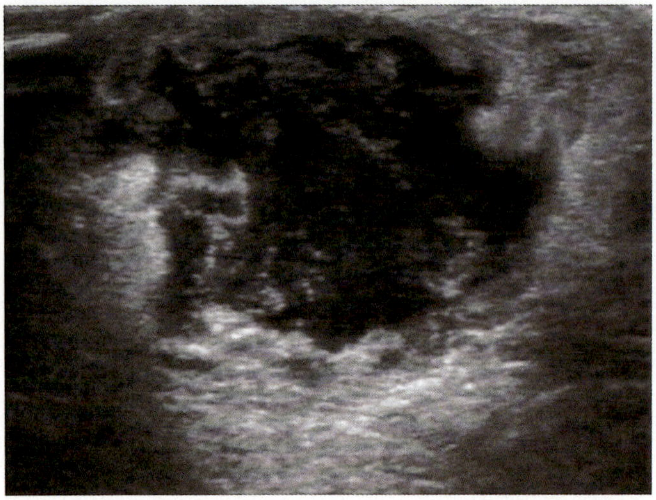

Used with permission from Dr. Emily Adhikari.

a. Intravenous antibiotics, supportive care, suspend breast feeding on the affected side for 48–72 hours

b. Oral antibiotics, discontinuation of breast feeding on the affected side, follow up with OB/GYN next week

c. Intravenous antibiotics, drainage of abscess, culture, pumping or breast feeding continued for both breasts

d. Milk culture, discharge home with pain medication, encourage breast feeding on that side, antibiotics if the milk culture is positive

CHAPTER 37 ANSWER KEY

Question number	Letter answer	Page cited	Header cited
37–1	a	p. 666	Puerperal Fever
37–2	d	p. 666	Puerperal Fever
37–3	a	p. 667	Puerperal Fever
37–4	a	p. 667	Uterine Infection
37–5	a	p. 667	Uterine Infection
37–6	c	p. 668	Uterine Infection
37–7	a	p. 668	Uterine Infection
37–8	d	p. 668	Uterine Infection
37–9	b	p. 668	Choice of Antimicrobials
37–10	d	p. 669	Table 37-2 Antimicrobial regimens for pelvic infections following cesarean delivery
37–11	a	p. 669	Perioperative Prophylaxis
37–12	d	p. 669–670	Perioperative Prophylaxis
37–13	c	p. 670	Complications of Uterine and Pelvic Infections
37–14	c	p. 670–671	Vacuum-Assisted Wound Closure
37–15	d	p. 671	Abdominal Incisional Infections
37–16	a	p. 671	Necrotizing Fasciitis
37–17	d	p. 671	Adnexal Abscesses and Peritonitis
37–18	c	p. 672	Adnexal Abscesses and Peritonitis
37–19	c	p. 672	Figure 37-3
37–20	d	p. 672	Parametrial Phlegmon
37–21	c	p. 673	Septic Pelvic Thrombophlebitis
37–22	b	p. 673	Septic Pelvic Thrombophlebitis
37–23	d	p. 674	Perineal Infections
37–24	d	p. 675	Early Repair of Infected Episiotomy
37–25	c	p. 675	Toxic Shock Syndrome
37–26	d	p. 675	Toxic Shock Syndrome
37–27	c	p. 675	Toxic Shock Syndrome
37–28	b	p. 675	Breast Infections
37–29	c	p. 675	Breast Infections
37–30	c	p. 675	Breast Infections
37–31	d	p. 675	Breast Infections
37–32	c	p. 676	Breast Abscess

CHAPTER 38

Contraception

38–1. According to the World Health Organization, with no contraceptive use, a sexually active woman has what risk for pregnancy over a year?

- **a.** 65%
- **b.** 70%
- **c.** 75%
- **d.** 85%

38–2. In contrast to the answer to Question 38–1, typical use of combination oral contraceptive pills by a sexually active woman has what risk for pregnancy over the first year of use?

- **a.** 3%
- **b.** 9%
- **c.** 13%
- **d.** 17%

38–3. Which of the following is not considered a long-acting reversible contraceptive method?

- **a.** Levonorgestrel implant
- **b.** Copper intrauterine device
- **c.** Depot medroxyprogesterone acetate
- **d.** All of the above are long-acting reversible contraceptive methods

38–4. What is the purpose of the United States Medical Eligibility Criteria, published by the Centers for Disease Control and Prevention?

- **a.** Provides legal criteria for contraception provision to minors
- **b.** Provides codified data for insurance submission under the Affordable Care Act
- **c.** Provides financial stratification criteria for Medicaid contraception eligibility
- **d.** Provides guidance in contraceptive choice for women with various comorbidities

38–5. Which of the following statements properly describe the intrauterine device?

- **a.** Mirena is a levonorgestrel-eluting device, and it is approved for 5 years of use following insertion.
- **b.** Liletta contains 52 mg of levonorgestrel, and it is approved for 5 years of use following insertion.
- **c.** Skyla is the largest of the intrauterine devices, and it is approved for 3 years of use following insertion.
- **d.** ParaGard is not considered a "chemically active" intrauterine device, and it is approved for 7 years of use following insertion.

38–6. Contraceptive efficacy with the method pictured below is not believed to result from which of the following mechanisms?

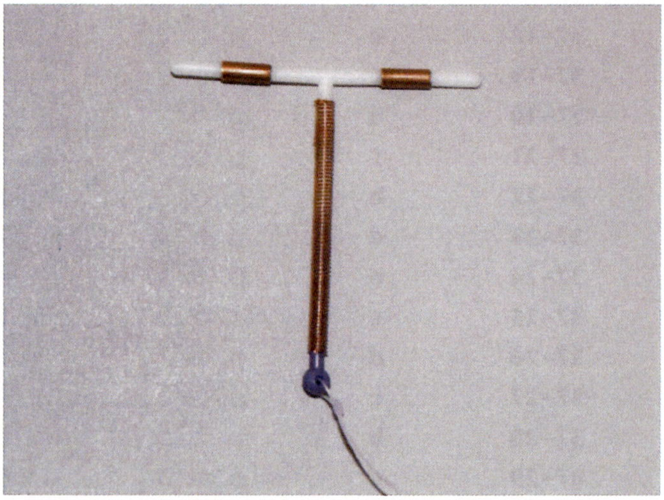

- **a.** Ovulation inhibition
- **b.** Decreased motility and viability of sperm
- **c.** Reduced viability of egg and sperm preventing fertilization
- **d.** Endometrial inflammation action directed toward a blastocyst, if formed

38–7. Which of the following statements properly characterizes expulsion of an intrauterine device?

a. The cumulative expulsion rate after 3 years is 20%.

b. Expulsion is most common in the final years of approved use.

c. If a woman is unable to palpate the trailing strings, she should be evaluated.

d. All of the above

38–8. Ms. Thomas calls complaining of dull lower abdominal pain for the last 2 months. You placed an intrauterine device (IUD) 3 months ago, and she has never attempted to palpate the strings. On speculum examination you see the picture below. Which of the following is the most appropriate next step?

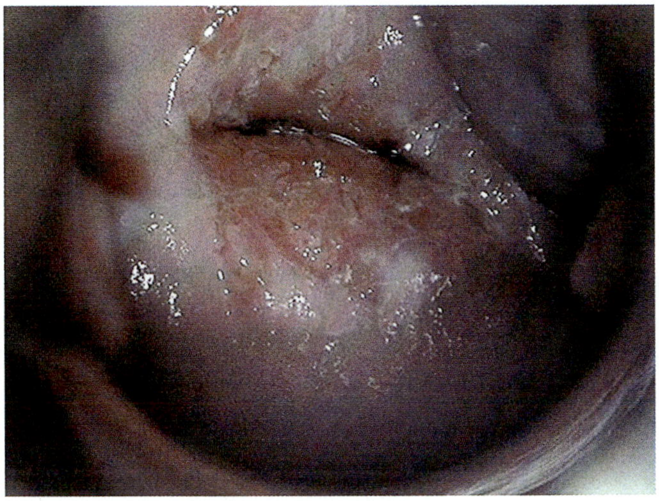

a. Obtain a β-hCG level

b. Obtain a KUB radiograph

c. Attempt IUD removal by means of an IUD hook or Randall stone clamp

d. Continue the exam by twirling a cytologic brush in her endocervical canal

38–9. Ms. Thomas in Question 38–8 has a negative β-hCG. Which of the following is the next best management step?

a. Diagnostic laparoscopy

b. Diagnostic hysteroscopy

c. Transvaginal ultrasound

d. Computed tomography scan

38–10. Ms. Thomas from Question 38–8 undergoes an ultrasound with the findings shown below. Which of the following is the next best clinical step?

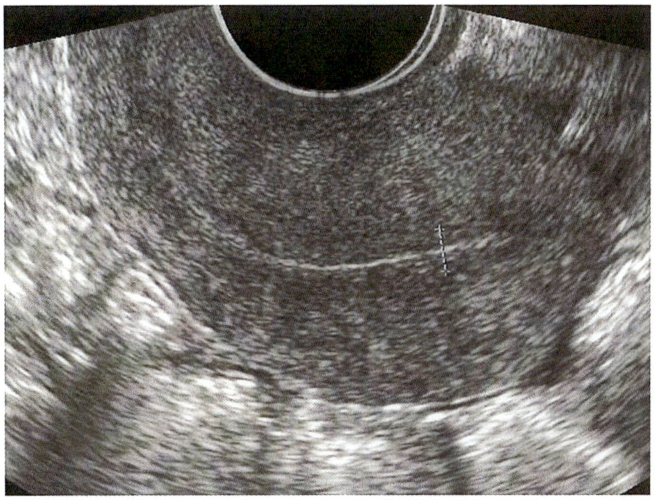

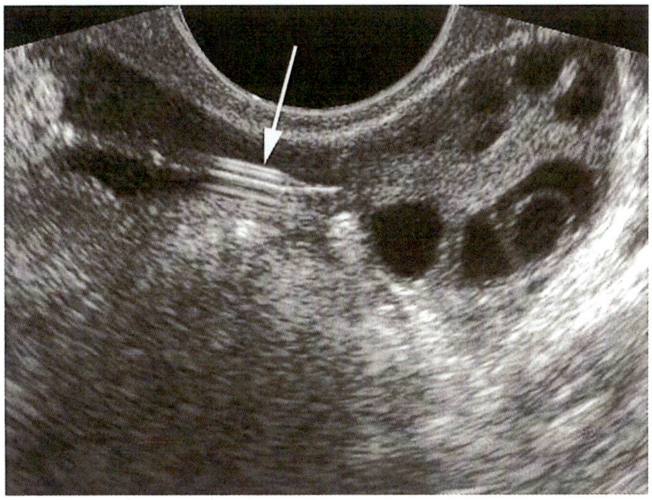

a. Hysterectomy

b. Dilation and curettage

c. Diagnostic laparoscopy

d. Operative hysteroscopy

38–11. You receive a phone call from an emergency medicine physician. She is seeing a patient who reports having a ParaGard in place. Which of the following imaging modalities is contraindicated in this patient?

a. Computed tomography scan

b. 3-tesla magnetic resonance imaging

c. 1.5-tesla magnetic resonance imaging

d. None of the above

CHAPTER 38

38–12. Which of the following is true regarding the intrauterine device–related complication pictured here?

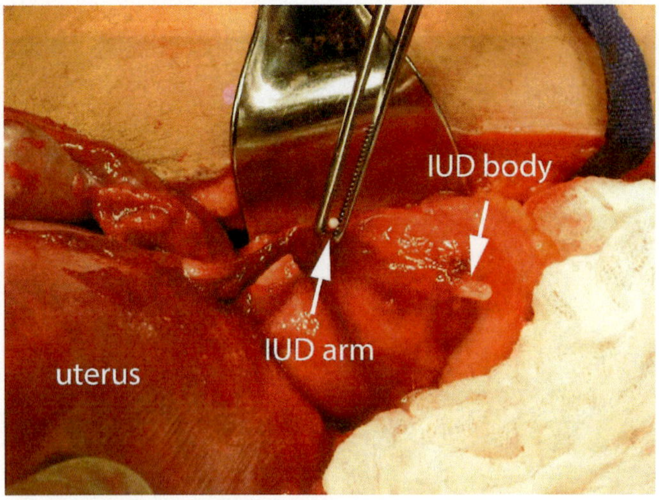

Used with permission from Dr. Seth Hawkins.

- **a.** Is more common with insertion during lactation
- **b.** Rate of occurrence is approximately 1 per 100 insertions
- **c.** Is suspected clinically when sound or insertion device will not travel as far as expected based on bimanual examination
- **d.** None of the above

38–13. Which of the following best characterizes the relationship between intrauterine device (IUD) use and ectopic pregnancy?

- **a.** Use of an IUD increases the risk for an ectopic pregnancy.
- **b.** IUD is contraindicated in women with a history of an ectopic pregnancy.
- **c.** Use of an IUD does not impact risk for an ectopic pregnancy because the overall risk for pregnancy is decreased.
- **d.** Compared to pregnancy after failure of combination oral contraceptive pills, a higher proportion of pregnancies after IUD failure will be ectopic pregnancies.

38–14. Which of the following is true regarding the risk for infection associated with an intrauterine device (IUD)?

- **a.** An IUD is not a safe method of contraception for women with human immunodeficiency virus.
- **b.** The risk for upper genital tract device-related infection increases in parallel with increasing time of device use.
- **c.** The American Heart Association recommends single dose antibiotic prophylaxis prior to IUD insertion for women at risk for bacterial endocarditis.
- **d.** An IUD may remain in situ for pelvic inflammatory disease that is responding to antibiotic therapy, but removal is indicated in the case of a tuboovarian abscess.

38–15. Ms. Cooper presents reporting 14 weeks of amenorrhea and she is found to have a positive pregnancy test. Strings of her intrauterine device (IUD) are visible at the cervical os, and her ultrasound findings are shown below. Which of the following is the correct course of action in this case?

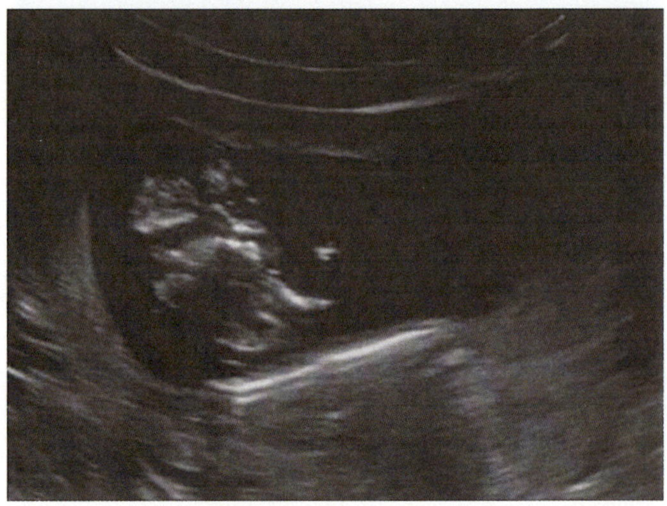

- **a.** IUD removal
- **b.** IUD removal and laparoscopy
- **c.** IUD removal and 10-day course of doxycycline
- **d.** IUD remains in place, and continue routine prenatal care

38–16. Which of the following is most accurate regarding pregnancy with an intrauterine device (IUD) in situ?

a. Risk for spontaneous abortion is approximately four times as high if the device is left in situ.

b. Retention of an IUD during pregnancy increases risk for fetal malformation and preterm delivery.

c. After viability has been reached, data is definitive that the IUD should be left in place even if strings are visible.

d. Evidence of pelvic infection during a pregnancy with a retained IUD should be treated with antibiotics and uterine evacuation.

38–17. Which of the following is true regarding insertion of an intrauterine device (IUD)?

a. Implanon cannot be easily identified for removal with ultrasound and has lost approval by the Food and Drug Administration.

b. For placement unrelated to pregnancy, the only recommended time is near the end of menstruation as it is easier, and pregnancy is excluded.

c. With immediate postabortion or postdelivery placement, fewer women will receive and retain their IUD compared to those scheduled to return for traditionally timed placement.

d. All of the above

38–18. Which of the following is true regarding progestin implants?

a. Implanon cannot be easily identified for removal with ultrasound and has lost approval by the Food and Drug Administration.

b. Nexplanon provides 3 years of contraception by releasing etonogestrel, and it is implanted in the upper, medial surface of the arm.

c. The first implantable progestin contraceptive was Norplant, which released etonogestrel from six subdermal rods, but it is no longer manufactured.

d. All of the above

38–19. Ms. Bradley calls your office a few weeks after insertion of her Nexplanon and reports that she has had numbness and tingling in her arm. Which of the following characterizes the most likely approximate region of her symptoms?

a. Anterior and posterior portions of her shoulder

b. Lateral surface of her forearm extending inferiorly to the base of her thumb

c. Anterior and posterior portions of her 5th digit and the medial half of her 4th digit

d. Medial aspect of her forearm extending superiorly to the anterior surface of her upper arm

38–20. Which of the following is true regarding placement of the progestin implant?

a. For women who are certain they are not pregnant, insertion can occur at any time with no need for backup contraception.

b. For women transitioning from combination oral contraceptives, it is inserted on what would be the first day of a new pack.

c. Insertion can occur prior to discharge home following miscarriage, abortion, or delivery with no impairment of lactation.

d. For women not currently using hormonal contraception, it is ideally inserted 5 days prior to expected menses onset with contraception established within 24 hours.

38–21. Which of the following is a suspected method of efficacy for all progestin-only contraceptive methods?

a. Endometrial atrophy

b. Inhibition of ovulation

c. Thickening of cervical mucus

d. All of the above

38–22 Ms. Hubbard is a 28-year-old G6P5 who is seeing you for her postpartum exam. She had a repeat cesarean delivery 2 weeks ago and desires reversible contraception. Her pregnancy was complicated by gestational diabetes requiring insulin. She also takes medication for depression. She asks about Nexplanon. Which of the following is an appropriate statement as part of her contraceptive counseling?

a. Nexplanon will further increase your risk for overt diabetes due to weight gain and increased insulin resistance.

b. Nexplanon is a good choice, but may increase your depression, so I would like you to call me if you notice changes.

c. According to the United Stated Medical Eligibility Criteria, depression is a contraindication to progestin only contraceptive methods.

d. Nexplanon will reduce your breast milk production, but if you choose this method we should insert it today before ovulation can resume.

38–23. Which of the following statements most accurately describes the injectable progestin contraceptive depot medroxyprogesterone acetate (DMPA)?

a. When injection is given within 5 days of the onset of menses, a backup method is needed for 7 days.

b. Although irregular bleeding leads to 25% of users discontinuing within the first year, amenorrhea develops in 80% of users after 1 year.

c. For women desiring only a brief period of contraception, DMPA is not a good choice due to prolonged anovulation after discontinuation.

d. All of the above

38–24. Combination oral contraceptive (COC) pills differ from progestin-only "mini-pills" in which of the following ways?

a. COC pills primarily inhibit ovulation, and progestin only pills do not reliably inhibit ovulation.

b. COC pills are contraindicated in women with breast cancer, but progestin only pills are not.

c. When one COC dose is missed, a barrier method should be used for 7 days. Whereas, when one progestin pill is taken >4 hours late, a barrier method needs to be used for 48 hours.

d. All of the above

38–25. The combination oral contraceptive pill's mechanism of action is best described by which of the following statements?

a. The estrogen component suppresses luteinizing hormone.

b. Overall mechanism is stimulation of the hypothalamic gonadotropin-releasing factors.

c. Pituitary secretion of follicle-stimulating hormone and luteinizing hormone are blocked, and ovulation is inhibited

d. All of the above

38–26. Undesirable effects attributed to the estrogen component of combination oral contraceptive pills include all except which of the following?

a. Headache

b. Hirsutism

c. Weight gain

d. Breast tenderness

38–27. Which of the following statements is true regarding patient-specific factors that impact choice of combination oral contraceptive (COC) pill?

a. Ongoing irregular bleeding may improve from using a pill with a higher estrogen dose.

b. Women with significant menstrual symptoms may benefit from an extended cycle formulation.

c. Patients on heparin should have their potassium monitored in the first month of using a COC with the progestin drospirenone.

d. All of the above

38–28. Which of the following is not true regarding the relationship of combination oral contraceptive (COC) pills and thrombotic events?

a. Etonogestrel-containing COCs are linked to greater risk.

b. Highest risk is in women with a co-morbid thrombophilia.

c. COCs are contraindicated for women over 35 years of age who smoke.

d. Thrombotic events are increased with COC use in the 4 weeks prior to a major operation and in the first weeks postpartum.

38–29. Relative risk is increased for which of the following cancers with combination oral contraceptive (COC) pill use?

a. Ovarian

b. Cervical

c. Endometrial

d. Hepatocellular carcinoma

38–30. With use of the contraceptive method pictured, how frequently should it be replaced?

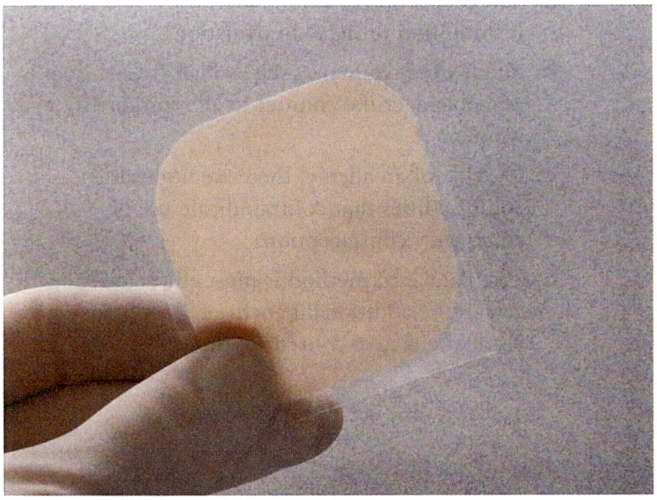

- **a.** Daily
- **b.** Weekly
- **c.** Every 9 days
- **d.** Every 3 weeks

38–31. Ms. Adams is a 35-year-old multigravida who is seeing you for her annual exam. She has hypertension that is well controlled with a single agent. You are encouraged that three times per week she is still doing the water aerobics you recommended last year. Her blood pressure is 130/78 mm Hg and weight is 92 kg, which is down from 98 kg at last year's visit. She inquires about starting the contraceptive patch for her birth control method. Which characteristic below is not a reason she cannot use the patch?

- **a.** Patient weight may reduce efficacy
- **b.** Regular immersion in water limits patch efficacy
- **c.** A 35-year-old with hypertension presents excess cardiac risk
- **d.** All of the above make this a poor choice

38–32. In counseling a woman who is considering the contraceptive method pictured here, which of the following is not true?

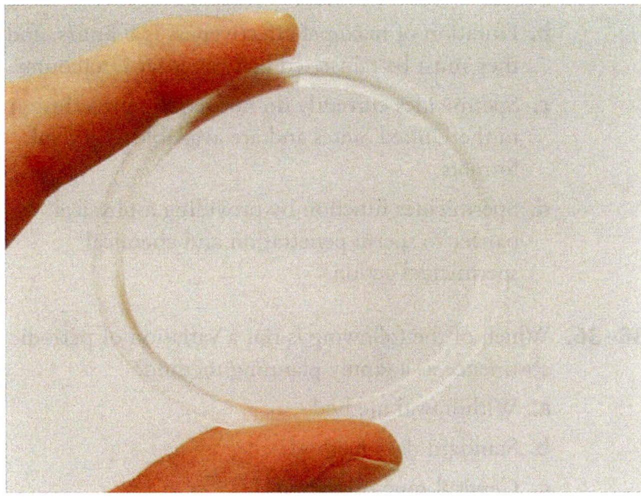

- **a.** The ring must be carefully inserted such that it remains in an oblique lie around the cervix.
- **b.** The ring can be removed during intercourse but should be replaced within 3 hours of removal.
- **c.** The ring is more forgiving than combination oral contraceptive pills, as it remains efficacious if left in place for a fourth week.
- **d.** The ring is placed within 5 days of menses onset and stays in place for 3 weeks with removal prompting withdrawal bleeding.

38–33. Contraceptive efficacy of the male latex condom is enhanced by which of the following?

- **a.** Reservoir tip
- **b.** Oil-based spermicide
- **c.** Concurrent female condom use
- **d.** All of the above

38–34. Ms. Burns is a 26-year-old G1P1001 with a partner who has a history of herpes. She desires contraception, and advice on how she can reduce the risk for getting genital herpes. In addition to counseling her regarding symptoms and lesions, you discuss which of the following?

- **a.** The female condom is not an option if she is allergic to latex.
- **b.** The female condom has a lower contraceptive failure rate than the male condom.
- **c.** The female condom is a single-use barrier method that provides both contraception and protection against sexually transmitted diseases.
- **d.** All of the above should be considered.

38–35. Which of the following is not true regarding spermicide use?

a. Spermicide enhances the contraceptive efficacy of other barrier methods.

b. Duration of maximal effectiveness is 6 hours, and they must be reinserted before repeat intercourse.

c. Spermicides currently do not require prescription in the United States and are available in several formats.

d. Spermicides function by providing a physical barrier to sperm penetration and chemical spermicidal action.

38–36. Which of the following is not a variation of periodic abstinence as a family planning method?

a. Withdrawal method

b. Standard days method

c. Cervical mucus method

d. Temperature rhythm method

38–37. Ms. Polly is a 24-year-old recently engaged G0 who presents to discuss contraceptive methods in advance of her wedding. She and her fiancé have not been sexually active and do not intend to be until after the wedding. She has no medical comorbidities and has a normal body mass index. She has always had irregular menstrual cycles ranging from 28 to 40 days. She is sure that they do not desire pregnancy for 1 to 2 years, and she has a religious objection to any method that has prevention of implantation of a fertilized embryo as a major mechanism of action. Taking all these factors into account, what is the most efficacious method you can recommend for this patient?

a. Male condom

b. Intrauterine device

c. Fertility awareness-based method

d. Combination oral contraceptive pill

38–38. Which of the following is false regarding emergency contraception?

a. The major mechanism of action with all methods is inhibition or delay in ovulation.

b. Single dose regimen, such as Plan B One-Step is available over the counter to all reproductive aged women.

c. Outside of an allergy, there are no health comorbidities that contraindicate use of emergency contraception.

d. The ParaGard method is most efficacious and carries the additional benefit of 10 subsequent years of effective contraception.

CHAPTER 38 ANSWER KEY

Question number	Letter answer	Page cited	Header cited
38–1	d	p. 680	Table 38-1
38–2	b	p. 680	Table 38-1
38–3	c	p. 681	Introduction
38–4	d	p. 681	Introduction
38–5	a	p. 682	Intrauterine Devices
38–6	a	p. 683	Intrauterine Devices
38–7	c	p. 683	Intrauterine Devices
38–8	a	p. 683	Intrauterine Devices
38–9	c	p. 683	Intrauterine Devices
38–10	c	p. 683	Intrauterine Devices
38–11	d	p. 683	Intrauterine Devices
38–12	a	p. 683	Intrauterine Devices
38–13	d	p. 683	Intrauterine Devices
38–14	d	p. 684	Intrauterine Devices
38–15	a	p. 684	Intrauterine Devices
38–16	d	p. 684	Intrauterine Devices
38–17	a	p. 685	Intrauterine Devices
38–18	b	p. 687	Progestin Implants
38–19	d	p. 688	Progestin Implants
38–20	c	p. 688	Progestin Implants
38–21	d	p. 689	Progestin-Only Contraceptives
38–22	b	p. 689	Progestin-Only Contraceptives
38–23	c	p. 693	Injectable Progestin Contraceptives
38–24	a	p. 690 p. 693	Combination Oral Contraceptive Pills Progestin-Only Pills
38–25	c	p. 689	Combination Hormonal Contraceptives Mechanism of Action
38–26	b	p. 690	Combination Oral Contraceptive Pills
38–27	d	p. 690	Combination Oral Contraceptive Pills
38–28	a	p. 691	Combination Oral Contraceptive Pills
38–29	b	p. 692	Combination Oral Contraceptive Pills
38–30	b	p. 692	Transdermal Patch
38–31	b	p. 692	Transdermal Patch
38–32	a	p. 693	Transvaginal Ring
38–33	a	p. 694	Barrier Methods
38–34	c	p. 680 p. 694	Table 38-1 Barrier Methods
38–35	b	p. 695	Spermicides
38–36	a	p. 695	Fertility Awareness-Based Methods
38–37	d	p. 680 p. 683 p. 689 p. 695	Table 38-1 Contraceptive Action Actions and Side Effects Fertility Awareness-Based Methods
38–38	c	p. 696	Emergency Contraception

CHAPTER 39

Sterilization

39–1. Among women using contraception, what percentage use sterilization?

- **a.** 10%
- **b.** 15%
- **c.** 20%
- **d.** 33%

39–2. A 28-year-old G4P3 presents for prenatal care at 8 weeks' gestation and reports she does not want any more children. She asks for a postpartum bilateral tubal ligation. All except which of the following are accurate and should be included in your counseling?

- **a.** It is permanent
- **b.** There are failure rates
- **c.** It can be reversed without consequence
- **d.** An explanation of alternative options for contraception

39–3. Which of the following aspects of postpartum anatomy are advantageous for a puerperal sterilization?

- **a.** A noninvoluted uterus
- **b.** Laxity of the abdominal wall
- **c.** Fallopian tubes directly beneath the abdominal wall
- **d.** All of the above

39–4. All except which of the following aspects of the intrapartum and postpartum periods should be accounted for when considering a puerperal tubal sterilization?

- **a.** Status of the newborn
- **b.** Postpartum hemorrhage
- **c.** Patient's ability to ambulate
- **d.** Utilization of neuraxial anesthesia placed for labor

39–5. Which of the following methods of puerperal sterilization carries the greatest morbidity?

- **a.** Hysterectomy
- **b.** Salpingectomy
- **c.** Uchida method
- **d.** Parkland method

39–6. A 36-year-old G3P2 desires permanent sterilization after delivery. She has read recently that the entire fallopian tube should be removed when performing a tubal ligation. What is the rationale for this recommendation?

- **a.** Decrease cancer risks
- **b.** Decrease the failure rate
- **c.** Decrease bleeding complications
- **d.** Decrease the risk for an ectopic pregnancy

39–7. What method of tubal ligation is displayed below?

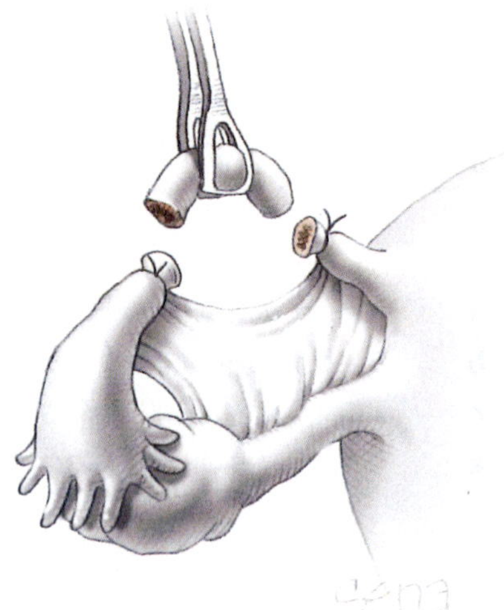

Reproduced with permission from Cunningham FG, Leveno KJ, Bloom SL, et al (eds): Sterilization. In Williams Obstetrics, 25th ed. New York, McGraw-Hill, 2018, Figure 39-1B.

- **a.** Uchida
- **b.** Pomeroy
- **c.** Parkland
- **d.** Modified Pomeroy

39–8. Sterilization in the puerperium is typically performed using which of the following anesthetic methods?

- **a.** Spinal anesthesia
- **b.** General anesthesia
- **c.** Incision infiltration
- **d.** Transverse abdominis plane block

39–9. You are seeing a 33-year-old G3P2 for prenatal care. She had two prior vaginal deliveries and desires a bilateral tubal ligation after this pregnancy. She anticipates having another vaginal delivery and wants to know what type of incision she will have for her tubal ligation. Which of the answer choices below depicts the best incision for a puerperal tubal ligation?

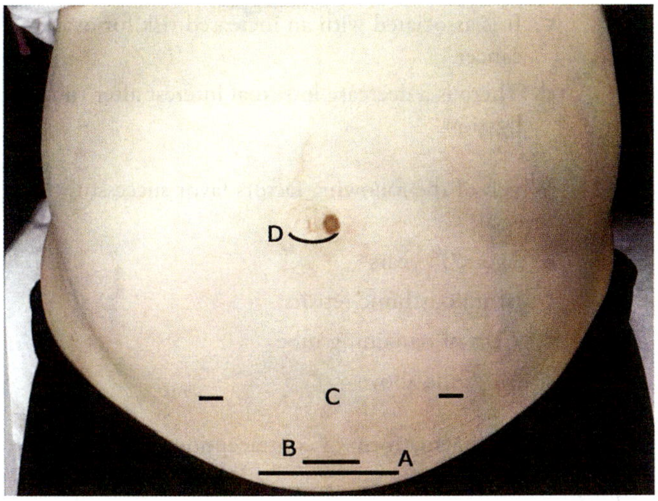

- **a.** A
- **b.** B
- **c.** C
- **d.** D

39–10. Why is an infraumbilical incision the most favorable for a puerperal tubal ligation?

- **a.** Smallest incision
- **b.** Yields better cosmesis
- **c.** Decreased risk for bleeding complications
- **d.** It's the thickest portion, which improves the integrity of the incision.

39–11. Which of the following are reasonable options to provide adequate exposure during a puerperal tubal ligation?

- **a.** A larger incision
- **b.** Reverse Trendelenburg
- **c.** Elevate the abdominal wall with your fingers
- **d.** Tilt the table to same side as the tube being exposed

39–12. Which of the following is true regarding identification of the structure being ligated?

- **a.** The distal fimbria must be seen prior to ligation.
- **b.** Common reason for failure of sterilization is ligation of the wrong structure.
- **c.** The midportion of the fallopian tube can be confused with that of the round ligament.
- **d.** All of the above

39–13. What is the most common approach to the nonpuerperal tubal ligation?

- **a.** Colpotomy
- **b.** Laparotomy
- **c.** Laparoscopy
- **d.** Minilaparotomy

39–14. What type of suture is typically used to complete the tubal ligation picture below?

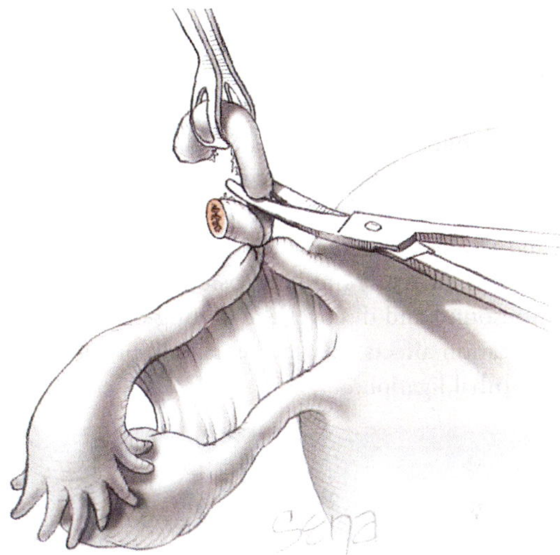

Reproduced with permission from Cunningham FG, Leveno KJ, Bloom SL, et al (eds): Sterilization. In Williams Obstetrics, 25th ed. New York, McGraw-Hill, 2018, Figure 39-2.

- **a.** Vicryl
- **b.** Chromic
- **c.** Monocryl
- **d.** Plain catgut

39–15. Why should that particular suture be used in Question 39–14?

- **a.** Quick absorption allows separation of the severed ends
- **b.** Easier to tie knots with this suture compared to others
- **c.** Quick absorption leads to decreased adhesion formation
- **d.** Delayed absorption decreases the risk for bleeding complications

39–16. What is the cumulative failure rate for tubal sterilization?

a. 0.5%
b. 1%
c. 3%
d. 5%

39–17. Which of the following are reasons for failure of tubal sterilization?

a. Spontaneous reanastomosis
b. Transection of the round ligament
c. Partial transection of the fallopian tube
d. All of the above

39–18. What benefits, other than contraception, does a tubal ligation provide?

a. Decrease risk for menorrhagia
b. Decrease risk for breast cancer
c. Decrease risk for ovarian cancer
d. All of the above

39–19. A 37-year-old G3P3 underwent a bilateral tubal ligation 2 years ago at the time of her third cesarean section. She now presents with amenorrhea and nausea and vomiting for the last month. You perform a urine pregnancy test and it is positive. You perform an ultrasound and discover the finding below. This complication affects what percentage of pregnancies after a tubal ligation?

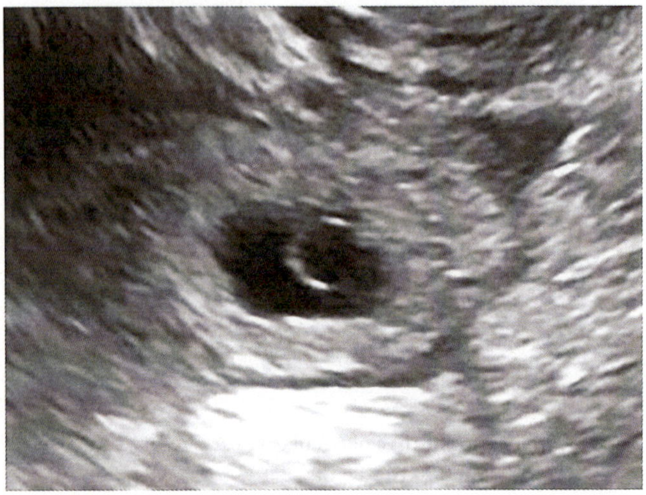

a. 10%
b. 20%
c. 30%
d. 70%

39–20. A 27-year-old multigravida tells you at her 28-week prenatal care visit that she desires a tubal ligation after delivery. For which of the following reasons do you counsel her on the permanence of the procedure and encourage her to seek another method of contraception?

a. It is associated with early menopause.
b. Younger women have increased risk for regret.
c. It is associated with an increased risk for ovarian cancer.
d. There is a decrease in sexual interest after tubal ligation.

39–21. Which of the following factors favor successful tubal reversal?

a. Age <35 years
b. Isthmic-isthmic repairs
c. 7 cm of remaining tube
d. All of the above

39–22. The following form of contraception is made of what material?

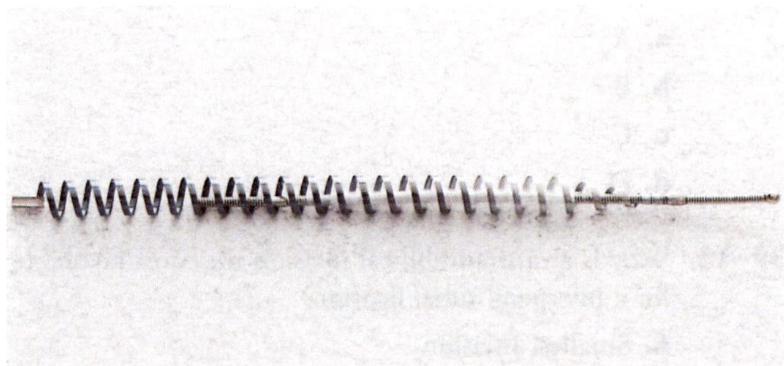

a. Zinc
b. Copper
c. Progesterone
d. Nickel and titanium alloy

39–23. How does Essure work as a form of contraception?

a. Prevents ovulation
b. Alters cervical mucous
c. Tubal lumen occlusion
d. Thinning of the endometrium

39–24. What adverse effects are associated with Essure use?

a. Perforation
b. Allergic reactions
c. Abnormal bleeding
d. All of the above

39–25. When after Essure placement should confirmation with a hysterosalpingography be performed?

a. 3 weeks
b. 6 weeks
c. 12 weeks
d. 16 weeks

39–26. During a vasectomy, which of the following structures is ligated?

a. Epididymis
b. Spermatic cord
c. Efferent ductile
d. Ductus deferens

39–27. Compared with tubal ligation, which of the following is an advantage of vasectomy?

a. Less invasive
b. Easily reversed
c. Immediately effective
d. Does not require confirmation

39–28. How long does it take for sperm to be completely removed from the reproductive tract?

a. 1 week
b. 4 weeks
c. 12 weeks
d. 16 weeks

39–29. Which of the following is a reason why pregnancy after a vasectomy may occur?

a. Recanalization
b. Incomplete occlusion
c. Unprotected intercourse too soon
d. All of the above

39–30. Pregnancy rates after vasectomy reversal increase with all except which of the following?

a. Microsurgical technique
b. Younger female partner age
c. Longer duration from vasectomy to reversal
d. Normal sperm quality during reversal procedure

39–31. Compared to a traditional tubal ligation, which of the following is increased with a salpingectomy?

a. Risk for bleeding
b. Risk for postoperative ileus
c. Risk for adhesion formation
d. All of the above

39–32. Why should the bladder be emptied prior to a puerperal tubal ligation?

a. Avoid bladder injury
b. Prevent postop urinary retention
c. Prevent the fundus from dropping to the pubic symphysis
d. All of the above

CHAPTER 39 ANSWER KEY

Question number	Letter answer	Page cited	Header cited
39–1	**d**	p. 702	Introduction
39–2	**c**	p. 702	Introduction
39–3	**d**	p. 702	Timing
39–4	**c**	p. 702	Timing
39–5	**a**	p. 703	Technique
39–6	**a**	p. 703	Technique
39–7	**c**	p. 703	Figure 39-1
39–8	**a**	p. 703	Technique
39–9	**d**	p. 703	Technique
39–10	**b**	p. 703	Technique
39–11	**a**	p. 703	Technique
39–12	**d**	p. 703	Technique
39–13	**c**	p. 704	Nonpuerperal Tubal Sterilization
39–14	**d**	p. 704	Figure 39-2
39–15	**a**	p. 704	Figure 39-2
39–16	**a**	p. 704	Contraceptive Failure
39–17	**d**	p. 705	Contraceptive Failure
39–18	**c**	p. 705	Other Effects
39–19	**c**	p. 705	Contraceptive Failure
39–20	**b**	p. 705	Other Effects
39–21	**d**	p. 705	Tubal Sterilization Reversal
39–22	**d**	p. 705	Transcervical Sterilization
39–23	**c**	p. 705	Transcervical Sterilization
39–24	**d**	p. 705	Transcervical Sterilization
39–25	**c**	p. 705	Transcervical Sterilization
39–26	**d**	p. 706	Vasectomy
39–27	**a**	p. 706	Vasectomy
39–28	**c**	p. 706	Vasectomy
39–29	**d**	p. 706	Vasectomy
39–30	**c**	p. 706	Vasectomy
39–31	**a**	p. 704	Technique
39–32	**a**	p. 703	Technique

SECTION 11

OBSTETRICAL COMPLICATIONS

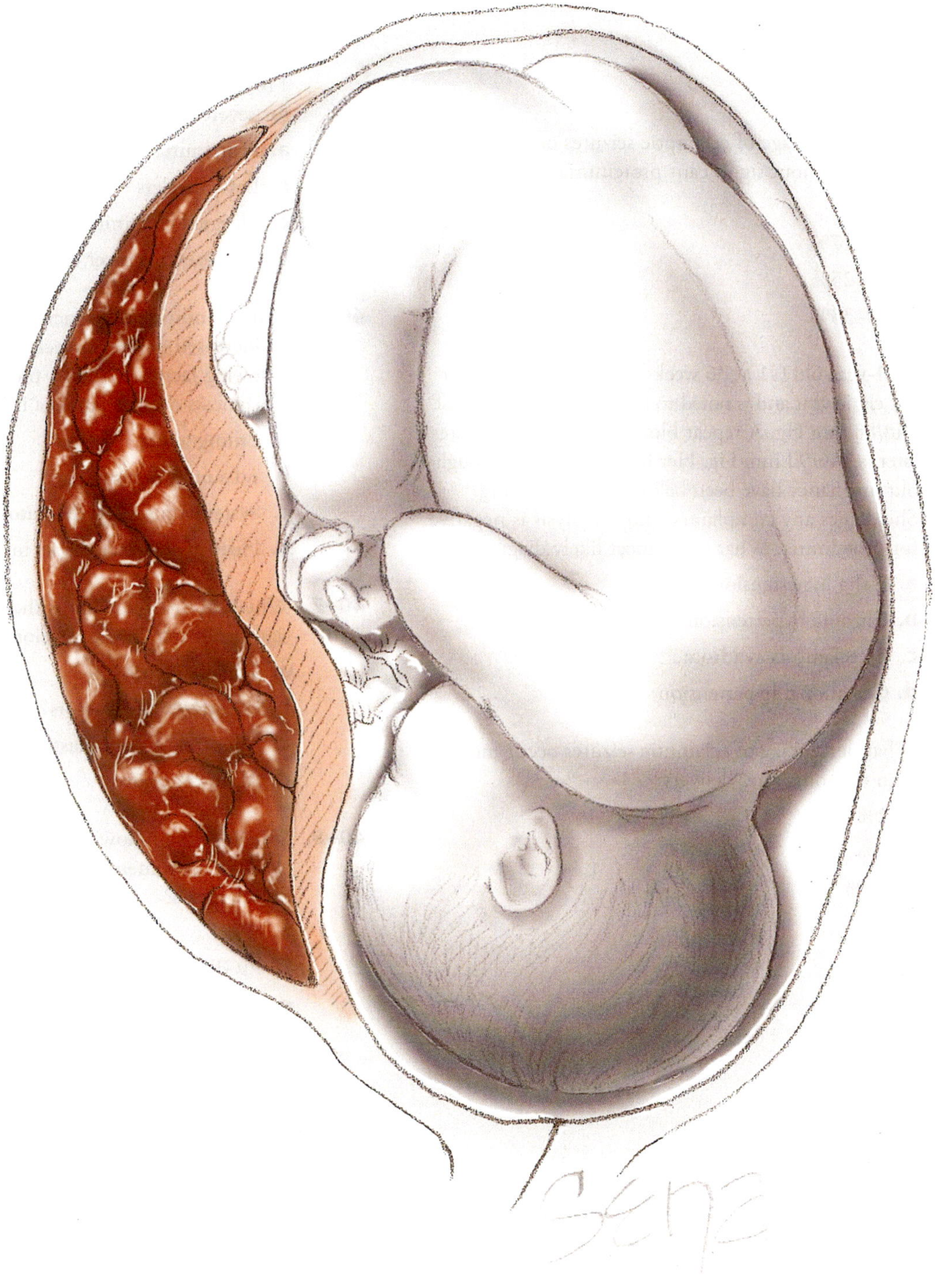

CHAPTER 40

Hypertensive Disorders

40–1. What percentage of pregnancies are complicated by hypertension?

a. 2–3%

b. 4–5%

c. 5–10%

d. 10–20%

40–2. What percentage of eclamptic seizures occur in women without significant proteinuria?

a. 5–9%

b. 10–17%

c. 20–25%

d. 30–33%

40–3. A 21-year-old G1 at 36 weeks' gestation presents for her clinic visit and is noted to have a blood pressure of 148/88 mm Hg. A repeat blood pressure 30 minutes later is 146/92 mm Hg. Her blood pressures throughout pregnancy have been below 140/90 mm Hg. She denies any complaints, and urinalysis is negative for proteinuria. What is the most likely diagnosis?

a. Delta hypertension

b. Chronic hypertension

c. Preeclampsia syndrome

d. Gestational hypertension

40–4. What percentage of eclamptic seizures occur more than 48 hours after delivery?

a. 2%

b. 5%

c. 10%

d. 20%

40–5. A 28-year-old G1 at 38 weeks' gestation presents with complaint of contractions. Her blood pressure is noted to be 148/90 mm Hg and 152/96 mm Hg. She has a urine protein:creatinine ratio of 0.4, a creatinine of 1.04 mg/dL (baseline 0.48 mg/dL), normal AST and ALT, and platelet count of 110,000/μL. She denies any symptoms. What criteria for severe preeclampsia does this patient meet?

a. Proteinuria

b. Low platelets

c. Elevated creatinine

d. She does not meet criteria for severe preeclampsia.

40–6. Many conditions and factors are associated with an increased risk for preeclampsia. Which of the following factors results in the greatest relative risk for a diagnosis of preeclampsia in the current pregnancy?

a. Primigravida

b. Advanced maternal age

c. Systemic lupus erythematous

d. History of preeclampsia in a prior pregnancy

40–7. Which of the following is thought to play a significant role in the development of preeclampsia?

a. Genetic factors

b. Immunological factors

c. Abnormal trophoblastic invasion

d. All of the above

40–8. Which of the following angiogenic factors are elevated in women who proceed to develop preeclampsia?

a. sFlt-1

b. PIGF

c. VEGF

d. TGF-β

40–9. Which of the following is not a pathophysiological change to the cardiovascular system seen in the setting of preeclampsia?

a. Increased preload

b. Decreased preload

c. Increased afterload

d. Endothelial activation

40–10. A 25-year-old primigravida at 36 weeks' gestation presents with scotomata and headache, a blood pressure of 168/102 mm Hg, and proteinuria. A diagnosis of severe preeclampsia is made. On the below schematic, which position best describes her hemodynamic state?

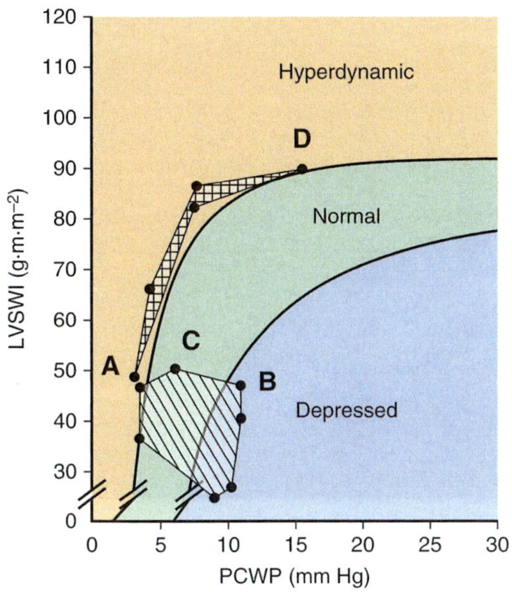

Reproduced with permission from Cunningham FG, Leveno KJ, Bloom SL, et al (eds): Hypertensive disorders. In Williams Obstetrics, 25th ed. New York, McGraw-Hill, 2018, Figure 40-5.

a. A

b. B

c. C

d. D

40–11. The patient Question 40–10 has a prolonged induction receiving over 5 liters of intravenous fluids. She requires 4 liters supplemental oxygen via nasal cannula. On the below schematic, which position best describes her hemodynamic state at this time?

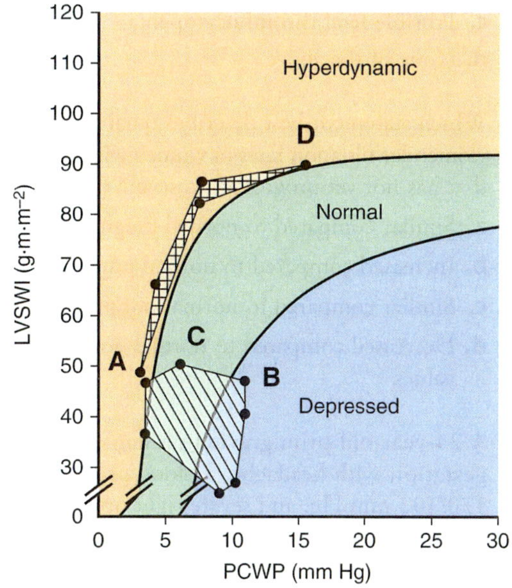

Reproduced with permission from Cunningham FG, Leveno KJ, Bloom SL, et al (eds): Hypertensive disorders. In Williams Obstetrics, 25th ed. New York, McGraw-Hill, 2018, Figure 40-5.

a. A

b. B

c. C

d. D

40–12. A 21-year-old primigravida presents at 36 weeks' gestation with new-onset headache. Her blood pressure is 150/90 mm Hg, her serum creatinine is 0.8 mg/mL, AST is 32 U/L, and platelet count is 28,000/μL. Which of the following criteria for severe preeclampsia is met?

a. Hypertension

b. Liver dysfunction

c. Thrombocytopenia

d. Elevated serum creatinine

40–13. For the patient Question 40–12, which of the following is an indication for primary cesarean delivery without an attempt at induction?

a. Malpresentation
b. Unfavorable cervix
c. Possible fetal thrombocytopenia
d. None of the above

40–14. Which statement best describes renal perfusion and glomerular filtration rates in women with preeclampsia that has not yet progressed to severe disease?

a. Similar compared to normal pregnant values
b. Increased compared to normal pregnant values
c. Similar compared to normal nonpregnant values
d. Decreased compared to normal nonpregnant values

40–15. A 24-year-old primigravida presents at 37 weeks' gestation with headache, a blood pressure of 170/102 mm Hg, and severe right upper quadrant pain. She is diagnosed with HELLP syndrome and undergoes an uncomplicated induction of labor. Her right upper quadrant pain persists, and a computed tomography scan of her abdomen/pelvis is completed with the findings as shown below. What is denoted by the asterisk (*)?

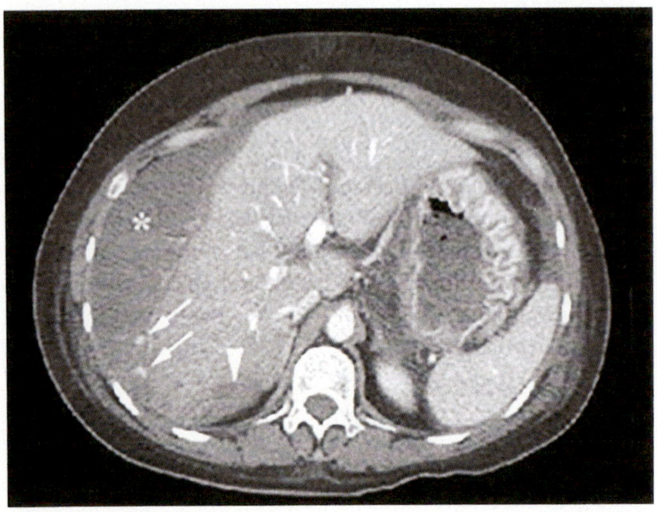

a. Splenic infarction
b. Intrahepatic infarction
c. Subcapsular hematoma
d. Periportal hemorrhagic necrosis

40–16. What proportion of maternal deaths can be attributed to hypertensive disorders in pregnancy?

a. 1 in 2
b. 1 in 6
c. 1 in 10
d. 1 in 20

40–17. A G3P2 at 16 weeks' gestation presents to the emergency department complaining of vaginal bleeding. Her blood pressure is 148/96 mm Hg and she has 3+ proteinuria on a specimen obtained during bladder catheterization. Which of the following may explain the development of preeclampsia in this patient?

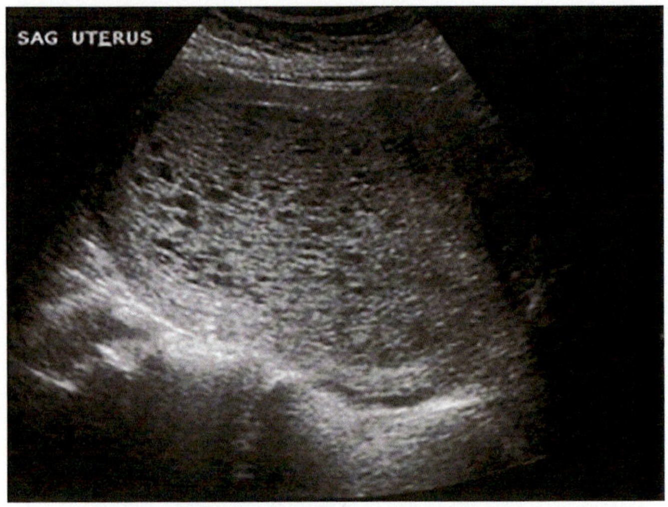

a. Increased volume of chorionic villi
b. Extensive remodeling of the spiral arterioles
c. Increased invasion of extravillous trophoblastic tissue
d. None of the above

40–18. What is the underlying etiology of the proteinuria seen with preeclampsia?

a. Increased capillary permeability
b. Increased renal artery resistance
c. Increased glomerular filtration rate
d. Increased systemic vascular resistance

41–15. The following picture unfortunately depicts a maternal death after postpartum hemorrhage. Which of the following are possible contributors?

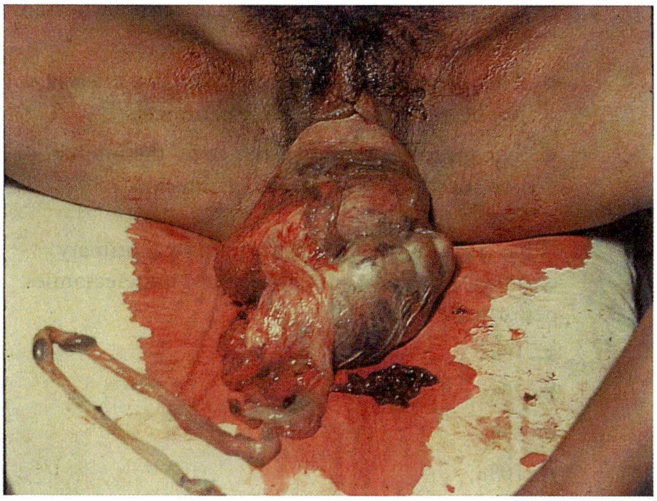

Reproduced with permission from Cunningham FG, Leveno KJ, Bloom SL, et al (eds): Obstetrical hemorrhage. In Williams Obstetrics, 25th ed. New York, McGraw-Hill, 2018, Figure 41-7.

a. Placenta previa
b. Uterine rupture
c. Uterine inversion
d. Chorioamnionitis

41–16. What percentage of women have lacerations at the time of vaginal delivery?

a. 50%
b. 90%
c. 80%
d. 65%

41–17. Which maneuvers below should be performed when repairing a cervical laceration?

a. Operator grasps lips of cervix with ring forceps.
b. Second assistant can provide better exposure with vaginal wall retractors.
c. Assistant place downward pressure on the uterus to expose the cervix better for the operator.
d. All of the above

41–18. What is the appropriate management of vulvovaginal hematomas?

a. Surgical exploration in all cases
b. To prevent infection they should all undergo ultrasound guided drainage.
c. In a small hematoma, if pain is severe then ice packs and analgesia are appropriate.
d. If bleeding ceases, small to moderate-sized hematomas can be treated expectantly.

41–19. The hematoma in the following picture is in which location?

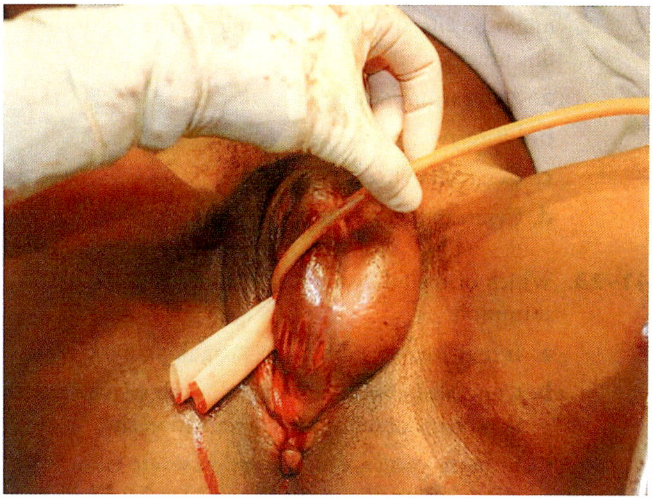

a. Ischiorectal hematoma
b. Periurethral hematoma
c. Supralevator hematoma
d. Left-sided anterior perineal triangle

41–20. The following picture represents which of the following?

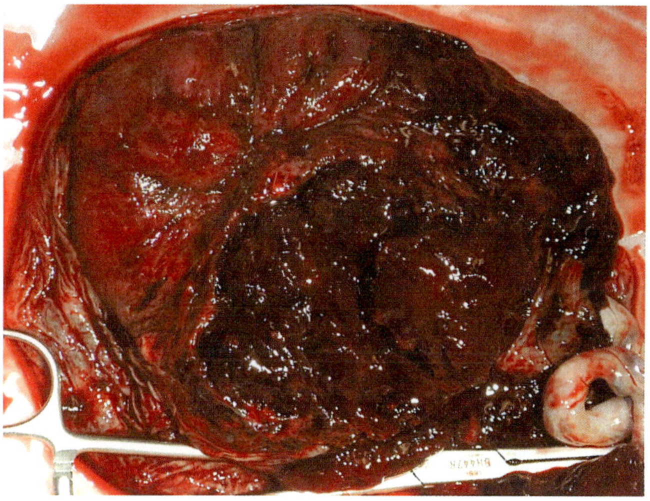

Used with permission from Dr. Ed Wells.

a. Molar gestation
b. Placenta accreta
c. Acute abruption
d. Partial abruption

41–21. Which of the following are risk factors for recurrent abruption?

a. Prior abruption
b. Low birthweight
c. Preterm rupture of membranes
d. None of the above

41–22. Your patient is a 22-year-old G2P1 at 36 weeks' gestation with a history of prior abruption during a spontaneous vaginal delivery. Which of the following might be effective for preventing recurrence during this pregnancy?

a. Antepartum testing
b. Delivery at 38 weeks
c. Cesarean delivery at 38 weeks
d. Cesarean delivery at 39 weeks

41–23. Which of the following is true concerning placental abruption?

a. It may lead to a dilutional coagulopathy.
b. Concealed abruption forces thromboplastin into large veins draining the implantation site.
c. In most women with abruption severe enough to kill the fetus, the plasma fibrinogen level will be less than 150 mg/dL.
d. All of the above

41–24. What is depicted in the following picture?

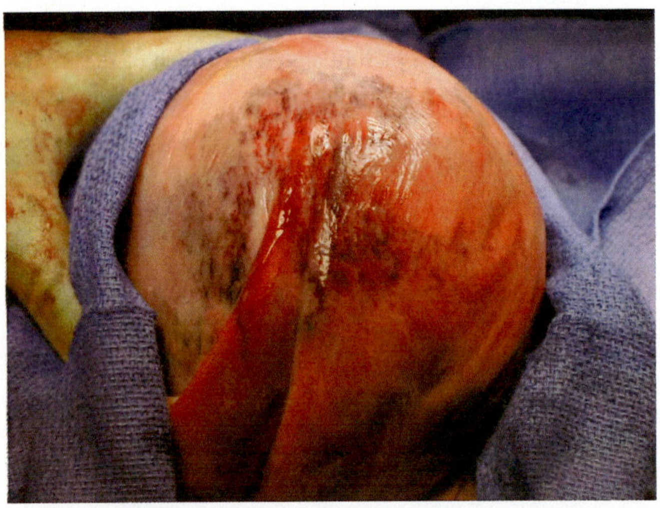

a. Placenta previa
b. Placenta accreta
c. Couvelaire uterus
d. None of the above

41–25. A 22-year-old G2P1 at 28 weeks' gestation presents with rupture of membranes about 2 hours ago. What is true about this patient concerning abruption?

a. She has a 5% risk for abruption.
b. She has a 17% risk for abruption.
c. Her risk for abruption is not increased.
d. None of the above

41–26. How is a low-lying placenta defined?

a. The placenta is implanted in the lower uterine segment.
b. The placental edge covers the internal os, but not completely.
c. The placental edge does not cover the internal os but lies within a 1-cm wide perimeter.
d. The placental edge does not cover the internal os but lies within a 2-cm wide perimeter.

41–27. What percentage of women who have a primary cesarean with a placenta previa have hysterectomies performed?

a. 1%
b. 2%
c. 6%
d. 10%

41–28. Which of the following statements are true concerning morbidly adherent placentas?

a. Cesarean-scar pregnancies are a precursor to a morbidly adherent placenta.
b. Placenta villi attach to smooth muscle fibers rather than to decidual cells.
c. Abnormal placental adherence is in part due to partial or total absence of Nitabuch layer.
d. All of the above

41–29. The picture below represents which of the following placental pathologies?

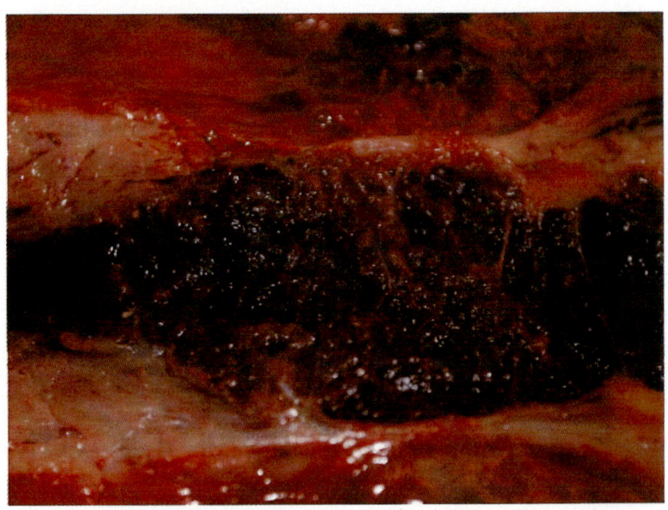

Used with permission from Dr. Ed Wells.

a. Placenta increta
b. Placenta accreta
c. Placenta percreta
d. Placental abruption

41–30. From the following graph, which of the following statements concerning morbidly adherent placenta (MAP) is accurate?

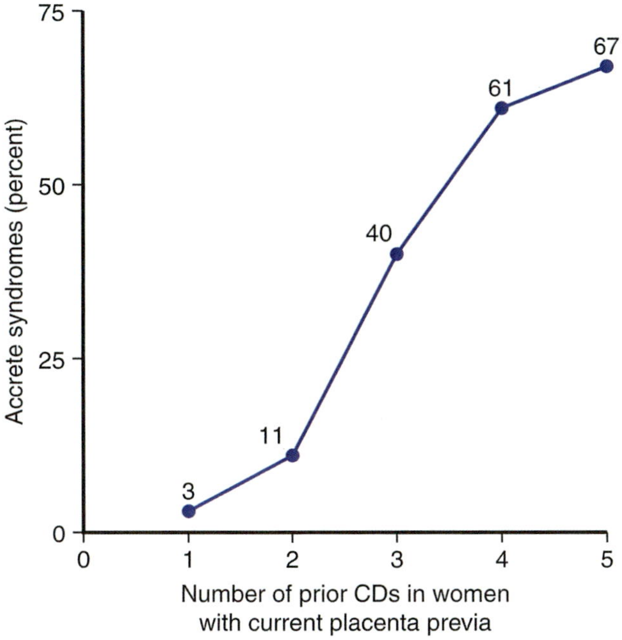

Reproduced with permission from Cunningham FG, Leveno KJ, Bloom SL, et al (eds): Obstetrical hemorrhage. In Williams Obstetrics, 25th ed. New York, McGraw-Hill, 2018, Figure 41-26.

a. The highest risk for placenta previa is with your 5th pregnancy.
b. Most women with MAP have had more than 3 previous cesareans.
c. With placenta previa, the more cesareans a woman has had, the higher her risk for MAP.
d. All of the above

41–31. Which of the following can be seen in the ultrasound picture below?

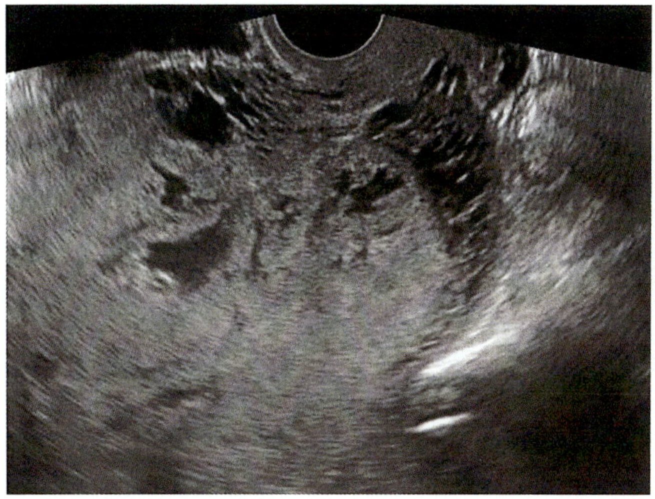

a. Lacunae
b. Bridging vessels
c. Intraabdominal placental implantation
d. None of the above

41–32. Which of the statements below accurately depicts the difference between consumptive coagulopathy and disseminated intravascular coagulation?

a. Abruption best represents a consumptive coagulopathy.
b. Loss of procoagulants with massive hemorrhage is the basis of dilutional coagulopathy.
c. A concealed abruption forces thromboplastin into the circulation and leads to the consumption of procoagulants.
d. All of the above

41–33. The slide pictured below is consistent with a fatal syndrome. Which of the following proposed diagnostic criteria are required to make the diagnosis?

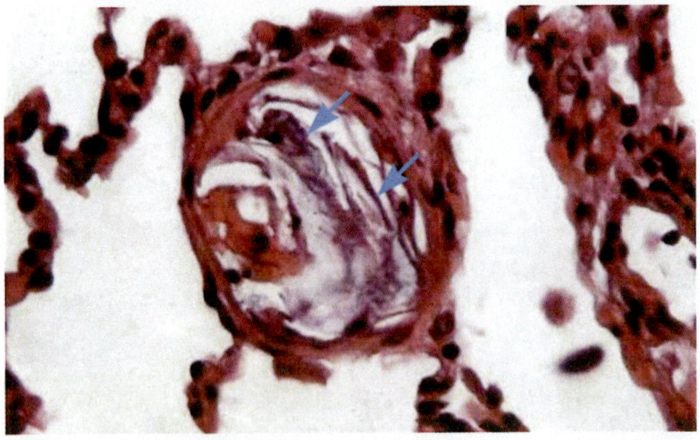

Reproduced with permission from Cunningham FG, Leveno KJ, Bloom SL, et al (eds): Obstetrical hemorrhage. In Williams Obstetrics, 25th ed. New York, McGraw-Hill, 2018, Figure 41-31a.

- **a.** Clinical onset during labor or within 30 minutes of placental delivery.
- **b.** Abrupt onset of cardiorespiratory arrest, or both hypotension and respiratory compromise.
- **c.** Documentation of overt disseminated intravascular coagulopathy must be detected prior to enough blood loss to cause dilutional coagulopathy.
- **d.** All of the above

41–34. Which of the bacteria below are associated with consumptive coagulopathy?

- **a.** *Escherichia coli*
- **b.** *Klebsiella pneumoniae*
- **c.** Group A streptococcus
- **d.** Group B streptococcus

41–35. The use of whole blood for massive hemorrhage is supported by which of the following?

- **a.** Less renal failure
- **b.** Less pulmonary edema
- **c.** Fewer intensive care unit admissions
- **d.** All of the above

41–36. Viral infection risks from transfusion are accurately depicted in which of the following statements?

- **a.** Hepatitis B risk is <1 per 100,000 units
- **b.** Hepatitis C risk is 1 per 1–2 million units
- **c.** Human immunodeficiency virus risk is 1 per 1–2 million units
- **d.** All of the above

41–37. Which hemostatic surgical procedure is to be performed in the picture below?

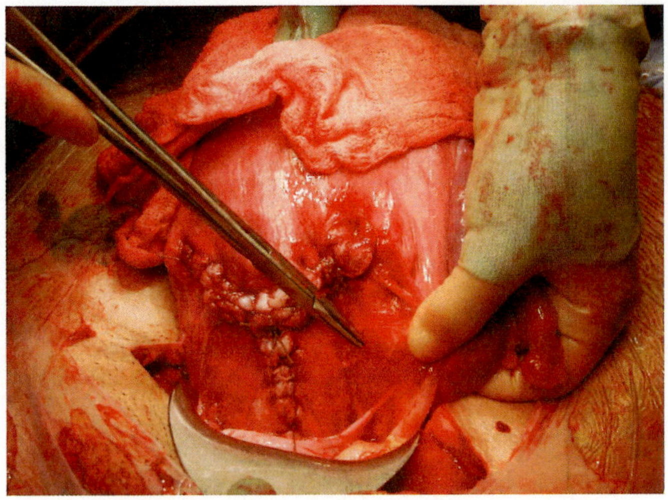

- **a.** B-Lynch procedure
- **b.** Uterine artery ligation
- **c.** Vaginal artery ligation
- **d.** Ovarian artery ligation

41–38. Which hemostatic surgical procedure is demonstrated in the picture below?

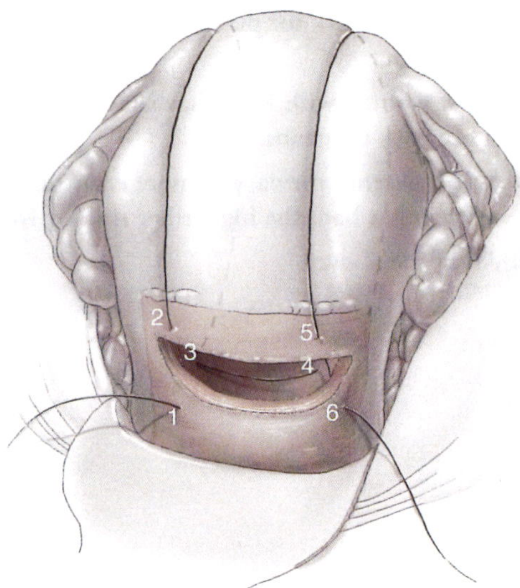

Reproduced with permission from Cunningham FG, Leveno KJ, Bloom SL, et al (eds): Obstetrical hemorrhage. In Williams Obstetrics, 25th ed. New York, McGraw-Hill, 2018, Figure 41-34b.

- **a.** B-Lynch procedure
- **b.** Uterine artery ligation
- **c.** Vaginal artery ligation
- **d.** Ovarian artery ligation

41–39. Ligation at which of the following labeled vessel points in the retroperitoneum will decrease the pulse pressure in the uterine artery?

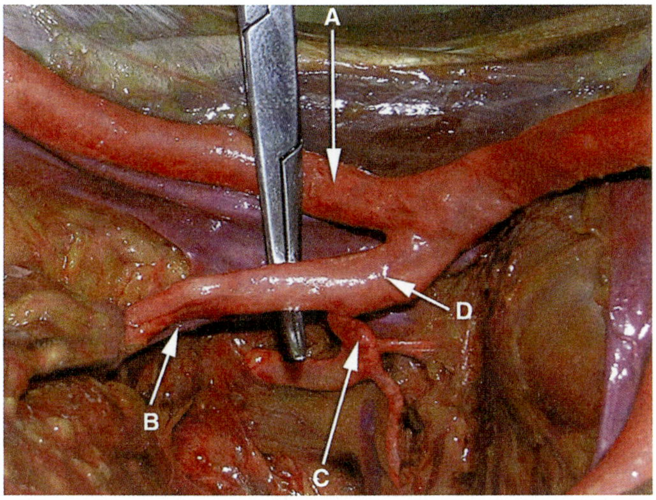

Reproduced with permission from Cunningham FG, Leveno KJ, Bloom SL, et al (eds): Obstetrical hemorrhage. In Williams Obstetrics, 25th ed. New York, McGraw-Hill, 2018, Figure 41-35.

- **a.** Posterior division
- **b.** Internal iliac vein
- **c.** Internal iliac artery
- **d.** External iliac artery

CHAPTER 41 ANSWER KEY

Question number	Letter answer	Page cited	Header cited
41-1	**b**	p. 755	Introduction
41-2	**b**	p. 756	Definition and Incidence
41-3	**d**	p. 756	Definition and Incidence
41-4	**a**	p. 756	Table 41-1
41-5	**b**	p. 756	Table 41-1
41-6	**c**	p. 757	Table 41-2
41-7	**d**	p. 757	Antepartum Hemorrhage
41-8	**d**	p. 758	Postpartum Hemorrhage
41-9	**a**	p. 759	Uterotonic Agents
41-10	**d**	p. 760	Bleeding Unresponsive to Uterotonic Agents
41-11	**d**	p. 760	Clinical Correlation
41-12	**b**	p. 761	Clinical Correlation
41-13	**b**	p. 761	Clinical Correlation
41-14	**b**	p. 761	Recognition and Management
41-15	**c**	p. 762	Recognition and Management
41-16	**c**	p. 763	Vulvovaginal Lacerations
41-17	**d**	p. 763	Cervical Lacerations
41-18	**d**	p. 763	Vulvovaginal Lacerations
41-19	**d**	p. 763	Vulvovaginal Lacerations
41-20	**d**	p. 767	Abruption
41-21	**a**	p. 769	Predisposing Factors
41-22	**b**	p. 770	Prior Abruption
41-23	**b**	p. 771	Hypovolemic Shock and Consumptive Coagulopathy
41-24	**c**	p. 771	Couvelaire Uterus
41-25	**a**	p. 770	Preterm Prematurely Ruptured Membranes
41-26	**d**	p. 774	Classification
41-27	**c**	p. 773	Placenta Previa
41-28	**d**	p. 777	Morbidly Adherent Placenta
41-29	**c**	p. 778	Classification
41-30	**a**	p. 779	Risk Factors
41-31	**a**	p. 780	Clinical Presentation and Diagnosis
41-32	**d**	p. 782	Obstetrical Coagulopathies
41-33	**d**	p. 784	Diagnosis
41-34	**c**	P. 787	Sepsis Syndrome
41-35	**d**	p. 788	Blood Component Products
41-36	**d**	p. 791	Transfusion Complications
41-37	**b**	p. 792	Uterine Artery Ligation
41-38	**a**	p. 793	Uterine Compression Sutures
41-39	**c**	p. 792	Internal Artery Ligation

CHAPTER 42

Preterm Birth

42–1. What is the definition of very low birthweight?

a. <500 grams
b. 500 to 1000 grams
c. 1000 to 1500 grams
d. 1500 to 2500 grams

42–2. What is the approximate preterm birth rate in the United States based on the most recently available data (2015)?

a. 9.5%
b. 10.0%
c. 10.5%
d. 11.0%

42–3. You deliver a 17-year-old G1 at 28 weeks' gestation following preterm labor. She gives birth to a female infant weighing 1090 grams who is immediately taken to the neonatal intensive care unit for evaluation. What would you tell her is the approximate survival rate for her infant?

a. 85%
b. 90%
c. 95%
d. 99%

42–4. An infant born at 25 weeks' gestation is at risk for all except which of the following complications?

a. Asthma
b. Blindness
c. Blood cancers
d. Pulmonary hypertension

42–5. What percentage of infants born at 22 weeks' gestation is expected to survive without neurodevelopmental impairment?

a. 0.5%
b. 1.0%
c. 1.5%
d. 2.0%

42–6. At what gestational age does the Obstetric Care Consensus document recommend consideration of neonatal resuscitation?

a. 21 weeks' gestation
b. 22 weeks' gestation
c. 23 weeks' gestation
d. 24 weeks' gestation

42–7. A 25-year-old G2P1 presents at 23 weeks and 3 days' gestation with painful contractions. Her cervix is dilated to 3 cm. Which interventions should be considered based on her presentation?

a. Magnesium sulfate
b. Corticosteroid therapy
c. Cesarean delivery for fetal indications
d. All of the above

42–8. Approximately what percentage of all preterm births in the United States occurs after 34 weeks' gestation?

a. 30%
b. 50%
c. 70%
d. 90%

42–9. Of the responses listed below, which complication is least commonly associated with preterm delivery?

a. Hypertension
b. Fetal complications
c. Placental abruption
d. None of the above

42–10. A 26-year-old G3P2 presents for pregnancy confirmation at 10 weeks' gestation. She is noted to have the ultrasound findings pictured. What is her risk for preterm birth based on the findings?

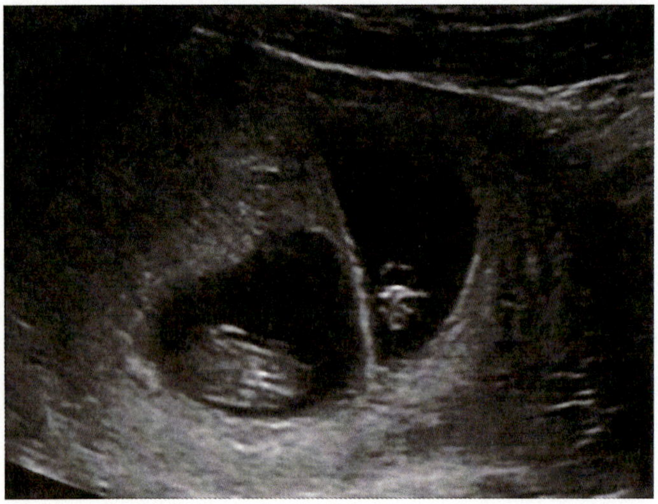

a. 30%
b. 50%
c. 70%
d. 90%

42–11. Which of the following placental hormones may play a role in preterm birth caused by maternal–fetal stress?

a. Estrogen
b. Human placental lactogen
c. Insulin-like growth hormone
d. Corticotropin-releasing hormone

42–12. Which of the following bacteria may enhance the risk for preterm birth by secretion of hyaluronidase?

a. *Escherichia coli*
b. *Peptostreptococcus*
c. Bacterial vaginosis
d. Group B streptococcus

42–13. Which of the following enzymes is not involved in the inflammatory cascade by which infection induces preterm labor?

a. IL-4
b. IL-8
c. Tumor-necrosis factor alpha
d. All of the above are involved

42–14. Which of the following bacteria is frequently detected in the amnionic fluid of women with preterm labor?

a. *Mycoplasma hominis*
b. *Gardnerella vaginalis*
c. *Ureaplasma urealyticum*
d. All of the above

42–15. Which of the following lifestyle factors is not associated with preterm birth?

a. Poverty
b. Short stature
c. Vitamin D deficiency
d. Advanced maternal age

42–16. A 32-year-old G2P1 presents at 16 weeks' gestation for prenatal care. She describes a history of preterm premature rupture of membranes in her last pregnancy with delivery at 31 weeks' gestation. How significantly increased is her preterm birth risk in her current pregnancy based on this history?

a. 2-fold increase
b. 3-fold increase
c. 4-fold increase
d. Her recurrent preterm birth risk is not increased

42–17. A 22-year-old G2P1 at 14 weeks' gestation complains of malodorous vaginal discharge. A saline preparation of the discharge is performed, and the findings are illustrated in the image below. What do you tell her regarding her diagnosis?

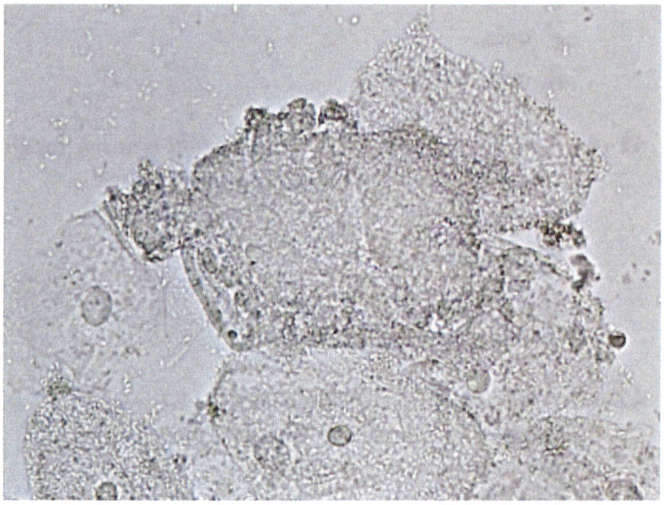

a. The condition is associated with frequent douching.
b. There is an association with preeclampsia and placental abruption.
c. Women with this diagnosis and a susceptible genotype have a 6-fold increased risk for preterm birth.
d. All of the above

42–18. You perform a routine cervical exam on a 39-year-old G3P2 at 30 weeks' gestation. You find her cervix to be 2 to 3 cm dilated. She denies having any contractions, discharge, pelvic pain or pressure. What is her chance of a preterm delivery before 34 weeks' gestation?

a. 5%

b. 15%

c. 25%

d. 35%

42–19. Which of the following is true regarding transvaginal sonographic evaluation of the cervix as a part of the assessment for preterm labor?

a. It can be performed any time after 14 weeks' gestation.

b. It is not affected by maternal obesity, cervix position, or shadowing.

c. The American College of Obstetricians and Gynecologists recommends it for all women with a history of a spontaneous preterm birth.

d. All of the above

42–20. Your patient is found to have the sonographic finding shown below during her anatomy ultrasound at 22 weeks' gestation. Her last pregnancy was complicated by spontaneous preterm birth at 33 weeks' gestation. Which of the following interventions could be recommended based on her history and current findings?

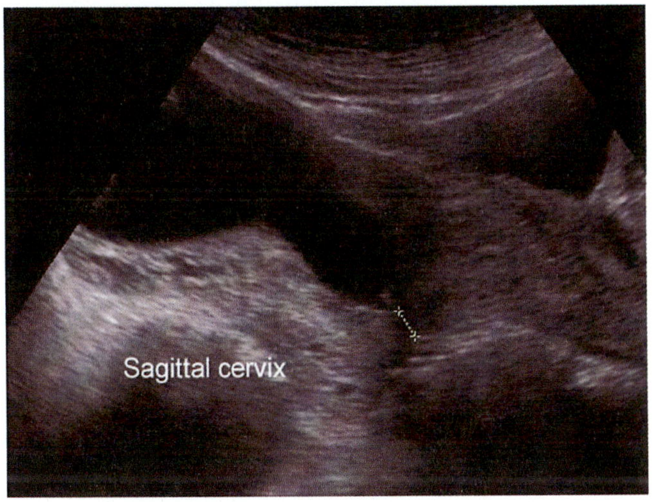

a. Cerclage placement

b. Aspirin 81 mg daily

c. Vaginal progesterone

d. None of the above

42–21. The Food and Drug Administration approved 17-hydroxyprogesterone caproate for the prevention of recurrent preterm birth based on a 2003 Maternal-Fetal Medicine Units (MFMU) Network study performed by Meis et al. What was one of the major criticisms of this study?

a. It was underpowered

b. Injections were not initiated until 16 weeks' gestation

c. There was an unexpectedly high preterm delivery rate in the placebo arm

d. All of the above

42–22. A recent study by Nelson et al showed that which of the following complications might be increased in pregnant women using 17-hydroxyprogesterone caproate to prevent recurrent preterm birth?

a. Depression

b. Hypertension

c. Gestational diabetes

d. Urinary tract infections

42–23. A 23-year-old G1 is incidentally noted to have a cervical length of 18 mm at 21 weeks' gestation. According to available research, which of the following therapies could be offered to potentially decrease her chance of preterm birth?

a. Cerclage

b. Vaginal progesterone

c. 17-hydroxyprogesterone caproate

d. None of the above

42–24. In women who experience preterm premature rupture of membranes between 24 and 34 weeks' gestation, what percentage might be expected to still be pregnant 48 hours after rupture?

a. 5–10%

b. 10–15%

c. 15–20%

d. 20–25%

42–25. A pregnant woman presents at 32 weeks and 5 days' gestation complaining of mild contractions and heavy discharge. You perform a speculum exam, which demonstrates pooling in the posterior fornix. Which of the following interventions would not be considered based on the clinical presentation?

a. Antimicrobials

b. Corticosteroids

c. Magnesium sulfate

d. Expectant management

42–26. What appears to be the gestational age threshold for lung hypoplasia in women with early membrane rupture?

a. 19 weeks' gestation
b. 21 weeks' gestation
c. 23 weeks' gestation
d. 25 weeks' gestation

42–27. Which of the following neonatal outcomes was potentially improved following antimicrobial therapy for pregnant woman with premature rupture of membranes before 35 weeks' gestation?

a. Improved survival
b. Decreased risk for sepsis
c. Decreased risk for intracranial hemorrhage
d. Decreased risk for respiratory distress syndrome

42–28. Which of the following drugs would not be recommended either alone or in combination for treatment of preterm premature rupture of membranes?

a. Amoxicillin
b. Erythromycin
c. Ampicillin-sulbactam
d. None of the above

42–29. A pregnant patient is transferred to your facility because of concerns for preterm labor at 35 weeks' gestation. She received a single course of corticosteroids prior to transfer. What neonatal complication is her infant potentially at greater risk for?

a. Sepsis
b. Hypothermia
c. Hypoglycemia
d. Transient tachypnea of the newborn

42–30. Treatment with magnesium sulfate is often used for neuroprotection for women at risk for delivery prior to 32 weeks' gestation. Approximately how many women need to be treated with magnesium to prevent one case of cerebral palsy?

a. 65
b. 70
c. 75
d. 80

42–31. Which of the following is a potential consequence of bed rest for suspected preterm labor?

a. Bone loss
b. Venous thromboembolism
c. Increased risk for preterm delivery
d. All of the above

42–32. An 18-year-old G1 African American female presents to the emergency department at 19 weeks' gestation complaining of pelvic pressure. She is found to be 2 cm dilated with membranes prolapsing beyond the os. No contractions are noted after extended monitoring. You perform a rescue cerclage as pictured in the image below. Which of the following factors is not associated with a decreased chance of pregnancy continuation after cerclage placement?

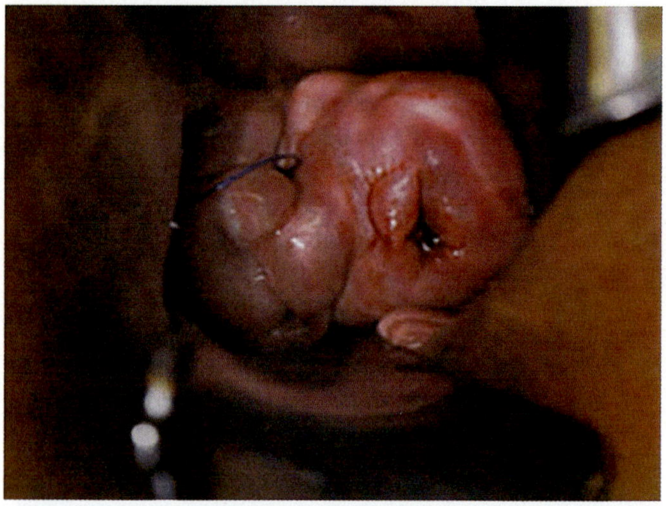

a. Nulligravida
b. African American race
c. Membrane prolapse beyond the external os
d. Cerclage placement before 22 weeks' gestation

42–33. A 28-week pregnant woman presents to labor and delivery with preterm contractions and is treated with terbutaline. Two days after the initiation of therapy, she begins complaining of shortness of breath and cough. A chest radiograph is obtained and shown in the image below. Which of the following risk factors is associated with development of this complication?

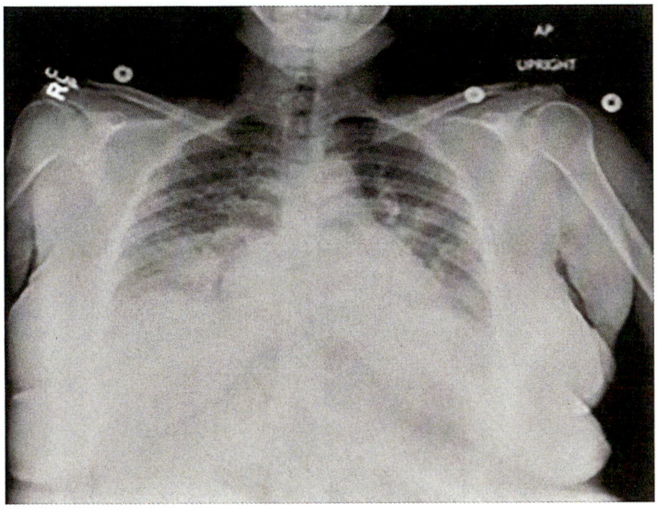

a. Asthma
b. Gestational diabetes
c. Concurrent corticosteroid therapy
d. All of the above

42–34. Which of the following is true regarding indomethacin use in pregnancy?

a. It can only be administered orally
b. It can lead to reversible oligohydramnios
c. It lowers the risk for necrotizing enterocolitis
d. All of the above

42–35. Cesarean delivery would be expected to decrease the risk for intracranial hemorrhage in which of the following scenarios?

a. Estimated fetal weight <1000 grams
b. Estimated fetal weight <1500 grams
c. Estimated fetal weight <2000 grams
d. None of the above

CHAPTER 42 ANSWER KEY

Question number	Letter answer	Page cited	Header cited
42–1	**c**	p. 803	Definition of Preterm Birth
42–2	**a**	p. 804	Preterm Birth Rate Trends
42–3	**c**	p. 805	Preterm Newborn Morbidity
42–4	**c**	p. 805	Table 42-2
42–5	**b**	p. 806	Periviable Neonatal Survival
42–6	**b**	p. 807	Table 42-4
42–7	**d**	p. 807	Clinical Management
42–8	**c**	p. 807	Late Preterm Birth
42–9	**c**	p. 808	Late Preterm Birth
42–10	**b**	p. 809	Causes of Late Preterm Birth
42–11	**d**	p. 810	Maternal–Fetal Stress
42–12	**d**	p. 810	Cervical Dysfunction
42–13	**a**	p. 810	Inflammatory Responses
42–14	**d**	p. 811	Origin of Cytokines
42–15	**c**	p. 812	Lifestyle Factors
42–16	**b**	p. 813	Prior Preterm Birth
42–17	**a**	p. 813	Bacterial Vaginosis
42–18	**c**	p. 814	Cervical Change
42–19	**b**	p. 815	Cervical Length Measurement
42–20	**a**	p. 815	Cervical Cerclage
42–21	**c**	p. 816	Prior Preterm Birth and Progestogen Compounds
42–22	**c**	p. 817	Use of 17-OHP-C at Parkland Hospital
42–23	**b**	p. 818	Progesterone Use without Prior Preterm Birth
42–24	**a**	p. 819	Natural History
42–25	**c**	p. 820	Table 42-9
42–26	**c**	p. 821	Considerations for Expectant Management
42–27	**b**	p. 822	Antimicrobial Therapy
42–28	**d**	p. 822	Antimicrobial Therapy
42–29	**c**	p. 823	Women at Risk for Late-Preterm Delivery
42–30	**a**	p. 824	Magnesium for Neuroprotection
42–31	**d**	p. 825	Bed Rest
42–32	**b**	p. 825	Emergency or Rescue Cerclage
42–33	**c**	p. 826	β-Adrenergic Receptor Agonists
42–34	**b**	p. 826	Prostaglandin Inhibitors
42–35	**d**	p. 827	Prevention of Intracranial Hemorrhage

CHAPTER 43

Postterm Pregnancy

43–1. A pregnancy is considered prolonged after how many completed weeks?

a. 39 weeks
b. 40 weeks
c. 41 weeks
d. 42 weeks

43–2. What is the most accurate way of dating a pregnancy?

a. Last menstrual period
b. 1st-trimester ultrasound
c. 2nd-trimester ultrasound
d. Last menstrual period and a 2nd-trimester ultrasound

43–3. In the United States in 2013, what percentage of pregnancies were considered postterm?

a. 3%
b. 5%
c. 8%
d. 10%

43–4. Rare fetal–placental factors associated with postterm pregnancy include which of the following?

a. Anencephaly
b. Wilms tumor
c. Adrenal hyperplasia
d. Autosomal-recessive placental sulfatase deficiency

43–5. What is a major cause of perinatal mortality associated with pregnancy duration beyond 41 weeks?

a. Birth injuries
b. Gestational hypertension
c. Hypoxic-ischemic encephalopathy
d. All of the above

43–6. Which of the following have been found to be increased in the setting of postterm pregnancies?

a. Neonatal seizures and deaths
b. Neonatal intensive care admissions
c. Cesarean delivery for fetal distress
d. All of the above

43–7. Maternal risks of postterm pregnancy include all except which of the following?

a. Preeclampsia
b. Perineal lacerations
c. Postpartum hemorrhage
d. Morbidly adherent placenta

43–8. What are the best estimates for the frequency of postmaturity syndrome in gestations that have completed 42 weeks?

a. 1%
b. 5%
c. 10–20%
d. 25%

43–9. Which of the following is true the syndrome afflicting this infant?

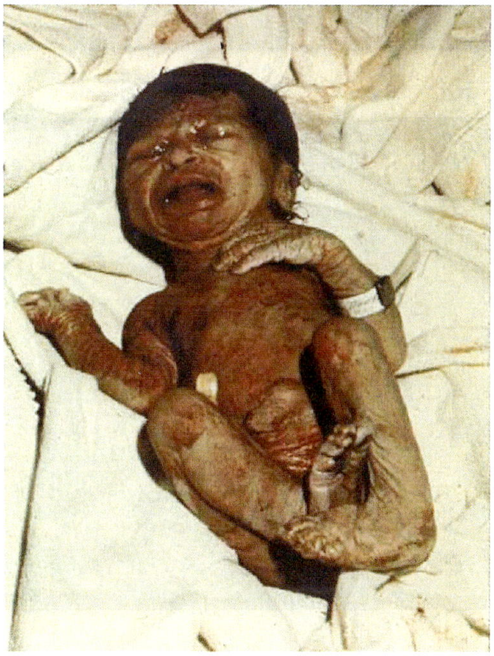

Reproduced with permission from Cunningham FG, Leveno KJ, Bloom SL, et al (eds): Postterm pregnancy. In Williams Obstetrics, 25th ed. New York, McGraw-Hill, 2018, Figure 43-2.

a. Neurological deficits are found in 33%
b. Majority have birthweights <10th percentile
c. Features include simian crease and low-set ears
d. Oligohydramnios increases its likelihood at 42 weeks

43–10. Which of the following characterizes the placenta in a postterm pregnancy?

a. Decreased rate of apoptosis

b. Increased rates of placental separation

c. Downregulation of the kisspeptin gene

d. Increased levels of cord erythropoietin levels

43–11. A 33-year-old multigravida presents in labor at 43 weeks' gestation. She is 3 cm dilated and approximately 2 hours after arrival undergoes an emergent cesarean delivery due to fetal heart rate abnormalities. Which of the following was most likely her tracing prior to delivery?

a.

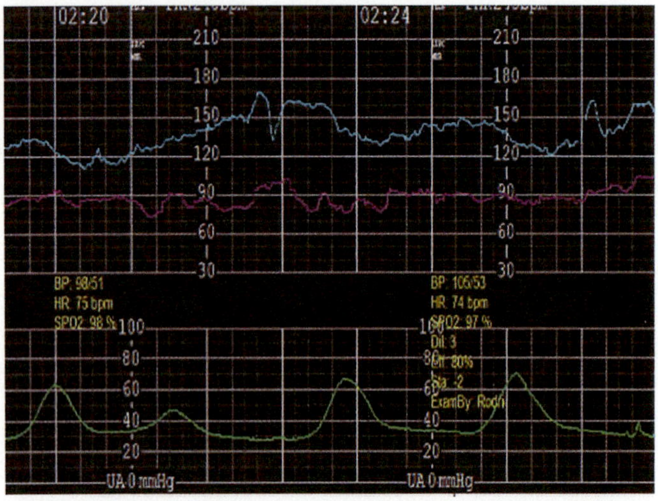

b.

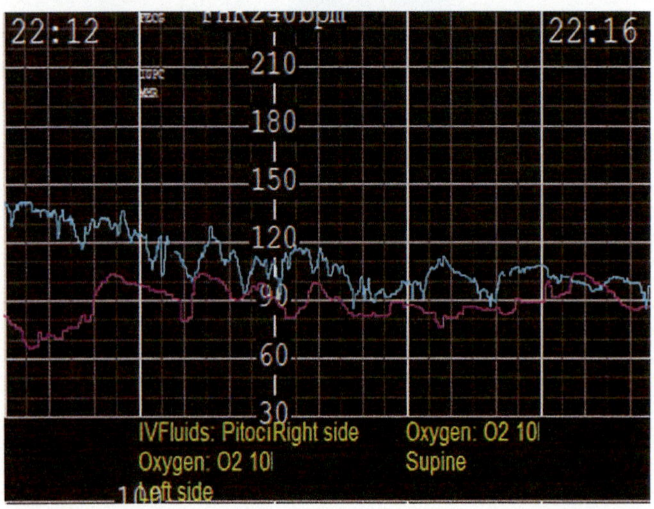

c.

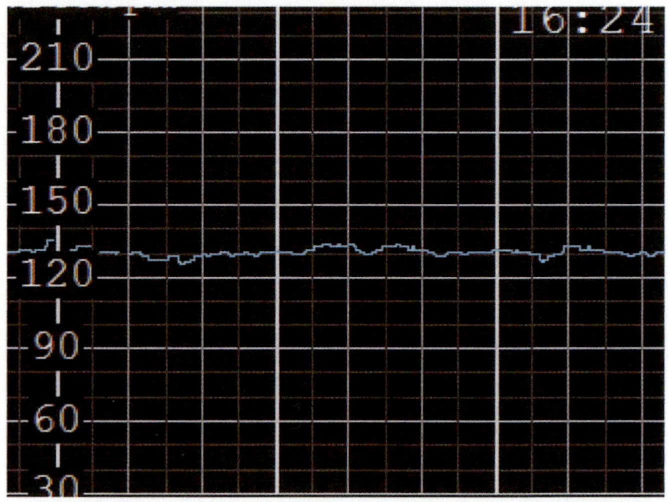

d.

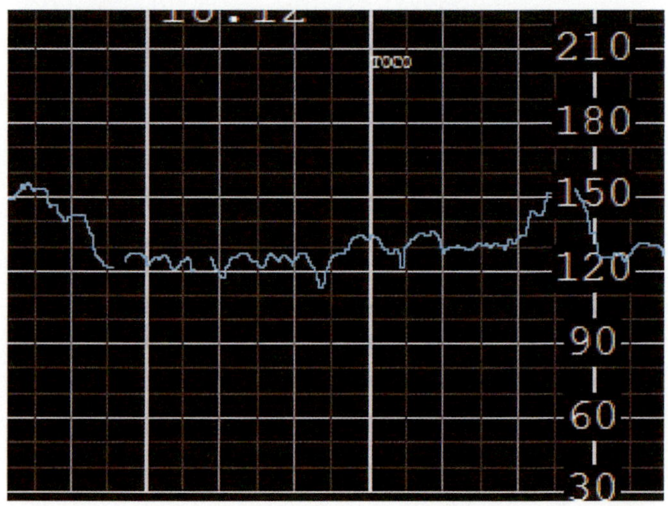

43–12. At the time of cesarean delivery in Question 43–11, which of the following was likely present?

- **a.** Meconium
- **b.** Polyhydramnios
- **c.** Short umbilical cord
- **d.** Bloody amnionic fluid

43–13. When does the volume of amnionic fluid begin to decline?

- **a.** After 36 weeks
- **b.** After 37 weeks
- **c.** After 38 weeks
- **d.** After 39 weeks

43–14. In which of the following conditions in pregnancy is it generally recommended to be delivered at less than 42 weeks?

- **a.** Diabetes
- **b.** Gestational hypertension
- **c.** Previous cesarean delivery
- **d.** All of the above

43–15. Most stillbirths in prolonged pregnancies are associated with which of the following?

- **a.** Oligohydramnios
- **b.** Late prenatal care
- **c.** Fetal growth restriction
- **d.** Shortened pregnancy interval

43–16. A 24-year-old primigravida presents to clinic at 42 weeks' gestation after missing several clinic visits. An ultrasound image of the deepest vertical pocket is displayed below. She is at risk for having which of the following outcomes?

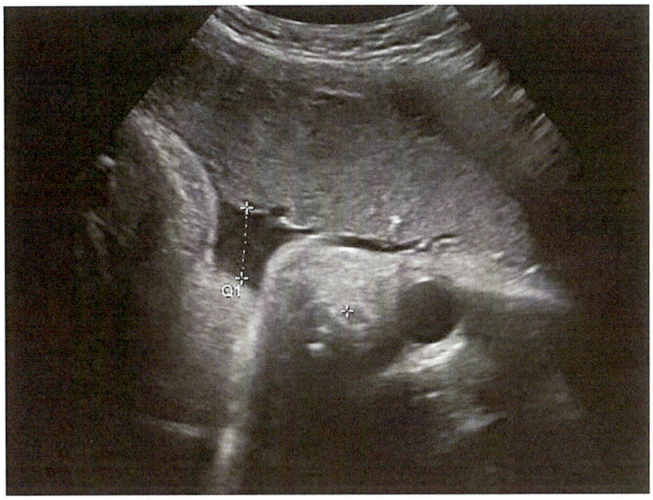

- **a.** Meconium
- **b.** Macrosomia
- **c.** Shoulder dystocia
- **d.** 5-minute Apgar ≤ 6

43–17. Which of the following statements concerning decreased amnionic fluid is false?

- **a.** Associated with fetal distress during labor
- **b.** Amnionic fluid index <5 cm is associated with more adverse outcomes than largest vertical pocket <2 cm.
- **c.** Amnionic fluid index is the best method by which to estimate the occurrence of oligohydramnios.
- **d.** All of the above

43–18. According to the American College of Obstetricians and Gynecologists, at what estimated fetal weight is it reasonable to offer cesarean delivery to a nondiabetic gravida at term?

- **a.** 4250 grams
- **b.** 4500 grams
- **c.** 4750 grams
- **d.** 5000 grams

43–19. Routine membrane sweeping on cervical exam at 38–40 weeks' gestation has been shown to be associated with which of the following?

a. Increased pain

b. Increased bleeding

c. Lower rate of postterm pregnancies

d. All of the above

43–20. In primigravidas undergoing induction of labor at 41 weeks' gestation, what beginning fetal station was associated with the highest rate of cesarean section?

a. 0

b. –1

c. –2

d. –4

43–21. Which of the following is predictive of a successful induction of labor?

a. Cervical length <3 cm

b. Cervical length <2.5 cm

c. Cervical dilation prior to induction

d. All of the above

43–22. Comparing induction of labor at 41 weeks' gestation to prolonging pregnancies with fetal testing, research supports which of the following statements?

a. Induction increases the rate of cesarean delivery.

b. Induction increases the rate of postpartum hemorrhage.

c. Induction increases the rate of anesthesia complications.

d. Induction decreases the rate of meconium aspiration syndrome.

43–23. What are considerations when considering amniotomy during a postterm induction?

a. Increase risk for cord compression

b. Allows more precise fetal heart rate monitoring

c. Aids in identification of thick meconium in amnionic fluid

d. All of the above

43–24. When used during labor, amnioinfusion does which of the following?

a. Prevents placental abruption

b. Decreases the occurrence of variable decelerations

c. Decreases the incidence of meconium aspiration syndrome

d. None of the above

43–25. With thick meconium early in the labor process, which of the following is true?

a. Cesarean delivery is likely

b. Chances for vaginal delivery are diminished

c. If delivery is remote, some obstetricians elect to perform cesarean delivery

d. All of the above

43–26. The American College of Obstetricians and Gynecologists recommends which of the following in the setting of meconium-stained amnionic fluid?

a. Intubation if the baby is depressed

b. Amnioinfusion only during active labor

c. The pediatrician should immediately perform bulb suction on the warmer.

d. The obstetrician should perform bulb suction after delivery of the baby.

43–27. A 44-year-old primigravida presents to clinic at 40 weeks' gestation. She wants to go into labor naturally, and therefore wants to wait as long as possible to be induced. Based on the American College of Obstetricians and Gynecologists, when should she be induced?

a. 40 weeks' gestation

b. 41 weeks' gestation

c. 42 weeks' gestation

d. When the patient is ready

43–28. The patient in Question 43–27 inquires about the risks of going past 41 weeks' gestation. What are the risks she is concerned about?

a. Macrosomia

b. Cesarean delivery

c. Postmaturity syndrome

d. Anesthesia complications

43–29. The patient in Question 43–27 agrees to induction of labor at 41 weeks' gestation. How will you manage her pregnancy during this week?

a. Fetal surveillance

b. Anesthesia consult

c. Weekly prenatal care visit only, as usual

d. Cancel her clinic visit and see her on the day of her induction

43–30. The patient in Question 43–27 presents for her nonstress test, and her tracing is pictured below. Given the fetal heart rate tracing, what are you worried about?

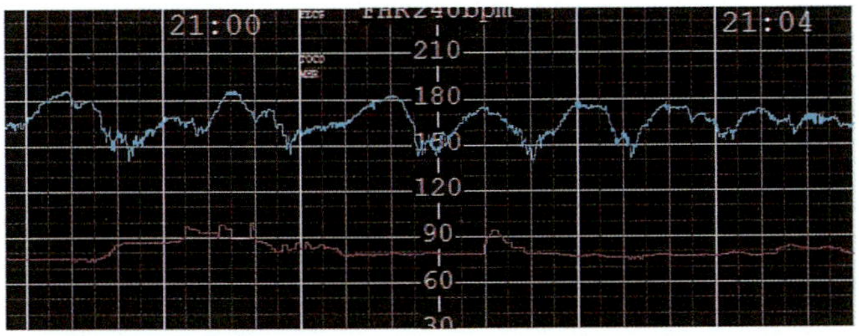

a. Meconium

b. Fetal acidemia

c. Oligohydramnios

d. Placental insufficiency

43–31. A 27-year-old primigravida presents to labor and delivery reporting contractions. She reports scant prenatal care, and based on her last menstrual period she is 41 weeks pregnant. Bedside ultrasound is consistent with her last menstrual period. She is not in labor, but 1 cm dilated, and she would like to be induced. What is the next best step?

a. Delivery

b. Follow-up in clinic in 1 week

c. Amniocentesis for fetal lung maturity

d. Schedule for induction at 42 weeks' gestation

43–32. The patient in Question 43–31 delivers a male infant, and the neonatologist at delivery suspects postmaturity syndrome. Her suspicion is based on which of the findings below?

a. Peeling skin

b. Long, thin body

c. Unusually old in appearance

d. All of the above

CHAPTER 43 ANSWER KEY

Question number	Letter answer	Page cited	Header cited
43–1	**d**	p. 835	Introduction
43–2	**b**	p. 835	Estimated Gestational Age
43–3	**c**	p. 836	Incidence
43–4	**a**	p. 836	Incidence
43–5	**d**	p. 836	Perinatal Morbidity and Mortality
43–6	**d**	p. 836	Perinatal Morbidity and Mortality
43–7	**d**	p. 836	Perinatal Morbidity and Mortality
43–8	**c**	p. 837	Postmaturity Syndrome
43–9	**d**	p. 837	Postmaturity Syndrome
43–10	**d**	p. 837	Placental Dysfunction
43–11	**b**	p. 838	Fetal Distress and Oligohydramnios
43–12	**a**	p. 838	Fetal Distress and Oligohydramnios
43–13	**c**	p. 838	Fetal Distress and Oligohydramnios
43–14	**d**	p. 839	Complications
43–15	**c**	p. 839	Fetal Growth Restriction
43–16	**d**	p. 839	Figure 43-5
43–17	**d**	p. 839	Oligohydramnios
43–18	**d**	p. 839	Macrosomia
43–19	**d**	p. 840	Induction Factors
43–20	**d**	p. 840	Induction Factors
43–21	**d**	p. 840	Induction Factors
43–22	**d**	p. 840	Induction versus Fetal Testing
43–23	**d**	p. 841	Intrapartum Management
43–24	**b**	p. 841	Intrapartum Management
43–25	**d**	p. 841	Intrapartum Management
43–26	**a**	p. 842	Intrapartum Management
43–27	**c**	p. 840	Induction versus Fetal Testing
43–28	**b**	p. 840	Induction versus Fetal Testing
43–29	**a**	p. 841	Figure 43-6
43–30	**c**	p. 838	Figure 43-4
43–31	**a**	p. 841	Management Strategies
43–32	**d**	p. 836	Postmaturity Syndrome

CHAPTER 44

Fetal-Growth Disorders

44–1. What is true about the extremes of fetal growth in the United States?

a. In 2015, 8.1% of newborns weighed less than 2500 grams.

b. In 2015, 8% of newborns weighed more than 4000 grams.

c. 20% of the almost 4 million neonates born in the United States are at the low and high extremes of fetal growth.

d. All of the above

44–2. In the diagram below, fetal growth rates are depicted. Which of the following is correct?

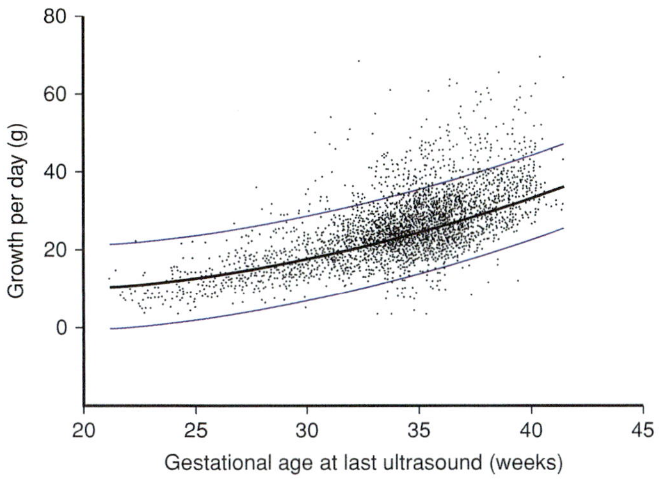

Reproduced with permission from Cunningham FG, Leveno KJ, Bloom SL, et al (eds): Fetal-growth disorders. In Williams Obstetrics, 25th ed. New York, McGraw-Hill, 2018, Figure 44-1.

a. 10 g/d at 15 weeks' gestation

b. 10 to 15 g/d at 24 weeks' gestation

c. 20 to 30 g/d at 35 weeks' gestation

d. 30 to 35 g/d at 34 weeks' gestation

44–3. Which of the following is a risk factor for poor fetal growth?

a. Malaria

b. Tuberculosis

c. Cytomegalovirus

d. All of the above

44–4. Which of the following statements is closely associated with the characteristics of human fetal growth?

a. Need a narrow pelvis to walk upright

b. A large head is needed for a large brain

c. The ability to growth restrict may be adaptive

d. All of the above

44–5. Referencing the graphic below, what can be said about dating and ultrasonography in obstetrics?

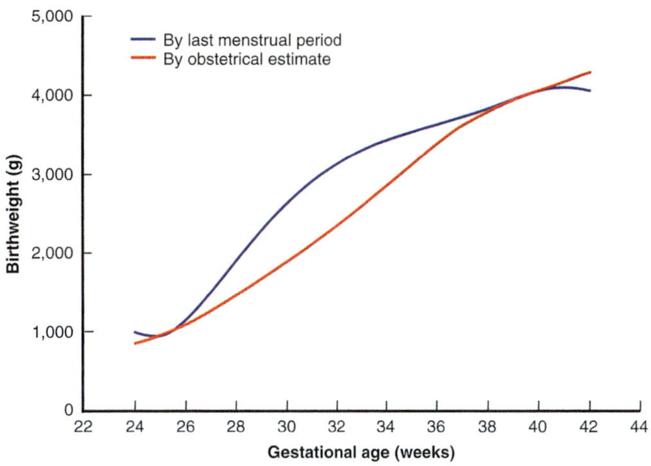

Reproduced with permission from Cunningham FG, Leveno KJ, Bloom SL, et al (eds): Fetal-growth disorders. In Williams Obstetrics, 25th ed. New York, McGraw-Hill, 2018, Figure 44-2.

a. Postterm birthweights were relatively lower using menstrual dating.

b. Best obstetric estimates were mainly based on menstrual dating.

c. Preterm birthweights were overestimated prior to the use of best obstetric estimates.

d. All of the above

44–6. How is symmetrical versus asymmetrical growth restriction differentiated?

a. Symmetrically growth restricted fetuses were proportionately small.

b. The abdominal circumference to head circumference ratio is used to differentiate between the two.

c. Asymmetrically growth restricted fetuses had a disproportionately lagging head compared with abdominal growth.

d. All of the above

44–7. Which of the following statements is true regarding brain sparing and growth restriction?

a. Brain sparing is restricted to symmetrically growth restricted fetuses.

b. With limited nutrients, there is preferential shunting of oxygen and nutrients to the brain.

c. During the last 12 weeks of growth in the growth restricted infant, brain sparing is demonstrated by a brain-to-liver weight ratio of 3:1 instead of the normal 2:1.

d. All of the above

44–8. Growing evidence suggests that fetal growth restriction affects organ development, especially which of the following?

a. Brain

b. Heart

c. Kidney

d. Thyroid

44–9. Risk factors for impaired fetal growth are divided into mother, fetus, and placenta. Which of the following is a common risk factor to all three sources?

a. Infection

b. Drugs and teratogens

c. Genetic abnormalities

d. Maternal medical conditions

44–10. Which of the following markers is associated with fetal overgrowth?

a. IGF-1

b. Hyperglycemia

c. Hyperinsulinemia

d. All of the above

44–11. What risk factors are associated with fetal growth restriction in women with pre-gestational diabetes?

a. Maternal vascular disease

b. Congenital malformations

c. Worsening White classification

d. All of the above

44–12. Compared to women who do not undergo psychosocial risk factor screening during pregnancy, those that do have which of the following?

a. Lower preterm birth rates

b. More appropriate interventions

c. Lower rates of low-birthweight newborns

d. All of the above

44–13. The presence of which of the following vascular diseases during pregnancy leads to the highest perinatal morbidity rates?

a. Class F diabetes

b. Valvular heart disease

c. Ischemic heart disease

d. Chronic hypertension

44–14. Which of the following conditions is associated with chronic hypoxia?

a. Chronic hypertension

b. Living in Dallas, Texas

c. Sporadic marijuana smoking

d. None of the above

44–15. Given the graphic below, at what gestational age does growth begin to differentiate due to order of multifetal gestation?

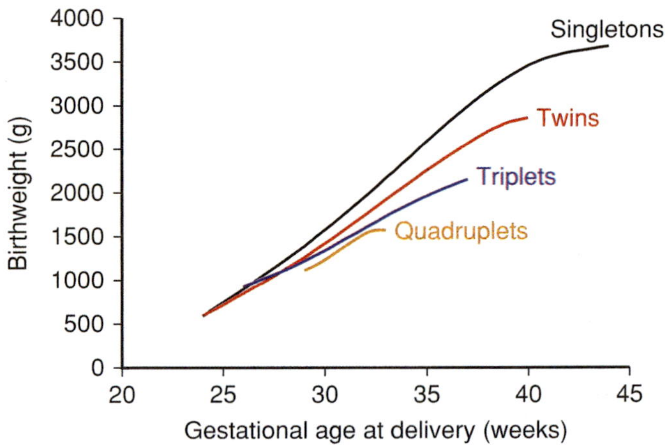

Reproduced with permission from Cunningham FG, Leveno KJ, Bloom SL, et al (eds): Fetal-growth disorders. In Williams Obstetrics, 25th ed. New York, McGraw-Hill, 2018, Figure 44-5.

a. 15–20 weeks

b. 20–25 weeks

c. 25–30 weeks

d. After 30 weeks

44–16. Between 18 and 30 weeks, which of the following fundal height measurements would suggest that fetal growth should be checked by ultrasound?

a. Current gestational age of 16 weeks and fundal height measuring 18 cm

b. Current gestational age of 22 weeks and fundal height measuring 20 cm

c. Current gestational age of 25 weeks and fundal height measuring 22 cm

d. Current gestational age of 13 weeks and fundal height measuring 32 cm

44–17. Which of the following antiphospholipid antibodies are associated with fetal growth restriction?

- **a.** G20210A mutation
- **b.** Lupus anticoagulant
- **c.** Anti-$\beta 2$ glycoprotein antibodies
- **d.** All of the above

44–18. Which of the following is true regarding oligohydramnios?

- **a.** It is associated with fetal growth restriction.
- **b.** It is associated with a higher cesarean delivery rate.
- **c.** It is associated with congenital fetal malformations.
- **d.** All of the above

44–19. What can be said concerning sonographic diagnosis of fetal growth restriction?

- **a.** First-trimester ultrasound is superior for predicting small-for-gestational-age infants.
- **b.** Second-trimester ultrasound is superior to first-trimester ultrasound for predicting small-for-gestational-age infants.
- **c.** The most common method for identifying poor fetal growth is standard indexing of weights to gestational age by femur length.
- **d.** None of the above

44–20. What can be said about the following Doppler waveforms of the umbilical artery?

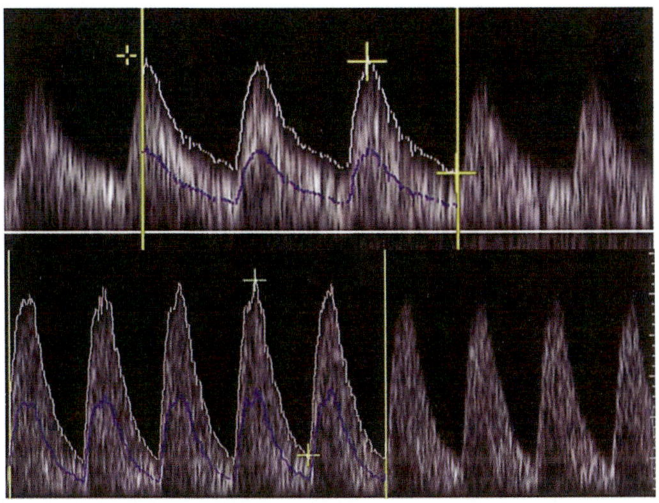

Reproduced with permission from Cunningham FG, Leveno KJ, Bloom SL, et al (eds): Fetal-growth disorders. In Williams Obstetrics, 25th ed. New York, McGraw-Hill, 2018, Figure 44-8.

- **a.** The S/D ratio in B is abnormal.
- **b.** The S/D ratio is greater in B than A.
- **c.** The S/D ratio is greater in A than B.
- **d.** None of the above

44–21. What can be said about the following Doppler waveform of the umbilical artery?

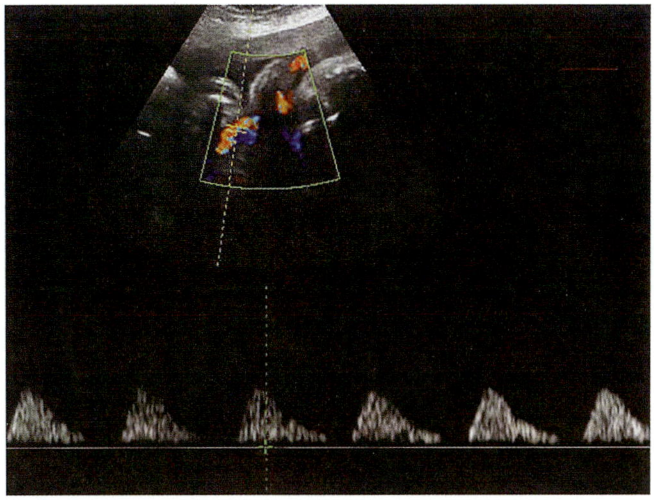

- **a.** The S/D ratio is between 2 and 4.
- **b.** This represents reversed end-diastolic flow.
- **c.** This is only considered clinically useful in an infant with growth restriction.
- **d.** None of the above

44–22. Your patient arrives late in her care. She brought a copy of her ultrasound from 12 weeks' gestation which matched her dates of 32 weeks. Ultrasound performed in your office reveals an estimated fetal weight <3rd percentile for gestational age. Doppler velocimetry of the umbilical artery reveals the waveform below. Continuous fetal monitor detects a fetal baseline heart rate of 150, minimal variability, and repetitive late decelerations. What is your next course of action?

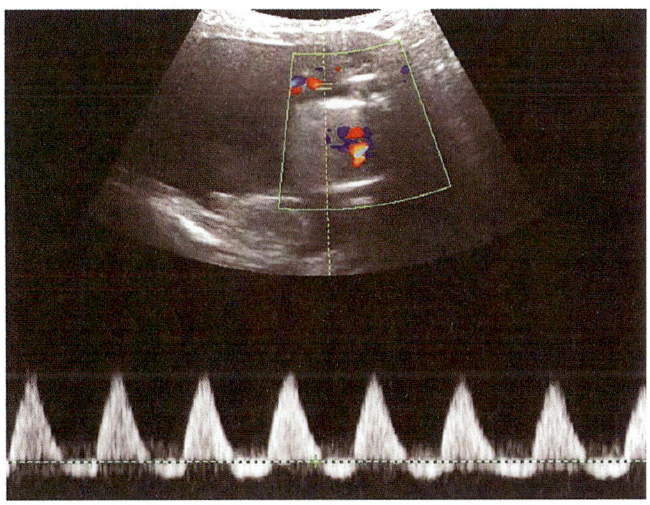

- **a.** Proceed with primary cesarean delivery
- **b.** Give betamethasone, wait 48 hours, and deliver
- **c.** Admit to the floor for daily fetal surveillance
- **d.** Any of the above would be reasonable

44–23. In which chromosomal aneuploidy is fetal-growth restriction virtually always present?

a. 45,X
b. Trisomy 13
c. Trisomy 18
d. Trisomy 21

44–24. Which of the following drugs and chemicals is capable of limiting fetal growth?

a. Alcohol
b. Cocaine
c. Cigarettes
d. All of the above

44–25. Which of the following practices may prevent or limit fetal growth restriction?

a. Smoking cessation
b. Increase caloric requirements for women with a growth restricted infant.
c. Even with normal fundal height and presumed growth, it is reasonable to perform Doppler velocimetry and fetal surveillance on the current pregnancy if the woman had an infant with growth restriction previously.
d. All of the above

44–26. Ms. Smith is a 37-year-old multigravida who presents to your office at 32 weeks' gestation as calculated by her last menstrual period. Her hematocrit is 29%, and she has sickle-cell trait. During sonographic evaluation, the fetus has biometric values that correlate with a 28-week fetus. What is the most likely explanation?

a. Aneuploidy
b. Chronic hypoxia
c. Poor pregnancy dating
d. First-trimester cytomegalovirus infection

44–27. For the patient in Question 44–26, when will you reevaluate fetal growth?

a. 1 week
b. 2 weeks
c. 3 weeks
d. 6 weeks

44–28. What is the major risk factor for fetal overgrowth?

a. Genetics
b. Multiparity
c. Maternal obesity
d. Gestational diabetes

44–29. For the prediction of macrosomia, how does clinical estimation of fetal weight compare with sonographic estimation?

a. Less accurate
b. Similar accuracy
c. Modestly more accurate
d. Significantly more accurate

44–30. Which of the following is accurate regarding prophylactic labor induction for suspected fetal macrosomia?

a. Increased rate of cesarean delivery
b. Improves maternal and neonatal outcomes
c. Decreases the risk for postpartum hemorrhage
d. All of the above

44–31. At what estimated fetal weight is a cesarean delivery indicated in a woman without diabetes?

a. ≥4000 grams
b. ≥4250 grams
c. ≥4500 grams
d. ≥5000 grams

CHAPTER 44 ANSWER KEY

Question number	Letter answer	Page cited	Header cited
44–1	**d**	p. 844	Introduction
44–2	**d**	p. 845	Fetal Growth
44–3	**d**	p. 849	Risk Factors and Etiologies
44–4	**d**	p. 844	Pathophysiology
44–5	**c**	p. 845	Normal Birthweight
44–6	**a**	p. 847	Symmetrical versus Asymmetrical Growth Restriction
44–7	**b**	p. 847	Brain Sparing
44–8	**b**	p. 848	Fetal Undergrowth
44–9	**a**	p. 849	Risk Factors and Etiologies
44–10	**d**	p. 849	Fetal Overgrowth
44–11	**d**	p. 850	Pre-gestational Diabetes
44–12	**d**	p. 850	Social Issues
44–13	**c**	p. 850	Vascular and Renal Disease
44–14	**a**	p. 850	Chronic Hypoxia
44–15	**d**	p. 851	Multifetal Gestation
44–16	**c**	p. 852	Uterine Fundal Height
44–17	**c**	p. 851	Antiphospholipid Antibody Syndrome
44–18	**d**	p. 853	Amnionic Fluid Volume Measurement
44–19	**b**	p. 852	Sonographic Measurement
44–20	**b**	p. 853	Doppler Velocimetry
44–21	**c**	p. 853	Doppler Velocimetry
44–22	**a**	p. 854	Doppler Velocimetry
44–23	**c**	p. 852	Chromosomal Aneuploidies
44–24	**d**	p. 851	Drugs with Teratogenic and Fetal Effects
44–25	**a**	p. 854	Prevention
44–26	**c**	p. 849	Risk Factors and Etiologies
44–27	**c**	p. 855	Management
44–28	**c**	p. 857	Risk Factors
44–29	**b**	p. 858	Diagnosis
44–30	**a**	p. 858	Prophylactic Labor Induction
44–31	**d**	p. 859	Elective Cesarean Delivery

CHAPTER 45

Multifetal Gestation

45–1. All except which of the following complications are increased in multifetal gestations?

a. Preeclampsia
b. Hysterectomy
c. Maternal death
d. Postterm delivery

45–2. Which of the following mechanisms may result in monozygotic twins being discordant for malformations or traits?

a. Prezygotic mutation
b. Variable expression of the same genetic disease
c. Skewed lyonization in male fetuses with differential expression of X-linked traits or diseases
d. All of the above

45–3. A 37-year-old G1 comes to establish prenatal care with you after being discharged from her reproductive endocrinologist. This pregnancy was conceived via single embryo transfer in vitro fertilization. Which one of the following is true regarding her situation?

a. Assisted reproductive technology increases the incidence of monozygotic twins two- to fivefold.
b. If a single zygote splits 8 days post fertilization, a monochorionic diamnionic twin gestation results.
c. Because this pregnancy is known to have begun with one embryo, you can be certain that she will have monochorionic twins, but amnionicity depends on timing of split.
d. All of the above

45–4. A 29-year-old G1P1 conceived dichorionic twins via gonadotropin stimulation and intrauterine insemination (IUI) with her husband's semen. Her blood type is O-negative, so prior to receiving anti-D immune globulin the neonates' blood type is assessed. One neonate is A-positive and the other is O-negative. Her husband is A-positive. This finding can be explained to the parents by describing which of the following phenomena?

a. Superfetation
b. Superfecundation
c. This is not atypical for dichorionic twins
d. This cannot be explained without alleging infidelity or poor technique by her reproductive endocrinologist's office.

45–5. The first trimester ultrasound image shown here shows two fetal heads arising from a shared body. How many days after fertilization must the division of this zygote have occurred to lead to the finding shown?

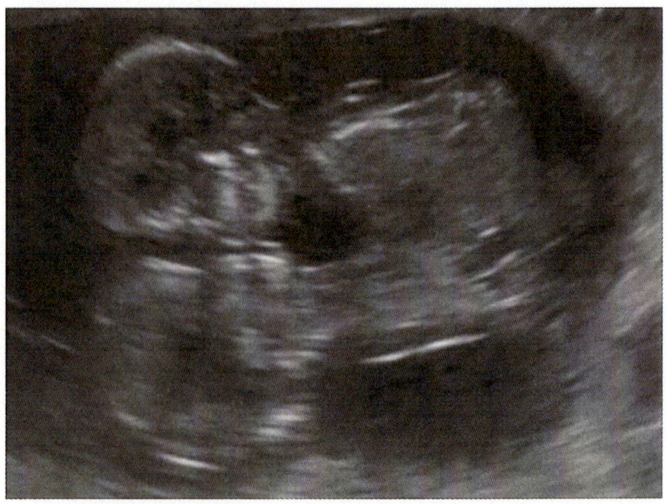

a. 0–3 days
b. 4–7 days
c. 8–12 days
d. ≥13 days

45–6. Which of the following factors increases the risk for monozygotic twinning?

a. Maternal age
b. Increased parity
c. Race and family history
d. None of the above

45–7. Which hormone is the most likely underlying cause of increased twinning seen in some racial and ethnic groups?

a. Estrogen
b. Progesterone
c. Luteinizing hormone
d. Follicle-stimulating hormone

45–8. Which of the following statements regarding atypical twinning is not true?

a. Monochorionic twins are never dizygotic.
b. Twins of opposite sex are not always dizygotic.
c. Monochorionic twins are not always the same sex.
d. None of the above is true

45–9. A 23-year-old G1 is found to have a twin gestation on ultrasound. How would you describe the image shown below?

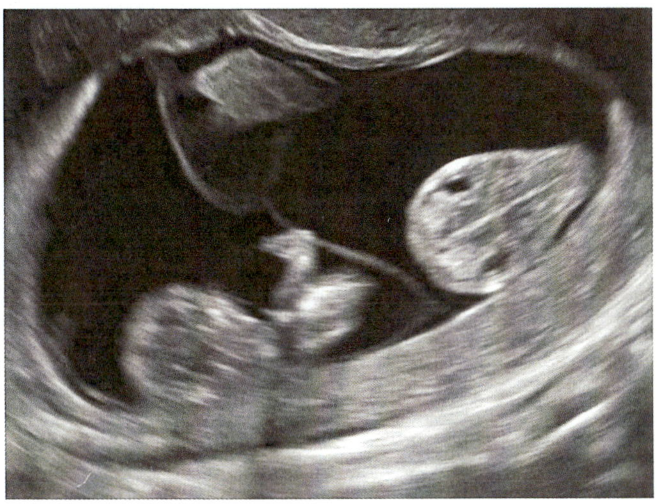

a. Two placentas are seen.
b. The twins must be monozygotic.
c. This is a monoamnionic twin gestation.
d. Without ability to visualize the yolk sac in this image, you cannot make a comment regarding placental number at this gestational age.

45–10. The finding shown in this ultrasound image facilitates accurate identification of a dichorionic gestation. Which of the following statements is true regarding ultrasound determination of chorionicity?

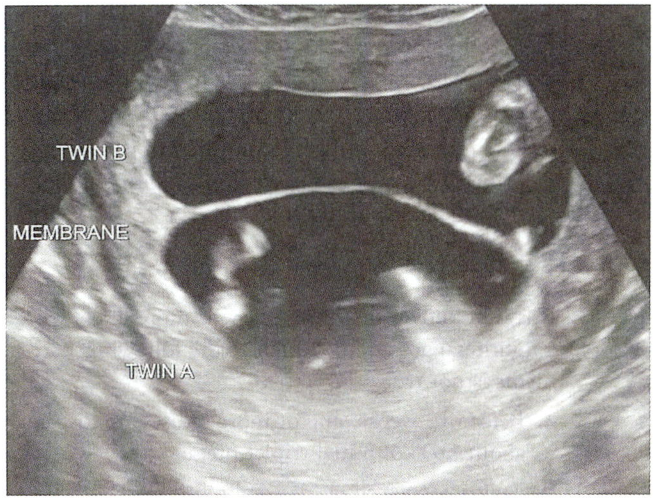

a. Dichorionic intervening membrane may not be easily seen prior to 10 weeks.
b. Accuracy in ultrasound classification of chorionicity improves with advancing gestation.
c. Risk for misclassification of chorionicity decreases by 1% for each additional week from 15 to 20 weeks.
d. Accuracy in ultrasound classification of chorionicity is 98% in the first trimester and diminishes with advancing gestational age.

45–11. What can be confirmed about the placenta being examined in the image shown here?

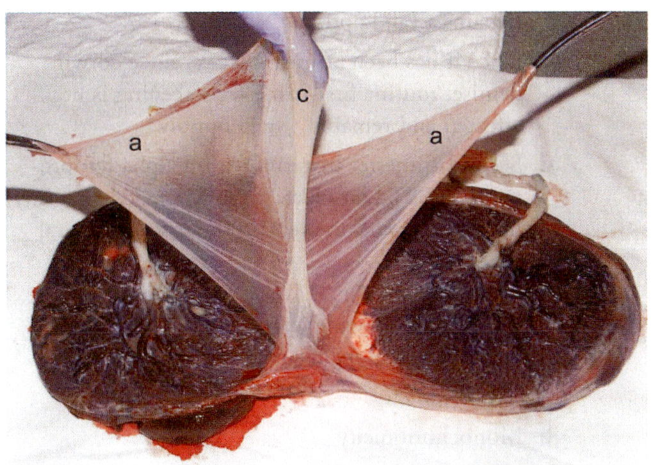

Reproduced with permission from Cunningham FG, Leveno KJ, Bloom SL, et al (eds): Multifetal pregnancy. In Williams Obstetrics, 25th ed. New York, McGraw-Hill, 2018, Figure 45–6.

a. Dizygosity
b. Monozygosity
c. One chorion, two amnions
d. Two chorions, two amnions

45–12. Maternal physiological adaptation to twin pregnancy in comparison to a singleton pregnancy is accurately described in which of the following statements?

- **a.** Cardiac output increases 40% above that of a woman carrying a singleton fetus.
- **b.** Blood volume expansion averages 70%, which is greater than the 40–50% seen in women carrying a singleton.
- **c.** The increased cardiac output in twin gestation is primarily due to increased stroke volume rather than increased heart rate.
- **d.** All of the above

45–13. It is well known that miscarriage is more likely with a multifetal gestation. Which of the following statements is not true?

- **a.** Before 12 weeks, one or more fetuses are lost in about 50% of initial triplet pregnancies.
- **b.** Twins conceived via assisted reproductive techniques are at greater risk for spontaneous loss.
- **c.** Spontaneous loss of a cotwin before the second trimester occurs in 10–40% of all twin gestations.
- **d.** None of the above is true.

45–14. A 34-year-old G2P1 at 12 weeks' gestation presents to discuss aneuploidy screening. This pregnancy started out with dichorionic twins, but spontaneously reduced to singleton at 7–8 weeks' gestation. Which of the following is the most appropriate?

- **a.** First-trimester screening is not recommended.
- **b.** Since the cotwin demise occurred prior to 9 weeks, routine first-trimester screening is not affected and remains a valid option.
- **c.** Since it has been at least 4 weeks since cotwin demise, routine first-trimester screening is not affected and remains a valid option.
- **d.** Second-trimester maternal serum alpha fetoprotein will be falsely elevated, so a detailed anatomy ultrasound is recommended to assess for neural tube defect.

45–15. Which of the following is associated with increased risk for congenital malformation?

- **a.** Dichorionicity
- **b.** Monochorionicity
- **c.** Conception via assisted reproductive technology
- **d.** All of the above

45–16. Ultrasound estimation of fetal weight is 2000 g for twin A, one of a dichorionic pair, at 33 weeks' gestation. Which of the following is an appropriate impression from this information?

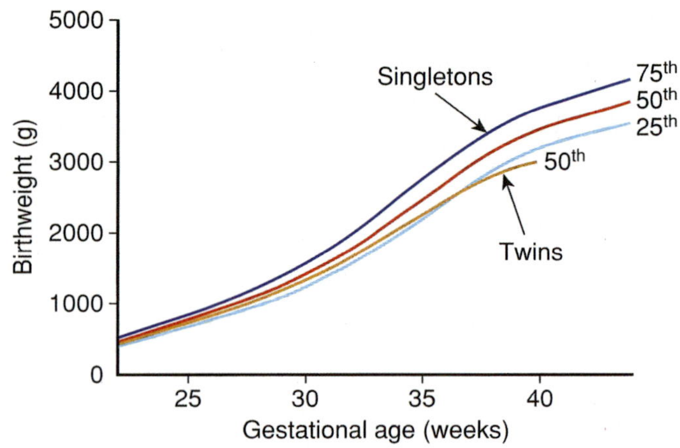

Reproduced with permission from Cunningham FG, Leveno KJ, Bloom SL, et al (eds): Multifetal pregnancy. In Williams Obstetrics, 25th ed. New York, McGraw-Hill, 2018, Figure 45–8.

- **a.** The fetus will be growth restricted at term.
- **b.** The fetus already shows growth restriction.
- **c.** The fetal growth is appropriate for gestational age.
- **d.** Without information for twin B, it is not feasible to form an impression about the adequacy of the growth of this twin.

45–17. The increased risk for hypertensive disorders of pregnancy seen with multifetal gestation is related to which of the following?

- **a.** Increased levels of placental growth factor
- **b.** Greater placental mass relative to singleton gestation
- **c.** Soluble fms-like tyrosine kinase-1 levels are half those seen in singleton gestation
- **d.** All of the above

45–18. A 22-year-old G2P1 presents to you for establishment of prenatal care at 14 weeks. What can you summarize about pregnancy outcome from her ultrasound images shown here?

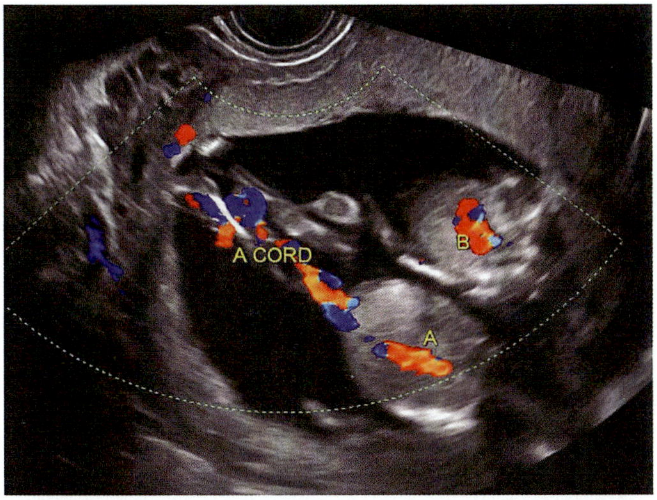

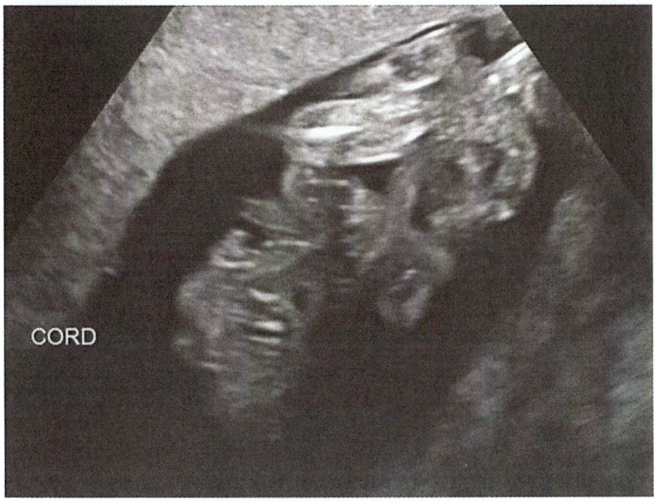

a. Initial rate of fetal demise is low, but the risk increases exponentially in the third trimester.
b. There is a lower rate of twin-twin transfusion syndrome than that seen in monochorionic-diamnionic twins.
c. Fetal and neonatal mortality rate is higher than for dichorionic-diamnionic, but similar to monochorionic-diamnionic twins.
d. None of the above

45–19. The patient in Question 45–18 asks for a "best case scenario" explanation of her care plan. Which of the following is not a reasonable recommendation for the care of a monochorionic-monoamnionic pregnancy?
a. Admission for fetal surveillance around 26–28 weeks' gestation.
b. Daily extended fetal monitoring and continued serial observation of fetal growth.
c. Elective induction of labor at 32–34 weeks' gestation in the absence of a prior indication.
d. Administration of corticosteroid course for fetal lung maturity at 26–28 weeks' gestation.

45–20. Among the complications that may be seen in twin pregnancies, which of the following may be seen in dichorionic twin pregnancies?
a. Fetus-in-fetu
b. Acardiac twin
c. Twin-twin transfusion syndrome
d. Complete mole with coexisting normal twin

45–21. A 29-year-old G2P1 has a twin pregnancy at 11 weeks' gestation consisting of an apparently normal fetus and a coexisting complete mole. Which of the following is not an evidence-based reason to counsel her against expectant management?
a. Increased risk for hemorrhage
b. Increased risk for hyperemesis gravidarum with thyrotoxicosis
c. Increased risk for early-onset preeclampsia with resultant preterm birth
d. Increased risk for persistent trophoblastic disease with pregnancy prolongation

45–22. Which is the most common form of vascular anastomoses seen in monochorionic twin placentas?
a. Deep vein-to-vein
b. Deep artery-to-vein
c. Superficial artery-to-vein
d. Superficial artery-to-artery

45–23. A pair of monochorionic twins present at 20 weeks' gestation with sonographic findings that suggest twin-twin transfusion syndrome. There is significant growth and fluid discordance, no bladder is visualized in the smaller twin, neither twin has abnormal umbilical artery Doppler studies, and neither twin has ascites or hydrops. How would you assign Quintero stage based on this information?
a. Stage I
b. Stage II
c. Stage III
d. Stage IV

45–24. What percentage of Quintero stage I twin-twin transfusion syndrome cases will remain stable without intervention?

a. 35%

b. 50%

c. 75%

d. 90%

45–25. Which of the following are not beneficial interventions for complicated monochorionic twin pregnancies?

a. Immediate delivery of surviving twin to prevent neurological damage after finding of cotwin demise.

b. Intentional septostomy to equalize fluid and pressure for Quintero stage II twin-twin transfusion syndrome.

c. Selective feticide via intracardiac injection of potassium chloride when lethal anomaly is found in one twin.

d. All of the above

45–26. Evaluation for twin anemia-polycythemia sequence (TAPS) is performed via the Doppler study shown here. Which of the following statements best characterize this condition?

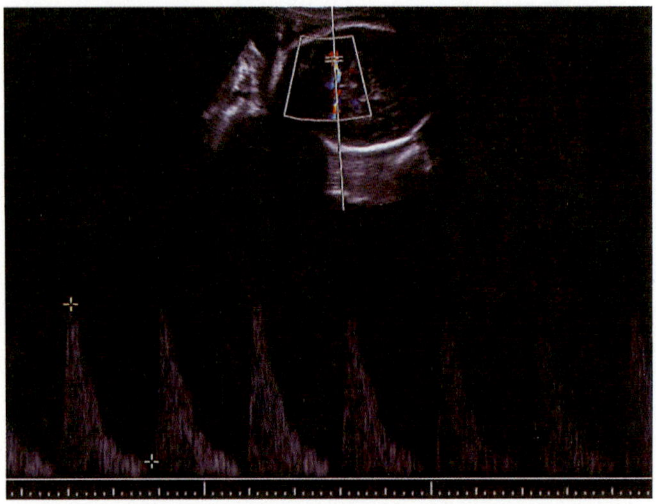

a. Can occur spontaneously or after laser photocoagulation of the placenta

b. Middle cerebral artery Doppler peak systolic velocity is <1.5 multiples of the median in the donor

c. Middle cerebral artery Doppler peak systolic velocity is >1.5 multiples of the median in the recipient

d. All of the above

45–27. A patient is referred for suspected twin gestation with early cotwin demise due to absent cardiac motion and lag in crown-rump length. Although you confirm no cardiac motion, you do observe retrograde color Doppler flow in the umbilical artery of the *acardius acephalus*. Images of your ultrasound findings are shown here. How do you counsel this patient?

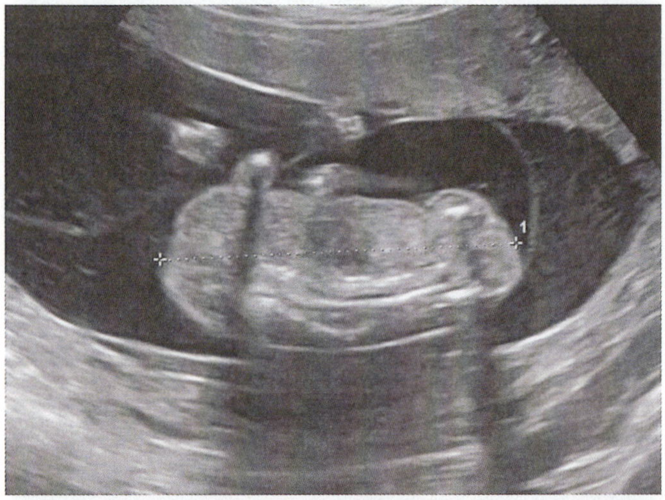

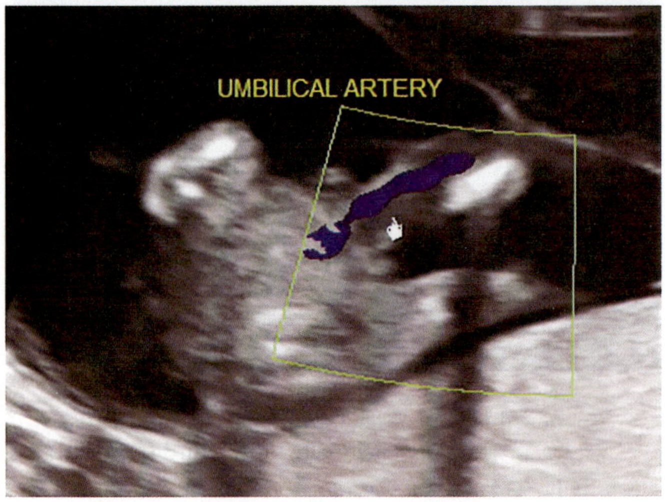

a. The recipient twin is at risk for high-output heart failure.

b. Expectant management of this condition with close surveillance may be an option.

c. If the recipient twin volume exceeds 35% of the donor twin, intervention with radiofrequency ablation will be recommended.

d. All of the above

45–28. What is the calculated fetal growth discordance of a twin pair where the estimated fetal weight of twin A is 800 g and that of twin B is 600 g?

a. 20%

b. 25%

c. 33%

d. 75%

45–29. At their next ultrasound, the twin pair described in Question 45–28 shows 27% discordance (twin A > twin B). One fetus is male and one is female. Which mechanism is not the likely cause of their discordance?

a. Unequal placental sharing

b. Histological placental abnormality

c. Different inherent growth potential

d. Suboptimal implantation site for the placenta of twin B

45–30. Which of the following methods of antepartum fetal surveillance is the most evidence-based strategy to improve outcome in a twin pregnancy?

a. Nonstress test

b. Biophysical profile

c. Doppler velocimetry of the umbilical artery

d. Sonographic evaluation of monochorionic twins at least every 2 weeks

45–31. Which of the following is the most important predictor of neurological outcome of the survivor after death of a cotwin?

a. Chorionicity

b. Gestational age at the time of demise

c. Whether malformations are present in the deceased twin

d. Length of time between demise of the cotwin and delivery of the survivor

45–32. Which of the following modalities provide reassurance of a lower risk for preterm birth in a twin gestation?

a. Closed cervix on digital examination

b. Cervical length over 20 mm, measured at 22–24 weeks by transvaginal ultrasound

c. Cervical length over 20 mm, measured serially in the second trimester by transvaginal ultrasound

d. All of the above

45–33. Which of the following interventions has been shown to decrease preterm birth in twin pregnancies?

a. Tocolysis of preterm labor

b. Prophylactic cerclage placement in the early second trimester

c. Weekly intramuscular injection of 17 alpha-hydroxyprogesterone caproate when initiated prior to 18 weeks

d. None of the above

45–34. Many aspects of the care of a twin pregnancy differ from that of a singleton. Which of the following is different for a twin gestation?

a. Guidelines for administration of corticosteroids for fetal lung maturity

b. Administration of antibiotics for latency after preterm premature rupture of membranes

c. Gestational age at which delivery is recommended for a pregnancy that has been uncomplicated

d. None of the above

45–35. Planned cesarean delivery has not been shown to improve neonatal outcome and is not advocated above vaginal delivery for which of the following clinical scenarios?

a. Vertex-vertex diamnionic twin gestation

b. Breech-vertex diamnionic twin gestation

c. Vertex-vertex monoamnionic twin gestation

d. Vertex-vertex-transverse triamnionic triplet gestation

45–36. A 34-year-old G1 presents with spontaneous conception of a trichorionic-triamnionic triplet gestation. Which of the following is not an appropriate aspect of her early pregnancy counseling?

a. Selective fetal reduction can be performed with ultrasound-guided intracardiac injection of potassium chloride.

b. She is counseled that elective fetal reduction from triplet to twin gestation carries a 4.5% risk for loss of the entire pregnancy.

c. She is counseled that elective reduction should be performed because it will result in a lower rate of maternal complications, preterm birth, and neonatal death.

d. All of the above are appropriate aspects of your counseling.

CHAPTER 45 ANSWER KEY

Question number	Letter answer	Page cited	Header cited
45–1	**d**	p. 864	Introduction
45–2	**b**	p. 864	Dizygotic vs Monozygotic Twinning
45–3	**a**	p. 864	Genesis of Monozygotic Twins
45–4	**c**	p. 864	Superfetation and Superfecundation
45–5	**d**	p. 865	Figure 45-1
45–6	**d**	p. 865	Factors Affecting Twinning
45–7	**d**	p. 866	Demographics
45–8	**a**	p. 864 p. 867	Genesis of Monochorionic Twins Determining Zygosity
45–9	**b**	p. 867	Sonographic Determination
45–10	**d**	p. 867	Sonographic Determination
45–11	**d**	p. 869	Placental Examination
45–12	**c**	p. 870	Maternal Physiological Adaptations
45–13	**b**	p. 871	Spontaneous Abortion
45–14	**b**	p. 871	Spontaneous Abortion
45–15	**d**	p. 871	Congenital Malformations
45–16	**c**	p. 872	Low Birthweight; Figure 45-8
45–17	**b**	p. 872	Hypertension
45–18	**b**	p. 873	Monoamnionic Twins
45–19	**c**	p. 873	Monoamnionic Twins
45–20	**d**	p. 875 p. 881	Unique and Aberrant Twinning Hydatidiform Mole with Coexisting Normal Fetus
45–21	**d**	p. 881	Hydatidiform Mole with Coexisting Normal Fetus
45–22	**d**	p. 876	Monochorionic Twins and Vascular Anastomoses
45–23	**b**	p. 879	Diagnosis; Twin-Twin Transfusion Syndrome
45–24	**c**	p. 879	Management and Prognosis; Twin-Twin Transfusion Syndrome
45–25	**d**	p. 878 p. 879	Fetal Brain Damage Management and Prognosis
45–26	**a**	p. 880	Twin Anemia-Polycythemia Sequence
45–27	**b**	p. 880	Twin Reversed Arterial Perfusion Sequence
45–28	**b**	p. 882	Diagnosis; Discordant Growth of Twin Fetuses
45–29	**a**	p. 881	Etiopathogenesis
45–30	**d**	p. 882	Fetal Surveillance
45–31	**a**	p. 882	Death of One Fetus
45–32	**d**	p. 885	Prediction of Preterm Birth
45–33	**d**	p. 885 p. 886	Prevention of Preterm Birth Treatment of Preterm Labor
45–34	**c**	p. 886 p. 887	Treatment of Preterm Labor Timing of Delivery
45–35	**b**	p. 888	Delivery Route
45–36	**c**	p. 891	Selective Reduction or Termination

SECTION 12

MEDICAL AND SURGICAL COMPLICATIONS

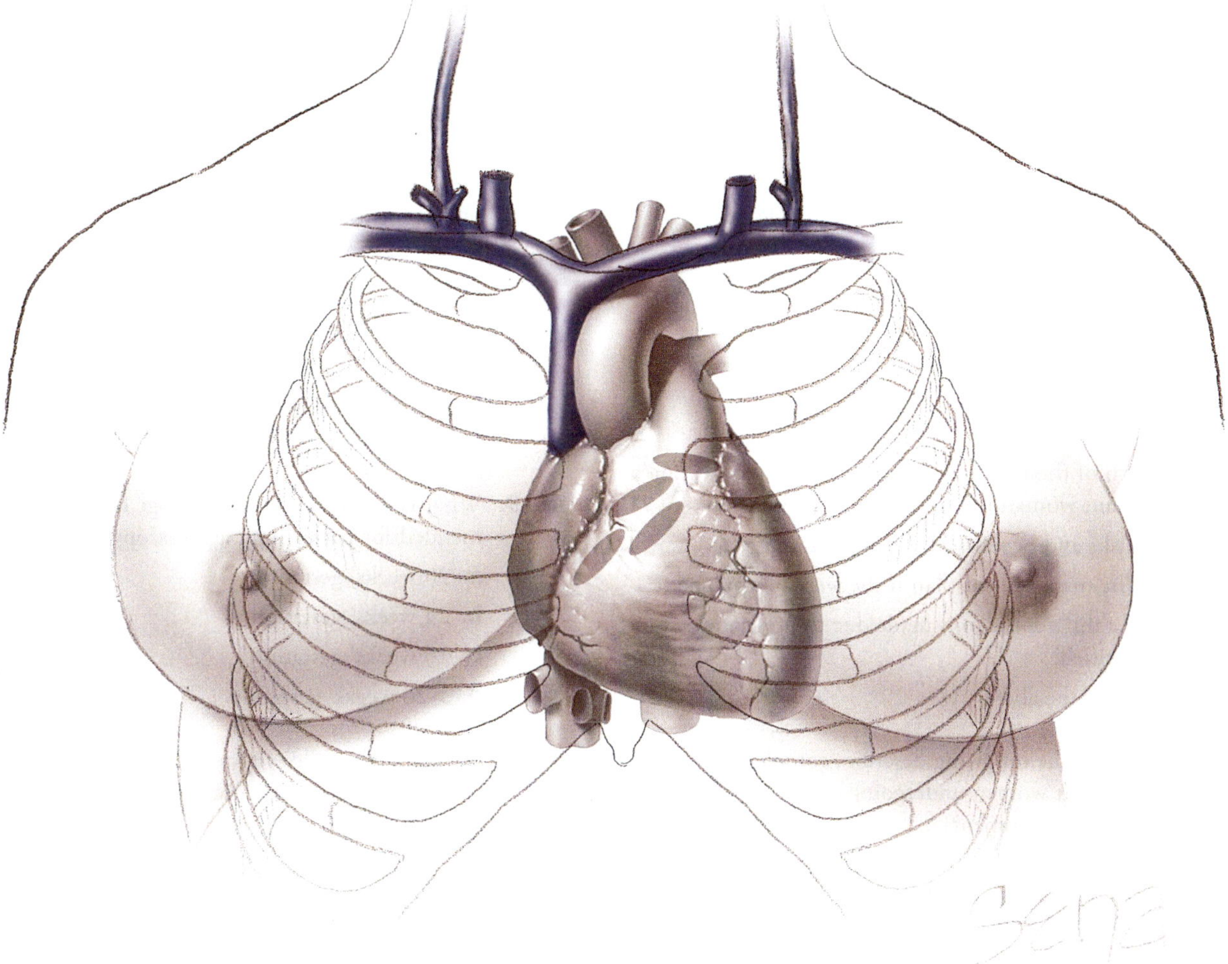

CHAPTER 46

General Considerations and Maternal Evaluation

46–1. What was the antenatal hospitalization rate in one managed-care population?

a. 5/100 deliveries
b. 10/100 deliveries
c. 20/100 deliveries
d. 35/100 deliveries

46–2. What percentage of antepartum hospitalizations are due to nonobstetrical conditions?

a. 15%
b. 20%
c. 33%
d. 50%

46–3. What percentage of pregnant women will undergo surgery?

a. 0.15%
b. 0.5%
c. 1%
d. 1.5%

46–4. Which of these should be considered when treating a pregnant woman for a nonobstetric condition?

a. Risks and benefits to the mother and fetus
b. The management plan if she were not pregnant
c. If a different plan is made due to pregnancy, is it justified?
d. All of the above

46–5. Which of the following describes complication rates in pregnant women undergoing surgery compared to nonpregnant women?

a. Increased
b. Decreased
c. Equivalent
d. Increased, but only in the first trimester

46–6. Nonobstetrical surgery performed beyond what gestational age results in higher rates of preterm birth?

a. 20 weeks' gestation
b. 23 weeks' gestation
c. 24 weeks' gestation
d. 26 weeks' gestation

46–7. Which of the following is the most common second-trimester procedure performed?

a. Appendectomy
b. Cholecystectomy
c. Ovarian cystectomy
d. All are performed at equal rates

46–8. All except which of the following morbidities are increased in women who undergo surgery during pregnancy?

a. Stillbirth
b. Preterm birth
c. Neonatal death by 7 days
d. Birthweight <1500 grams

46–9. What is the upper gestational-age limit recommended for performing laparoscopy in pregnancy?

a. 20 weeks' gestation
b. 24 weeks' gestation
c. 26 weeks' gestation
d. >26 weeks' gestation

46–10. Which of the following techniques is recommended when performing laparoscopy in pregnancy?

a. Open technique entry
b. Lateral recumbent position
c. Intraoperative capnography
d. All of the above

46–11. What should the maximum insufflation pressure be to prevent severe cardiorespiratory changes?

a. 10 mm Hg
b. 15 mm Hg
c. 20 mm Hg
d. 22 mm Hg

46–12. Which of the following hemodynamic changes as a result of insufflation of the peritoneal cavity is accurate?

a. Decreased pH
b. Decreased cardiac output
c. Increased cerebral blood flow
d. All of the above

46–13. Which of the following is accurate concerning laparoscopy in obese women compared to normal-weight women?

a. Better pain control
b. Increased risk for hemorrhage
c. Decreased risk for port-site hernias
d. Increased risk for conversion to laparotomy

46–14. Why does uteroplacental blood flow decrease when intraperitoneal insufflation pressures exceed 15 mm Hg?

a. Induces uterine contractions
b. Places pressure on the uterine wall
c. Increases placental vessel resistance
d. Leads to constriction of the umbilical arteries

46–15. Women undergoing laparoscopic procedures are at increased risk for which of the following perinatal outcomes compared to women undergoing laparotomy?

a. Preterm delivery
b. Low birthweight
c. Fetal-growth restriction
d. None of the above

46–16. Which of the following should be considered preoperatively in a pregnant patient?

a. Nasogastric decompression to reduce aspiration
b. Right lateral tilt to avoid aortocaval compression
c. Candy cane stirrups to allow access to the vagina
d. Clear liquid diet up to 2 hours prior to avoid vasovagal symptoms

46–17. All except which of the following techniques helps prevent uterine injury during laparoscopy?

a. Open entry
b. Slow insufflation
c. Left upper quadrant port
d. Use of only one secondary trocar

46–18. Which of the following forms of radiation have short wavelengths with high energy?

a. X-rays
b. Ultrasound
c. Microwaves
d. Radio waves

46–19. Which of the following regarding ionizing radiation is true?

a. It can create free radicals.
b. It can change the structure of DNA.
c. It can create ions capable of secondarily damaging tissue.
d. All of the above

46–20. Which of the following terms is used to measure the amount of energy in tissues?

a. Dose
b. Exposure
c. Quantity
d. Relative effective dose

46–21. All except which of the following is a potential harmful effect of radiation exposure?

a. Cancer
b. Abortion
c. Microcephaly
d. Growth restriction

46–22. What is the *no observed adverse effect level* in pregnancy?

a. 0.05 rad
b. 2 rad
c. 5 rad
d. 20 rad

46–23. During what period is the risk for mental retardation the greatest?

a. First 10 days
b. 6–8 weeks' gestation
c. 6–10 weeks' gestation
d. 8–15 weeks' gestation

46–24. What happens to the estimated risk for childhood cancer after exposure to 3 rad?

a. Doubles
b. Triples
c. Quadruples
d. Increases by 10×

46–25. Which radiograph results in the lowest dose exposure for the fetus?

a. Hip
b. Mammogram
c. Lumbosacral spine
d. Intravenous pyelogram

46–26. Which of the following affects the amount of fetal exposure during fluoroscopy?

a. Total fluoroscopy time
b. Number of radiographs
c. Fluoroscopy time with fetus in the radiation field
d. All of the above

46–27. What is the fetal exposure of the imaging study seen below?

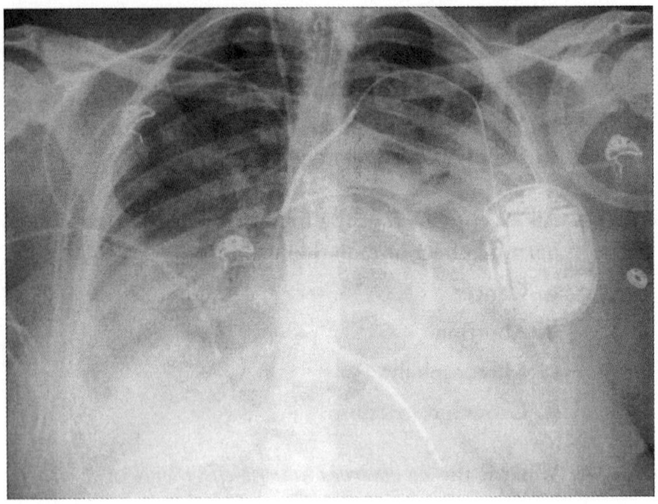

a. 5 mrad
b. 50 mrad
c. 70 mrad
d. 100 mrad

46–28. Computed tomography of which organ system is most common in pregnancy?

a. Head
b. Chest
c. Pelvis
d. Abdomen

46–29. A 26-year-old woman at 29 weeks' gestation is an unrestrained passenger in a motor vehicle accident. She is confused and complaining of a headache. Computer tomographic scanning of her head is ordered to exclude acute bleeding. What should her family be told about the risk to her fetus from the imaging study?

a. The risk is negligible
b. Computed tomography does not involve ionizing radiation, thus there is no risk.
c. There is a small risk for ionizing radiation causing childhood cancer with this study, but it is balanced by the necessity of the test.
d. None of the above

46–30. At 14 weeks' gestation, a patient presents with chest pain and shortness of breath. Using standard protocols for pulmonary embolus evaluation, which of the following statements is the most accurate regarding dosimetry exposure when comparing ventilation-perfusion scans and computed tomography scans?

a. Exposure is equivalent for the two types of scans.
b. Exposure is greater with computed tomography scans.
c. Exposure is greater with ventilation-perfusion scans.
d. None of the above

46–31. An obstetrician discovers a breast mass in a woman who is having her first prenatal visit at 10 weeks' gestation. The biopsy is positive for cancer, and the breast surgeon would like to perform a sentinel lymphoscintigram during the surgical procedure. Which of the following is an accurate statement?

a. Pregnancy does not alter the use of ^{99m}Tc-sulfur colloid.
b. ^{99m}Tc-sulfur should not be used at all during pregnancy.
c. Surgery and the sentinel lymphoscintigram should be delayed until after 15 weeks' gestation.
d. Because of fetal concerns, use of the sentinel lymphoscintigram with ^{99m}Tc-sulfur should be based on the individual's risk for tumor spread.

46–32. What are the preferred imaging modalities in pregnancy?

a. Ultrasound and x-ray
b. X-ray and magnetic resonance
c. Sonography and magnetic resonance
d. Sonography and computed tomography

CHAPTER 46 ANSWER KEY

Question number	Letter answer	Page cited	Header cited
46–1	b	p. 901	Introduction
46–2	c	p. 901	Introduction
46–3	a	p. 901	Introduction
46–4	d	p. 901	Introduction
46–5	c	p. 902	Pregnancy Outcomes
46–6	b	p. 902	Pregnancy Outcomes
46–7	a	p. 902	Pregnancy Outcomes
46–8	a	p. 902	Perinatal Morbidity
46–9	d	p. 902	Laparoscopic Surgery
46–10	d	p. 903	Table 46-2
46–11	b	p. 903	Hemodynamic Effects
46–12	d	p. 903	Table 46-3
46–13	d	p. 904	Obesity
46–14	c	p. 904	Perinatal Outcomes
46–15	d	p. 904	Perinatal Outcomes
46–16	a	p. 904	Technique
46–17	d	p. 904	Technique
46–18	a	p. 905	Ionizing Radiation
46–19	d	p. 905	Ionizing Radiation
46–20	a	p. 906	Ionizing Radiation
46–21	a	p. 906	Deterministic Effects
46–22	c	p. 906	Deterministic Effects
46–23	d	p. 906	Deterministic Effects
46–24	a	p. 906	Stochastic Effects
46–25	b	p. 906	Table 46-5
46–26	d	p. 907	Diagnostic Radiation
46–27	c	p. 907	Diagnostic Radiation
46–28	a	p. 908	Diagnostic Radiation
46–29	a	p. 908	Diagnostic Radiation
46–30	a	p. 908	Diagnostic Radiation
46–31	a	p. 910	Diagnostic Radiation
46–32	c	p. 912	Table 46-9

CHAPTER 47

Critical Care and Trauma

47–1. Which is not an indication for transfer of a pregnant patient to an intensive care unit?

a. Need for invasive monitoring
b. Impending respiratory failure
c. Thyrotoxicosis with normotensive tachycardia
d. Refractory hypotension despite adequate resuscitation

47–2. According to the American College of Obstetricians and Gynecologists, which is universally required during the transport of a pregnant patient?

a. Telemetry
b. Central venous access
c. Continuous pulse oximetry
d. Continuous fetal heart rate monitoring

47–3. What is the most common indication for admission to an obstetrical intermediate care unit?

a. Sepsis
b. Hemorrhage
c. Hypertension
d. Cardiopulmonary disease

47–4. Why does ventricle performance, measured with the use of pulmonary artery catheters, remain within normal range in term pregnant women?

a. Increased pulse rate
b. Decreased vascular resistance
c. Increased blood volume and cardiac output
d. All of the above

47–5. Which of the following changes would cause an increase in stroke volume?

a. Increase in heart rate
b. Increase in cardiac output
c. Increase in systemic vascular resistance
d. Decrease in pulmonary vascular resistance

47–6. What is the most common cause of pulmonary edema in a pregnant patient?

a. Sepsis
b. Cardiac failure
d. Hypertensive disorders
c. Iatrogenic fluid overload

47–7. A 32-year-old primigravida at 36 weeks' gestation is undergoing induction of labor for severe preeclampsia. She experiences tachysystole with recurrent fetal heart rate decelerations and is given terbutaline. The fetal heart rate decelerations improve, but the patient develops shortness of breath with an oxygenation saturation of 94% and crackles on lung exam. The chest radiograph is shown below. What is the best first step in treatment?

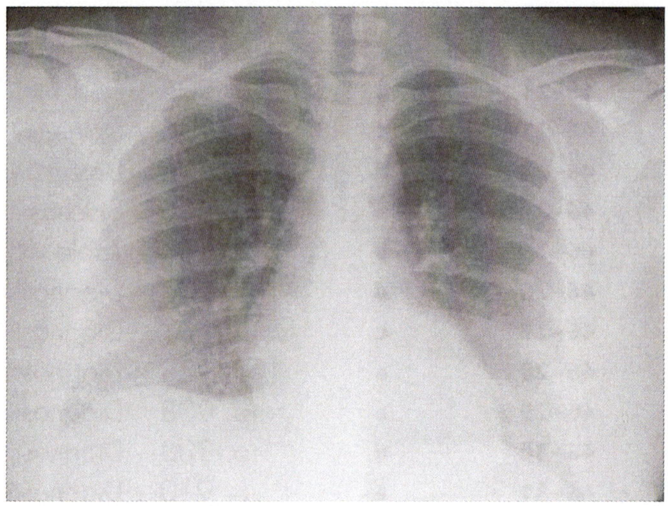

a. Anticoagulation
b. Intubation to protect the airway
c. Administer intravenous furosemide
d. Initiation of broad-spectrum antibiotics

47–8. When diagnosing acute respiratory distress syndrome, which criteria is necessary?

a. PaO_2:FiO_2 <300
b. Evidence of heart failure
c. Chest radiograph with pulmonary infiltrates
d. All these criteria are necessary

47–9. When managing pregnant women with severe acute lung injury, which intervention is most effective for improving oxygen delivery?

a. Maximizing FiO_2

b. Antibiotic therapy

c. Delivery of the fetus

d. Transfusion to correct anemia

47–10. In order to maintain placental perfusion during pregnancy a hemoglobin oxygen saturation of at least 90% is preferred. What is the goal PaO_2 in the management of acute respiratory distress syndrome in pregnancy?

a. >40 mm Hg

b. >60 mm Hg

c. >80 mm Hg

d. >100 mm Hg

47–11. Positive end-expiratory pressure is sometimes increased to 5–15 mm Hg to accomplish adequate ventilation in cases of severe lung injury. Which is a possible complication of using high levels of positive end-expiratory pressure in pregnancy?

a. Barotrauma

b. Decreased cardiac output

c. Decreased uteroplacental perfusion

d. All of the above

47–12. During pregnancy the concentration of 2,3-diphosphoglycerate in maternal erythrocytes increases by 30% to improve oxygen delivery to the fetus and maternal tissues. Which direction is the maternal oxygen-dissociation curve shifted in pregnancy, and how does this affect hemoglobin affinity for oxygen?

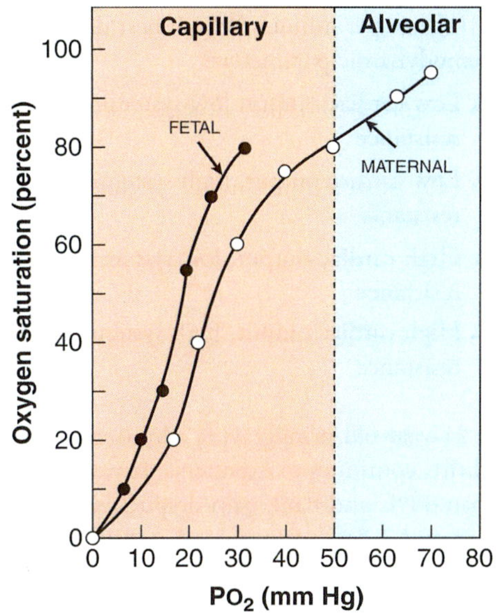

Reproduced with permission from Cunningham FG, Leveno KJ, Bloom SL, et al (eds): Critical care and trauma. In Williams Obstetrics, 25th ed. New York, McGraw-Hill, 2018, Figure 47-2.

a. To the left, increased affinity

b. To the left, decreased affinity

c. To the right, increased affinity

d. To the right, decreased affinity

47–13. At what wedge pressure gradient would a pregnant woman begin to experience pulmonary edema?

a. <4 mm Hg

b. >4 mm Hg

c. <10 mm Hg

d. >10 mm Hg

47–14. A 21-year-old primigravida presents at 18 weeks' gestation with fever, flank pain, and dysuria for 2 days. On arrival she has costovertebral angle tenderness, a temperature of 39.0°C, a heart rate of 120 beats per minute, and a blood pressure of 84/48 mm Hg. After administration of 2 liters of crystalloid and intravenous antibiotics, her blood pressure is 90/50 mm Hg and her heart rate is 110 beats per minute. Which best describes her hemodynamic parameters?

- **a.** Low cardiac output, low systemic vascular resistance
- **b.** Low cardiac output, high systemic vascular resistance
- **c.** High cardiac output, low systemic vascular resistance
- **d.** High cardiac output, high systemic vascular resistance

47–15. A 21-year-old primigravida admitted for pyelonephritis continues to experience temperatures greater than 38°C and flank pain despite adequate hydration and 3 days of parenteral ampicillin and gentamicin. Her urine culture demonstrated *Escherichia coli* resistant to ampicillin but sensitive to gentamicin. What is the next best step in management?

- **a.** Renal sonogram
- **b.** Urology consult
- **c.** Broaden antibiotic coverage
- **d.** Continue current management plan

47–16. A 30-year-old primigravida presents at term with rupture of membranes. She undergoes induction of labor, receives epidural anesthesia, and has an uncomplicated vaginal delivery. In the first hour after delivery she experiences the onset of rigors with a temperature of 40.1°C and heart rate of 140 beats per minute. Which of the below medication regimens is most appropriate?

- **a.** Ampicillin and gentamicin
- **b.** Ampicillin, gentamicin, and clindamycin
- **c.** Vancomycin and piperacillin/tazobactam
- **d.** Tylenol and repeat temperature in 15 minutes

47–17. Which obstetrical complication has been associated with domestic violence?

- **a.** Uterine rupture
- **b.** Preterm delivery
- **c.** Placental abruption
- **d.** All of the above

47–18. A 22-year-old woman at 20 weeks' gestation presents to the emergency department complaining of sexual assault 4 days ago by a male relative. Which medication is recommended for prophylaxis?

- **a.** Antiretroviral therapy
- **b.** Hepatitis B immunoglobulin
- **c.** Ceftriaxone, azithromycin, and metronidazole
- **d.** All of the above

47–19. Which type of traumatic injury is less common in pregnancy?

- **a.** Bowel injury
- **b.** Orthopedic injury
- **c.** Retroperitoneal hemorrhage
- **d.** None of the above

47–20. Which finding is more common in the setting of traumatic abruption as compared to nontraumatic abruption?

- **a.** Vaginal bleeding
- **b.** Uterine tenderness
- **c.** Fetal heart rate abnormalities
- **d.** Clinically significant fetomaternal hemorrhage

47–21. A 34 year-old-woman at 32 weeks' gestation was a restrained passenger in a moderate-speed motor vehicle collision 2 hours ago. She sustained minor injuries and is without abdominal pain or vaginal bleeding. She reports good fetal movement, external fetal monitoring is category I, and she is experiencing contractions every 5–6 minutes. Which is the best course of action?

- **a.** Discharge home
- **b.** Administer tocolytics
- **c.** Immediate cesarean delivery
- **d.** Expectant management and external fetal monitoring

47–22. One of the first steps to ensure adequate cardiopulmonary resuscitation in the third trimester is uterine displacement as shown below. In addition, which of the following special considerations is most appropriate when beginning cardiopulmonary resuscitation of a woman in the third trimester of pregnancy?

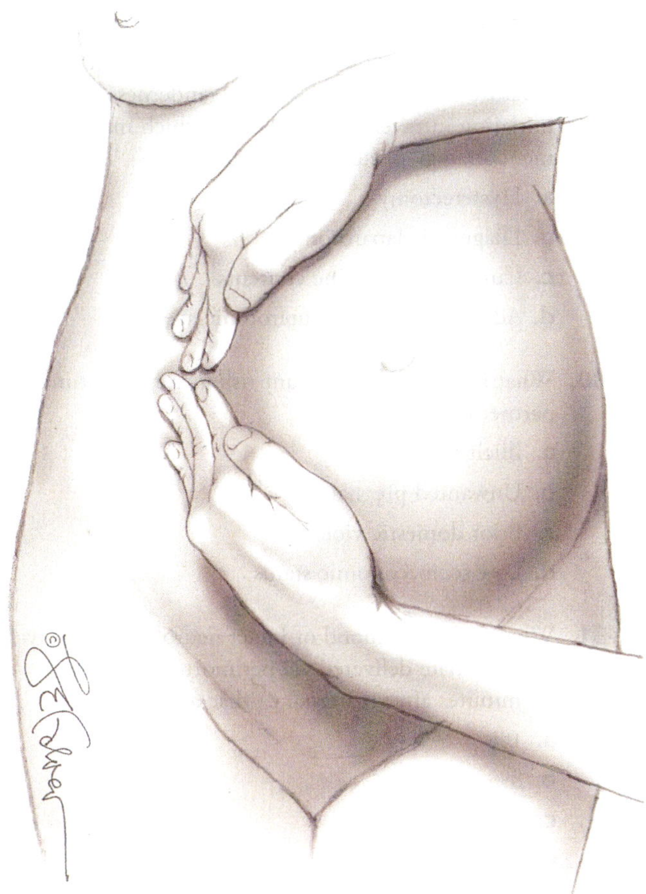

Reproduced with permission from Yeomans ER, Hoffman BL, Gilstrap LC, et al (eds): Critical illness in pregnancy. In Operative Obstetrics, 3rd ed. New York, McGraw-Hill, 2017, Figure 7-4.

a. Administration of 100% oxygen
b. Establish venous access via femoral line
c. Immediate initiation of cesarean delivery
d. All of the above

47–23. Which of the following statements is true of obstetrical patients who require intensive care?

a. The highest use is prior to delivery.
b. The associated mortality rate can reach 10%.
c. Pulmonary embolism is the most common indication.
d. All of the above

47–24. Which of the following statements is true regarding pulmonary artery catheter monitoring in the acutely ill gravida?

a. It has been shown to improve survival.
b. Its use in critically ill patients is of limited value.
c. It is essential for the care of patients with pulmonary edema.
d. It aids in the management of patients with low injury-severity scores.

47–25. Which infectious process is least likely to be the cause of acute respiratory distress syndrome in pregnancy?

a. Pneumonia
b. Appendicitis
c. Pyelonephritis
d. Chorioamnionitis

47–26. A woman experienced an uncomplicated vaginal delivery at term, followed by overwhelming sepsis requiring a total abdominal hysterectomy and bilateral salpingo-oophorectomy. Which of the following pathogens is known for its exotoxin that can cause rapid and extensive tissue necrosis and gangrene?

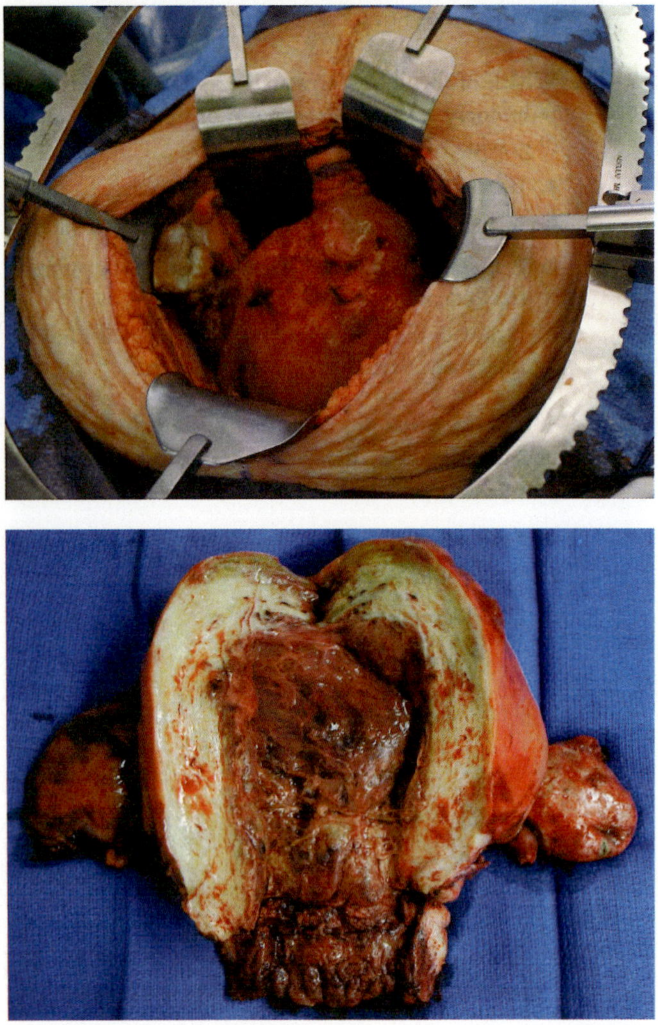

Used with permission from Dr. Sarah Happe.

- **a.** *Escherichia coli*
- **b.** *Bacteroides fragilis*
- **c.** *Klebsiella pneumoniae*
- **d.** Group A beta-hemolytic streptococcus

47–27. Which of the following clinical signs define progression from the warm phase to the cold phase of septic shock?

- **a.** Oliguria
- **b.** Tachypnea
- **c.** Leukocytosis
- **d.** Pulmonary hypertension

47–28. Which intervention is least likely to be beneficial in the treatment of early sepsis?

- **a.** Correction of anemia
- **b.** Colloid administration
- **c.** Crystalloid administration
- **d.** Broad-spectrum antimicrobials

47–29. A 23-year-old primigravida presents with an incomplete abortion at 12 weeks' gestation and a temperature of 38.5°C with uterine tenderness. After initiating intravenous antibiotics, which management strategy is most appropriate?

- **a.** Hysterectomy
- **b.** Diagnostic laparotomy
- **c.** Curettage of uterine contents
- **d.** Administration of a uterotonic agent

47–30. What is the most important risk factor for intimate partner homicide?

- **a.** Illicit drug use
- **b.** Unwanted pregnancy
- **c.** Prior domestic violence
- **d.** Low socioeconomic status

47–31. What is the likelihood of intact neurological survival for a neonate delivered via perimortem cesarean 30 minutes after maternal cardiac arrest?

- **a.** 1%
- **b.** 8%
- **c.** 15%
- **d.** 25%

47–32. A pregnant patient presents after a gunshot wound to the abdomen. She undergoes assessment by the trauma team including a FAST exam with significant hemoperitoneum as demonstrated in the image below. Exploratory laparotomy is deemed necessary. Which of the following would make you more likely to deliver the fetus at the time of surgery?

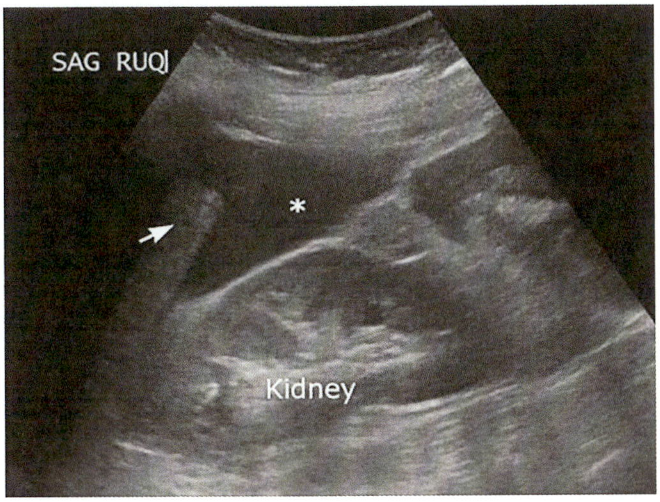

Reproduced with permission from Cunningham FG, Leveno KJ, Bloom SL, et al (eds): Critical care and trauma. In Williams Obstetrics, 25th ed. New York, McGraw-Hill, 2018, Figure 47-11.

a. Gestational age of 34 weeks
b. Reassuring fetal heart rate tracing
c. Uterine contractions every 20 minutes
d. Limited evaluation of the injury due to the gravid uterus

47–33. A woman at 22 weeks' gestation presents via ambulance after a high-speed motor vehicle collision. She has altered mental status and hypotension with concern for both head and intraabdominal injuries. She undergoes computed tomography as shown below. What is the most likely diagnosis?

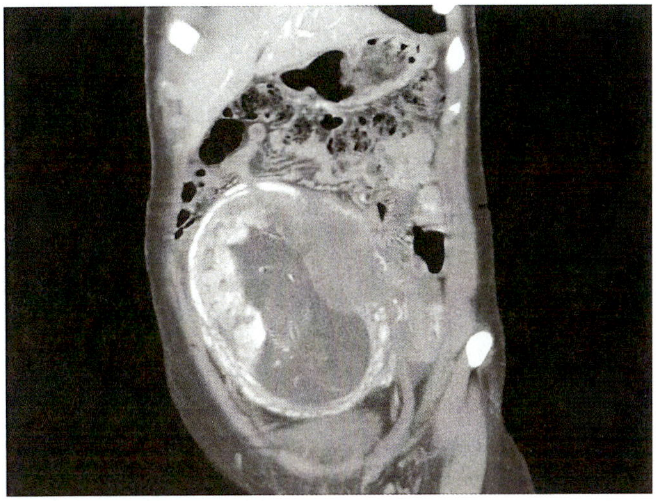

a. Uterine rupture
b. Fetal skull fracture
c. Placental abruption
d. Grade 4 liver laceration

CHAPTER 47 ANSWER KEY

Question number	Letter answer	Page cited	Header cited
47–1	**c**	p. 916	Obstetrical Critical Care
47–2	**c**	p. 916	Obstetrical Critical Care
47–3	**c**	p. 916	Obstetrical Critical Care
47–4	**d**	p. 917	Hemodynamic Changes in Pregnancy
47–5	**b**	p. 917	Hemodynamic Changes in Pregnancy
47–6	**d**	p. 917	Acute Pulmonary Edema
47–7	**c**	p. 918	Acute Pulmonary Edema
47–8	**c**	p. 918	Acute Respiratory Distress Syndrome
47–9	**b**	p. 919	Acute Respiratory Distress Syndrome
47–10	**b**	p. 920	Acute Respiratory Distress Syndrome
47–11	**d**	p. 920	Acute Respiratory Distress Syndrome
47–12	**d**	p. 920	Acute Respiratory Distress Syndrome
47–13	**a**	p. 921	Acute Respiratory Distress Syndrome
47–14	**c**	p. 922	Sepsis Syndrome
47–15	**a**	p. 922	Sepsis Syndrome
47–16	**b**	p. 925	Sepsis Syndrome
47–17	**d**	p. 926	Trauma
47–18	**c**	p. 926	Trauma
47–19	**a**	p. 927	Trauma
47–20	**d**	p. 929	Trauma
47–21	**d**	p. 930	Trauma
47–22	**a**	p. 931	Cardiopulmonary Resuscitation
47–23	**b**	p. 916	Obstetrical Intensive Care
47–24	**b**	p. 917	Obstetrical Critical Care
47–25	**b**	p. 918	Acute Respiratory Distress Syndrome
47–26	**d**	p. 922	Sepsis Syndrome
47–27	**a**	p. 923	Sepsis Syndrome
47–28	**b**	p. 923	Sepsis Syndrome
47–29	**c**	p. 923	Sepsis Syndrome
47–30	**c**	p. 925	Trauma
47–31	**d**	p. 931	Cardiopulmonary Resuscitation
47–32	**d**	p. 929	Trauma
47–33	**c**	p. 929	Trauma

CHAPTER 48

Obesity

48–1. The calculation for body mass index is:

a. pounds/foot^3

b. pounds/inches^2

c. kilograms/meter^2

d. kilograms × meters

48–2. The definition of supermorbid obesity is:

a. Body mass index $\geq$30 kg/m^2

b. Body mass index $\geq$35 kg/m^2

c. Body mass index $\geq$40 kg/m^2

d. Body mass index $\geq$50 kg/m^2

48–3. What percentage of women are obese?

a. 12%

b. 27%

c. 36%

d. 48%

48–4. Which of the following does not cause insulin resistance?

a. IL-6

b. Leptin

c. TNF-α

d. Adiponectin

48–5. A 22-year-old primigravida at 6 weeks' gestation presents for prenatal care. She is 150 pounds and 5 feet 7 inches tall. What is her body mass index classification based on the figure provided below?

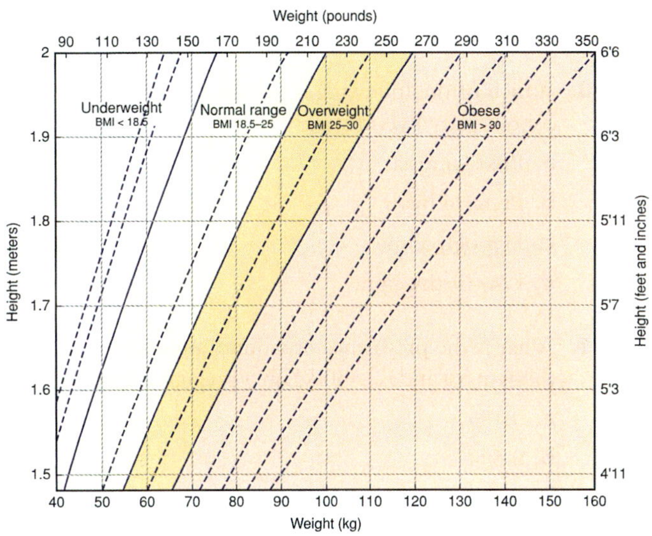

Reproduced with permission from Cunningham FG, Leveno KJ, Bloom SL, et al (eds): Obesity. In Williams Obstetrics, 25th ed. New York, McGraw-Hill, 2018, Figure 48-1.

a. Normal

b. Overweight

c. Class 1 obesity

d. Class 2 obesity

48–6. Which of the following is not a constituent of the metabolic syndrome?

a. Dyslipidemia

b. Hypertension

c. Type 2 diabetes

d. Chronic renal disease

48–7. To diagnose metabolic syndrome, a patient must have at least 3 diagnostic criteria. Which of the following is not one of the criteria?

a. Elevated waist circumference

b. HDL >50 mg/dL in females

c. Fasting glucose $\geq$100 mg/dL

d. Systolic blood pressure $\geq$130 mm Hg

48–8. What percentage of patients with type 2 diabetes who undergo bariatric surgery fail to maintain the weight loss long term?

a. <10%

b. Up to 50%

c. 75%

d. 100%

48–9. Obesity increases the risk for maternal death by how much?

a. 2-fold

b. 4-fold

c. 10-fold

d. It does not increase the risk

48–10. Which of the following is not associated with nonalcoholic fatty liver disease?

a. Preeclampsia

b. Preterm birth

c. Hypoglycemia

d. Low birthweight

48–11. What is the prevalence of wound infection in obese (body mass index >30 kg/m^2) pregnant women?

a. 0.1%

b. 0.5%

c. 1.0%

d. 5.0%

48–12. What is the odds ratio for preeclampsia in obese (body mass index >30 kg/m^2) pregnant women?

a. 1

b. 2

c. 3

d. 5

48–13. What is the highest ranking modifiable risk factor for stillbirth?

a. Obesity

b. Cocaine use

c. Mental illness

d. Vitamin deficiencies

48–14. Which of the following is more common in obese pregnant women?

a. Macrosomia

b. Neural tube defect

c. Congenital heart defect

d. All of the above

48–15. A 25-year-old primigravida at 20 weeks' gestation presents for her anatomy ultrasound. The patient has a body mass index of 45 kg/m^2. Which of the following statements should be part of this patient's counseling?

a. Obesity limits the accuracy of the ultrasound, but obesity does not increase the risk for birth defects.

b. Obesity does not limit the accuracy of the ultrasound nor does it increase the risk for birth defects.

c. Obesity increases the risk for certain birth defects, but ultrasound remains excellent at identifying these problems.

d. Obesity increases the risk for certain birth defects, and obesity limits the accuracy of the ultrasound done to identify those problems.

48–16. A 30-year-old primigravida at 12 weeks' gestation presents for prenatal care. She has a body mass index of 35 kg/m^2. How much weight should she gain this pregnancy?

a. 5–10 pounds

b. 11–20 pounds

c. 15–25 pounds

d. 25–40 pounds

48–17. A 26-year-old primigravida at 10 weeks' gestation presents for prenatal care. She is 5 feet 7 inches tall and 170 pounds. How much weight should she gain this pregnancy?

a. 5–10 pounds

b. 11–20 pounds

c. 15–25 pounds

d. 25–40 pounds

48–18. Why have lifestyle interventions such as exercise in obese pregnant women not been shown to significantly improve neonatal outcomes?

a. Endorphin release with exercise increases insulin resistance

b. Early gene expression within the placenta has already been programmed

c. Patients are not capable of changing as dramatically as needed to make a significant difference

d. Increased physical activity increases hunger disproportionately, which results in increased weight gain

48–19. You are following a 28-year-old G3P2 pregnant woman. She has a body mass index of 55 kg/m^2. You question the accuracy of the fundal heights you are measuring. What is the best management plan to ensure appropriate fetal growth?

- **a.** Serial ultrasounds for rate of growth
- **b.** Do not measure fundal heights and instead perform weekly NSTs
- **c.** Measure the fundal height three times each visit and average the results
- **d.** Follow the change in fundal height each visit instead of the absolute number

48–20. Which of the following statements about labor induction in the obese pregnant woman is true?

- **a.** Degree of obesity does not impact induction success
- **b.** Obese women are twice as likely to have a failed induction
- **c.** Obese women are 10 times more likely to undergo a labor induction
- **d.** Every study has shown improved maternal and neonatal outcomes with elective induction at term

48–21. Which of the following statements about anesthesia in obese women is true?

- **a.** Spinal is better than combined spinal-epidural
- **b.** Combined spinal-epidural is better than spinal
- **c.** General anesthesia is better than regional anesthesia
- **d.** Combined spinal-epidural and spinal anesthesia can be placed with equal expediency and function

48–22. What is the likely reason that obese pregnant women who become hypotensive from anesthesia more frequently have acidotic neonates than normal weight pregnant women?

- **a.** Delayed delivery
- **b.** Increased macrosomia
- **c.** Increased placenta size
- **d.** Reduced maternal tidal volume

48–23. According to the authors, what is the optimal location for placement of the skin incision for cesarean section in a morbidly obese pregnant woman? See the image below.

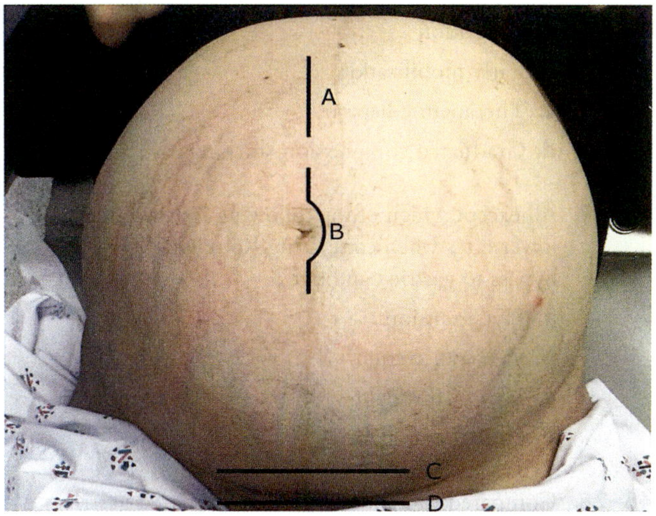

Used with permission from Dr. Tommy Hyslop.

- **a.** A
- **b.** B
- **c.** C, above the pannus
- **d.** D, below the pannus

48–24. What is the increase in risk for wound infection in supermorbidly obese pregnant women compare to nonobese pregnant women?

- **a.** 2-fold
- **b.** 3-fold
- **c.** 4-fold
- **d.** 5-fold

48–25. You are going to perform a cesarean section on a woman with a body mass index of 40 kg/m^2. You want to minimize her risk for wound infection. Which of the following interventions has not been shown to help with this?

- **a.** Exercising good sterile technique
- **b.** Prophylactic negative-pressure wound therapy
- **c.** Increasing perioperative prophylactic antibiotics
- **d.** Closing subcutaneous tissue when it is $\geq$2 cm deep

48–26. You perform a cesarean section on a 23-year-old woman whose body mass index is 45 kg/m^2. You want to avoid thromboembolic complications. You order all except which of the following postoperatively?

- **a.** Hydration
- **b.** Early mobilization
- **c.** Therapeutic heparin
- **d.** Graduated compression stockings

48–27. All except which of the following is associated with lower rates when comparing Roux-en-Y gastric bypass to gastric banding?

- **a.** Hypertension
- **b.** Cesarean section
- **c.** Low birthweight
- **d.** Gestational diabetes

48–28. Compared to maintenance of an inflated gastric band during pregnancy, full deflation of a gastric band results in all except which of the following?

- **a.** Increased macrosomia
- **b.** Increased birthweight
- **c.** Increased mean weight gain
- **d.** Increased fetal cerebral hemorrhage

48–29. What is the most common procedure for gastric restriction and selective malabsorption?

- **a.** REALIZE
- **b.** LAPBAND
- **c.** Gastric sleeve
- **d.** Roux-en-Y gastric bypass

48–30. The surgical procedure depicted in the image below is frequently associated with which of the following symptoms in pregnancy?

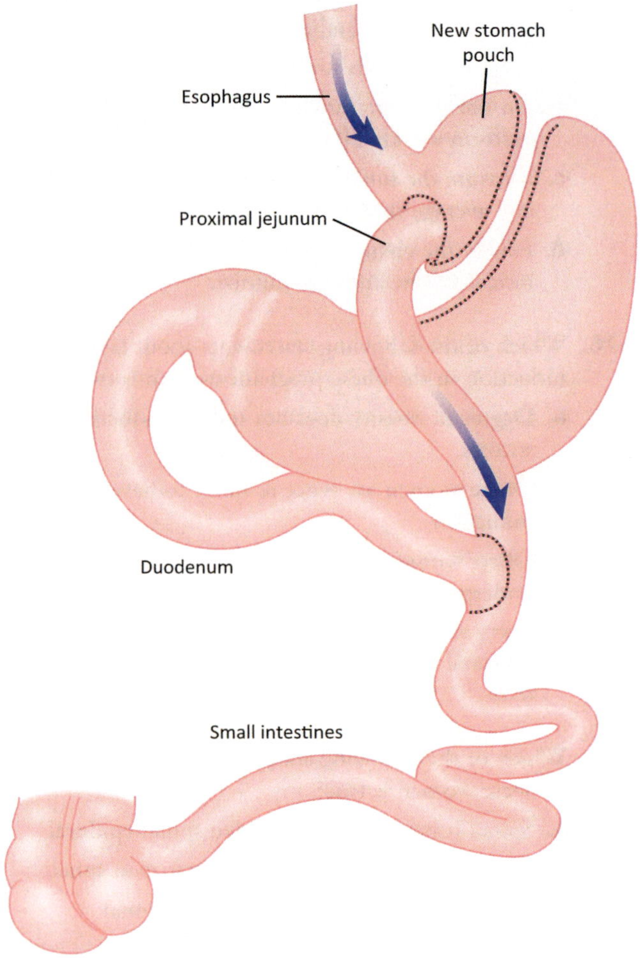

Reproduced with permission from Cunningham FG, Leveno KJ, Bloom SL, et al (eds): Obesity. In Williams Obstetrics, 25th ed. New York, McGraw-Hill, 2018, Figure 48-9.

- **a.** Headache
- **b.** Constipation
- **c.** Lower abdominal pain
- **d.** Upper abdominal pain

48–31. In women hoping to become pregnant after bariatric surgery, counseling should include all except which of the following points?

- **a.** Fertility rates are increased.
- **b.** Obstetric complications are reduced.
- **c.** Large-for-gestational-age neonates are less common.
- **d.** Rates of small-for-gestational-age neonates remain the same.

48–32. Which of the following vitamins is of least concern in pregnant women who have undergone bariatric surgery?

- **a.** Folic acid
- **b.** Vitamin D
- **c.** Vitamin C
- **d.** Vitamin B_{12}

CHAPTER 48 ANSWER KEY

Question number	Letter answer	Page cited	Header cited
48–1	c	p. 936	Definitions and Prevalence
48–2	d	p. 936	Definitions and Prevalence
48–3	c	p. 936	Definitions and Prevalence
48–4	d	p. 936	Adipose Pathophysiology
48–5	a	p. 937	Figure 48-1
48–6	d	p. 937	Metabolic Syndrome
48–7	b	p. 938	Table 48-1
48–8	b	p. 938	Obesity Treatment
48–9	b	p. 939	Maternal Morbidity
48–10	c	p. 939	Maternal Morbidity
48–11	c	p. 939	Table 48-2
48–12	c	p. 939	Table 48-2
48–13	a	p. 940	Perinatal Mortality
48–14	d	p. 941	Perinatal Morbidity
48–15	d	p. 941	Perinatal Morbidity
48–16	b	p. 941	Maternal Weight Gain
48–17	c	p. 941	Maternal Weight Gain
48–18	b	p. 942	Dietary Intervention
48–19	a	p. 942	Prenatal Care
48–20	b	p. 942	Labor Induction
48–21	d	p. 942	Anesthesia Risks
48–22	a	p. 942	Anesthesia Risks
48–23	b	p. 943	Figure 48-8
48–24	b	p. 943	Surgical Concerns
48–25	b	p. 943	Surgical Concerns
48–26	c	p. 943	Surgical Concerns
48–27	c	p. 944	Table 48-3
48–28	d	p. 944	Restrictive Procedures
48–29	d	p. 944	Restrictive Malabsorptive Procedures
48–30	d	p. 944	Restrictive Malabsorptive Procedures
48–31	d	p. 944	Pregnancy
48–32	c	p. 945	Pregnancy

CHAPTER 49

Cardiovascular Disorders

49–1. What percentage of pregnancy-related deaths in the United States were attributable to cardiovascular diseases between 2011 and 2013?

a. 10–15%
b. 15–20%
c. 20–25%
d. 25–30%

49–2. Which of the following does not contribute to the 40% increase in cardiac output seen during normal pregnancy?

a. Increased heart rate
b. Increased left ventricular contractility
c. Decreased systemic vascular resistance
d. All of the above contribute to increased cardiac output in pregnancy

49–3. You are caring for a 24-year-old G1 with severe aortic stenosis. When in pregnancy are you most concerned about cardiac decompensation?

a. Peripartum
b. During the first trimester
c. During the second trimester
d. During the third trimester

49–4. Which of the following best describes the remodeling of the heart that occurs in normal pregnancy?

a. Eccentric left ventricular mass expansion with spherical remodeling
b. Concentric left ventricular mass expansion with spherical remodeling
c. Eccentric left ventricular mass expansion with longitudinal remodeling
d. Concentric left ventricular mass expansion with longitudinal remodeling

49–5. Regarding diagnostic studies, which of the following correctly describes a normal change that is characteristic of pregnancy?

a. Improved systolic function on echocardiographic assessment
b. A decrease in the cardiac silhouette size on chest radiograph
c. An average 15-degree left axis deviation on electrocardiogram
d. All of the above

49–6. A 32-year-old G2P1 presents to your office at 17 weeks' gestation. She reports a history of tetralogy of Fallot, which was repaired in infancy. She appears comfortable on the exam table with a heart rate of 92 beats per minute and a blood pressure of 96/62 mm Hg. However, she does report significant palpitations and dyspnea when climbing the two flights of stairs to her apartment on the third floor. Which New York Heart Association class best describes her functional disability?

a. Class I
b. Class II
c. Class III
d. Class IV

49–7. You are caring for a pregnant patient with mitral stenosis. She is able to perform most activities of daily living without significant limitation. On echocardiogram, her ejection fraction is 50% and her mitral valve area measures 1.8 cm^2. Which of the following variables is most predictive of a high risk for cardiac complications during this pregnancy?

a. Her ejection fraction
b. Her functional capacity
c. Her degree of left-sided obstruction
d. None of the above

49–8. The World Health Organization identifies which of the following conditions as prohibitive of pregnancy?

a. Heart transplantation
b. Cyanotic heart disease
c. Pulmonary artery hypertension
d. Systemic ventricular dysfunction with left ventricular ejection fraction of 35%

49–9. For which of the following cardiac conditions is conduction analgesia highly recommended?

a. Severe aortic stenosis
b. Pulmonary artery hypertension
c. Repaired hypoplastic left heart syndrome
d. All of the above

49–10. You are caring for a 28-year-old G1 with a history of moderate mitral stenosis who presented in active labor and is now 8 cm dilated. She desires a natural labor and declines pain medications during labor. As her contractions get closer together, she reports increasing pain, is visibly uncomfortable, and intermittently becomes tachycardic to 130 beats per minute. She suddenly begins complaining of shortness of breath and her oxygen saturation declines to 90% on room air. What is your best course of action?

a. Administer metoprolol
b. Administer intravenous Lasix
c. Request immediate anesthesia assessment
d. All of the above

49–11. A 30-year-old G2P0A1 presents at 11 weeks' gestation to establish care. She has a history of rheumatic heart disease and had a mechanical valve replacement at age 20. She was previously on warfarin 7.5 mg daily, but stopped taking her medication when she found out she was pregnant 1 week ago. What is her risk for warfarin embryopathy based on her warfarin dosing?

a. 1%
b. 3%
c. 5%
d. 8%

49–12. You obtain a chest radiograph for the patient in Question 49–11 at 14 weeks' gestation because of a persistent cough and shortness of breath. Her chest x-ray is shown. What is her mortality risk in pregnancy based on her history of mechanical valve replacement?

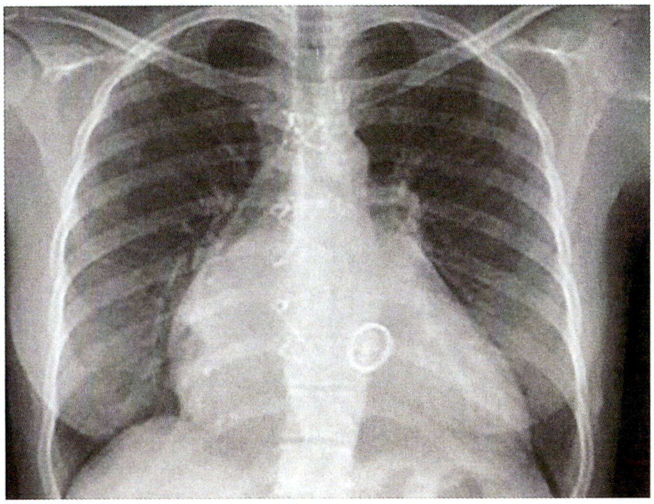

a. 0.1–0.5%
b. 1–2%
c. 3–4%
d. 5–6%

49–13. In a pregnant woman who has previously undergone a heart transplantation, what is the approximate risk for suffering a rejection episode during pregnancy?

a. 10%
b. 20%
c. 30%
d. 40%

49–14. At 32 weeks' gestation, an uncomplicated primigravida you are caring for complains of shortness of breath and chest pain with minimal exertion. You obtain an echocardiogram, which demonstrates a mitral valve surface area of 2.1 cm^2, a dilated left atrium, an aortic valve area of 3.7 cm^2, a right ventricular systolic pressure of 20 mm Hg, and an ejection fraction of 55%. You also obtain a chest x-ray, which is shown. What is the likely underlying cause of her symptoms?

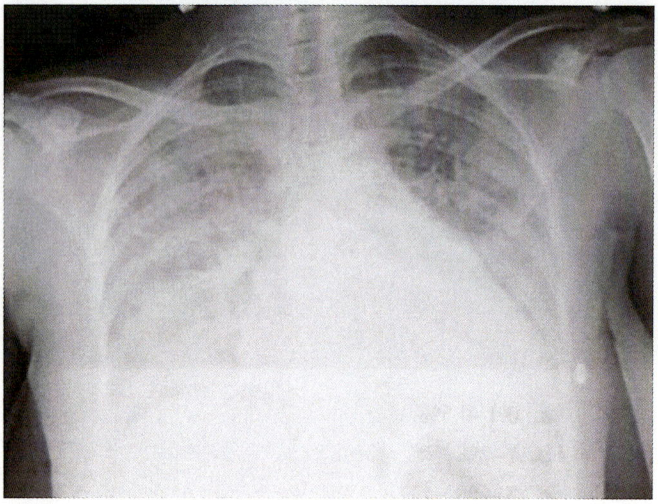

a. Aortic stenosis

b. Mitral stenosis

c. Left ventricular heart failure

d. Pulmonary artery hypertension

49–15. How would you manage the patient in Question 49–14?

a. Administer diuretics

b. Initiate anticoagulation

c. Recommend immediate labor induction

d. All of the above

49–16. A graphic of pulmonary capillary wedge pressure (red line) is shown for a woman with mitral stenosis. "A" represents the first stage of labor, "B" marks the second stage of labor, "C" demonstrates the immediate postpartum period, and "D" shows the period 4–6 hours postdelivery. What accounts for the rise in pulmonary capillary wedge pressure immediately following delivery?

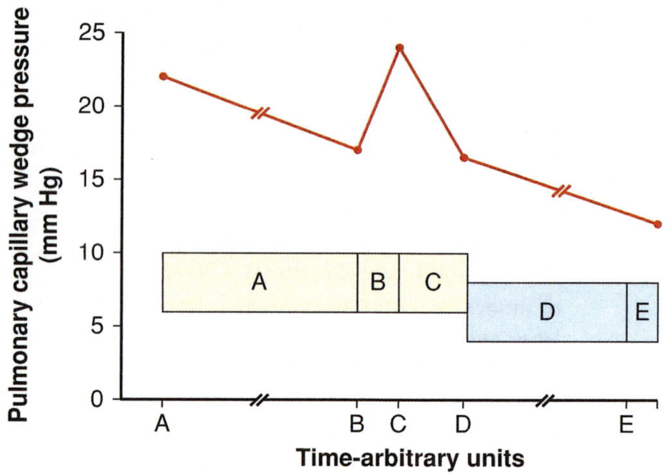

Reproduced with permission from Cunningham FG, Leveno KJ, Bloom SL, et al (eds): Cardiovascular disorders. In Williams Obstetrics, 25th ed. New York, McGraw-Hill, 2018, Figure 49-3.

a. Heart rate normalization

b. Placental autotransfusion

c. Increase in systemic vascular resistance

d. Pitocin-induced increase in cardiac output

49–17. The patient whose heart is shown in this image has systemic lupus erythematosus and has a history of a prior stroke. The left atrium (LA) and left ventricle (LV) are identified, and the arrows point to noninfectious vegetations on the mitral leaflets. Which of the following is the likely condition associated with her mitral insufficiency?

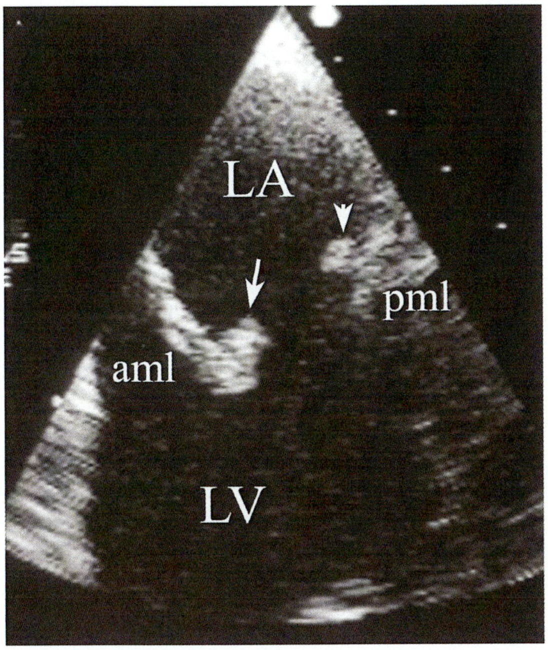

a. Antiphospholipid antibodies
b. Infarction of the papillary muscle
c. Calcification of the mitral annulus
d. None of the above

49–18. Which of the following conditions usually improves during pregnancy due to pregnancy-induced hypervolemia?

a. Aortic stenosis
b. Mitral stenosis
c. Mitral valve prolapse
d. All of the above

49–19. In the United States, what is the most common cause of aortic stenosis?

a. Idiopathic
b. Bicuspid aortic valve
c. Infectious endocarditis
d. Rheumatic heart disease

49–20. A patient with a term gestation and a history of critical aortic stenosis presents in active labor. Which of the following management strategies is advisable while caring for her in her labor course?

a. Assisted second stage delivery
b. Slow-dose epidural anesthesia
c. Generous fluid administration
d. All of the above

49–21. You are caring for a patient with an unrepaired ventricular septal defect who is considering pregnancy. You perform an echocardiogram to assess her future risks. Which of the following parameters would indicate an extremely elevated maternal and fetal risk during pregnancy?

a. A septal defect measuring 0.7 cm^2
b. Presence of left ventricular hypertrophy
c. A left ventricular ejection fraction of 50%
d. A right ventricular systolic pressure of 75 mm Hg

49–22. What associated condition is the patient in Question 49–21 at high risk for developing based on her history?

a. Embolic stroke
b. Bacterial endocarditis
c. Venous thromboembolism
d. None of the above

49–23. A schematic of Eisenmenger syndrome due to a ventricular septal defect is depicted. What is the most common cause of death in pregnant women with this condition?

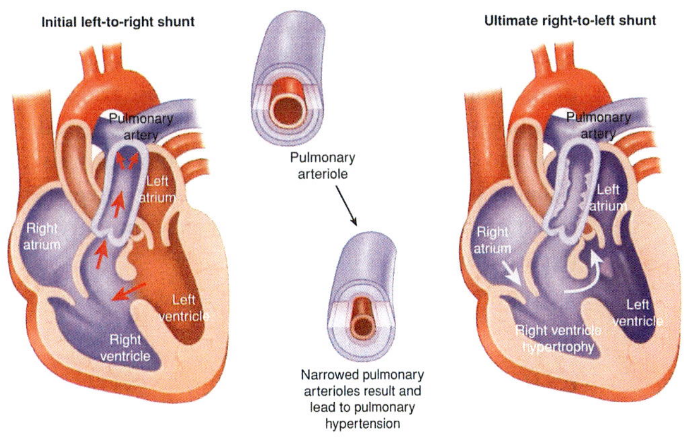

Reproduced with permission from Cunningham FG, Leveno KJ, Bloom SL, et al (eds): Cardiovascular disorders. In Williams Obstetrics, 25th ed. New York, McGraw-Hill, 2018, Figure 49–4.

a. Sepsis
b. Cardiac tamponade
c. Left ventricular failure
d. Right ventricular failure

49–24. In a pregnant population, what is the most common cause of the condition portrayed in the chest x-ray image below?

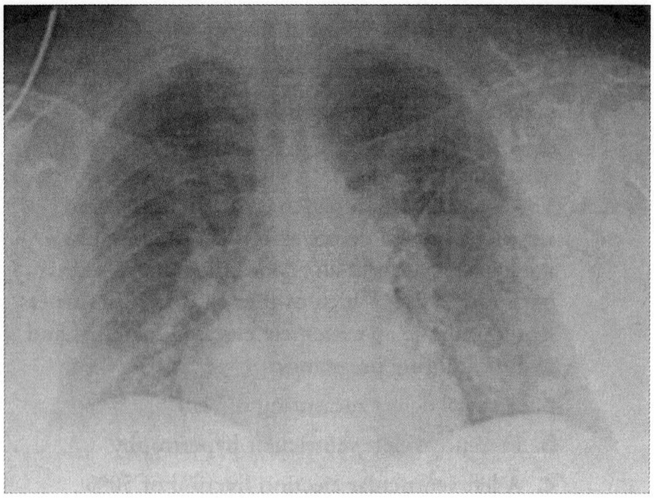

a. Idiopathic
b. Left-sided heart disease
c. Obstructive sleep apnea
d. Connective tissue disease

49–25. What is the gold standard for diagnosis of the condition in Question 49–24?

a. Echocardiography
b. Chest radiography
c. Electrocardiography
d. Right heart catheterization

49–26. A 32-year-old G2P1 transfers to your care at 18 weeks' gestation. She has a history of pulmonary hypertension due to chronic thromboembolic disease. She was told by her previous obstetrician that pregnancy was contraindicated with her condition and is very concerned about her mortality risk. What is her approximate mortality risk in pregnancy based on the underlying cause of her pulmonary hypertension?

a. 1%
b. 5%
c. 10%
d. 20%

49–27. At 24 weeks' gestation the patient in Question 49–26 begins to develop orthopnea and dyspnea on exertion. What treatment would you consider to decrease her symptoms?

a. Diuretics
b. Supplemental oxygen
c. Pulmonary vasodilator drugs
d. All of the above

49–28. You are caring for a primigravida with known hypertrophic cardiomyopathy. She tells you her mother also suffered from the condition and passed away at an early age. The patient is concerned about her child's future risk for developing the same condition. What do you tell her is the most likely risk for passing the condition to her child?

a. <1%
b. 25%
c. 50%
d. 100%

49–29. You are the on-call hospitalist when you receive an urgent call from the postpartum floor about a patient who is complaining of chest pain and shortness of breath. She had an uncomplicated vaginal delivery the previous day and has no significant past medical or surgical history. You obtain a stat chest x-ray, which is shown. Based on the findings, what are you most concerned for?

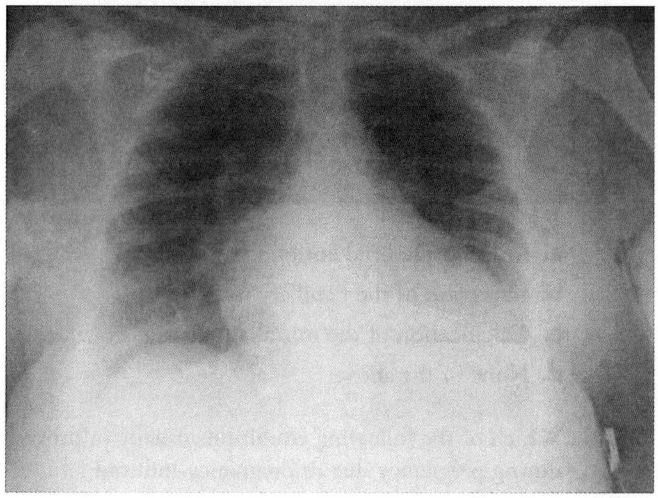

Reproduced with permission from Cunningham FG, Leveno KJ, Bloom SL, et al (eds): Cardiovascular disorders. In Williams Obstetrics, 25th ed. New York, McGraw-Hill, 2018, Figure 49-5.

a. Pneumonia
b. Cardiomyopathy
c. Pulmonary edema
d. Pulmonary hypertension

49–30. You obtain an echocardiogram on the patient in Question 49–29. Her ejection fraction is found to be 20% with no significant structural or valvular disease noted. Which hormone has been implicated in the development of this condition?

a. Estrogen
b. Prolactin
c. Progesterone
d. Human placental lactogen

49–31. Based on her diagnosis and assuming a recovery of systolic function by 6 months postpartum, what is the patient in Question 49–30's risk for suffering a relapse of the same condition in a future pregnancy?

a. 5%

b. 10%

c. 20%

d. 30%

49–32. What is the most common cause of heart failure in pregnancy?

a. Idiopathic

b. Severe preeclampsia

c. Chronic hypertension

d. Chronic hypertension with superimposed preeclampsia

49–33. A pregnant woman presents to the emergency room in an obtunded state. She has a fever to 102.6°F. On exam, a 4/6 murmur is noted, she withdraws from pain during her abdominal exam, and track marks are noted on her arms and legs. Her fundal height is approximately 32 cm. An emergent echocardiogram is obtained, which demonstrates a mitral valve vegetation. What is the most likely organism underlying her diagnosis?

a. *Enterococcus*

b. *Staphylococcus aureus*

c. *Neisseria gonorrhoeae*

d. *Staphylococcus epidermidis*

49–34. Which of the following patients do not have an indication for endocarditis prophylaxis?

a. A patient with a porcine mitral valve

b. A patient with a history of endocarditis

c. A patient with Eisenmenger syndrome due to an atrial septal defect

d. A patient with a ventricular septal defect repaired with a synthetic patch without a current defect

49–35. You are caring for a patient with Marfan syndrome who just found out she is 13 weeks pregnant. You obtain an echocardiogram which demonstrates an aortic root measurement of 4.5 cm. Based on these findings, what would you recommend?

a. Beta blocker initiation

b. Bimonthly echocardiograms

c. Consideration of pregnancy termination

d. All of the above

49–36. Which of the following therapies is safe in pregnancy to treat acute supraventricular tachycardia?

a. Valsalva maneuver

b. Intravenous adenosine

c. Synchronized cardioversion

d. All of the above

CHAPTER 49 ANSWER KEY

Question number	Letter answer	Page cited	Header cited
49–1	**a**	p. 948	Introduction
49–2	**b**	p. 948	Cardiovascular Physiology
49–3	**a**	p. 949	Cardiovascular Physiology
49–4	**a**	p. 949	Ventricular Function in Pregnancy
49–5	**c**	p. 949	Diagnostic Studies
49–6	**b**	p. 951	Classification of Functional Heart Disease
49–7	**c**	p. 951	Classification of Functional Heart Disease
49–8	**c**	p. 952	Table 49-3
49–9	**c**	p. 953	Analgesia and Anesthesia
49–10	**d**	p. 953	Intrapartum Heart Failure
49–11	**d**	p. 954	Anticoagulation
49–12	**b**	p. 954	Valve Replacement before Pregnancy
49–13	**b**	p. 955	Pregnancy after Heart Transplantation
49–14	**b**	p. 955	Mitral Stenosis
49–15	**a**	p. 956	Mitral Stenosis
49–16	**b**	p. 956	Mitral Stenosis
49–17	**a**	p. 957	Mitral Insufficiency
49–18	**d**	p. 957	Mitral Insufficiency
49–19	**b**	p. 957	Aortic Stenosis
49–20	**d**	p. 957	Aortic Stenosis
49–21	**d**	p. 958	Ventricular Septal Defects
49–22	**b**	p. 959	Ventricular Septal Defects
49–23	**d**	p. 960	Eisenmenger Syndrome
49–24	**c**	p. 960	Pulmonary Hypertension
49–25	**d**	p. 961	Pulmonary Hypertension
49–26	**b**	p. 962	Pulmonary Hypertension
49–27	**d**	p. 962	Pulmonary Hypertension
49–28	**c**	p. 962	Hypertrophic Cardiomyopathy
49–29	**b**	p. 963	Peripartum Cardiomyopathy
49–30	**b**	p. 963	Peripartum Cardiomyopathy
49–31	**d**	p. 964	Peripartum Cardiomyopathy
49–32	**d**	p. 964	Heart Failure
49–33	**b**	p. 965	Infective Endocarditis
49–34	**d**	p. 965	Endocarditis Prophylaxis
49–35	**d**	p. 967	Marfan Syndrome
49–36	**d**	p. 966	Supraventricular Tachycardias

CHAPTER 50

Chronic Hypertension

50–1. Which of the following factors does not impact resting blood pressure reading?

a. Race

b. Gender

c. Activity level

d. Age and weight

50–2. The threshold of 140/90 mm Hg as the upper limit of normal is based on which of the following?

a. Actuarial tables based on data from white adult males

b. A large, widely sampled international population of men and women of various ages with no known health complications

c. The discrete point at which risk for myocardial infarction, stroke, renal failure, and peripheral artery disease sharply increases

d. None of the above

50–3. A 37-year-old G2P2 with no medical diagnoses and a normal body mass index saw your partner for an annual well woman exam. Her blood pressure was 142/92 mm Hg, and after checking several times over the next week at home, she calls with a blood pressure log that ranges from 140–154/90–100 mm Hg. Your partner is now out on maternity leave, so prior to calling her back you ask your nurse to confirm that patient's ethnicity. Why is her ethnicity important in your recommendations to initiate an antihypertensive agent?

a. Beta blockers are recommended as initial therapy in the Asian population.

b. Beta blockers are not recommended as initial therapy in the Asian population.

c. Angiotensin-converting enzyme inhibitors and angiotensin-receptor blockers are recommended as initial therapy in the black population.

d. Angiotensin-converting enzyme inhibitors and angiotensin-receptor blockers are not recommended as initial therapy in the black population.

50–4. Regarding the patient in Question 50–3, according to the recommendations of the Eighth Joint National Committee, what is your goal blood pressure with therapy?

a. <120/80 mm Hg

b. <130/85 mm Hg

c. <140/90 mm Hg

d. <150/100 mm Hg

50–5. Ms. Thomas presents for a preconception counseling visit. She is a 37-year-old G0 with a body mass index of 38 kg/m^2, 4-year history of chronic hypertension treated with amlodipine 5 mg per day, and a 2-year history of diabetes which she manages with diet and exercise. Her blood pressure range is 128–144/80–94 mm Hg from the week prior. What workup would you like to pursue referent to her diagnosis of chronic hypertension and prepregnancy risk stratification?

a. Serum creatinine and urine protein-to-creatinine ratio

b. Serum creatinine, urine protein-to-creatinine ratio, electrocardiogram, and maternal echocardiogram

c. Serum creatinine, 24-hour urine collection for protein and creatinine clearance, electrocardiogram, and cardiac stress test

d. No further evaluation is indicated, as she has only had a diagnosis of hypertension for 4 years and her blood pressure is well controlled on a single medication.

50–6. The patient in Question 50–5 has a copy of her records from her primary care physician. Review of the records shows a recent serum creatinine of 0.9 mg/dL, urine protein-to-creatinine ratio of 0.22, a normal electrocardiogram, and she had a normal exercise stress test performed 3 months ago. Fasting glucose was 93 mg/dL this morning, and her hemoglobin A_{1C} was 6.0 last month. Which of the following is the most appropriate recommendation?

a. You do not yet have adequate information from which to make a recommendation.

b. Risk for adverse outcome in pregnancy is unacceptably high, and you recommend that she consider gestational surrogacy or adoption.

c. There is no contraindication to pregnancy, but she can further reduce her risk with weight loss and regular, moderate intensity aerobic exercise 3–4 times per week.

d. There is no contraindication to pregnancy, but you recommend converting to an alternative antihypertensive agent in advance of pursuing pregnancy to reduce teratogenic risk.

50–7. For a woman who does not enter pregnancy with a known diagnosis, the diagnosis of chronic hypertension is supported when hypertension is present prior to what gestational age threshold?

a. 14 weeks' gestation

b. 20 weeks' gestation

c. 24 weeks' gestation

d. 28 weeks' gestation

50–8. A 28-year-old G3P1102 at 9 weeks' gestation presents for establishment of prenatal care. Her first pregnancy was complicated by gestational hypertension at term, and her second was complicated by iatrogenic preterm delivery at 36 weeks' gestation for preeclampsia. Her blood pressure was normal at her postpartum visit 2 years ago but has not been assessed since. Today her body mass index is 46 kg/m^2 and her blood pressure is 158/96 mm Hg. As instructed, she calls back 2 days after her visit to report that blood pressures have been in the 146–160/94–100 mm Hg range at home. In addition to initiation of an antihypertensive agent, what is the next step in management of her blood pressure in this pregnancy?

a. Baseline serum creatinine

b. Renal ultrasound with Doppler

c. Baseline 24-hour urine collection for protein, creatinine clearance, and urinary metanephrines

d. All of the above

50–9. According to the Nationwide Patient Sample data, which of the following is the most frequent comorbidity associated with chronic hypertension?

a. Depression

b. Hypothyroidism

c. Pregestational diabetes

d. Systemic lupus erythematosus

50–10. Pregnancy is associated with which of the following blood pressure changes in women with chronic hypertension?

a. Blood pressure decreases from baseline in early pregnancy

b. Blood pressure reaches its nadir at approximately 20 weeks' gestation

c. In pregnancy, women with chronic hypertension have persistently elevated vascular resistance

d. All of the above

50–11. Among women with chronic hypertension, which of the following is true regarding risk for adverse maternal and perinatal outcome?

a. Chronic hypertension is associated with a twofold increased risk for maternal death.

b. The risk is inversely proportional to the severity and duration of hypertension prior to pregnancy.

c. Complications are more likely with severe range hypertension at baseline and the presence of end-organ damage.

d. All of the above

50–12. Ms. Clamp is a 30-year-old G1 presenting for initiation of prenatal care at 12 weeks' gestation. Her medical history is notable for chronic hypertension, and she has been on antihypertensive therapy for 3 years. Her blood pressure is 148/94 mm Hg. How would you best counsel her regarding the risk for developing superimposed preeclampsia?

a. The risk for developing superimposed preeclampsia is in the 7–9% range.

b. The risk is highest if workup reveals proteinuria or other end-organ impact.

c. The risk for superimposed preeclampsia is not related to the severity of her baseline hypertension.

d. Maternal serum markers yield a high positive predictive value in discriminating who will and will not develop superimposed preeclampsia.

50–13. Which of the following is not true regarding the complication shown here, in the computerized tomography scan image?

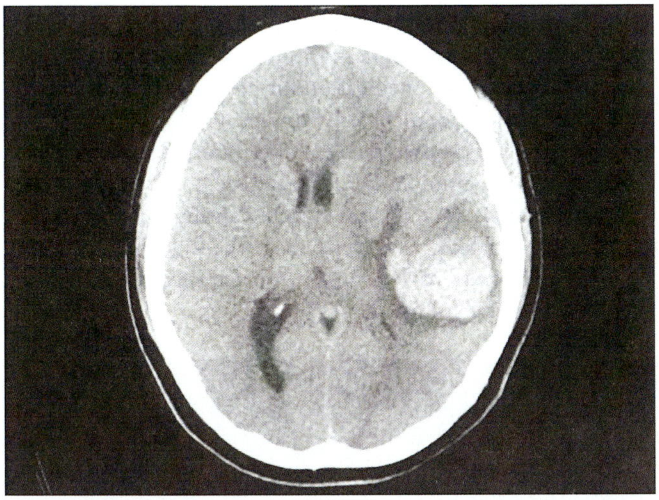

a. This occurs during pregnancy in approximately 3 per 1000 women with chronic hypertension.

b. The risk is not increased among women with chronic hypertension in the absence of superimposed preeclampsia.

c. Systolic blood pressure ≥160 mm Hg or diastolic blood pressure ≥110 mm Hg can rapidly result in the finding shown here.

d. None of the above

50–14. Which of the following interventions is recommended by the American College of Obstetricians and Gynecologists in their 2016 Clinical Update to reduce risk for developing preeclampsia in women with chronic hypertension?

a. At least 3 months of preconception supplementation with vitamins C and E.

b. Initiation of low dose aspirin as early as possible and continuation until 28 weeks' gestation.

c. Initiation of low dose aspirin from 12–28 weeks' gestation with continuation until delivery.

d. No intervention has shown benefit over preconception and early pregnancy folic acid supplementation.

50–15. In addition to chronic hypertension, which of the following conditions are considered high-risk for developing preeclampsia by the American College of Obstetricians and Gynecologists in their 2016 Clinical Update guidelines?

a. Asthma

b. Systemic lupus erythematosus

c. History of gestational diabetes

d. Elevated maternal serum alpha-fetoprotein

50–16. Risk for the complication pictured below is increased in pregnancies complicated by chronic hypertension. How would you best characterize the risk?

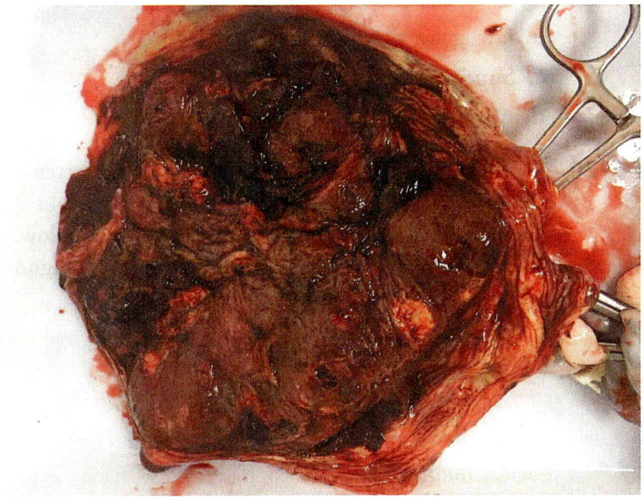

Used with permission from Dr. Patricia Santiago-Munoz.

a. Incidence not impacted by the severity of blood pressure

b. 2-3-fold increase over the general obstetric population

c. 5-6-fold increase over the general obstetric population

d. Incidence not impacted by development of superimposed preeclampsia

50–17. For women with chronic hypertension, which modifiable factor further increases the risk for the complication referenced in Question 50–16?

a. Obesity

b. Exercise

c. Smoking

d. Marijuana use

50–18. Which of the following approximates the risk for perinatal mortality in pregnancies complicated by chronic hypertension?

a. Approximately 3% of births in women with mild hypertension

b. Approximately 10% of births in women with severe hypertension

c. 3- to 4-fold increase over pregnancies not complicated by chronic hypertension

d. All of the above

50–19. Which of the following is a major factor contributing to the incidence of perinatal mortality noted in pregnancies complicated by chronic hypertension?

a. Fetal growth restriction

b. Iatrogenic preterm birth

c. Superimposed preeclampsia

d. All of the above

50–20. A 36-year-old multigravida with chronic hypertension presents for a growth ultrasound at 36 weeks' gestation. The ultrasound report is displayed below. Which of the following is true regarding the diagnosis made on the growth ultrasound?

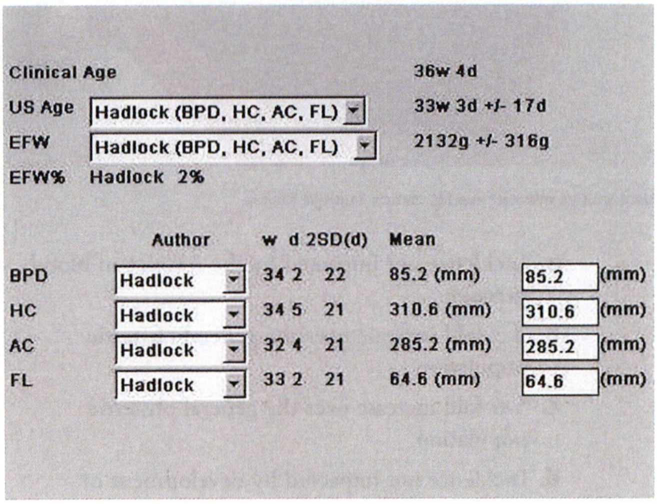

a. The risk is reduced with administration of the antioxidants, vitamin C and vitamin E.

b. The risk is not modified by whether a woman with chronic hypertension requires treatment.

c. The risk is approximately 20% in women with chronic hypertension, and approximately 50% if women with chronic hypertension develop superimposed preeclampsia.

d. All of the above

50–21. You are seeing Ms. Blanche for prenatal care. She is a 37-year-old G1 at 8 weeks' gestation. She has been your patient for several years, and chart review shows former blood pressure readings have been 110–120/70–80 mm Hg at prior visits. The blood pressure noted at her first obstetric visit is 150/96 mm Hg. Which of the following is the most appropriate next step?

a. Order maternal cardiac echocardiogram.

b. Recommend low-sodium diet and recheck her blood pressure in 2 weeks.

c. Request that she have her blood pressure measured a few times over the next 2 weeks and return with her log for review.

d. Counsel regarding the risks of preexisting hypertension in pregnancy and recommend initiation of a daily baby aspirin to reduce the risk for preeclampsia.

50–22. A 43-year-old G5P3013 presents to labor and delivery at 32 weeks' gestation with contractions. She only recently realized she was pregnant and has not been able to establish prenatal care. She reports a history of chronic hypertension and type 2 diabetes. Her blood pressure is 136/80 mm Hg. She is taking an unknown medication for her hypertension and manages her diabetes with diet. Her fetal heart rate tracing is shown below. An ultrasound is performed, and the amnionic fluid index is 2.4 cm. You suspect that this may be related to the antihypertensive agent she is taking. Use of which of the following classes of antihypertensive agents is contraindicated during all trimesters of pregnancy?

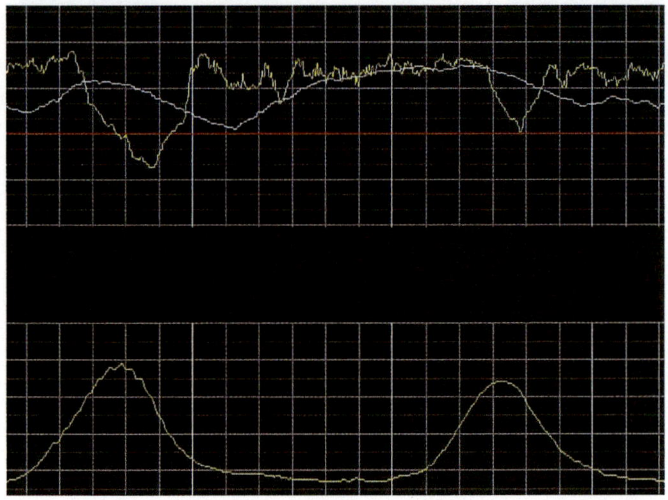

a. Those that act centrally to reduce sympathetic outflow

b. Those that interfere with binding sites on voltage-dependent calcium channels.

c. Those that act to inhibit the conversion of angiotensin-I to angiotensin-II.

d. Those that act peripherally to reduce sympathetic tone and decrease cardiac output

50–23. A 24-year-old G1 with chronic hypertension has required medication for 2 years. She is being induced at 29 weeks' gestation for superimposed severe preeclampsia. Which of the following characterizes the relationship between chronic hypertension and superimposed preeclampsia?

a. Approximately 30% of women with severe range hypertension will develop superimposed preeclampsia.

b. Approximately 40% of women with severe range hypertension will develop superimposed preeclampsia.

c. Approximately 80% of those who also have at least 300 mg/day of proteinuria at baseline will develop severe preeclampsia

d. None of the above

50–24. Ms. Aldo is a 30-year-old G3P2 who presents for establishment of prenatal care at 9 weeks' gestation. Her prior pregnancies have both been complicated by gestational hypertension near term. Her blood pressure was 146/88 mm Hg, which she states is concordant with other recent measurements. Which of the following is the most appropriate next step in her management?

a. Continued routine observation

b. Initiate antihypertensive therapy

c. Recommend that she keep a log of her blood pressures and bring them to her appointments

d. None of the above

50–25. For Ms. Aldo in Question 50–24, which of the following complications is reduced with use of antihypertensive therapy during pregnancy?

a. Preterm birth

b. Fetal growth restriction

c. Development of severe hypertension

d. All of the above

50–26. Guidelines provided by the American College of Obstetricians and Gynecologists in 2013 and the Society for Maternal-Fetal Medicine in 2015 state that antihypertensive therapy is mandatory for which of the following women during pregnancy?

a. 30-year-old G3P2 with a blood pressure of 160/110 mm Hg and a history of asthma

b. 42-year-old G2P1 with a blood pressure of 130/88 mm Hg and a history of myocardial infarction

c. 28-year-old G2P1 with a blood pressure of 146/94 mm Hg and history of preeclampsia in her last pregnancy

d. 38-year-old G4P3 with a blood pressure of 148/96 mm Hg and history of transient renal insufficiency 3 years ago when she had an obstructive nephrolithiasis

50–27. All except which of the following support the diagnosis of superimposed preeclampsia?

a. Decreased platelet count

b. Increased serum creatinine level

c. Elevated serum alkaline phosphatase level

d. Elevated serum aspartate aminotransferase level

50–28. According to the American College of Obstetricians and Gynecologists, which of the following methods of antenatal fetal surveillance has been conclusively shown to be of benefit in the management of pregnancies complicated by chronic hypertension?

a. Nonstress testing

b. Biophysical profile

c. Umbilical artery Doppler studies

d. Serial sonographic evaluations of fetal growth

50–29. A 33-year-old G1 at 32 weeks' gestation has been diagnosed with chronic hypertension with superimposed preeclampsia via worsening hypertension. She is asymptomatic with normal labs and normal fetal growth. An increase in the dose of her antihypertensive medication has resulted in nonsevere blood pressures. She asks you about expectant management of superimposed preeclampsia. Which of the following is the most appropriate, evidence-based response?

a. Preeclampsia mandates immediate delivery, so you recommend proceeding with cesarean.

b. Inpatient expectant management is reasonable, and with close surveillance, adverse outcome would not be expected.

c. It is reasonable, with very close inpatient surveillance, to pursue expectant management, but there are risks for adverse outcomes.

d. None of the above

50–30. For women with chronic hypertension without superimposed preeclampsia, when is delivery recommended?

a. 37 weeks 0 days to 38 weeks 6 days

b. 38 weeks 0 days to 39 weeks 6 days

c. 39 weeks 0 days to 40 weeks 0 days

d. There are no guidelines for a specific recommendation

50–31. Which intravenous antihypertensive drug commonly used to treat intrapartum severe range hypertension is properly matched with its most notable side effect?

a. Hydralazine—fetal arrhythmia

b. Labetalol—neonatal tachycardia

c. Hydralazine—maternal tachycardia

d. Labetalol—neonatal rebound hypertension

50–32. Which of the following statements is not true regarding intrapartum management of a woman with chronic hypertension with superimposed preeclampsia?

a. Trial of labor is not contraindicated.

b. Magnesium sulfate is the neuroprophylactic agent of choice to prevent eclampsia.

c. These women are more sensitive to the acute hypotensive effects of epidural anesthesia.

d. Postpartum analgesia should include scheduled nonsteroidal antiinflammatory drugs for at least 72 hours to reduce narcotic use.

50–33. Ms. Edwards is a 26-year-old G2P2, now 3 days postpartum from a vaginal delivery. She has chronic hypertension and developed superimposed severe preeclampsia at 36 weeks' gestation. She did well initially, but in the last 12 hours her blood pressure has been trending up. Most recent blood pressure was 156/90 mm Hg. The nurse has called you because Ms. Edwards is feeling short of breath. A representative chest radiograph is shown here. What is the appropriate treatment for this condition?

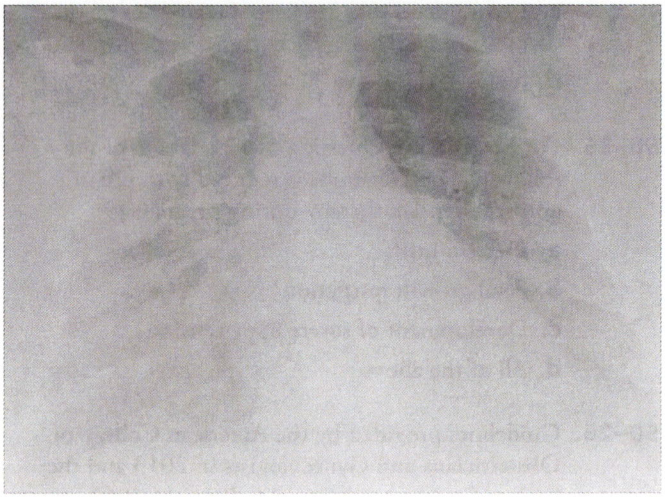

Used with permission from Dr. Barbara Hoffman.

a. Lovenox anticoagulation

b. Albuterol via metered dose inhaler

c. Incentive spirometer and ambulation

d. Intravenous furosemide administration

CHAPTER 50 ANSWER KEY

Question number	Letter answer	Page cited	Header cited
50–1	c	p. 975	General Considerations
50–2	a	p. 976	Definition and Classification
50–3	d	p. 976	Table 50-1
50–4	c	p. 976	Table 50-1
50–5	b	p. 976	Preconception Counseling
50–6	c	p. 977	Table 50-2
50–7	b	p. 977	Diagnosis and Evaluation in Pregnancy
50–8	a	p. 977	Diagnosis and Evaluation in Pregnancy
50–9	c	p. 977	Associated Risk Factors
50–10	d	p. 977	Effects of Pregnancy on Chronic Hypertension
50–11	c	p. 978	Maternal Morbidity and Mortality
50–12	b	p. 978	Superimposed Preeclampsia
50–13	b	p. 978	Maternal Morbidity and Mortality
50–14	c	p. 979	Prevention
50–15	b	p. 979	Prevention
50–16	b	p. 979	Placental Abruption
50–17	c	p. 979	Placental Abruption
50–18	d	p. 979	Perinatal Morbidity and Mortality
50–19	d	p. 979	Perinatal Morbidity and Mortality
50–20	c	p. 980	Perinatal Morbidity and Mortality
50–21	c	p. 980	Management During Pregnancy
50–22	c	p. 980	Antihypertensive Drugs
50–23	c	p. 981	Severe Chronic Hypertension
50–24	c	p. 981	Mild or Moderate Hypertension
50–25	c	p. 982	"Tight Control"
50–26	a	p. 982	Recommendations for Therapy
50–27	c	p. 983	Pregnancy-Aggravated Hypertension or Superimposed Preeclampsia
50–28	d	p. 983	Fetal Assessment
50–29	c	p. 983	Expectant Management of Early-Onset Preeclampsia
50–30	b	p. 983	Delivery
50–31	c	p. 984	Intrapartum Considerations
50–32	d	p. 983 p. 984 p. 984	Delivery Intrapartum Considerations Postpartum Care
50–33	d	p. 984	Postpartum Care

CHAPTER 51

Pulmonary Disorders

51–1. What happens to vital capacity in pregnancy?

a. Increases by 20%
b. Increases by 40%
c. Decreases by 25%
d. Decreases by 45%

51–2. What effect does progesterone have on tidal volume?

a. Increases by 20%
b. Increases by 40%
c. Decreases by 25%
d. Decreases by 45%

51–3. What happens to carbon dioxide production in pregnancy?

a. Increases by 20%
b. Increases by 30%
c. Decreases by 25%
d. Decreases by 35%

51–4. What happens to residual volume in pregnancy?

a. Increases by 20%
b. Increases by 30%
c. Decreases by 20%
d. Decreases by 35%

51–5. Which of the following is not a hallmark of asthma?

a. Mucosal edema
b. Tenacious mucus
c. Vascular congestion
d. Bronchial smooth muscle relaxation

51–6. A 20-year-old G1P0 at 18 weeks' gestation presents for prenatal care. She reports a history of asthma. On further questioning, you find out that she has symptoms about once per week. She does not wake up at night. She uses her albuterol inhaler once per week on average. She does not feel that she has trouble with daily activities. You test her FEV_1, which is 90%. What is the severity of this patient's asthma?

a. Intermittent
b. Mild persistent
c. Severe persistent
d. Moderate persistent

51–7. A 22-year-old G2P1 presents at 6 weeks' gestation. She has a history of asthma for which she takes albuterol daily. She feels symptoms every day, and she moved with her family to a first-floor apartment to avoid stairs. She does manage to care for her 2-year-old daughter without issue. Her baseline FEV_1 is 65% of predicted. You label this patient's asthma as:

a. Intermittent
b. Mild persistent
c. Severe persistent
d. Moderate persistent

51–8. Which of the following is not a characteristic of mild persistent asthma?

a. Normal FEV_1/FVC
b. FEV_1 60–70% of predicted
c. Minor limitation with normal activity
d. Nocturnal awakenings 3–4 times per month

51–9. The fetal response to maternal hypoxemia includes which of the following?

a. Increased cardiac output
b. Decreased umbilical blood flow
c. Decreased systemic vascular resistance
d. Decreased pulmonary vascular resistance

51–10. A pregnant woman in the late second trimester is being evaluated in the emergency room for an asthma exacerbation. An arterial blood gas is sent. Her PCO_2 is 42 mm Hg, and her pH is 7.29. This is consistent with:

a. Hypoventilation with CO_2 retention
b. Hyperventilation with CO_2 retention
c. Hypoventilation without CO_2 retention
d. Hyperventilation without CO_2 retention

51–11. Which of the following is the best measure of asthma severity?

a. FEV_1
b. Chest x-ray
c. Arterial blood gas
d. Echocardiography

51–12. Treatment of moderate persistent asthma includes low-dose inhaled corticosteroids and which of the following?

a. Azithromycin
b. Oral corticosteroids
c. Long-acting beta agonist
d. High-dose inhaled corticosteroids

51–13. The recommended treatment for severe persistent asthma includes a short-acting beta agonist and which of the following?

a. No other agents
b. Low-dose inhaled corticosteroids
c. Low-dose inhaled corticosteroids and a long-acting beta agonist
d. High-dose inhaled corticosteroids and a long-acting beta agonist

51–14. Which of the following is used for treating asthma acutely?

a. Zileuton
b. Cromolyn
c. Terbutaline
d. Montelukast

51–15. A 25-year-old G3P2 at 20 weeks' gestation presents to the emergency room for an asthma exacerbation. Her FEV_1 is 40%. She receives inhaled corticosteroids and 3 doses of an inhaled beta agonist. Her FEV_1 is now 50%. She has an oxygen saturation of 95%. What is the next best step in management of this patient?

a. Intubation
b. Discharge home with a short-acting beta agonist inhaler and an oral steroid taper.
c. Discharge home with a short-acting beta agonist inhaler and a course of azithromycin.
d. Admission for continued inhaled beta agonists, intravenous steroids, and close observation.

51–16. Which asthmatic patients should receive stress-dose corticosteroids in labor?

a. All asthmatic patients regardless of their treatment regimen
b. Those who received systemic corticosteroid therapy within the preceding 4 weeks
c. Those who received inhaled corticosteroid therapy within the preceding 8 weeks
d. Those who received systemic corticosteroid therapy anytime during the pregnancy

51–17. Which of the following medications is contraindicated in pregnant patients with asthma?

a. Oxytocin
b. Prostaglandin E_1
c. Prostaglandin E_2
d. Prostaglandin $F_{2\alpha}$

51–18. How long does the cough associated with acute bronchitis last?

a. 1–2 days
b. 3–5 days
c. 5–7 days
d. 10–20 days

51–19. Which of the following is essential for the diagnosis of pneumonia in pregnancy?

a. Chest x-ray
b. Blood cultures
c. Sputum cultures
d. Complete blood count

51–20. This chest x-ray suggests that this pregnant woman should be admitted to the hospital for treatment of pneumonia. What criterion for admission is demonstrated in this image?

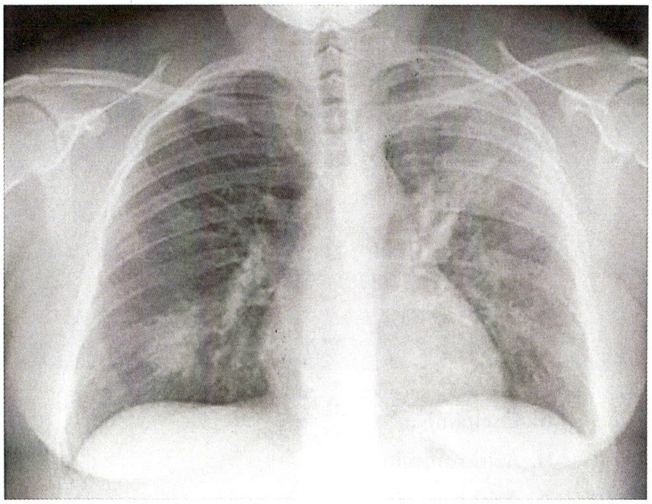

Reproduced with permission from Cunningham FG, Leveno KJ, Bloom SL, et al (eds): Pulmonary disorders. In Williams Obstetrics, 25th ed. New York, McGraw-Hill, 2018, Figure 51-3.

a. Cardiomegaly
b. Pleural effusions
c. Tracheal deviation
d. Multilobar infiltrates

51–21. Which of the following is not a criterion for severe community-acquired pneumonia?

a. Uremia

b. Core temperature <36°C

c. Platelet count <100,000/μL

d. White blood cell count >10,000/μL

51–22. A 34-year-old G4P3 presents to the emergency room at 27 weeks' gestation. She reports a 1-week history of cold symptoms with worsening cough. She believes she's had a fever, but she did not take her temperature at home. Her children have also been sick. Everyone in the family received a flu shot this season. The patient's vitals are: temperature 38.7°C, heart rate 102 beats per minute, blood pressure 110/70 mm Hg, and respiratory rate 30 breaths per minute. Her oxygen saturation is 93% on room air. A rapid test for influenza and respiratory syncytial virus is negative. The patient has a chest x-ray, which is provided below. It is consistent with right lower lobe pneumonia. You admit her for treatment. Which of the following is the most appropriate choice of medications?

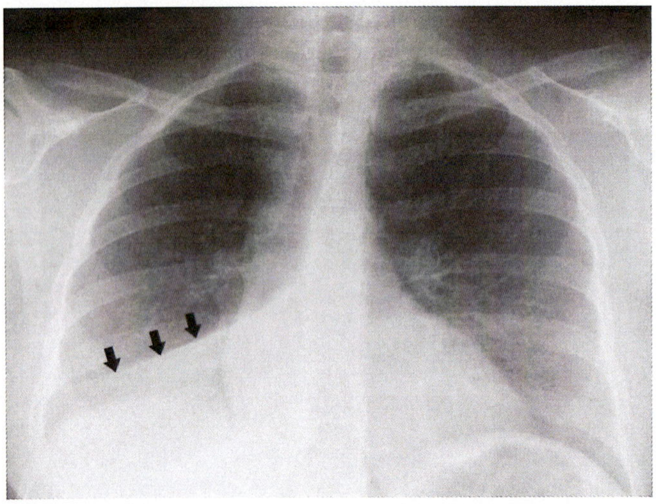

a. Oseltamivir

b. Azithromycin

c. Azithromycin and oseltamivir

d. Azithromycin and ceftriaxone

51–23. Regarding the patient in Question 51–22, for how long should she be treated with antibiotics, provided she responds to therapy?

a. 1–2 days

b. 2–3 days

c. 5–7 days

d. 10–14 days

51–24. How long is it expected to take for the chest x-ray findings for the patient in Question 51–22 to resolve?

a. 2–3 days

b. 5–7 days

c. 2 weeks

d. Up to 6 weeks

51–25. The patient in Question 51–22 does not show improvement. She continues to have fever and tachypnea. Her respiratory status deteriorates, and she is transferred to the intensive care unit. Her repeat chest x-ray is provided below. A sputum culture comes back with methicillin-resistant *Staphylococcus aureus*. What antibiotic should she be given?

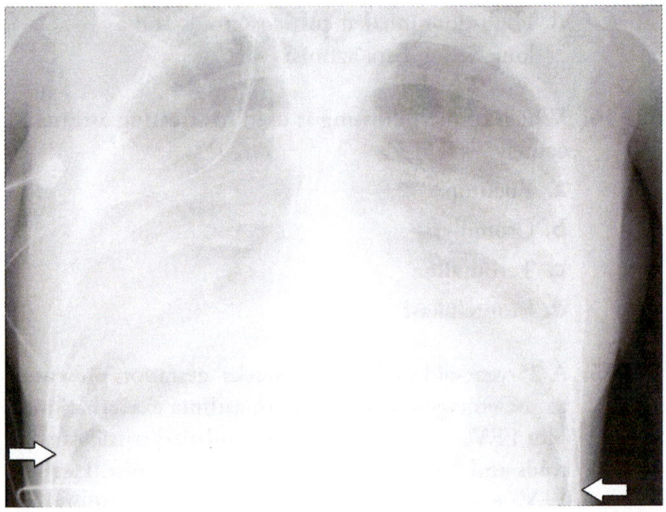

Reproduced with permission from Cunningham FG, Leveno KJ, Bloom SL, et al (eds): Pulmonary disorders. In Williams Obstetrics, 25th ed. New York, McGraw-Hill, 2018, Figure 53-2A.

a. Doxycycline

b. Vancomycin

c. Clarithromycin

d. Amoxicillin/clavulanate

51–26. What is the most common complication of influenza?

a. Epistaxis

b. Pneumonia

c. Renal failure

d. Thrombocytopenia

51–27. What is the treatment of choice for influenza?

a. Ceftriaxone

b. Oseltamivir

c. Amantadine

d. Azithromycin

51–28. Which of the following is the best choice for treatment of pneumocystis pneumonia?

a. Ceftriaxone for 7–10 days
b. Azithromycin for 5–7 days
c. Moxifloxacin for 10–14 days
d. Trimethoprim-sulfamethoxazole for 14–21 days

51–29. A 35-year-old G2P1 presents at 10 weeks' gestation for prenatal care. The patient is a recent immigrant from India. You want to test her for tuberculosis. She reports that she received the *bacille Calmette-Guérin* (BCG) vaccination. How should you evaluate the patient for latent tuberculosis?

a. Chest x-ray
b. Sputum culture
c. Tuberculin skin test
d. Interferon-gamma release assay

51–30. In which group of pregnant patients can treatment of latent tuberculosis be postponed to the postpartum period?

a. Known recent skin-test convertors
b. Human immunodeficiency virus positive women
c. Skin-test positive women exposed to active infection
d. Healthy women incidentally identified with no known tuberculosis contacts

51–31. A 25-year-old G3P2 at 18 weeks' gestation is evaluated for persistent cough. She is a recent immigrant. Her T-SPOT is positive, and her chest x-ray is as you see below. Which of the following is the recommended initial treatment for active tuberculosis in pregnant women?

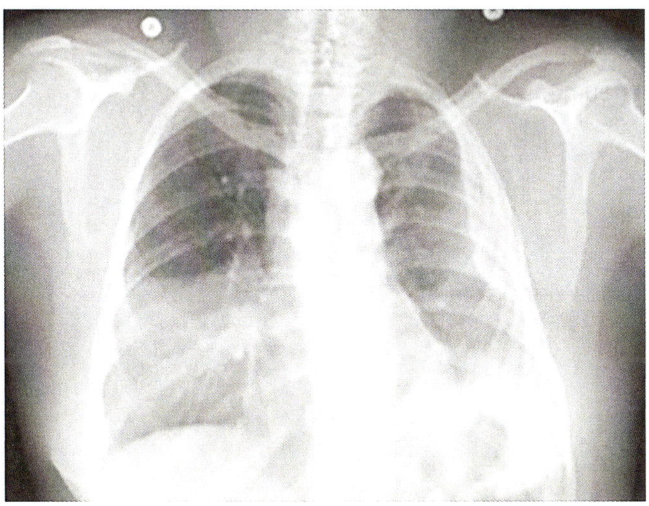

a. Isoniazid
b. Isoniazid and rifampin
c. Isoniazid and ethambutol
d. Isoniazid, rifampin, ethambutol, and pyrazinamide

51–32. Which of the following is the most common organism to cause chronic inflammation in the lungs of patients with cystic fibrosis?

a. *Burkholderia cepacia*
b. *Staphylococcus aureus*
c. *Pseudomonas aeruginosa*
d. *Haemophilus influenzae*

51–33. Which of the following statements about cystic fibrosis (CF) and pregnancy is true?

a. CF is not a risk factor for preterm birth.
b. The natural course of CF is worsened by pregnancy.
c. If the woman has an FEV_1 of at least 50%, pregnancy should be well tolerated.
d. Up to 25% of CF patients develop diabetes by age 20, so these pregnant patients must be closely monitored for this.

51–34. A 25-year-old G4P3 at 19 weeks' gestation and in good health is brought to the emergency room for altered mental status. She is somnolent with complaints of headache and dizziness. She vomited in the ambulance. The patient's spouse reports that she was sleeping alone in the back of the house when he found her like this. The emergency medical technicians report that she had two space heaters in the room with her and no ventilation. You are concerned that she is suffering from carbon monoxide poisoning. Which of the following is your initial treatment?

a. Dialysis
b. 100% oxygen
c. Plasma exchange
d. Blood transfusion

CHAPTER 51 ANSWER KEY

Question number	Letter answer	Page cited	Header cited
51–1	**a**	p. 987	Pulmonary Disorders
51–2	**b**	p. 987	Pulmonary Disorders
51–3	**b**	p. 987	Pulmonary Disorders
51–4	**c**	p. 987	Pulmonary Disorders
51–5	**d**	p. 988	Pathophysiology
51–6	**a**	p. 988	Table 51-1
51–7	**d**	p. 988	Table 51-1
51–8	**b**	p. 988	Table 51-1
51–9	**b**	p. 990	Fetal Effects
51–10	**b**	p. 990	Clinical Evaluation
51–11	**a**	p. 990	Clinical Evaluation
51–12	**c**	p. 990	Figure 51-2
51–13	**d**	p. 990	Figure 51-2
51–14	**c**	p. 991	Management of Acute Asthma
51–15	**d**	p. 991	Management of Acute Asthma
51–16	**b**	p. 991	Labor and Delivery
51–17	**d**	p. 991	Labor and Delivery
51–18	**d**	p. 991	Acute Bronchitis
51–19	**a**	p. 992	Diagnosis
51–20	**d**	p. 993	Table 51-3
51–21	**d**	p. 993	Table 51-3
51–22	**d**	p. 993	Table 51-4
51–23	**c**	p. 993	Management
51–24	**d**	p. 993	Management
51–25	**b**	p. 993	Management
51–26	**b**	p. 994	Clinical Presentation
51–27	**b**	p. 994	Management
51–28	**d**	p. 994	Pneumocystis Pneumonia
51–29	**d**	p. 996	Diagnosis
51–30	**d**	p. 996	Treatment
51–31	**d**	p. 996	Active Infection
51–32	**c**	p. 998	Pathophysiology
51–33	**d**	p. 998	Prenatal Care and Management
51–34	**b**	p. 999	Treatment

CHAPTER 52

Thromboembolic Disease

52–1. What has led to a decrease in the frequency of venous thromboembolism in the puerperium?

a. Anticoagulation

b. Early ambulation

c. Decrease in cesarean deliveries

d. Sequential compression devices

52–2. What percentage of pregnancy-related deaths are due to pulmonary embolism?

a. 9%

b. 15%

c. 25%

d. 30%

52–3. Which of the following statements is accurate regarding the timing of venous thrombosis?

a. Deep-vein thrombosis is more common during the antepartum period.

b. An equal number occur during the antepartum period and puerperium.

c. Pulmonary embolism is more common in the first 6 weeks postpartum.

d. All of the above

52–4. All except which of the following is an aspect of Virchow's triad?

a. Stasis

b. Local trauma

c. Immobilization

d. Hypercoagulability

52–5. Which of the following pregnancy-related factors contributes to an increased risk for venous thromboembolism?

a. Enhanced synthesis of clotting factors

b. Endothelial cell injury during delivery

c. Compression of the pelvic veins and inferior vena cava

d. All of the above

52–6. A 33-year-old G4P5 presents to the hospital on POD #15 from a cesarean delivery due to a twin gestation complaining of right lower extremity swelling. She reports the swelling started 2 days ago but has not improved with leg elevation. She reports she had a blood clot in her left leg 10 years ago. The only medication she is taking is iron because her hemoglobin was 8 mg/dL on discharge. Which of the following risk factors for venous thromboembolism is most important in pregnancy?

a. Anemia

b. Cesarean delivery

c. Multifetal gestation

d. Personal history of thrombosis

52–7. The patient in Question 52–6 reports she was never tested for a thrombophilia. What percentage of women with venous thrombosis during pregnancy have an underlying thrombophilia?

a. 10%

b. 20%

c. 50%

d. 90%

52–8. Which of the following is not an inherited thrombophilia?

a. Protein S deficiency

b. Antiphospholipid syndrome

c. Antithrombin III deficiency

d. Activated protein C resistance

52–9. Which of the following statements regarding antithrombin III deficiency is accurate?

a. Autosomal dominant

b. Inactivates thrombin and factor Xa

c. The most thrombogenic inheritable coagulopathy

d. All of the above

52–10. What happens to protein S levels in pregnancy?

a. Increase

b. Decrease

c. Stay the same

d. Decrease in the first trimester and then increase

52–11. Why does the presence of a factor V Leiden mutation lead to increased risk for venous thromboembolism?

- **a.** Increased levels of factor V are produced
- **b.** Decreased levels of factor V are produced
- **c.** Factor V is resistant to inactivation by protein C
- **d.** Factor V is more sensitive to inactivation by protein C

52–12. How does the prothrombin G20210A mutation promote clot formation?

- **a.** Leads to increased prothrombin production
- **b.** Leads to decreased prothrombin production
- **c.** Accelerates prothrombin inactivation by protein S
- **d.** Yields prothrombin resistant to inactivation by protein S

52–13. Which of the following adverse pregnancy outcomes is linked to factor V Leiden mutation?

- **a.** Preeclampsia
- **b.** Fetal-growth restriction
- **c.** First-trimester pregnancy loss
- **d.** None of the above

52–14. Which of the following is an acquired thrombophilia?

- **a.** Cancer
- **b.** Antiphospholipid syndrome
- **c.** Heparin-induced thrombocytopenia
- **d.** All of the above

52–15. Which of the following is in the clinical criteria for antiphospholipid syndrome?

- **a.** At least one spontaneous preterm birth
- **b.** Three unexplained fetal losses before 12 weeks' gestation
- **c.** At least one unexplained fetal death beyond 20 weeks' gestation
- **d.** At least 1 preterm birth before 34 weeks' gestation due to severe preeclampsia, eclampsia, or placental insufficiency

52–16. A 34-year-old G1P1 presents for preconception counseling because her last pregnancy ended in delivery at 27 weeks' gestation due to preeclampsia with severe features. She brings documentation of lab results showing she is positive for anti-β_2-glycoprotein I IgM. A minimum of how many weeks after the initial labs are the confirmatory labs drawn?

- **a.** 8 weeks
- **b.** 10 weeks
- **c.** 12 weeks
- **d.** 16 weeks

52–17. Which of the following antiphospholipid antibodies is associated with the lowest live birth rate?

- **a.** Lupus anticoagulant
- **b.** Anti-β_2-glycoprotein I
- **c.** Anticardiolipin antibody
- **d.** All are equal

52–18. A 32-year-old G3P0 presents for preconception counseling after suffering three first-trimester pregnancy losses. She reports her obstetrician performed a workup and she has a genetic blood clotting disorder. Which inherited thrombophilia has been associated with adverse pregnancy outcomes, including first-trimester loss?

- **a.** Prothrombin G20210A
- **b.** Factor V Leiden mutation
- **c.** 5,10-Methylene-tetrahydrofolate reductase (MTHFR) mutation
- **d.** None of the above

52–19. As you discuss her results, for which thrombophilia do you encourage the patient in Question 52–18 to undergo testing?

- **a.** Protein S deficiency
- **b.** Protein C deficiency
- **c.** Antiphospholipid syndrome
- **d.** All of the above

52–20. The American College of Obstetricians and Gynecologists recommends screening in which of the following situations?

- **a.** Personal history of an unprovoked deep-vein thrombosis
- **b.** Personal history of a deep-vein thrombosis after knee surgery
- **c.** Family history consisting of a sister with a pulmonary embolus during pregnancy at age 25
- **d.** Family history of an aunt with a deep-vein thrombosis while undergoing treatment for breast cancer at the age of 62

52–21. Which one of the following thrombophilias can be tested for while on treatment for a venous thrombosis?

- **a.** Protein S deficiency
- **b.** Protein C deficiency
- **c.** Antithrombin III deficiency
- **d.** Prothrombin G20210A mutation

52–22. Which of the following thrombophilias is tested for using DNA analysis?

a. Protein S deficiency
b. Protein C deficiency
c. Antithrombin III deficiency
d. Prothrombin G20210A mutation

52–23. In pregnancy, why is a left leg deep-vein thrombosis more common than a right leg deep-vein thrombosis?

a. Natural leftward tilt of the gravid uterus
b. Compression of the left iliac vein by the left iliac artery
c. Compression of the left iliac vein by the left ovarian artery
d. Compression of the left iliac vein by the right iliac artery

52–24. A 29-year-old G2P1 at 29 weeks' gestation presents for a routine prenatal care visit with complaints of lower extremity swelling. On examination her feet appear as pictured below. Which of the following is true regarding this condition in pregnancy?

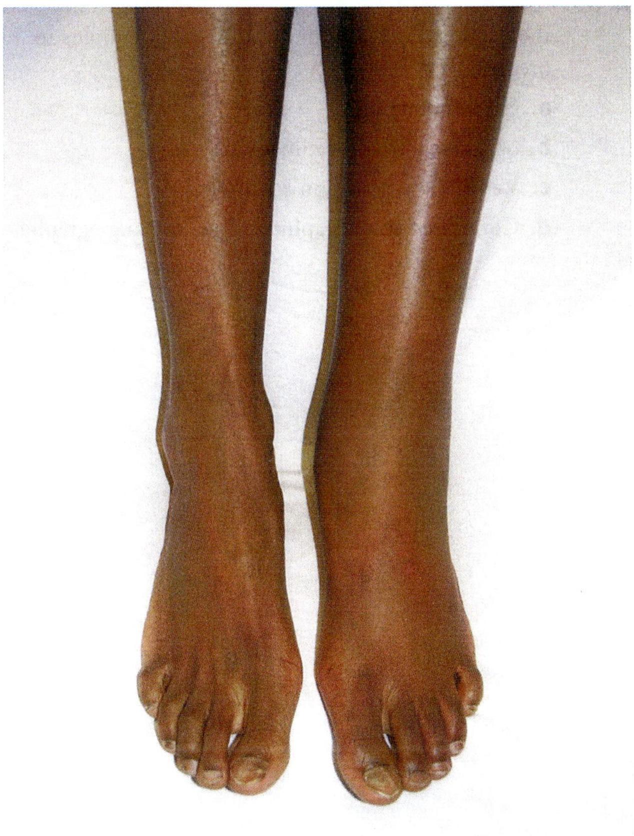

a. A positive Homans sign is virtually diagnostic
b. Most cases are located in the iliofemoral veins
c. Associated with a pulmonary embolism in 30–60% of cases
d. Pain more than swelling correlates with the degree of vessel involvement

52–25. The patient in Question 52–24 undergoes compression ultrasonography with the findings shown below. What is the next best step in the management of this patient?

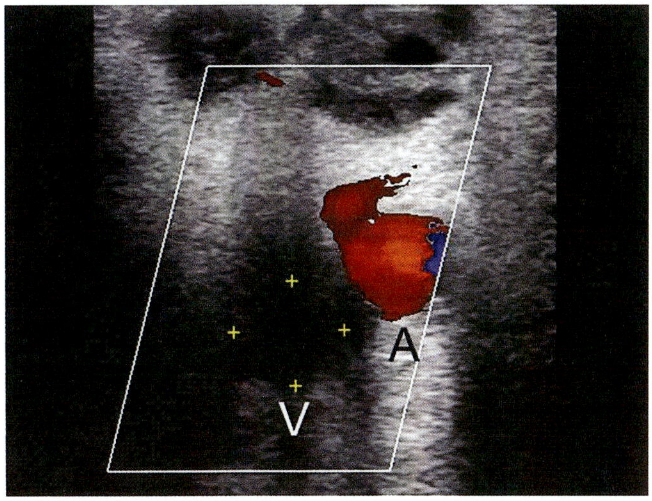

a. Serum D-dimer
b. Initiate anticoagulation
c. Magnetic resonance imaging
d. Ventilation-perfusion scintigraphy

52–26. Serum D-dimer is unreliable in pregnancy because it is affected by all except which of the following?

a. Preeclampsia
b. Cesarean delivery
c. Multifetal gestation
d. All of the above

52–27. What are the advantages of low-molecular-weight heparin in pregnancy?

a. Shorter half-life
b. Easily reversible
c. Better bioavailability
d. Increased dosing leads to more predictable response

52–28. What is the risk of pulmonary embolism in the setting of a treated deep-vein thrombosis?

a. 2%
b. 5%
c. 10%
d. 15%

52–29. A 33-year-old G3P2 is on prophylactic low-molecular-weight heparin due to history of venous thromboembolism and factor V Leiden mutation. She inquires as to why she has to be switched to a medication that requires injections twice daily at 36 weeks' gestation. What is your response?

a. Heparin has a shorter half-life and is more easily reversible.

b. Heparin has a lower rate of heparin-induced thrombocytopenia.

c. Heparin does not cross the placenta as low-molecular-weight heparin does.

d. Fetal exposure to low-molecular-weight heparin close to delivery increases the risk for intraventricular hemorrhage.

52–30. What medication is used to reverse the effects of heparin?

a. Calcium

b. Vitamin K

c. Protamine sulfate

d. Fresh frozen plasma

52–31. When switching from therapeutic heparin to warfarin, how are paradoxical thrombosis and skin necrosis from the anti–protein C effects of warfarin avoided?

a. Watch the patient in the hospital for the first 5 days.

b. Give the patient a test dose and watch for these side effects.

c. Overlap of heparin and warfarin for at least 3 days and until the INR is therapeutic for 1 day.

d. Overlap of heparin and warfarin for at least 5 days and until the INR is therapeutic for 2 days.

52–32. Superficial venous thrombophlebitis is treated with all except which of the following?

a. Heat

b. Analgesia

c. Elastic support

d. Anticoagulation

52–33. What percentage of maternal deaths are caused by pulmonary embolism?

a. 1%

b. 5%

c. 10%

d. 20%

52–34. What is the most common presenting symptom in patients with a pulmonary embolus?

a. Cough

b. Syncope

c. Dyspnea

d. Chest pain

52–35. All except which of the following is included in the diagnostic algorithm of pulmonary embolus in pregnancy?

a. Chest radiograph

b. Magnetic resonance imaging

c. Ventilation-perfusion scintigraphy

d. Computed-tomographic pulmonary angiography

CHAPTER 52 ANSWER KEY

Question number	Letter answer	Page cited	Header cited
52-1	**b**	p. 1004	Introduction
52-2	**a**	p. 1004	Introduction
52-3	**d**	p. 1004	Introduction
52-4	**c**	p. 1004	Pathophysiology
52-5	**d**	p. 1004	Pathophysiology
52-6	**d**	p. 1005	Pathophysiology
52-7	**c**	p. 1005	Pathophysiology
52-8	**b**	p. 1006	Table 52-2
52-9	**d**	p. 1006	Antithrombin Deficiency
52-10	**b**	p. 1007	Protein S Deficiency
52-11	**c**	p. 1007	Activated Protein C Resistance-Factor V Leiden Mutation
52-12	**a**	p. 1007	Prothrombin G20210A Mutation
52-13	**d**	p. 1007	Activated Protein C Resistance-Factor V Leiden Mutation
52-14	**d**	p. 1008	Acquired Thrombophilias
52-15	**d**	p. 1008	Antiphospholipid Syndrome
52-16	**c**	p. 1008	Antiphospholipid Syndrome
52-17	**b**	p. 1008	Antiphospholipid Syndrome
52-18	**d**	p. 1009	Thrombophilias and Pregnancy Complications
52-19	**c**	p. 1010	Thrombophilia Screening
52-20	**a**	p. 1010	Thrombophilia Screening
52-21	**d**	p. 1010	Table 52-4
52-22	**d**	p. 1010	Table 52-4
52-23	**d**	p. 1010	Clinical Presentation
52-24	**b**	p. 1010	Clinical Presentation
52-25	**b**	p. 1011	Diagnosis
52-26	**d**	p. 1011	D-Dimer Screening Tests
52-27	**c**	p. 1012	Management
52-28	**b**	p. 1012	Management
52-29	**a**	p. 1014	Labor and Delivery
52-30	**c**	p. 1014	Labor and Delivery
52-31	**d**	p. 1015	Anticoagulation with Warfarin Compounds
52-32	**d**	p. 1016	Superficial Venous Thrombophlebitis
52-33	**c**	p. 1016	Pulmonary Embolism
52-34	**c**	p. 1016	Clinical Presentation
52-35	**b**	p. 1017	Figure 52-5

CHAPTER 53

Renal and Urinary Tract Disorders

53–1. Which of the following is not a physiological change in pregnancy that contributes to the findings in the image below?

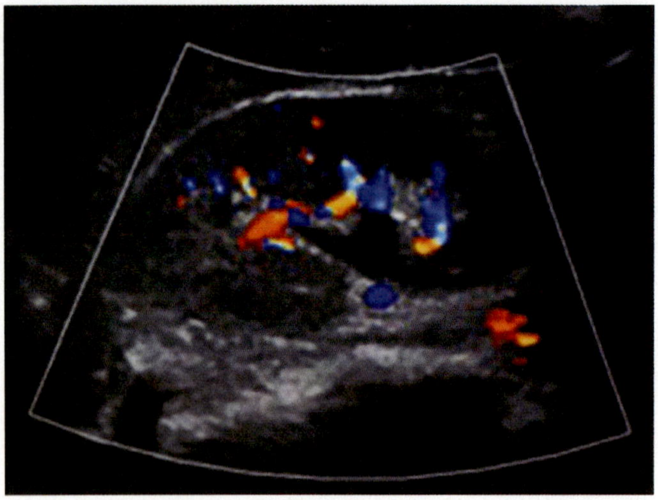

a. Vesicoureteral reflux
b. Glomerular hypertrophy
c. Distal ureteral compression by the uterus
d. Progesterone-induced relaxation of the muscularis

53–2. Which of the following statements regarding physiological changes in pregnancy is true?
a. Glomerular filtration decreases.
b. Effective renal plasma flow increases.
c. Serum creatinine concentration increases.
d. The number of glomerular cells increases.

53–3. A 35-year-old G5P3 presents at 24 weeks' gestation. She has a history of chronic hypertension, but she is noncompliant with medication. You would like to do a baseline 24-hour urine collection. The patient is of low health literacy, and you are concerned she will not complete the collection as an outpatient, but she refuses to be admitted for it. You decide to do a urinary protein-to-creatinine ratio on a spot urine sample so you can gather additional information about the patient's renal status. What is the cutoff for abnormal?
a. 0.1
b. 0.2
c. 0.3
d. 0.5

53–4. Which of the following is the threshold for proteinuria in pregnancy, above which levels are considered abnormal?
a. 100 mg/d
b. 250 mg/d
c. 300 mg/d
d. 1000 mg/d

53–5. Which of the following values is not a normal serum creatinine in pregnancy?
a. 0.4 mg/dL
b. 0.6 mg/dL
c. 0.8 mg/dL
d. 1.0 mg/dL

53–6. A pregnant patient who previously donated a kidney and now has only one healthy kidney is at risk for which of the following obstetric complications?
a. Placenta previa
b. Normocytic anemia
c. Gestational hypertension
d. Preterm premature rupture of membranes

53–7. A 28-year-old G1P0 at 20 weeks' gestation presents to the emergency room complaining of frequency, urgency, and dysuria. She is afebrile with no costovertebral angle tenderness. On review of her prenatal records, you see that she had a urine culture at her first prenatal visit with >100,000 colony-forming units/mL gram-negative rods that was never treated. What percentage of pregnant women with asymptomatic bacteriuria develop a symptomatic infection if left untreated?
a. 5%
b. 10%
c. 25%
d. 50%

53–8. Which of the following is an acceptable treatment regimen for newly diagnosed asymptomatic bacteriuria in pregnancy?

a. Nitrofurantoin 100 mg by mouth at bedtime for 10 days

b. Ampicillin 250 mg by mouth four times per day for one day

c. Trimethoprim-sulfamethoxazole 160/800 mg by mouth one time

d. Nitrofurantoin 100 mg by mouth four times daily for 21 days

53–9. You are consulted about a 19-year-old primigravida at 18 weeks' gestation. The patient was diagnosed at her first prenatal care visit with asymptomatic bacteriuria. Her provider treated her with nitrofurantoin 100 mg twice daily for 7 days. The patient was seen a month after treatment, and her repeat urine culture was negative. But now, a urine culture sent in error is positive for >100,000 colony-forming units/mL gram-negative rods again. She remains asymptomatic. Her provider is not sure what to do. What is the best response to this consult?

a. Single-dose treatment is more successful, so give the patient nitrofurantoin 200 mg by mouth one time.

b. The patient likely has a highly resistant organism, so she should be admitted for intravenous antibiotics.

c. The urine culture is probably a false-positive given it was negative after treatment, so she does not need any further antibiotics.

d. Recurrence of asymptomatic bacteriuria is 30% regardless of antibiotic regimen and it may indicate covert upper tract infection, so treat the patient with nitrofurantoin 100 mg by mouth at bedtime for 21 days.

53–10. Lower urinary tract symptoms with pyuria but a sterile urine culture are likely due to which pathogen?

a. *Escherichia coli*

b. *Proteus mirabilis*

c. *Klebsiella pneumoniae*

d. *Chlamydia trachomatis*

53–11. What is the leading cause of septic shock during pregnancy?

a. Pneumonia

b. Breast abscess

c. Pyelonephritis

d. Chorioamnionitis

53–12. In the setting of aggressive fluid hydration, what percentage of pregnant women with pyelonephritis develop acute kidney injury?

a. 5%

b. 10%

c. 15%

d. 20%

53–13. An 18-year-old G1P0 presents at 30 weeks' gestation with fever, chills, vomiting, dysuria, and frequency for 3 days. She is also experiencing contractions. You diagnose her with pyelonephritis based on her symptoms, fever of 39°C, and urinalysis. She is transferred to labor and delivery for monitoring of contractions. The patient is given intravenous (IV) antibiotics, IV fluids, acetaminophen, and a β-agonist because of the contractions. What complication is more likely in the setting of β-agonist use in patients with pyelonephritis?

a. Anemia

b. Abruption

c. Pulmonary edema

d. Acute kidney injury

53–14. Once you have treated a pregnant patient for pyelonephritis as an inpatient, for how long should you continue oral therapy as an outpatient?

a. 1–3 days

b. 3–5 days

c. 7–14 days

d. 14–21 days

53–15. What percentage of pregnant women experience a recurrent urinary tract infection after completion of treatment for pyelonephritis?

a. 5–10%

b. 10–20%

c. 30–40%

d. 50–60%

53–16. A 24-year-old G1P0 presents at 24 weeks' gestation complaining of back pain that radiates forward. She reports that the pain is intense, and she looks very uncomfortable. She has not been febrile. A urinalysis is significant only for red blood cells. An image from her renal ultrasound is provided below. You diagnose the patient with a kidney stone. Which of the following is the best management option for the patient at this time?

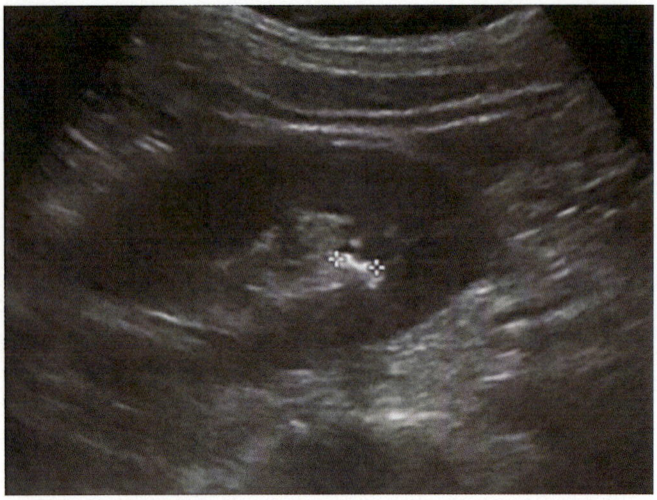

a. Analgesia

b. Analgesia and intravenous hydration

c. Analgesia, intravenous hydration, and intravenous antibiotics

d. Analgesia, intravenous hydration, intravenous antibiotics, and ureteral stenting

53–17. The patient in Question 53–16 asks how many pregnant women actually pass their stone with the management plan you selected. What is your response?

a. 50–60%

b. 65–80%

c. 90–95%

d. 95–100%

53–18. A 25-year-old G1P0 at 16 weeks' gestation presents for prenatal care. She has a history of a kidney transplant 3 years ago. She is stable on prednisone and azathioprine. The patient has not experienced any rejection, and her blood pressure is well controlled. The patient is concerned about how her pregnancy will be affected by her transplant and vice versa. Which of the following statements would not be part of your counseling?

a. Opportunistic infections are common, so there must be proper surveillance for that.

b. It is a good prognostic indicator that she has been stable and in good health for the past several years.

c. She would be expected to have a better outcome than someone with end-stage renal disease on dialysis.

d. It is unfortunate that she is on azathioprine as it has a much higher rate of fetal malformation than mycophenolate.

53–19. Which of the following obstetric complications is not increased in women who have undergone a kidney transplant?

a. Preeclampsia

b. Preterm birth

c. Fetal-growth restriction

d. Peripartum cardiomyopathy

53–20. Which of the following is not a recommended requisite for renal transplant patients who want to attempt pregnancy?

a. Proteinuria <300 mg/day

b. Serum creatinine <2 mg/dL

c. No evidence of graft rejection for 6 months

d. No identifiable pyelocalyceal distention by urography

53–21. Which of the following statements about polycystic kidney disease is true?

a. It is usually X-linked inheritance.

b. Renal complications are more common in women than men.

c. The majority of cases are due to the PKD3 mutation on chromosome 4.

d. 10% of those with this disease die from rupture of an intracranial berry aneurysm.

53–22. Which of the following is a pulmonary-renal syndrome?

a. Berger disease

b. Goodpasture syndrome

c. Minimal change disease

d. Focal segmental glomerulosclerosis

53–23. Which of the following does not characterize nephrotic syndromes?

a. Edema
b. Heavy proteinuria
c. Hyperalbuminemia
d. Hypercholesterolemia

53–24. Which of the following complications is not increased in pregnant patients with nephrotic syndrome?

a. Anemia
b. Preeclampsia
c. Renal insufficiency
d. Postterm pregnancy

53–25. Which of the following is most likely to lead to end-stage renal disease?

a. Diabetes
b. Hypertension
c. Glomerulonephritis
d. Polycystic kidney disease

53–26. By what creatinine does one define moderate renal impairment in patients with chronic renal disease?

a. 1–1.5 mg/dL
b. 1.5–3.0 mg/dL
c. 3.0–4.5 mg/dL
d. 5–7 mg/dL

53–27. Which of the following plans in a pregnant patient on dialysis is correct?

a. If the patient's creatinine is less than 7 mg/dL, the dialysis can be held.
b. Change from peritoneal dialysis to hemodialysis because outcomes are worse in cases of peritoneal dialysis.
c. Increase the frequency of dialysis to avoid the abrupt volume changes which could result in hypotension.
d. Decrease the frequency of dialysis because the glomerular filtration rate will increase with increasing blood volume, making dialysis less necessary.

53–28. When managing a patient with postpartum acute kidney injury, which of the following medications does not need to have its dose adjusted?

a. Gentamycin
b. Clindamycin
c. Magnesium sulfate
d. Ketorolac tromethamine

53–29. What is the most common reason for acute kidney injury in obstetrics?

a. Sepsis
b. Acute blood loss
c. Use of loop diuretics
d. Ureteral injury at cesarean section

53–30. A pregnant woman presents with flank pain. She is afebrile but tachycardic from pain. Her serum creatinine is elevated to 5 mg/dL. Images from her magnetic resonance imaging are presented below. Which of the following is the best plan of care?

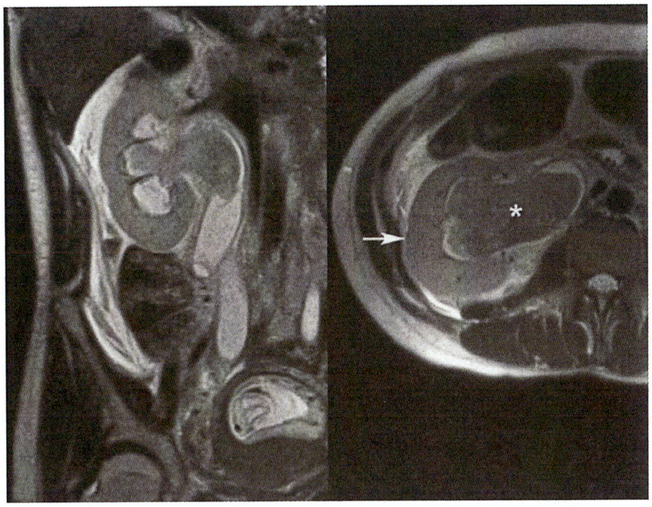

Reproduced with permission from Cunningham FG, Leveno KJ, Bloom SL, et al (eds): Renal and urinary tract disorders. In Williams Obstetrics, 25th ed. New York, McGraw-Hill, 2018, Figure 53-6A and 53-6B.

a. Renal biopsy
b. Nephrectomy
c. Percutaneous nephrostomy tube
d. Intravenous antibiotics and aggressive fluid hydration

53–31. Which of the following is not commonly found in patients with a urethral diverticulum?

a. Pain
b. Palpable mass
c. Urinary retention
d. Recurrent urinary infections

53–32. Which of the following circumstances is most likely to lead to fistula formation?

a. Rupture of a posterior wall fibroid
b. Prolonged obstructed labor in a resource-poor country
c. A fetus being at +1 station for the week leading up to labor
d. A cesarean section done for breech presentation at term and complicated by a 2-cm extension

CHAPTER 53 ANSWER KEY

Question number	Letter answer	Page cited	Header cited
53–1	**b**	p. 1026	Pregnancy-Induced Urinary Tract Changes
53–2	**b**	p. 1026	Pregnancy-Induced Urinary Tract Changes
53–3	**c**	p. 1026	Assessment of Renal Function During Pregnancy
53–4	**c**	p. 1026	Assessment of Renal Function During Pregnancy
53–5	**d**	p. 1026	Assessment of Renal Function During Pregnancy
53–6	**c**	p. 1026	Pregnancy after Unilateral Nephrectomy
53–7	**c**	p. 1027	Asymptomatic Bacteriuria
53–8	**a**	p. 1027	Table 53-1
53–9	**d**	p. 1027	Treatment
53–10	**d**	p. 1027	Cystitis and Urethritis
53–11	**c**	p. 1028	Acute Pyelonephritis
53–12	**a**	p. 1028	Clinical Findings
53–13	**c**	p. 1028	Clinical Findings
53–14	**c**	p. 1029	Management
53–15	**c**	p. 1029	Outpatient Management
53–16	**b**	p. 1030	Management
53–17	**b**	p. 1030	Management
53–18	**d**	p. 1031	Pregnancy after Renal Transplantation
53–19	**d**	p. 1031	Pregnancy Outcomes
53–20	**a**	p. 1031	Pregnancy Outcomes
53–21	**d**	p. 1031	Polycystic Kidney Disease
53–22	**b**	p. 1032	Table 53-3
53–23	**c**	p. 1033	Nephrotic Syndromes
53–24	**d**	p. 1033	Pregnancy
53–25	**a**	p. 1034	Chronic Kidney Disease
53–26	**b**	p. 1034	Chronic Kidney Disease
53–27	**c**	p. 1036	Dialysis During Pregnancy
53–28	**b**	p. 1036	Diagnosis and Management
53–29	**b**	p. 1037	Prevention
53–30	**c**	p. 1037	Figure 53-6
53–31	**c**	p. 1037	Urethral Diverticulum
53–32	**b**	p. 1037	Urogenital Tract Fistulas

CHAPTER 54

Gastrointestinal Disorders

54–1. Which portion of the gastrointestinal tract is most difficult to visualize with endoscopy?

a. Stomach
b. Esophagus
c. Proximal ileum
d. Proximal jejunum

54–2. A 39-year-old woman at 28 weeks' gestation has experienced multiple episodes of rectal bleeding, and a colonic mass is suspected on abdominal imaging. The decision is made to proceed with colonoscopy for diagnosis. You recommend which of the following alterations to the standard management of patients undergoing endoscopy?

a. Forego bowel preparation
b. Decrease in the dose of IV sedation
c. Intravenous hydration preoperatively
d. Continuous fetal monitoring during the procedure

54–3. A 22-year-old woman at 18 weeks' gestation is admitted with hyperemesis gravidarum that is unresponsive to dietary modifications and antiemetics. She has lost 10 kilograms this pregnancy, and this is her third hospitalization in 6 weeks. You recommend enteral feeds with a nasogastric tube, but she declines requesting parenteral nutrition. You inform her that which of the following is the most common complication of total parenteral nutrition?

a. Hemothorax
b. Pneumothorax
c. Brachial plexus injury
d. Catheter-associated sepsis

54–4. A 24-year-old woman experiences persistent hyperemesis gravidarum throughout her pregnancy with an inability to tolerate most foods despite antiemetic use. She was never able to tolerate prenatal vitamin supplementation. Shortly following an uneventful vaginal delivery her term infant develops seizures. On head ultrasound exam the infant has an intracranial hemorrhage. What nutritional deficiency is most likely responsible?

a. Folic acid
b. Vitamin K
c. Vitamin B_6
d. Vitamin B_{12}

54–5. Which agent is considered first-line treatment for mild nausea and vomiting in pregnancy?

a. Ranitidine
b. Ondansetron
c. Promethazine
d. Doxylamine + pyridoxine

54–6. Which is the strongest risk factor for hyperemesis gravidarum requiring hospitalization?

a. Female fetus
b. Twin gestation
c. *Helicobacter pylori* infection
d. Hospitalization in a previous pregnancy for hyperemesis gravidarum

54–7. What is a potential downside to ondansetron use in pregnancy?

a. It causes sedation.
b. It may cause a prolonged QT.
c. It is teratogenic before 12 weeks' gestation.
d. It is less efficacious than doxylamine + pyridoxine.

54–8. Which should be added to the initial intravenous crystalloid given to correct dehydration in a woman who presents with significant nausea and vomiting of pregnancy?

a. Dextrose
b. Thiamine
c. Pyridoxine
d. Potassium chloride

54–9. Which medication for symptomatic esophageal reflux should not be prescribed during pregnancy?

a. Sucralfate
b. Omeprazole
c. Ranitidine
d. Misoprostol

54–10. Which normal physiological change in pregnancy provides a protective effect against the development of ulcer disease?

a. Decrease in motility
b. Increased mucus secretion
c. Reduced gastric acid secretion
d. All of the above

54–11. A 25-year-old woman at 20 weeks' gestation with hyperemesis gravidarum presents complaining of worsening vomiting (at least 10 episodes per day) with new-onset hematemesis. What is the most likely cause of the bright-red blood seen here on her upper endoscopy?

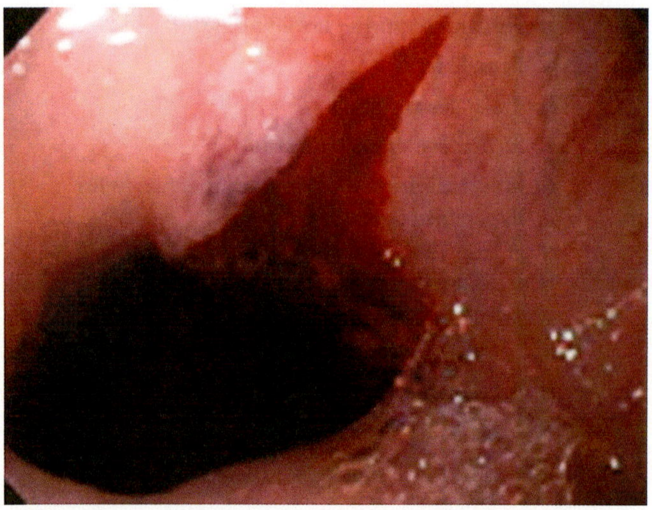

Reproduced with permission from Song LM, Topazian M: Gastrointestinal endoscopy. In Kasper DL, Fauci AS, Hauser SL, et al (eds): Harrison's Principles of Internal Medicine, 19th ed. New York, McGraw-Hill Education, 2015, Figure 345-27.

a Gastritis
b. Peptic ulcer
c. Mallory-Weiss tear
d. Boerhaave syndrome

54–12. A 34-year-old woman at 28 weeks' gestation is diagnosed with symptomatic *Helicobacter pylori* infection. She reports a history of anaphylaxis with penicillin administration in the past. Which is the most appropriate treatment regimen?

a. Omeprazole + amoxicillin + clarithromycin
b. Omeprazole + metronidazole + tetracycline
c. Omeprazole + metronidazole + doxycycline
d. Omeprazole + metronidazole + clarithromycin

54–13. Overall small bowel motility is decreased in pregnancy as compared to nonpregnant women. During which period is transit time slowest?

a. First trimester
b. Second trimester
c. Third trimester
d. Immediately postpartum

54–14. Which finding is an indication for further laboratory evaluation of a diarrheal illness?

a. Temperature >38°C
b. Grossly bloody stools
c. No improvement after >48 hours
d. All of the above

54–15. A 22-year-old woman at 32 weeks' gestation presents with 4–5 episodes daily of nonbloody diarrhea for the last 48 hours. She has moist mucous membranes, is normotensive with a heart rate of 110 beats per minute, has a temperature of 38°C, and has fecal leukocytes. Which of the following is an indication for empiric antibiotics in lieu of awaiting stool culture results?

a. Fecal WBC
b. Fever of 38°C
c. Mild tachycardia
d. Duration of illness

54–16. A 34-year-old woman at 18 weeks' gestation reports acute onset of profuse diarrhea and vomiting at 2 PM today following a group luncheon at work. She also reports multiple other coworkers are experiencing the same complaints. Which is the most likely pathogen?

a. Rotavirus
b. *Salmonella*
c. *Staphylococcus*
d. *Escherichia coli* O157:H7

54–17. Which antibiotic is not associated with subsequent *Clostridium difficile* infection?

a. Clindamycin
b. Metronidazole
c. Cephalosporins
d. Aminopenicillins

54–18. Which finding is more specific to Crohn disease as compared to ulcerative colitis?

a. Diarrhea
b. pANCA antibodies
c. Rectal involvement
d. Perianal involvement

54–19. Which medical morbidity is significantly more common with ulcerative colitis as compared to Crohn disease?

a. Colon cancer
b. Perirectal abscess
c. Arthritis and uveitis
d. Venous thromboembolism

54–20. A 32-year-old woman presents with recurrent episodes of abdominal pain, diarrhea, and fever. She undergoes colonoscopy with the finding of transmural lesions affecting the terminal ileum and colon. She asks what effect this disease will have on future pregnancies and whether there is benefit to undergoing treatment before attempting to conceive. Which of the following do you tell her?

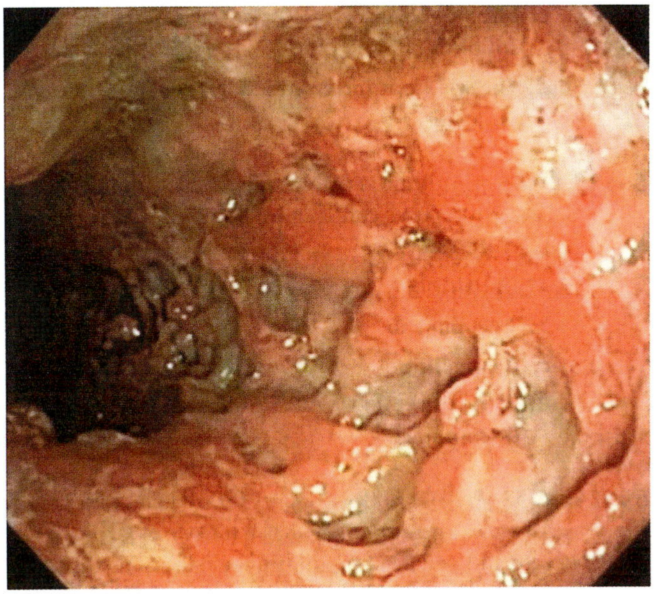

Reproduced with permission from Song LM, Topazian M: Gastrointestinal endoscopy. In Longo DL, Fauci AS, Kasper DL, et al (eds): Harrison's Principles of Internal Medicine, 18th ed. New York, McGraw-Hill, 2012, Figure 291-4B.

a. Proctocolectomy is curative.
b. Pregnancy increases her risk of a disease flare.
c. Infertility is to be expected, even if she enters remission.
d. If she requires bowel resection, laparoscopic surgery is associated with a higher subsequent fertility rate.

54–21. Which statement regarding inflammatory bowel disease and pregnancy is most accurate?

a. Surgery should be deferred until the postpartum period.
b. The incidence of disease flares increases during pregnancy.
c. Most treatment regimens should be discontinued in pregnancy.
d. Active disease in early pregnancy increases the likelihood of a poor pregnancy outcome.

54–22. A 31-year-old nulliparous woman with a history of ulcerative colitis with ileal pouch–anal anastomosis 3 years ago presents for preconception counseling. She asks if there are any complications to expect with pregnancy given her history. Which statement is most correct?

a. She will require a primary cesarean delivery.
b. She will be at increased risk for preterm birth.
c. She will be at increased risk for miscarriage and stillbirth.
d. She will be at increased risk for incontinence and pouchitis.

54–23. Which medication commonly used for moderate to severe ulcerative colitis should be discontinued during pregnancy?

a. Infliximab
b. Adalimumab
c. Azathioprine
d. None of the above medications should be discontinued

54–24. A 32-year-old G2P1 presents for prenatal care at 18 weeks' gestation. She has a history of Crohn disease and had been on multiple medications throughout the first trimester. Which medication is most likely responsible for the abnormality seen on her sonogram in this image?

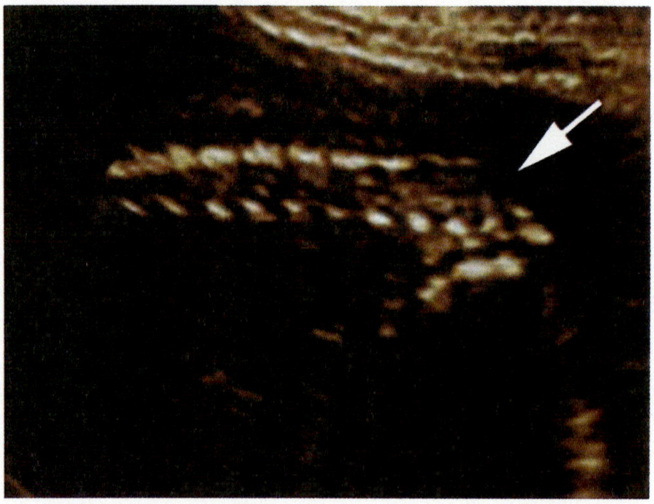

a. Cyclosporine
b. Sulfasalazine
c. 6-Mercaptopurine
d. Mycophenolate mofetil

54–25. Which statement regarding ostomies and pregnancy is true?

a. The majority of women require cesarean delivery.
b. Bowel obstruction is common, occurring in 30% of cases.
c. Long-term ostomy function is worsened by pregnancy.
d. Most women experience minimal ostomy dysfunction.

54–26. Which is the least common cause of bowel obstruction in pregnancy?

a. Volvulus
b. Malignancy
c. Intussusception
d. Prior abdominal surgery

54–27. Why is the diagnosis of appendicitis in pregnancy difficult?

a. A low-level leukocytosis is normal in pregnancy.
b. Nausea and vomiting are often experienced in pregnancy.
c. The anatomical location of the appendix changes with pregnancy progression.
d. All of the above

54–28. What is the preferred modality for the diagnosis of suspected appendicitis in pregnancy?

a. Computed tomography
b. Plain abdominal radiograph
c. Magnetic resonance imaging
d. Graded compression sonography

54–29. During what part of pregnancy is a patient most likely to be diagnosed with a ruptured appendix?

a. First trimester
b. Second trimester
c. Third trimester
d. Postpartum

54–30. What are the most reproducible findings in a pregnant woman with appendicitis?

a. Fever
b. Anorexia
c. Nausea and vomiting
d. Persistent abdominal pain and tenderness

54–31. A patient in the midtrimester presents with colicky abdominal pain, nausea, and vomiting. At laparotomy, surgical findings are similar to those shown here. What is her likely diagnosis?

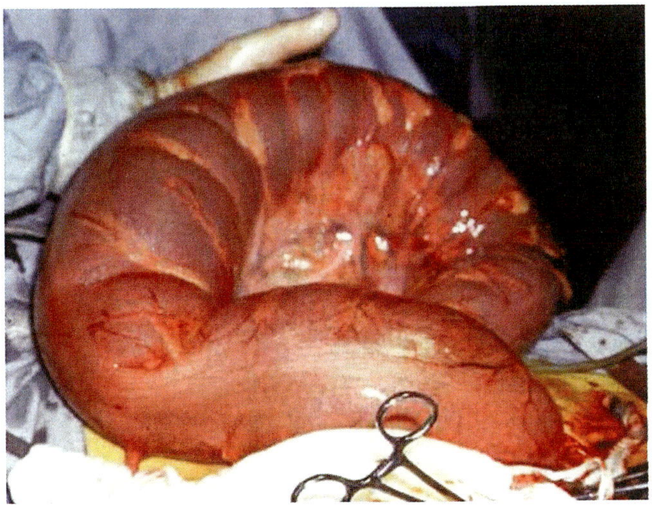

Reproduced with permission from Cunningham FG, Leveno KJ, Bloom SL, et al (eds): Gastrointestinal disorders. In Williams Obstetrics, 24th ed. New York, McGraw-Hill, 2014, Figure 54-4.

a. Volvulus
b. Perforation
c. Crohn disease
d. Ulcerative colitis

54–32. Which of the following diagnostic studies are considered safe to use in pregnancy?

a. Cystoscopy
b. Flexible sigmoidoscopy
c. Endoscopic retrograde cholangiopancreatography
d. All of the above

54–33. A pregnant patient with history of swallowing problems presents with dysphagia, chest pain, and vomiting. A barium swallow done just prior to pregnancy revealed these images. What is the patient's diagnosis?

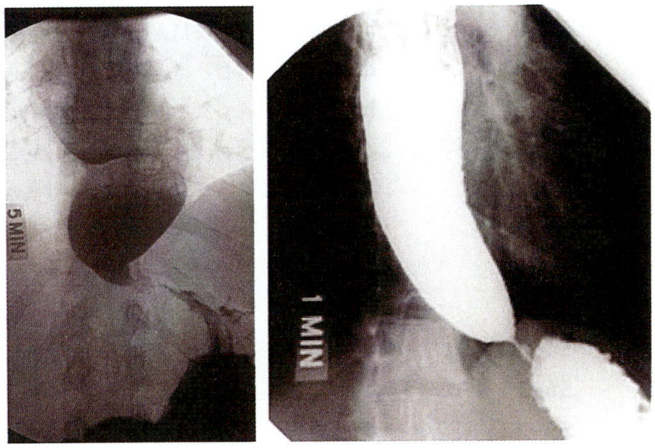

Reproduced with permission from Kahrilas PJ, Hirano I: Diseases of the esophagus. In Longo DL, Fauci AS, Kasper DL (eds): Harrison's Principles of Internal Medicine, 18th ed. New York, McGraw-Hill, 2012, Figure 292-5.

a. Achalasia
b. Hiatal hernia
c. Peptic ulcer disease
d. Congenital diaphragmatic hernia

54–34. Why is high-dose folic acid supplementation indicated in pregnant patients with inflammatory bowel disease?

a. To prevent fetal neural tube defects
b. Bowel inflammation may decrease absorption
c. To counteract the anti-folate actions of sulfasalazine
d. All of the above

54–35. What is the rate of hospital readmission in patients with hyperemesis gravidarum?

a. 5%
b. 15%
c. 30%
d. 45%

54–36. Cases of bowel obstruction in pregnancy are least likely to occur during which of the following timeframes?

a. Early first trimester
b. Midpregnancy
c. Third trimester
d. Immediately postpartum

CHAPTER 54 ANSWER KEY

Question number	Letter answer	Page cited	Header cited
54–1	**c**	p. 1042	Diagnostic Techniques
54–2	**c**	p. 1042	Diagnostic Techniques
54–3	**d**	p. 1043	Nutritional Support
54–4	**b**	p. 1044	Hyperemesis Gravidarum
54–5	**d**	p. 1044	Hyperemesis Gravidarum
54–6	**d**	p. 1044	Hyperemesis Gravidarum
54–7	**b**	p. 1045	Hyperemesis Gravidarum
54–8	**b**	p. 1045	Hyperemesis Gravidarum
54–9	**d**	p. 1046	Gastroesophageal Reflux Disease
54–10	**d**	p. 1047	Peptic Ulcer Disease
54–11	**c**	p. 1047	Upper Gastrointestinal Bleeding
54–12	**d**	p. 1047	Peptic Ulcer Disease
54–13	**c**	p. 1047	Small Bowel and Colon Disorders
54–14	**d**	p. 1048	Acute Diarrhea
54–15	**a**	p. 1048	Acute Diarrhea
54–16	**c**	p. 1048	Acute Diarrhea
54–17	**b**	p. 1048	*Clostridium difficile* Infection
54–18	**d**	p. 1049	Inflammatory Bowel Disease and Pregnancy
54–19	**a**	p. 1049	Inflammatory Bowel Disease and Pregnancy
54–20	**d**	p. 1050	Inflammatory Bowel Disease and Pregnancy
54–21	**d**	p. 1050	Inflammatory Bowel Disease and Pregnancy
54–22	**d**	p. 1050	Inflammatory Bowel Disease and Pregnancy
54–23	**d**	p. 1050	Inflammatory Bowel Disease and Pregnancy
54–24	**d**	p. 1051	Inflammatory Bowel Disease and Pregnancy
54–25	**d**	p. 1051	Ostomy and Pregnancy
54–26	**b**	p. 1052	Intestinal Obstruction
54–27	**d**	p. 1052	Appendicitis
54–28	**c**	p. 1053	Appendicitis
54–29	**c**	p. 1052	Appendicitis
54–30	**d**	p. 1053	Appendicitis
54–31	**a**	p. 1052	Intestinal Obstruction
54–32	**d**	p. 1042	Diagnostic Techniques
54–33	**a**	p. 1046	Achalasia
54–34	**d**	p. 1050	Inflammatory Bowel Disease and Pregnancy
54–35	**c**	p. 1044	Hyperemesis Gravidarum
54–36	**a**	p. 1052	Intestinal Obstruction

CHAPTER 55

Hepatic, Biliary, and Pancreatic Disorders

55–1. All except which of the following liver-related changes are physiological in pregnancy?
- **a.** Hypolipidemia
- **b.** Spider angiomas
- **c.** Palmar erythema
- **d.** Elevated serum alkaline phosphatase levels

55–2. The cytochrome P450 system is altered by which of the following during pregnancy?
- **a.** Estrogen levels
- **b.** Progesterone levels
- **c.** Placental expression
- **d.** All of the above

55–3. Which of the following pregnancy-related complications has the capacity to demonstrate the most prominent alterations of normal hepatic, renal, hematological, and coagulation laboratory studies?
- **a.** Preeclampsia
- **b.** Hyperemesis gravidarum
- **c.** Acute fatty liver of pregnancy
- **d.** Intrahepatic cholestasis of pregnancy

55–4. Which of the following findings can narrow the differential of elevated liver enzymes to exclude intrahepatic cholestasis of pregnancy?
- **a.** Jaundice
- **b.** AST 800 U/L
- **c.** Liver biopsy showing bile plugs in the hepatocytes
- **d.** All of the above

55–5. Which of the following viral infections has been associated with a marked increase in the risk for intrahepatic cholestasis of pregnancy?
- **a.** Hepatitis B
- **b.** Hepatitis C
- **c.** Cytomegalovirus
- **d.** Human immunodeficiency virus

55–6. A 27-year-old multigravida comes to you for her postpartum visit. Both of her pregnancies were complicated by intrahepatic cholestasis of pregnancy. She desires another child in about 2 years. Which of the following methods of contraception do you recommend?
- **a.** Vaginal ring
- **b.** Copper intrauterine device
- **c.** Combination oral contraceptive pills
- **d.** None of the above

55–7. Which of the following have the best data for treatment of intrahepatic cholestasis of pregnancy?
- **a.** Cholestyramine
- **b.** Dexamethasone
- **c.** Low-cholesterol diet
- **d.** Ursodeoxycholic acid

55–8. A 32-year-old G1 at 32 weeks' gestation is diagnosed with intrahepatic cholestasis of pregnancy. During the visit she inquires about whether this diagnosis will alter her prenatal care or delivery plans. What is the best evidence-based advice you can provide?
- **a.** We can avoid risk for stillbirth with weekly fetal nonstress testing.
- **b.** Since your bile acid levels are <10 μmol/L, delivery will be recommended before 39 weeks' gestation.
- **c.** If we pursue delivery at 38–39 weeks' gestation, we will avoid neonatal sequelae of intrahepatic cholestasis of pregnancy.
- **d.** None of the above

55–9. What is the incidence and recurrence risk of acute fatty liver of pregnancy?
- **a.** 1 in 10,000 pregnancies, and recurrence is rare
- **b.** 1 in 100,000 pregnancies, and recurrence is rare
- **c.** 1 in 100,000 pregnancies, and recurrence is common
- **d.** 1 in 1,000,000 pregnancies, and recurrence is rare

55–10. Maternal acute fatty liver of pregnancy is associated with all except with of the following recessively inherited abnormalities of mitochondrial fatty acid oxidation?

a. Carnitine palmitoyltransferase 1
b. Dihydrolipoamide dehydrogenase
c. Medium-chain acyl-CoA dehydrogenase
d. Long-chain-3-hydroxyacyl-CoA-dehydrogenase

55–11. From an etiopathogenesis perspective, the pregnancy-related complication pictured here is analogous to which childhood illness?

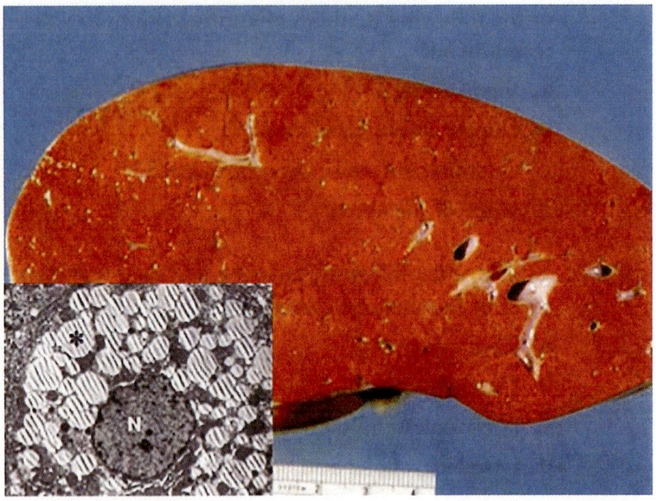

Reproduced with permission from Cunningham FC, Leveno KJ, Bloom SL, et al (eds): Hepatic, biliary, and pancreatic disorders. In Williams Obstetrics, 25th ed. New York, McGraw-Hill, 2018, Figure 55-1.

a. Biliary atresia
b. Reye-like syndromes
c. Autoimmune hepatitis
d. Epstein-Barr viral hepatitis

55–12. A 26-year-old primigravida presents at 34 weeks' gestation with nausea and vomiting, fatigue, and epigastric pain. All except which of the following are clinical characteristics that increase her risk for acute fatty liver of pregnancy as the underlying cause?

a. Nulliparity
b. Female fetus
c. Twin gestation
d. Third trimester

55–13. You know that nausea and vomiting in the third trimester is not something to be dismissed, so you start the work-up on the patient in Question 55–12. Which combination of laboratory findings below would be most concerning for acute fatty liver of pregnancy?

a. Hematocrit 34%, creatinine 1.1 mg/dL, platelets 190/L, AST 60 U/L, fibrinogen 450 mg/dL, and glucose 96 mg/dL
b. Hematocrit 32%, creatinine 2.0 mg/dL, platelets 90/L, AST 400 U/L, fibrinogen 130 mg/dL, and glucose 65 mg/dL
c. Hematocrit 39%, creatinine 1.2 mg/dL, platelets 90/L, AST 80 U/L, fibrinogen 450 mg/dL, and glucose 105 mg/dL
d. Hematocrit 30%, creatinine 1.0 mg/dL, platelets 200/L, AST 600 U/L, fibrinogen 420 mg/dL, and glucose 120 mg/dL

55–14. You send a peripheral blood smear on the patient in Question 55–12, and a representative slide is shown below. What is the underlying etiology of the blood smear findings?

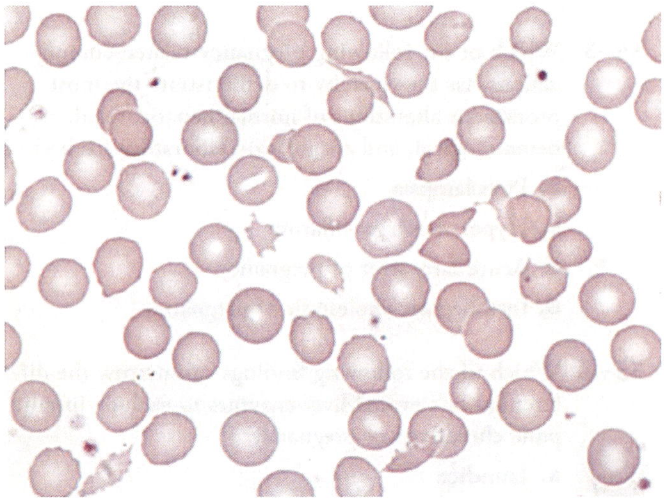

Reproduced with permission from Lichtman MA, Beutler E, Kipps TJ: Color Atlas III: Red cell morphology. In Williams Hematology, 7th ed. New York, McGraw-Hill, 2006, Plate III-3.

a. Autoimmune antibody binding
b. Decreased cholesterol production
c. Increased destruction in the spleen
d. Thrombotic microangiopathy in microvessels

55–15. Which imaging modality is recommended in discriminating acute fatty liver of pregnancy from other etiologies of elevated liver enzymes?

a. Computed tomography
b. Magnetic resonance imaging
c. Ultrasound with color Doppler
d. None of the above

55–16. Risk of maternal death with acute fatty liver is related to which of the following?

a. Sepsis
b. Hemorrhage
c. Renal failure
d. All of the above

55–17. After delivery, the liver function deterioration of acute fatty liver of pregnancy halted. Nonetheless, you recommend continued intensive maternal surveillance due to the approximately 20% risk of developing which of the following in the days after delivery?

a. Sepsis
b. Hemorrhage
c. Diabetes mellitus
d. Acute pancreatitis

55–18. Which of the following statements regarding acute viral hepatitis is correct?

a. Jaundice is usually the presenting symptom.
b. Low-grade fever is more common with hepatitis A.
c. Bilirubin levels typically fall as transaminase levels rise.
d. Serum transaminase levels correspond with disease severity.

55–19. Which of the following features are criteria for severe disease that should prompt hospitalization for acute viral hepatitis?

a. Hyperglycemia
b. AST over 500 U/L
c. Hyperalbuminemia
d. Hyperbilirubinemia

55–20. During the hospital care of a patient with acute viral hepatitis, which of the following personal protective equipment should be used at all times?

a. Gloves
b. N95 respiratory mask
c. Negative-pressure ventilation hospital room
d. All of the above

55–21. During a cesarean delivery you sustain a needle stick. The patient's prenatal record was not available at admission, so her infectious serologies are pending at the time of your contact. Immunization is not available for which of the following?

a. Hepatitis A
b. Hepatitis B
c. Hepatitis C
d. It is available for all three

55–22. The following viral serologies are resulted for the patient in Question 55–21. What is her diagnosis?

IgA Anti-Hepatitis B core antibody	+
Hepatitis B surface antibody	–
Hepatitis B e antigen	+

a. History of hepatitis B vaccination
b. Chronic hepatitis B infection, still active
c. History of hepatitis B infection, now latent
d. It is not possible to make a diagnosis from the serologies presented

55–23. How do you counsel the patient in Question 55–21 regarding her lab results?

a. She has a virus that can lead to cirrhosis and death, and you will refer her to a hepatologist for discussion of ribavirin therapy.
b. She does not need to be concerned. Her results represent vaccination for Hepatitis B, and she should have lifelong antibodies.
c. She has a virus that can lead to cirrhosis and death, but it appears dormant. You will refer her to a hepatologist for surveillance.
d. She has an active virus that can lead to cirrhosis and death, and you will refer her to a hepatologist for long-term management recommendations.

55–24. Lactation is contraindicated for women infected with which of the following?

a. Hepatitis A
b. Hepatitis B
c. Hepatitis C
d. None of the above

55–25. The Society for Maternal-Fetal Medicine recommended which of the following agents for women with high hepatitis B viral loads in pregnancy?

a. Ribavirin
b. Tenofovir
c. Lamivudine
d. Telbivudine

55–26. Chronic hepatitis B infection is most likely to develop after acquisition by which of the following patients?

a. 9-year-old child
b. Newborn infant
c. 28-year-old healthy woman
d. Risk is equivalent in all of the above

55–27. Which of the following combinations represents appropriate screening for hepatitis C in pregnancy?

a. 27-year-old woman with human immunodeficiency virus screened via anti-hepatitis C antibody

b. 26-year-old woman with a history of skin abscesses from heroin use screened via anti-hepatitis C antibody

c. 37-year-old woman with a history of blood transfusion after her last pregnancy in 2014 screened via hepatitis C RNA

d. 15-year-old woman whose mother was a chronic intravenous drug user and died of liver failure when the patient was 4 years old screened via hepatitis C RNA

55–28. A 29-year-old primigravida presents to you for prenatal care. She is known to have hepatitis C with no known risk factors, and your prenatal labs confirm presence of hepatitis C RNA and anti-hepatitis C antibody. Compared to a woman with anti-hepatitis C antibody who is RNA-negative, which of the following is more likely to complicate her pregnancy?

a. Preterm delivery

b. Fetal growth restriction

c. Vertical transmission of hepatitis C

d. None of the above

55–29. A 21-year-old nulligravida with Sjögren syndrome presents at 26 weeks' gestation with nausea, fatigue, and vague abdominal pain. On exam she has a blood pressure of 94/58 mmHg and you notice mild jaundice. Laboratory assessment shows severely elevated transaminases and anti-nuclear and anti-smooth muscle antibodies. Based on your primary diagnostic suspicion, how do you counsel her regarding complications of pregnancy?

a. She is at increased risk for preeclampsia.

b. She is at increased risk for preterm delivery.

c. She is at increased risk for cesarean delivery.

d. All of the above

55–30. A 23-year-old nulligravida and her husband present for preconception counseling. She has Wilson disease that is being treated with zinc sulfate. Which of the following should be included in your counseling?

a. Her husband should consider carrier testing.

b. Upon confirmation of pregnancy, she should discontinue her chelation therapy.

c. Available data suggests she should convert to penicillamine prior to conception, as it is a better chelating agent.

d. All of the above

55–31. A 36-year-old multigravida presents for preconception counseling. Her obstetric history includes two full-term vaginal deliveries after pregnancies complicated by gestational diabetes and a first-trimester pregnancy loss. She comes to you to discuss her recent diagnosis of nonalcoholic fatty liver disease (NAFLD) by her primary care physician. Diagnosis was based on imaging performed for an episode of abdominal pain. Her liver function tests are normal. Her medical history is otherwise notable for longstanding obesity (body mass index 34 kg/m^2) and diabetes (hemoglobin A_{1c} 8.2%) diagnosed 2 years ago. Which of the following should be included in your counseling?

a. The best interventions to reduce the risk to a future pregnancy are weight loss and optimizing her glucose control.

b. Compared to women of similar weight, because of the NAFLD, she has a much higher risk for liver-related adverse pregnancy outcome.

c. With normal liver enzymes, you question the diagnosis of NAFLD and recommend that she seek a second opinion from a gastroenterologist

d. All of the above

55–32. This image shows the typical nodular, fibrotic appearance of a cirrhotic liver. What is the most common cause of this condition in the general population?

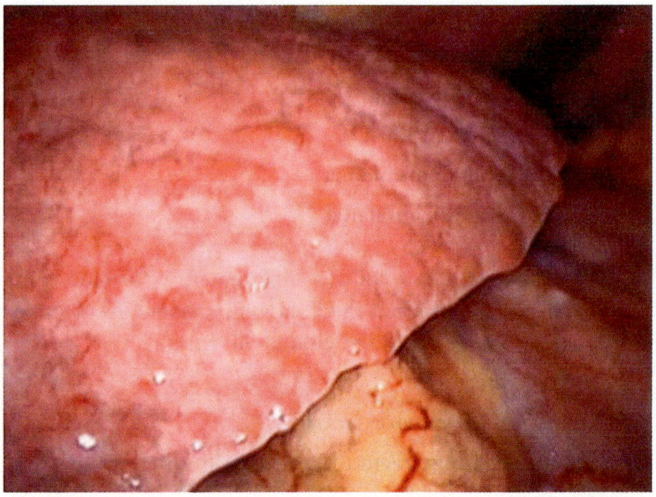

Reproduced with permission from Geller DA, Goss JA, Tsung A: Liver. In Brunicardi FC, Anderson DK, Billiar TR, et al (eds): Schwartz's Principles of Surgery, 9th ed. New York, McGraw-Hill, 2010, Figure 31-16a.

a. Viral hepatitis

b. Alcohol exposure

c. Autoimmune hepatitis

d. Nonalcoholic fatty liver disease

55–33. A 32-year-old nulligravida presents for preconception counseling due to cirrhosis with esophageal varices. Which of the following should be included in your counseling?

a. You do not recommend that she become pregnant.

b. 1/3 to 1/2 of women with varices will have bleeding in pregnancy and this carries an 18% mortality rate.

c. Without variceal rupture there is high risk for liver failure, preterm delivery, fetal growth restriction, and maternal death.

d. All of the above

55–34. A 27-year-old at 32 weeks' gestation is brought to the emergency room by ambulance after consuming 6 grams of acetaminophen. Which of the following is true?

a. The fetus is not at risk, so no monitoring is necessary.

b. *N*-Acetyl-*p*-benzoquinoneimine should be administered promptly.

c. This is the most common cause of acute liver failure in the United States.

d. All of the above

55–35. A 31-year-old at 20 weeks' gestation presents to the emergency room with complaints of right upper quadrant pain, fever, and vomiting. Exam reveals right upper quadrant tenderness, and she has a temperature of 38.7°C. One diagnostic image is shown here. Common bile duct obstruction is not suspected. What is the next most appropriate step in her management?

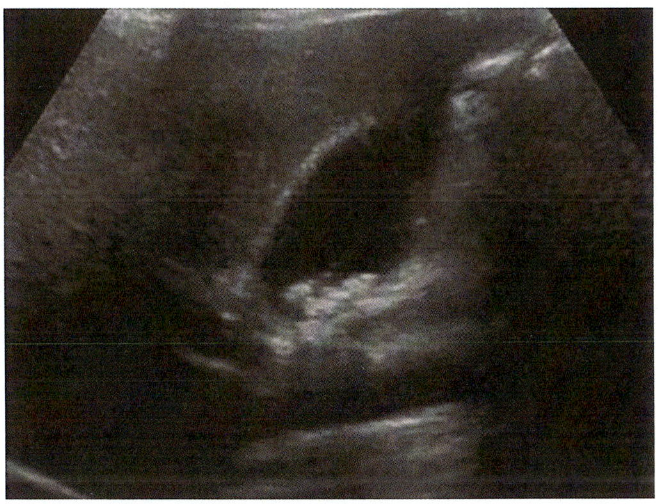

Used with permission from Dr. Barbara Hoffman.

a. Laparoscopic cholecystectomy

b. Endoscopic retrograde cholangiopancreatography

c. Admit for serial abdominal examinations and intravenous antibiotics

d. Discharge home with oral antibiotics, pain medication, and antiemetics

55–36. Which of the following is true regarding pancreatitis in pregnancy?

a. Severity is correlated to the degree of enzyme elevation.

b. The primary predisposing condition in pregnancy is cholelithiasis.

c. The Apache II scoring system is the most appropriate for pancreatitis in pregnancy.

d. Total parenteral nutrition is the preferred method of providing nutrition in severe pancreatitis.

55–37. A 32-year-old at 26 weeks' gestation has a 3.4-cm liver mass noted incidentally on a right upper quadrant ultrasound. She undergoes magnetic resonance imaging for further clarification. Which of the following is true?

a. Due to size and bleeding risk, surgical resection is indicated if it is a hepatic adenoma.

b. If it is a hepatic adenoma, there is a 5% risk of malignant transformation, so biopsy should be performed next.

c. If it is focal nodular hyperplasia, estrogen-containing birth control pills are not a good contraceptive option postpartum.

d. None of the above

CHAPTER 55 ANSWER KEY

Question number	Letter answer	Page cited	Header cited
55–1	**a**	p. 1058	Hepatic Disorders
55–2	**d**	p. 1058	Hepatic Disorders
55–3	**c**	p. 1059	Table 55-1
55–4	**b**	p. 1059	Pathogenesis Clinical Presentation
55–5	**b**	p. 1059	Clinical Presentation
55–6	**b**	p. 1059	Pathogenesis
55–7	**c**	p. 1059	Management
55–8	**d**	p. 1060	Pregnancy Outcomes
55–9	**a**	p. 1060	Acute Fatty Liver of Pregnancy
55–10	**b**	p. 1061	Etiopathogenesis
55–11	**b**	p. 1060	Etiopathogenesis
55–12	**b**	p. 1061	Clinical Findings
55–13	**b**	p. 1061	Clinical Findings
55–14	**b**	p. 1061	Clinical Findings
55–15	**d**	p. 1061	Clinical Findings
55–16	**d**	p. 1062	Management
55–17	**d**	p. 1062	Management
55–18	**b**	p. 1062	Acute Viral Hepatitis
55–19	**d**	p. 1062	Acute Viral Hepatitis
55–20	**a**	p. 1062	Acute Viral Hepatitis
55–21	**c**	p. 1062 p. 1063 p. 1065	Acute Viral Hepatitis Hepatitis A Pregnancy and Hepatitis B
55–22	**b**	p. 1064	Hepatitis B Figure 55-2
55–23	**d**	p. 1064	Hepatitis B
55–24	**d**	p. 1063 p. 1065 p. 1065	Hepatitis A Pregnancy and Hepatitis B Pregnancy and Hepatitis C
55–25	**b**	p. 1064	Pregnancy and Hepatitis B
55–26	**b**	p. 1064	Hepatitis B
55–27	**d**	p. 1065	Hepatitis C
55–28	**c**	p. 1065	Pregnancy and Hepatitis C
55–29	**b**	p. 1066	Autoimmune Hepatitis
55–30	**a**	p. 1067	Iron and Copper Overload
55–31	**a**	p. 1067	Nonalcoholic Fatty Liver Disease
55–32	**b**	p. 1067	Cirrhosis
55–33	**d**	p. 1067 p. 1068	Cirrhosis Portal Hypertension and Esophageal Varices
55–34	**c**	p. 1068	Acetaminophen Overdose Hepatotoxicity
55–35	**a**	p. 1070	Medical versus Surgical Management Endoscopic Retrograde Cholangiopancreatography
55–36	**b**	p. 1070 p. 1071 p. 1071	Pancreatitis Diagnosis Management
55–37	**d**	p. 1068 p. 1069	Focal Nodular Hyperplasia Hepatic Adenoma

CHAPTER 56

Hematological Disorders

56–1. What hemoglobin value is used to define anemia in the second trimester of pregnancy?

a. 9.5 g/dL
b. 10.0 g/dL
c. 10.5 g/dL
d. 11.0 g/dL

56–2. Which of the following adverse pregnancy outcomes is associated with anemia in pregnancy?

a. Stillbirth
b. Preeclampsia
c. Preterm birth
d. All of the above

56–3. What is the maternal iron requirement in pregnancy for a typical singleton gestation?

a. 500 mg
b. 800 mg
c. 1000 mg
d. 1200 mg

56–4. A 22-year-old G1 presents to your office at 32 weeks' gestation. Routine laboratory assessment reveals a hemoglobin of 8 g/dL with a mean corpuscular volume of 81 fL. As a part of the work-up for her anemia, a peripheral smear is performed, which is shown. What is the most likely diagnosis?

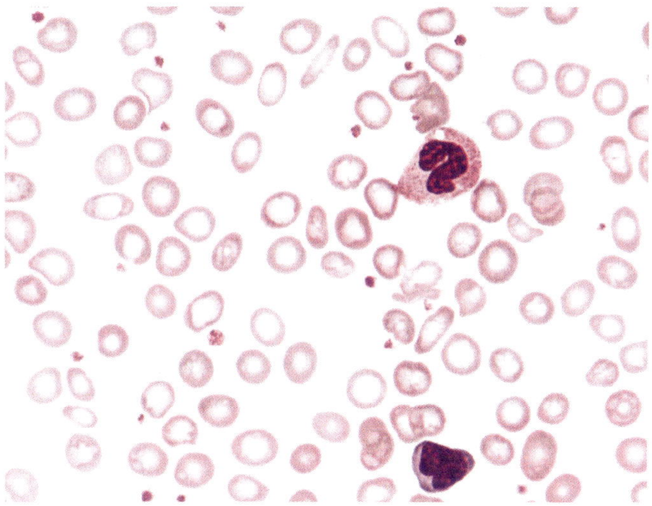

Reproduced with permission from Werner CL, Richardson DL, Chang SY, et al (eds): Perioperative Considerations. In Williams Gynecology Study Guide, 3rd ed. New York, McGraw-Hill Education, 2016, Q39-18.

a. Iron-deficiency anemia
b. Acute blood loss anemia
c. Anemia of chronic disease
d. Anemia resulting from folate deficiency

56–5. Your patient is diagnosed with severe iron-deficiency anemia at 34 weeks' gestation, for which you recommend ferrous sulfate supplementation three times daily. If you repeat a complete blood count one week after starting iron therapy, what would you expect to see if she is compliant with taking her iron?

a. A 20% rise in her hematocrit
b. An elevated reticulocyte count
c. An increase in red cell distribution width
d. An increase in the mean corpuscular volume

56–6. A 36-year-old G3P3 is postoperative day 3 following a repeat cesarean delivery with a 2-liter estimated blood loss due to lysis of adhesions. She reports feeling well and denies dizziness or palpitations when ambulating. Her blood pressure is 100/60 mmHg, her pulse is 92 beats per minute, and her postpartum hemoglobin is stable at 7.2 g/dL. Which of the following would you advise based on her clinical status?

a. Transfusion of 2 units of blood

b. Repeat a complete blood count emergently

c. Three months of iron supplementation at discharge

d. All of the above

56–7. You are caring for a 29-year-old G1 who suffers from long-standing type 1 diabetes and is currently 28 weeks pregnant. Her baseline creatinine at the beginning of pregnancy was 1.5 mg/dL. Her third-trimester complete blood count reveals a hematocrit of 19% with a ferritin of 150 ng/mL. She reports overall feeling well except for mild fatigue, and her vitals are as follows: pulse 82 beats per minute, blood pressure 128/78 mmHg, and temperature 36.8°C. What is the best next course of action for this patient?

a. Consult nephrology

b. Admit to the hospital for observation

c. Administer recombinant erythropoietin

d. All of the above

56–8. A 39-year-old G2P1 at 22 weeks' gestation complains of extreme fatigue. Laboratory evaluation reveals a hemoglobin of 7.3 g/dL, platelet count of 102,000/μL, and a mean corpuscular volume of 122 fL. A peripheral smear is performed for further evaluation and is shown below. Based on the findings, what additional symptom is she most likely to complain of?

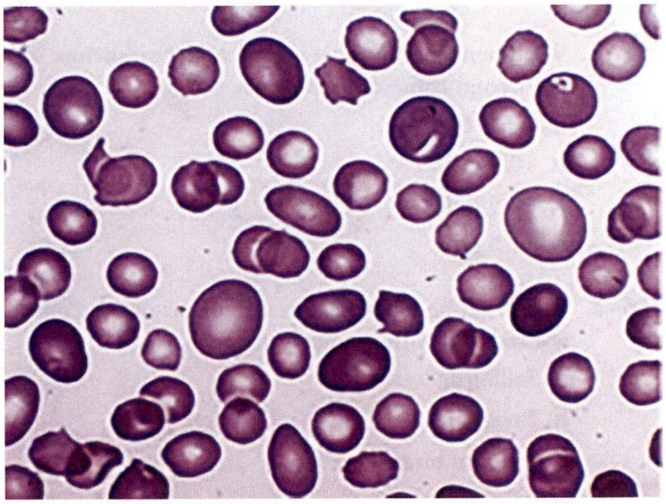

Reproduced with permission from Green R: Folate, cobalamin, and megaloblastic anemia. In Lichtman MA, Kipps TJ, Seligsohn U (eds): Williams Hematology, 8th ed. New York, McGraw-Hill, 2010, Figure 41-12A.

a. Dry skin

b. Anorexia

c. Hair loss

d. Excessive perspiration

56–9. Which of the following is not a cause of vitamin B_{12} deficiency encountered in pregnancy?

a. Crohn disease

b. Ulcerative colitis

c. History of Roux-en-Y gastric bypass

d. Prior ileal resection following trauma

56–10. One of your patients was recently diagnosed with mononucleosis while 20 weeks pregnant. Three weeks after her diagnosis, she complains that her fatigue is worsening rather than improving, although she denies shortness of breath or palpitations. Laboratory evaluation reveals a hemoglobin of 6.8 mg/dL and a positive direct Coombs test. What treatment could you consider offering?

a. Iron supplementation

b. Monoclonal antibody therapy

c. Intravenous immunoglobulin infusion

d. None of the above are indicated

56–11. Which of the following is true regarding paroxysmal nocturnal hemoglobinuria?

a. Hemoglobinuria develops at irregular intervals

b. Almost half of patients suffer venous thromboses

c. Often precipitated by transfusions, infection or surgery

d. All of the above

56–12. Your 25-weeks-pregnant patient has hereditary spherocytosis due to spectrin deficiency, which was diagnosed prior to pregnancy. Her electron micrograph demonstrating spherocytes is shown below. What is the chance she will pass this to her offspring, assuming her husband does not carry the disease?

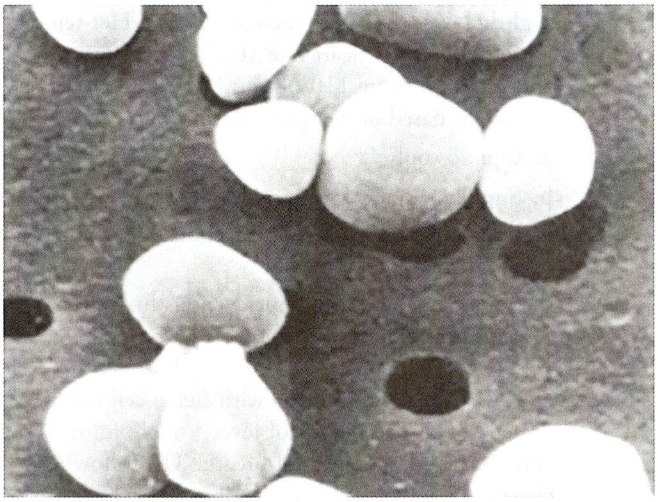

Reproduced with permission from Cunningham FG, Leveno KJ, Bloom SL, et al (eds): Hematological disorders. In Williams Obstetrics, 24th ed. New York, McGraw-Hill, 2014, Figure 56-2B.

a. 0%

b. 25%

c. 50%

d. This deficiency does not demonstrate germline inheritance

56–13. Which of the following erythrocyte enzyme deficiencies can result in hydrops fetalis in a fetus that is a homozygous carrier of the mutation?

a. Ankyrin

b. Pyruvate kinase

c. Glucose phosphate isomerase

d. Glucose-6-phosphate dehydrogenase

56–14. You are caring for a pregnant woman at 12 weeks' gestation with a history of Diamond-Blackfan anemia. What is true regarding this condition in pregnancy?

a. The major risks are hemorrhage and infection.

b. Steroid therapy should be continued in pregnancy.

c. Rates of preterm labor, preeclampsia, fetal-growth restriction, and stillbirth are increased.

d. All of the above

56–15. What therapy would you consider for a woman with polycythemia vera and no clot history who is now pregnant?

a. Aspirin alone

b. Heparin alone

c. Aspirin and heparin

d. None of the above

56–16. You are caring for an African American couple who are considering pregnancy. Neither of them has sickle-cell disease, but they are unsure if they are carriers of the sickle trait. Based on their race and origin, what would be their infant's risk of having sickle-cell disease?

a. 1/48

b. 1/144

c. 1/392

d. 1/576

56–17. In patients with sickle-cell disease, in which of the following conditions do red cells assume the shape shown in the peripheral smear below?

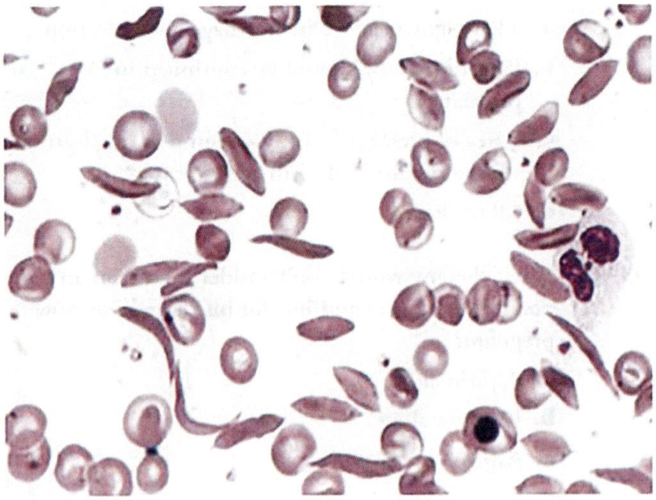

Reproduced with permission from Longo DL: Atlas of hematology and analysis of peripheral blood smears. In Longo DL, Fauci AS, Kasper DL, et al (eds): Harrison's Principles of Internal Medicine, 18th ed. New York, McGraw-Hill, 2012, Figure e17-12.

a. Hyperglycemia
b. Low oxygen tension
c. Dietary protein deficiency
d. Administration of certain antibiotics

56–18. You are caring for a 26-year-old G1 at 17 weeks' gestation with sickle-cell anemia. You order a routine echocardiogram which demonstrates a dilated pulmonary artery, right atrial dilation, and a right ventricular systolic pressure of 55 mmHg. What percentage of sickle-cell patients suffer the complication implied by these echocardiographic findings?

a. 2%
b. 5%
c. 10%
d. 20%

56–19. Which of the following obstetric complications is not increased in the context of sickle-cell disease in pregnancy?

a. Stillbirth
b. Preeclampsia
c. Gestational diabetes
d. Fetal-growth restriction

56–20. You are caring for a 30-year-old pregnant patient with hemoglobin SC disease who is 7 weeks along. She reports a remote history of a crisis as a child, but none since that time. What should you tell her regarding her risk of maternal sickle-cell complications such as sickle crises in the context of pregnancy?

a. No change in pregnancy
b. Increased risk in pregnancy
c. Decreased risk in pregnancy
d. Unpredictable risk in pregnancy

56–21. A 21-year-old G1 is admitted at 27 weeks' gestation with intense lower leg and back pain typical of her sickle crises. Her hematocrit is 21%, which is just slightly lower than her baseline of 24%. Her temperature is a 37.5°C, heart rate 102 beats per minute, and blood pressure 110/68 mmHg. What is the best treatment based on her presentation?

a. Opioids only
b. Supplemental oxygen and opioids
c. Supplemental oxygen, intravenous hydration, and opioids
d. Supplemental oxygen, intravenous hydration, opioids, and blood transfusion

56–22. A 21-year-old primigravida with sickle-cell disease presents with complaints of fever, cough, joint pain and increasing shortness of breath. The following chest radiograph is obtained. All except which of the following are precipitants of this condition?

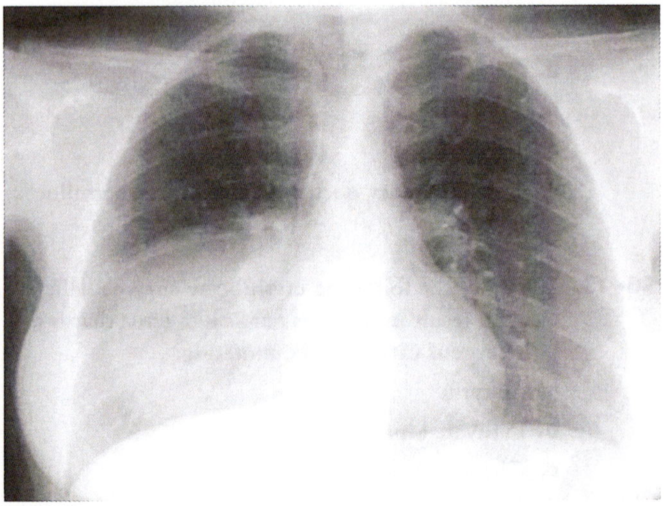

a. Infection
b. Atelectasis
c. Preterm labor
d. Marrow emboli

56–23. You are caring for a sickle-cell patient who is currently 16 weeks pregnant. Outside of pregnancy she is typically admitted every 3–4 months for a pain crisis. Her baseline hematocrit is 25% and her most recent complete blood count demonstrates a hematocrit of 23%. Which of the following interventions may decrease her risk of having a pain crisis this pregnancy?

a. Iron supplementation
b. Prophylactic red cell transfusion
c. Prophylactic antibiotic administration
d. None of these will decrease her risk of crisis

56–24. Which of the following complications is associated with sickle-cell trait in pregnancy?

a. Low birthweight
b. Perinatal mortality
c. Spontaneous abortion
d. Asymptomatic bacteruria

56–25. α-Thalassemia minor is more common in women of both Asian and African descent, although hemoglobin H disease and hemoglobin Bart disease are rare or unreported in women of African descent. Which of the following genotypes, which is found more commonly in women of African descent, explains this observation?

a. $-\alpha/-\alpha$
b. $-\alpha/\alpha\alpha$
c. $--/\alpha\alpha$
d. $--/-\alpha$

56–26. An infant born with hemoglobin H disease will have which of the following red cell types present at birth?

a. Hemoglobin A
b. Hemoglobin H (β_4)
c. Hemoglobin Bart (Υ_4)
d. All of the above

56–27. You are performing an anatomical survey on a 23-year-old primigravida at 20 weeks' gestation. Both she and her husband are of Asian descent. Her pregnancy has been uncomplicated thus far except for mild anemia. On ultrasound, you observe fetal hydrops with elevated middle cerebral artery velocities. Which of the following is the most likely explanation for the observed hydrops?

a. Turner syndrome
b. Parvovirus infection
c. Hemoglobin Bart disease
d. None of the above

56–28. Which of the following hemoglobin electrophoresis results is compatible with β-thalassemia minor?

a. Hemoglobin A2 2.5%, hemoglobin F 1%
b. Hemoglobin A2 3.5%, hemoglobin F 1%
c. Hemoglobin A2 2.5%, hemoglobin F 3%
d. Hemoglobin A2 3.5%, hemoglobin F 3%

56–29. Thrombocytopenia, defined as a platelet count <150,000/μL, complicates what percentage of pregnancies?

a. 1%
b. 3%
c. 5%
d. 10%

56–30. You are caring for a pregnant patient with known idiopathic thrombocytopenic purpura who is currently 29 weeks pregnant. Her platelet count returns at 21,000/μL. Which of the following treatments would you consider as first-line therapy?

a. Splenectomy
b. Azathioprine
c. Corticosteroids
d. Intravenous immune globulin

56–31. A 32-year-old G3P2 presents at 38 weeks' gestation complaining of mild fever and headache. Her temperature is 38.1°C, blood pressure measures 152/94 mmHg, and her heart rate is 112 beats per minute. Her laboratory results demonstrate a hematocrit of 21%, platelet count of 17,000/μL, and her creatinine is 1.4 mg/dL. A peripheral smear is performed, which demonstrates schistocytes. What is the most likely underlying cause of her clinical presentation?

a. Severe preeclampsia
b. Idiopathic thrombocytopenic purpura
c. Endothelial damage due to an underlying infection
d. Elevated levels of large von Willebrand factor multimers

56–32. What is the most appropriate treatment for the patient in Question 56–31?

a. Plasmapheresis
b. Labor induction
c. Magnesium sulfate infusion
d. All of the above

56–33. What determines the factor VIII activity level in women affected with hemophilia A?

a. Mosaicism

b. Lyonization

c. Co-dominance

d. None of the above

56–34. What is the incidence of postpartum hemorrhage in women with von Willebrand disease?

a. 10%

b. 30%

c. 50%

d. 70%

CHAPTER 56 ANSWER KEY

Question number	Letter answer	Page cited	Header cited
56–1	**c**	p. 1075	Definition and Incidence
56–2	**c**	p. 1076	Effects on Pregnancy Outcomes
56–3	**c**	p. 1076	Iron-Deficiency Anemia
56–4	**a**	p. 1077	Iron-Deficiency Anemia
56–5	**b**	p. 1077	Diagnosis
56–6	**c**	p. 1077	Anemia from Acute Blood Loss
56–7	**d**	p. 1077	Anemia Associated with Chronic Disease
56–8	**b**	p. 1078	Folic Acid Deficiency
56–9	**b**	p. 1078	Vitamin B_{12} Deficiency
56–10	**b**	p. 1078	Autoimmune Hemolysis
56–11	**d**	p. 1079	Paroxysmal Nocturnal Hemoglobinuria
56–12	**c**	p. 1079	Inherited Erythrocyte Membrane Defects
56–13	**b**	p. 1080	Erythrocyte Enzyme Deficiencies
56–14	**d**	p. 1080	Aplastic and Hypoplastic Anemia
56–15	**a**	p. 1081	Polycythemia Vera
56–16	**d**	p. 1081	Sickle-Cell Hemoglobinopathies
56–17	**b**	p. 1081	Sickle-Cell Hemoglobinopathies—Pathophysiology
56–18	**d**	p. 1081	Sickle-Cell Hemoglobinopathies—Pathophysiology
56–19	**c**	p. 1082	Pregnancy and Sickle-Cell Syndromes
56–20	**b**	p. 1082	Hemoglobin SC
56–21	**c**	p. 1082	Management During Pregnancy
56–22	**c**	p. 1082	Management During Pregnancy
56–23	**b**	p. 1083	Management During Pregnancy
56–24	**d**	p. 1083	Sickle-Cell Trait
56–25	**a**	p. 1085	Alpha Thalassemias—Frequency
56–26	**d**	p. 1085	Alpha Thalassemias—Pregnancy
56–27	**c**	p. 1085	Alpha Thalassemias—Pregnancy
56–28	**d**	p. 1085	Beta Thalassemias
56–29	**d**	p. 1086	Thrombocytopenia
56–30	**c**	p. 1087	Immune Thrombocytopenic Purpura—Diagnosis and Management
56–31	**d**	p. 1088	Thrombotic microangiopathies—Etiopathogenesis
56–32	**a**	p. 1088	Thrombotic microangiopathies—Pregnancy
56–33	**b**	p. 1089	Hemophilias A and B—Pregnancy
56–34	**c**	p. 1090	Von Willebrand Disease—Pregnancy

CHAPTER 57

Diabetes Mellitus

57–1. What does in utero exposure to hyperglycemia lead to?

a. Increase fetal fat cells

b. Fetal hyperinsulinemia

c. Insulin resistance in adolescence

d. All of the above

57–2. How is diabetes classified during pregnancy?

a. Type 1 or type 2

b. Pregestational or gestational

c. Type 1, type 2, or gestational

d. Using the White classification

57–3. Diabetes is the most common medical complication of pregnancy. The diagram below shows the increasing prevalence of gestational diabetes in the past 20 years. Which ethnic group is at highest risk for gestational diabetes?

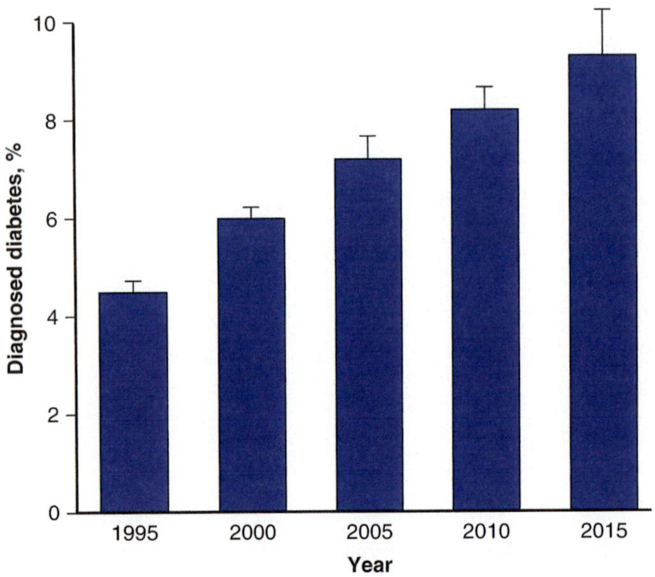

Reproduced with permission from Cunningham FG, Leveno KJ, Bloom SL, et al (eds): Diabetes mellitus. In Williams Obstetrics, 25th ed. New York, McGraw-Hill, 2018, Figure 57-1.

a. Asian

b. Native American

c. Ashkenazi Jewish

d. Eastern European

57–4. A 34-year-old woman was diagnosed with diabetes at the age of 20. Her initial prenatal care labs return with a 24-hour urine protein of 250 mg. She has benign retinopathy on ophthalmologic exam. What White classification does her pregnancy carry?

a. C

b. D

d. F

d. R

57–5. Which of the following findings are considered diagnostic for overt diabetes in pregnancy?

a. Hemoglobin A_{1C} >6%

b. Glucosuria on urine dip

c. Fasting plasma glucose ≥120 mg/dL

d. Random plasma glucose ≥200 mg/dL

57–6. Fetuses of overtly diabetic mothers have an increased risk for which of the following?

a. Preterm delivery

b. Spontaneous abortion

c. Congenital malformation

d. All of the above

57–7. The figure below illustrates the frequency of congenital malformations at given maternal hemoglobin A_{1C} levels early in pregnancy. What can be said regarding this relationship?

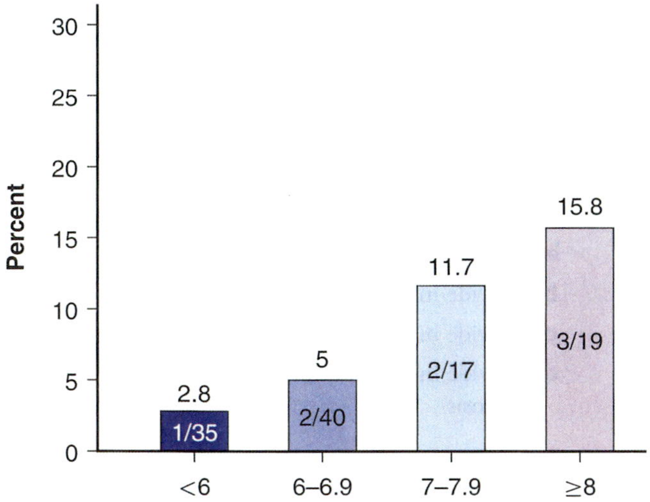

Reproduced with permission from Cunningham FG, Leveno KJ, Bloom SL, et al (eds): Diabetes mellitus. In Williams Obstetrics, 25th ed. New York, McGraw-Hill, 2018, Figure 57-2.

- **a.** If the hemoglobin A_{1C} is <7%, there is no increased risk.
- **b.** The highest risk for congenital malformation is seen with a hemoglobin A_{1C} level of 7–8%.
- **c.** As preconceptional glucose control worsens, the incidence of congenital malformation increases.
- **d.** All of the above

57–8. How does diminished fetal growth occur in pregestational diabetes?

- **a.** Substrate deprivation
- **b.** Fetal hyperinsulinemia
- **c.** Altered lipid metabolism
- **d.** All of the above

57–9. Compared to women without diabetes, which fetal condition occurs more often in the setting of pregestational diabetes?

- **a.** Stillbirth
- **b.** Perinatal death
- **c.** Postpartum hemorrhage
- **d.** Gestational hypertension

57–10. What might be said of the pregnancy yielding this 5000-g newborn?

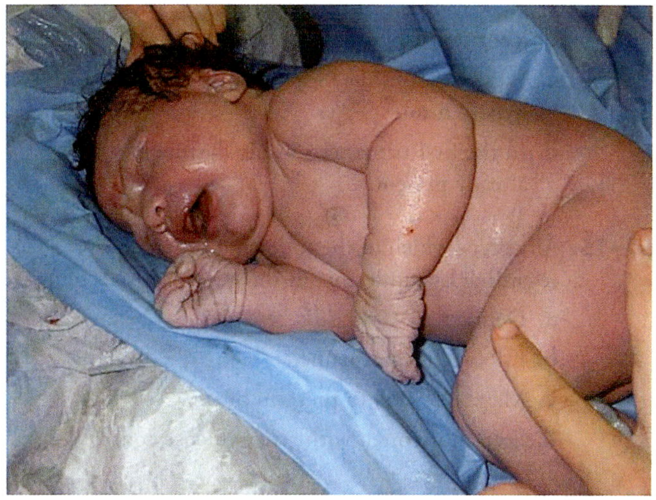

Used with permission from Dr. Patricia Santiago-Munoz.

- **a.** The mother likely had poor glycemic control.
- **b.** The baby was at risk for neonatal hypoglycemia.
- **c.** The mother had an increased risk for shoulder dystocia.
- **d.** All of the above

57–11. Which of the following are considered reasons for unexplained fetal demise in women requiring insulin during pregnancy?

- **a.** Nonketotic acidosis
- **b.** Elevated lactic acid levels
- **c.** Decreased fetal hematocrit
- **d.** None of the above

57–12. Which of the following is a reasonable explanation for hydramnios in a pregnancy complicated by diabetes?

- **a.** Maternal endothelial leak caused by hyperglycemia
- **b.** Glucose reabsorption by the fetal glomerular collecting system
- **c.** Osmotic gradient created by high glucose concentrations in the amnionic fluid
- **d.** All of the above

57–13. What is the most likely cause for the increased incidence of respiratory distress syndrome in the neonates of diabetic mothers?

- **a.** Indicated preterm delivery
- **b.** Delayed maturation of type II pneumocytes
- **c.** Decreased production of surfactant in a hyperglycemic environment
- **d.** All of the above

57–14. Which of the following statements regarding cardiomyopathy in infants of diabetic mothers is true?

a. Is reversible after birth

b. Ventricular hypertrophy is due to insulin excess

c. In severe cases may lead to pulmonary hypertension

d. In the first trimester systolic dysfunction is already present

57–15. All except which of the following statements regarding hypocalcemia in the newborn is accurate?

a. Defined as <9 mg/dL

b. Etiology is unexplained

c. May be related to preterm birth

d. Seen more often with strict glucose control

57–16. Maternal mortality in women with type 1 diabetes results from which of the following?

a. Infection

b. Hypertension

c. Diabetic ketoacidosis

d. All of the above

57–17. A 32-year-old primigravida present for preconception counseling regarding her class C diabetes. Given the diagram below, what can be said about her risk of developing preeclampsia in the setting of pregestational diabetes?

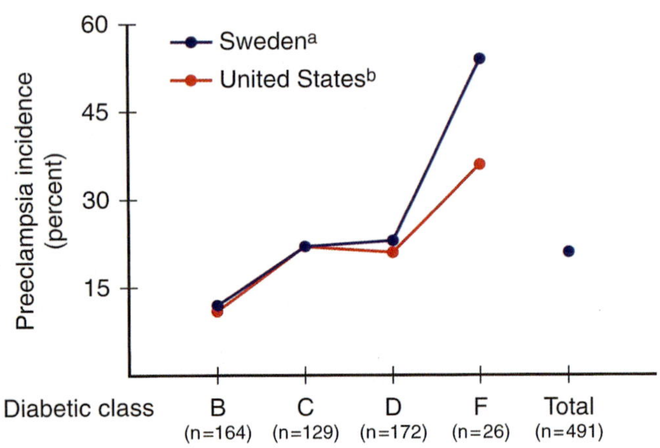

Reproduced with permission from Cunningham FG, Leveno KJ, Bloom SL, et al (eds): Diabetes mellitus. In Williams Obstetrics, 25th ed. New York, McGraw-Hill, 2018, Figure 57-5.

a. If she has good control, her risk is not increased.

b. She has the same risk as someone with class D diabetes.

c. The risk of preeclampsia increases with worsening vascular complications.

d. Her risk is increased when compared to someone who has underlying nephropathy due to diabetes.

57–18. The first and most common visible retinal lesions in diabetes are small microaneurysms followed by blot hemorrhages. This describes which of the following conditions?

a. Proliferative retinopathy

b. Nonproliferative retinopathy

c. Is irreversible with improved control

d. The etiology of cotton wool exudates

57–19. What is the most important component of diabetic ketoacidosis treatment in pregnancy?

a. Restore euglycemia

b. Provide intravenous hydration

c. Provide intravenous potassium repletion

d. Provide intravenous bicarbonate to correct acidosis

57–20. Which of the following infections is increased in pregnant women with overt diabetes?

a. Pyelonephritis

b. Respiratory infections

c. Wound infection after cesarean delivery

d. All of the above

57–21. The most difficult aspect of preconceptional control in women with diabetes is which of the following?

a. Resistance to insulin therapy

b. Unpredictable insulin requirements

c. Half of pregnancies in the United States are unplanned

d. All of the above

57–22. Women with type 1 diabetes should achieve glycemic control with which of the following during pregnancy?

a. Insulin

b. Diet alone

c. Insulin and diet

d. Oral hypoglycemic agents

57–23. Which of the following is associated with fasting blood glucose levels >120 mg/dL?

a. Preeclampsia

b. Cesarean delivery

c. Birthweight >90th percentile

d. All of the above

57–24. Which of the following is true concerning management of overt maternal diabetes in the second trimester?

a. Should undergo amniocentesis

b. Should undergo a fetal echocardiogram

c. Have higher rates of chromosomal abnormalities

d. Should be offered genetic screening if >35 years of age

57–25. The American College of Obstetricians and Gynecologists recommends which of the following regarding the management of women with overt diabetes during labor?

a. Morning dose of long-acting be held

b. Intravenous infusion of normal saline is given

c. Regular intravenous insulin is administered at an infusion rate of 1.25 U/h if glucose levels exceed 100 mg/dL

d. All of the above

57–26. Which of the following defines gestational diabetes?

a. Diabetes that is first detected in pregnancy

b. A hemoglobin A_{1C} level >6% found early in pregnancy

c. Diabetes that does not require insulin during pregnancy

d. None of the above

57–27. Concerning screening and diagnosis of gestational diabetes during pregnancy, which of the following statements is true?

a. The HAPO study supports the 1–step approach.

b. The American College of Obstetricians and Gynecologists recommends a 2–step approach.

c. Identifying the 10% of women in the 1–step approach who should not be screened would add unnecessary complexity to the diagnosis of gestational diabetes.

d. All of the above

57–28. Which of the following statements concerning the HAPO study research group are true?

a. Blood glucoses were measured fasting and then in 2 hours.

b. The reference group for plasma fasting glucose was ≤80 mg/dL.

c. Findings supported that increasing plasma glucose levels were associated with increasing adverse outcomes.

d. All of the above

57–29. In women with gestational diabetes, early fasting hyperglycemia is associated with increased rates of which of the following?

a. Cesarean delivery

b. Fetal macrosomia

c. Maternal hypertension

d. All of the above

57–30. Which of the following factors have been implicated in fetal macrosomia?

a. Leptin

b. C-peptide

c. Insulin-like growth factor

d. All of the above

57–31. What is the most correct distribution of nutritional intake concerning caloric intake as endorsed by the American College of Obstetricians and Gynecologists?

a. 30% fat

b. 30% protein

c. 40% carbohydrates

d. All of the above

57–32. The American College of Obstetricians and Gynecologists recommends which of the following concerning exercise in pregnancy for diabetics?

a. Weight lifting is contraindicated.

b. 30 minutes per day of aerobic exercise is recommended.

c. New York Heart Association Class I and II should participate in active aerobic programs.

d. Regular physical activity that incorporates aerobic and strength conditioning exercise is recommended during pregnancy.

57–33. Which of the following statements regarding treatment of gestational diabetes is accurate?

a. Insulin is the preferred medication in pregnancy.

b. Diet and exercise alone should not be used in pregnancy.

c. A trial of oral hypoglycemics can be used prior to initiating insulin therapy.

d. The starting dose of insulin is 0.6 mg/kg/day – 1.0 mg/kg/day in divided doses if insulin is needed.

57–34. Glyburide therapy for gestational diabetes is associated with which of the following?

a. Crosses the placenta and fetal levels are >2/3 maternal serum levels.

b. No studies have found increased rates of neonatal intensive care unit admissions.

c. Approved by Food and Drug Administration for the treatment of gestational diabetes.

d. All of the above

57–35. A multigravida with no prenatal care presents to labor and delivery at 39 weeks' gestation. Her last baby was born with forceps-assisted vaginal delivery, weighed 4200 grams, and she had a third-degree perineal laceration repaired. Her random glucose is 257 mg/dL and urinalysis reveals 3+ glycosuria. Bedside ultrasound reveals an estimated fetal weight of 4634 grams. On exam her cervix is 1 cm dilated. What course of action do you recommend?

a. Induction of labor

b. Return to clinic in 1 week

c. Amniocentesis for fetal lung maturity

d. Begin insulin and proceed with cesarean delivery

57–36. A 29-year-old primigravida with class B diabetes at 39 weeks' gestation presents to clinic. She has received parental care throughout pregnancy and her diabetes is under good control on split dose insulin. Her fetal anatomy ultrasound and echocardiogram were normal. The current estimated fetal weight is 4163 grams and her cervix is 1 cm dilated. What course of action do you recommend?

a. Cesarean delivery

b. Induction of labor

c. Return to clinic in 1 week

d. Amniocentesis for fetal lung maturity

57–37. A 17-year-old primigravida at 32 weeks' gestation arrives at your hospital in acute distress. Her mother informs you she has type 1 diabetes, has been acting strange, and started vomiting 2 hours ago. The fetal heart rate pattern is shown below. Diabetic ketoacidosis is diagnosed, and you begin treatment. How do you respond to this class III fetal heart rate tracing?

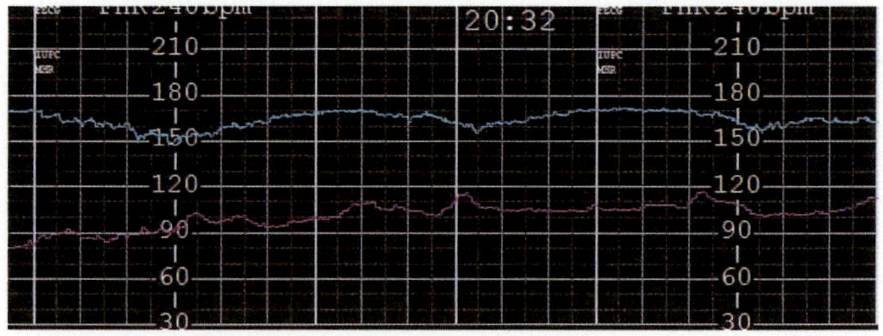

a. Induction with Foley bulb

b. Immediate cesarean delivery

c. Perform a biophysical profile

d. Do nothing and continue maternal treatment

57–38. After the patient in Question 57–37 is resuscitated and her acid–base status is normalized, the fetal heart rate tracing appears as shown below. What is your next action concerning the fetus?

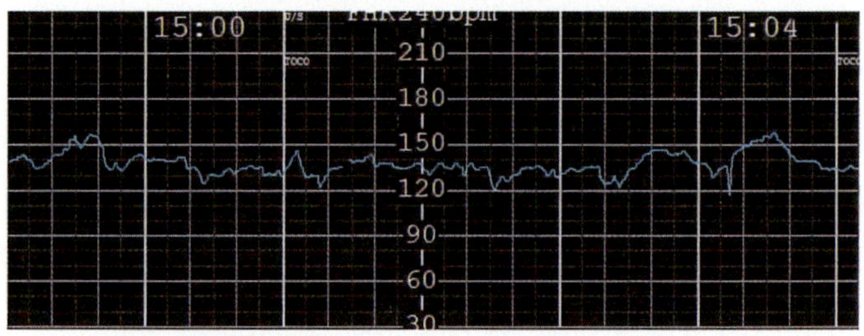

a. Extended fetal heart rate monitoring

b. Now with normalization, proceed with cesarean section

c. Now with normalization, place Foley bulb for induction

d. None of the above

CHAPTER 57 ANSWER KEY

Question number	Letter answer	Page cited	Header cited
57–1	**d**	p. 1097	Introduction
57–2	**c**	p. 1098	Classification During Pregnancy
57–3	**b**	p. 1098	Classification During Pregnancy
57–4	**b**	p. 1099	Table 57-2
57–5	**d**	p. 2200	Table 57-4
57–6	**d**	p. 1099	Fetal Effects
57–7	**c**	p. 1101	Figure 57-2
57–8	**a**	p. 1100	Altered Fetal Growth
57–9	**d**	p. 1100	Table 57-5
57–10	**d**	p. 1100	Altered Fetal Growth
57–11	**b**	p. 1101	Unexplained Fetal Demise
57–12	**c**	p. 1102	Hydramnios
57–13	**a**	p. 1102	Respiratory Distress Syndrome
57–14	**b**	p. 1102	Cardiomyopathy
57–15	**a**	p. 1102	Hypocalcemia
57–16	**d**	p. 1103	Maternal Effects
57–17	**c**	p. 1103	Figure 57-5
57–18	**b**	p. 1103	Diabetic Retinopathy
57–19	**b**	p. 1104	Diabetic Ketoacidosis
57–20	**d**	p. 1104	Infections
57–21	**c**	p. 1104	Preconceptional Care
57–22	**c**	p. 1105	Insulin Treatment
57–23	**d**	p. 1106	Hypoglycemia
57–24	**b**	p. 1106	Second Trimester
57–25	**d**	p. 1107	Table 57-10
57–26	**a**	p. 1107	Gestational Diabetes
57–27	**d**	p. 1108	Screening and Diagnosis
57–28	**c**	p. 1109	Screening and Diagnosis
57–29	**d**	p. 1110	Maternal and Fetal Effects (Fig. 57-6)
57–30	**d**	p. 1111	Fetal Macrosomia
57–31	**c**	p. 1112	Diabetic Diet
57–32	**d**	p. 1112	Exercise
57–33	**a**	p. 1112	Insulin Treatment
57–34	**a**	p. 1113	Oral Hypoglycemics
57–35	**d**	p. 1113	Obstetrical Management
57–36	**b**	p. 1113	Obstetrical Management
57–37	**d**	p. 1104	Diabetic Ketoacidosis
57–38	**d**	p. 1104	Diabetic Ketoacidosis

CHAPTER 58

Endocrine Disorders

58–1. During pregnancy TSH receptors are weakly cross stimulated by _____ which is produced in the _____.

a. AFP, trophoblast

b. β-hCG, trophoblast

c. AFP, syncytiotrophoblast

d. β-hCG, syncytiotrophoblast

58–2. When does the fetus begin to concentrate and synthesize thyroid hormone?

a. 8 weeks

b. 10 week

c. 12 weeks

d. 14 weeks

58–3. Thyroid-stimulating immunoglobulins are usually associated with which entity listed below?

a. Graves disease

b. Thyroid peroxidase

c. Fetal micro-chimerism

d. None of the above

58–4. The main cause of thyrotoxicosis in pregnancy is which of the following?

a. Graves disease

b. Type 1 diabetes

c. Multiple gestations

d. Methamphetamine toxicity

58–5. The American Thyroid Association recommends which of the following therapy strategies for hyperthyroidism?

a. 1st and 2nd trimesters: methimazole; 3rd trimester: propylthiouracil

b. 1st trimester: methimazole; 2nd and 3rd trimesters: propylthiouracil

c. 1st and 2nd trimesters: propylthiouracil; 3rd trimester: methimazole

d. 1st trimester: propylthiouracil; 2nd and 3rd trimesters: methimazole

58–6. After beginning propylthiouracil treatment, how often should you evaluate free T_4 levels?

a. Every 2 weeks

b. Every 3 weeks

c. Every trimester

d. Every 4–6 weeks

58–7. All except which of the following congenital defects are associated with methimazole embryopathy?

a. Aplasia cutis

b. Choanal atresia

c. Esophageal atresia

d. Posterior urethral valve

58–8. The International Commission on Radiological Protection has recommended that women avoid pregnancy for ___ months after radioablative therapy, and wait for ___ months after breastfeeding to have thyroid ablation done.

a. 3, 6

b. 6, 3

c. 9, 6

d. 6, 6

58–9. Which of the following adverse pregnancy outcomes is associated with inadequately treated thyroid disease?

a. Preeclampsia

b. Neonatal hearing loss

c. Maternal heart failure

d. All of the above

58–10. Concerning thyroid storm and heart failure, which of the following is true?

a. It is a dilated cardiomyopathy.

b. Pulmonary hypertension is common.

c. Decompensation can be precipitated with maternal anemia.

d. All of the above

58–11. During thyroid storm, what is the correct order of medication administration?

a. Dexamethasone, beta blocker, propylthiouracil, iodide

b. Iodide, propylthiouracil, beta blocker, dexamethasone

c. Propylthiouracil, beta blocker, iodide, dexamethasone

d. Beta blocker, iodide, propylthiouracil, dexamethasone

58–12. Which of the lab or clinical features listed below is consistent with subclinical hyperthyroidism?

a. Osteopenia

b. Normal free T_4

c. Elevated free T_4

d. Elevated thyroid-stimulating hormone

58–13. Which of the following is true of transient biochemical hyperthyroidism in early pregnancy?

a. Usually normalizes by mid-pregnancy

b. Should be treated with propylthiouracil

c. Occurs in about 25% of pregnant women

d. Have low thyroid-stimulating hormone and normal free T_4

58–14. What is the incidence of overt hypothyroidism in pregnancy?

a. 2%

b. 3%

c. 12%

d. 2–12 per thousand

58–15. A 32-year-old G2P1 presents with symptoms of weight gain and constipation. A picture of her neck is shown below. Labs return indicative of overt hypothyroidism. Which of the following is adequate therapy?

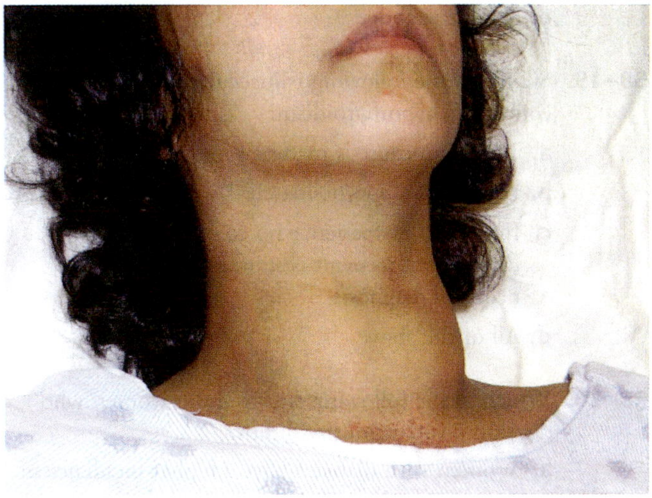

a. 50 μg per day

b. 100 μg per day

c. 250 μg per day

d. 1 to 2 μg/kg/day

58–16. The best data concerning subclinical hypothyroidism and treatment suggests which of the following?

a. About 3.3% of pregnant women have subclinical hypothyroidism.

b. There was no difference in maternal outcomes in thyroxine-treated women versus controls.

c. Treatment of these women demonstrates no differences in cognitive outcomes of their children at 5 years.

d. All of the above

58–17. Which of the following is true concerning isolated maternal hypothyroxinemia?

a. Incidence is about 3.1–4.5%

b. Thyroid-stimulating hormone is low, and thyroxine is high

c. These patients have a low incidence of antithyroid antibodies

d. All of the above

58–18. Iodine requirements during pregnancy are higher because of which of the following?

a. Increased renal losses

b. Fetal iodine requirements

c. Augmented thyroid hormone production

d. All of the above

58–19. Which of the following is inaccurate regarding congenital hypothyroidism?

a. The main cause is maternal iodine deficiency.

b. Develops in approximately 1 in 3000 newborns.

c. Infants will experience no cognitive deficits if thyroid replacement is started promptly after neonatal diagnosis.

d. All of the above

58–20. Which of the following is true about women who develop postpartum thyroiditis?

a. Women with diabetes have a higher incidence of postpartum thyroiditis.

b. Propylthiouracil will be effective against the initial phase of thyrotoxic symptomology.

c. The first phase of postpartum thyroiditis begins immediately after delivery and is usually recognizable at the time of discharge.

d. All of the above

58–21. Clinical manifestations of postpartum thyroiditis include which of the following?

a. Development of a large painless goiter.

b. The thyrotoxic phase lasts a few months.

c. The goiter will be replaced by diffuse nodularity.

d. Thyroxine replacement may be required for many years.

58–22. Sonographic characteristics of thyroid nodules associated with malignancy include which of the following?

a. Regular margins

b. Microcalcifications

c. Hyperechoic pattern

d. All of the above

58–23. Which of the following is true regarding hyperparathyroidism?

a. Hypercalcemia is caused by hyperparathyroidism and cancer in 90% of cases.

b. Almost 80% of hyperparathyroidism is caused by multiple adenomas in the parathyroid gland.

c. Hypercalcemic crisis is manifested as stupor, coma, vomiting, nausea, fatigue, and dehydration.

d. All of the above

58–24. What are the total calcium requirements during pregnancy?

a. 30 mg/day

b. 300 mg/day

c. 1800 mg/day

d. 2400 mg/day

58–25. Initial medical management of asymptomatic hyperparathyroidism includes which of the following?

a. Phosphate

b. Calcitonin

c. Normal saline

d. All of the above

58–26. Which of the following pregnant women are at risk for increased bone loss?

a. Breastfeeding

b. Multiple gestations

c. Low body mass index

d. All of the above

58–27. Pheochromocytomas are generally called the 10% tumor. Which of the following contributes to this description?

a. 10% are benign.

b. 10% are bilateral.

c. 10% are adrenal in origin.

d. All of the above

58–28. Which of the following is true regarding pheochromocytoma complicating pregnancy?

a. It is associated with fetal wastage about 20% of the time.

b. The preferred mode of diagnosis is with computed tomography scan.

c. Maternal death is more common if the diagnosis is made antepartum.

d. All of the above

58–29. Which of the following is considered appropriate in the treatment of pheochromocytoma in pregnancy?

a. α-blockade

b. Immediate α-and β-blockade

c. If diagnosed in the third trimester, then tumor excision

d. All of the above

58–30. In the picture below, which organ or structure is contiguous with the pheochromocytoma?

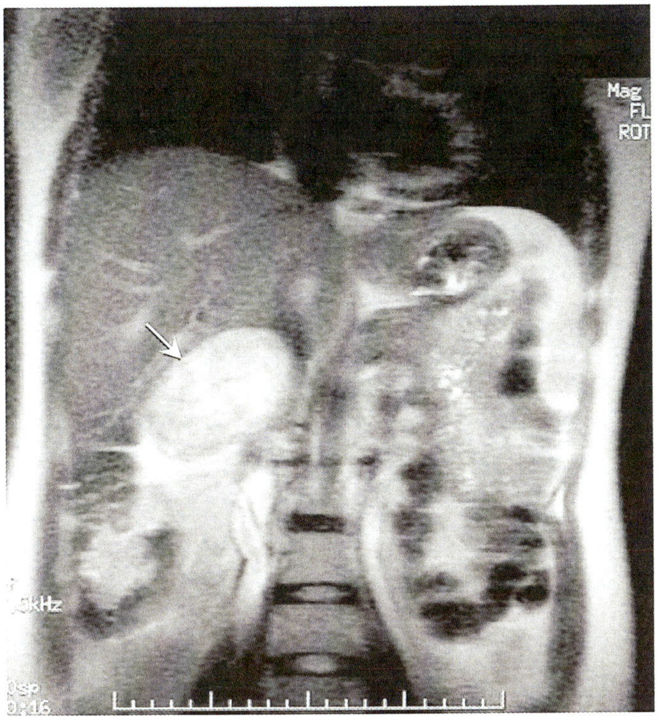

Reproduced with permission from Cunningham FG, Leveno KJ, Bloom SL, et al (eds): Endocrine disorders. In Williams Obstetrics, 25th ed. New York, McGraw-Hill, 2018, Figure 58-6.

a. Liver

b. Kidney

c. Gallbladder

d. Inferior vena cava

58–31. Which of the following is among the four most common maternal complications that occur in women with Cushing syndrome?

a. Diabetes

b. Cardiac failure

c. Psychiatric disorders

d. None of the above

58–32. Which of the following drugs is used to treat mild Cushing syndrome in pregnancy?

a. Cortisol

b. Metyrapone

c. Spironolactone

d. All of the above

58–33. Which of the following statements concerning Addison disease in pregnancy is true?

a. Patients are at increased risk for preterm birth.

b. Stress dose hydrocortisone therapy should be used during labor.

c. Glucocorticoid and mineralocorticoid replacement therapy should be continued.

d. All of the above

58–34. Which of the following statements is true regarding hyperaldosteronism?

a. Laparoscopic tumor resection is not curative.

b. Hypertension improves as pregnancy progresses.

c. It is primarily caused by bilateral adrenal hyperplasia.

d. Medical management includes potassium supplementation and antihypertensive agents.

58–35. Which of the following statements is true concerning prolactinoma?

a. Microadenomas are >10 mm.

b. Serum prolactin levels <25 ng/mL are considered normal in pregnant women.

c. It should be treated with bromocriptine in pregnancy to prevent enlargement.

d. Pregnant women with microadenomas should be queried regularly for headaches and visual symptoms.

58–36. A 34-year-old multigravida at 19 weeks' gestation presents with shortness of breath and tachycardia at 140 beats per minute. Which of the following is in the differential diagnosis?

b. Anemia

c. Thyroid storm

a. Pulmonary embolism

d. All of the above

58–37. The patient in Question 58–36 has a blood pressure of 145/90 mmHg, temperature of 37°C, and a respiratory rate of 24 breaths/minute. Which of the following tests might be helpful?

a. Hematocrit

b. Chest radiograph

c. Thyroid function tests

d. All of the above

58–38. The physical exam of the patient in Question 57–36 reveals mild exophthalmos, sweaty skin, and rales at the lung bases. Which of the tests ordered in Question 57–37 will give you the most specific result indicating the disease process?

a. Hematocrit

b. Chest radiograph

c. Thyroid function tests

d. None of the above

58–39. The patient in Question 57–36's thyroid function tests return, and the free T4 is 8.2 ng/dL. What do you expect the thyroid-stimulating hormone level to be?

a. Low normal

b. High normal

c. Pathologically low

d. Pathologically high

CHAPTER 58 ANSWER KEY

Question number	Letter answer	Page cited	Header cited
58–1	b	p. 1118	Thyroid Physiology and Pregnancy
58–2	c	p. 1118	Thyroid Physiology and Pregnancy
58–3	a	p. 1119	Autoimmunity and Thyroid Disease
58–4	a	p. 1120	Hyperthyroidism
58–5	d	p. 1120	Hyperthyroidism
58–6	d	p. 1120	Treatment
58–7	d	p. 1120	Treatment
58–8	b	p. 1120	Treatment
58–9	d	p. 1121	Pregnancy Outcome
58–10	d	p. 1122	Thyroid Storm and Heart Failure
58–11	c	p. 1123	Figure 58-4
58–12	b	p. 1124	Subclinical Hyperthyroidism
58–13	a	p. 1122	Hyperemesis Gravidarum and Gestational Transient Hyperthyroidism
58–14	d	p. 1123	Hypothyroidism
58–15	d	p. 1124	Treatment
58–16	d	p. 1126	Table 58-5
58–17	c	p. 1125	Isolated Maternal Hypothyroxinemia
58–18	d	p. 1126	Iodine Deficiency
58–19	b	p. 1127	Congenital Hypothyroidism
58–20	a	p. 1127	Postpartum Thyroiditis
58–21	b	p. 1127	Clinical Manifestations
58–22	b	p. 1128	Nodular Thyroid Disease
58–23	c	p. 1128	Parathyroid Diseases
58–24	b	p. 1128	Parathyroid Diseases
58–25	d	p. 1128	Hyperparathyroidism
58–26	d	p. 1129	Pregnancy-Associated Osteoporosis
58–27	b	p. 1130	Pheochromocytoma
58–28	a	p. 1130	Pheochromocytoma Complicating Pregnancy
58–29	a	p. 1131	Management
58–30	b	p. 1130	Figure 58-6
58–31	a	p. 1131	Table 58-7
58–32	b	p. 1131	Cushing Syndrome
58–33	d	p. 1132	Adrenal Insufficiency—Addison Disease
58–34	d	p. 1132	Primary Aldosteronism
58–35	d	p. 1132	Prolactinoma
58–36	d	p. 1122	Hyperthyroidism
58–37	d	p. 1122	Hyperthyroidism
58–38	c	p. 1122	Hyperthyroidism
58–39	c	p. 1122	Hyperthyroidism

CHAPTER 59

Connective Tissue Disorders

59–1. All except which of the following is an example of an immune-complex disease?

a. Marfan syndrome
b. Sjögren syndrome
c. Rheumatoid arthritis
d. Systemic lupus erythematosus

59–2. Which of the following is not an example of an inherited connective tissue disorder?

a. Marfan syndrome
b. Osteogenesis imperfecta
c. Ehlers-Danlos syndrome
d. Antiphospholipid syndrome

59–3. A 27-year-old G0 presents for preconception counseling. She reports she was diagnosed with arthritis after she had a rash but cannot remember her diagnosis. She does remember being told that her labs were positive for rheumatoid factor. Which of the following is in the differential diagnosis?

a. Scleroderma
b. Reiter disease
c. Psoriatic arthritis
d. Ankylosing spondylitis

59–4. How does pregnancy mitigate activity of autoimmune diseases?

a. Estrogen upregulates T-cell response
b. Progesterone has immunosuppressive properties
c. Pregnancy-induced predominance of T2 helper cells
d. All of the above

59–5. Women with immune-mediated diseases are at increased risk for all except which of the following obstetrical complications?

a. Preeclampsia
b. Preterm birth
c. Postpartum hemorrhage
d. Intrauterine growth restriction

59–6. Which of the following autoantibodies is specific to systemic lupus erythematosus?

a. Anti-Ro
b. Anti-Sm
c. Anti-RNP
d. Antihistone

59–7. Which of the following statements regarding systemic lupus erythematosus is inaccurate?

a. Stroke is a cause of death
b. Immunosuppression is impaired
c. Does not have a genetic component
d. Overactive B lymphocytes produce autoantibodies

59–8. A 25-year-old G1P0 at 8 weeks' gestation presents for initiation of prenatal care. She reports that she was diagnosed with lupus 2 years ago. Which of the following symptoms did she most likely have at presentation?

a. Rash
b. Arthralgias
c. Thrombocytopenia
d. Venous thrombosis

59–9. Which of the following can lead to a positive antinuclear antibody result?

a. Heart failure
b. Viral infection
c. Diabetes mellitus
d. Venous thrombosis

59–10. According to the diagnostic criteria for lupus, which of the following women would be diagnosed with lupus?

a. 23-year-old with diarrhea, arthritis, anemia, weight loss
b. 23-year-old with malar rash, anemia, oral ulcers, anti-Smith antibodies
c. 23-year-old with discoid rash, renal failure, elevated antinuclear antibody titers
d. 23-year-old with discoid rash, renal failure, elevated antinuclear antibody titers

59–11. Which of the following medications can induce a lupus-like syndrome?

a. Lisinopril
b. Prednisone
c. Oseltamivir
d. Atorvastatin

59–12. A 30-year-old nulligravida presents for preconception counseling. She reports she was diagnosed with lupus 6 years ago. Her last flare was 1 year ago, and her serum creatinine is 0.6 mg/dL. She tells you that part of her diagnosis was made by the presence of a protein that increases her risk for blood clots. Currently the only medication she is on is azathioprine. Which of the following aspects of her history places her at increased risk for an adverse pregnancy outcome?

a. Last flare 1 year ago
b. Current use of azathioprine
c. Serum creatinine of 0.6 mg/dL
d. Presence of antiphospholipid antibodies

59–13. Active lupus nephritis during pregnancy is associated with which of the following?

a. Preeclampsia
b. Maternal death
c. Preterm delivery
d. All of the above

59–14. A 37-year-old multigravida at 27 weeks' gestation presents to labor and delivery reporting a headache for 1 day. On admission her blood pressure is 162/98 mmHg. She reports some joint pain and believes she is having a flare. Urine dip reveals 3+ protein. Which of the following laboratory tests will help you distinguish a lupus flare from preeclampsia?

a. Creatinine
b. Hemoglobin
c. Complements
d. Transaminases

59–15. Anti-SS-A and anti-SS-B antibodies are associated with neonatal lupus syndrome. Which of the following components of neonatal lupus is not transient?

a. Hemolysis
b. Heart block
c. Cutaneous lupus
d. Thrombocytopenia

59–16. A 22-year-old primigravida is referred to your office by her rheumatologist. The patient informs you that she has lupus that was diagnosed 2 years ago and has never been under control. She says her kidney function is not good. Although she was told by her rheumatologist she should not get pregnant while she is being treated for active lupus, she is sexually active and denies using contraception. Which of the following medications is contraindicated in pregnancy?

a. Prednisone
b. Azathioprine
c. Hydroxychloroquine
d. Mycophenolate mofetil

59–17. Which of the following are safe and effective contraceptive methods for patients with systemic lupus erythematosus who do not have antiphospholipid antibodies?

a. Progesterone-only pills
b. Progesterone intrauterine device
c. Combination estrogen-progesterone pills
d. All of the above

59–18. Which of the following meets the clinical criteria for antiphospholipid syndrome?

a. Autoimmune hemolytic anemia
b. Early-onset preeclampsia necessitating delivery
c. Migraine headaches with more than 1 episode/month
d. Postpartum hemorrhage requiring blood transfusion

59–19. In women with antiphospholipid antibodies, which of the following portends an adverse pregnancy outcome?

a. Presence of all three antibody types
b. Presence of a systemic autoimmune disease
c. History of thrombosis or adverse pregnancy outcome
d. All of the above

59–20. Which of the following classes and titers of antiphospholipid antibodies are clinically important?

a. High IgA only
b. High IgG and IgM
c. High IgM and IgA
d. All of the above

59–21. In which of the following scenarios is anticoagulation recommended in the setting of antiphospholipid syndrome?

a. History of thromboembolic event

b. History of early-onset preeclampsia

c. History of thromboembolic event and adverse pregnancy outcome

d. All of the above

59–22. All except which of the following are true regarding aspirin in the setting of antiphospholipid syndrome?

a. Spares prostacyclin production

b. Blocks conversion of arachidonic acid to thromboxane A_2

c. Reduces the risk of adverse outcomes in women with antiphospholipid antibodies

d. Recommended by the American College of Obstetricians and Gynecologists for women with lupus

59–23. Which of the following is a neonatal consequence of in utero exposure to nonsteroidal anti-inflammatory drugs?

a. Thrombocytopenia

b. Gastritis and bleeding

c. Neonatal pulmonary hypertension

d. Prolonged patency of the ductus arteriosus

59–24. What score is necessary to meet the diagnostic criteria for rheumatoid arthritis?

a. 4

b. 6

c. 8

d. 9

59–25. Treatment of rheumatoid arthritis during pregnancy may involve all except which of the following?

a. Leflunomide

b. Glucocorticoids

c. Tumor necrosis factor-α inhibitors

d. Nonsteroidal anti-inflammatory agents

59–26. What percentage of women with rheumatoid arthritis will experience improvement in their disease during pregnancy?

a. 30%

b. 50%

c. 70%

d. 90%

59–27. In the setting of juvenile rheumatoid arthritis, the risk of which of the following pregnancy outcomes is increased?

a. Preeclampsia

b. Preterm birth

c. Postpartum hemorrhage

d. Venous thromboembolism

59–28. All except which of the following characterize scleroderma?

a. Microvascular damage

b. Immune system activation

c. Excessive collagen deposition

d. Typically affects 20- to 40-year-old individuals

59–29. Which of the following is not seen with scleroderma?

a. Cerebritis

b. Raynaud phenomenon

c. Esophageal involvement

d. Pulmonary hypertension

59–30. Which disorder is characterized by vasculitis affecting the respiratory tract and kidneys?

a. Systemic sclerosis

b. Takayasu arteritis

c. Wegener granulomatosis

d. Pulmonary hypertension

59–31. Which disorder is characterized by chronic inflammation of the great vessels?

a. Systemic sclerosis

b. Takayasu arteritis

c. Wegener granulomatosis

d. Ehlers-Danlos syndrome

59–32. A 28-year-old primigravida presents at 10 weeks' gestation for initiation of prenatal care. She informs you that she has type IV Ehlers-Danlos. Which of the following complications is she at risk for having during pregnancy?

a. Uterine rupture

b. Preterm delivery

c. Postpartum hemorrhage

d. All of the above

CHAPTER 59 ANSWER KEY

Question number	Letter answer	Page cited	Header cited
59–1	a	p. 1138	Introduction
59–2	d	p. 1138	Introduction
59–3	a	p. 1138	Immune-Mediated Connective Tissue Diseases
59–4	d	p. 1138	Immune-Mediated Connective Tissue Diseases
59–5	c	p. 1138	Immune-Mediated Connective Tissue Diseases
59–6	b	p. 1139	Table 59-1
59–7	c	p. 1139	Systemic Lupus Erythematosus
59–8	b	p. 1140	Table 59-2
59–9	b	p. 1139	Clinical Manifestations and Diagnosis
59–10	b	p. 1140	Table 59-3
59–11	d	p. 1140	Clinical Manifestations and Diagnosis
59–12	d	p. 1140	Lupus and Pregnancy
59–13	d	p. 1141	Lupus and Pregnancy
59–14	c	p. 1141	Lupus and Pregnancy
59–15	b	p. 1142	Perinatal Mortality and Morbidity
59–16	d	p. 1142	Management During Pregnancy
59–17	d	p. 1143	Long-Term Prognosis and Contraception
59–18	b	p. 1144	Table 59-5
59–19	d	p. 1145	Pregnancy and Antiphospholipid Antibodies
59–20	b	p. 1145	Pregnancy and Antiphospholipid Antibodies
59–21	a	p. 1145	Pregnancy and Antiphospholipid Antibodies
59–22	c	p. 1145	Pregnancy and Antiphospholipid Antibodies
59–23	c	p. 1147	Management
59–24	b	p. 1146	Rheumatoid Arthritis
59–25	a	p. 1147	Management
59–26	d	p. 1148	Pregnancy and Rheumatoid Arthritis
59–27	b	p. 1148	Juvenile Rheumatoid Arthritis
59–28	d	p. 1148	Systemic Sclerosis—Scleroderma
59–29	a	p. 1149	Clinical Course
59–30	c	p. 1150	Granulomatosis with Polyangiitis
59–31	b	p. 1148	Takayasu Arteritis
59–32	d	p. 1151	Ehlers-Danlos Syndrome

CHAPTER 60

Neurological Disorders

60–1. A 21-year-old primigravida at 32 weeks' gestation reports headaches occurring approximately every other day described as dull, located at the temporal and occipital region extending down into the neck and shoulders. Which of the below treatment strategies is least appropriate?

- **a.** Massage
- **b.** Ibuprofen as needed
- **c.** Acetaminophen as needed
- **d.** Local heat therapy and stress relief techniques

60–2. A 21-year-old primigravida at 26 weeks' gestation reports bothersome headaches, occurring once or twice per week. She describes unilateral temporal throbbing headaches accompanied by nausea. She does endorse that prior to the onset of the headache she has noted seeing "sparkles" on occasion. She has experienced similar headaches in the past prior to pregnancy, but feels they are increasing in severity and frequency. What is the most appropriate diagnosis?

- **a.** Chronic migraine
- **b.** Tension headache
- **c.** Migraine with aura
- **d.** Migraine without aura

60–3. For the patient in Question 60–2, which drug would be the most appropriate therapy to be prescribed to be taken when necessary?

- **a.** Propranolol
- **b.** Amitriptyline
- **c.** Magnesium oxide
- **d.** Acetaminophen, isometheptene, dichloralphenazone (Midrin)

60–4. Which of the following seizure types is least likely to demonstrate a postictal state?

- **a.** Focal
- **b.** Absence
- **c.** Eclamptic
- **d.** Generalized

60–5. A 22-year-old woman presents for her annual well-woman exam. She reports a history of generalized seizure disorder which is well-controlled on levetiracetam. She desires pregnancy and you recommend initiation of folic acid supplementation. What is the most appropriate dose for this patient?

- **a.** 1 mg
- **b.** 4 mg
- **c.** 400 μg
- **d.** 800 mg

60–6. The patient in Question 60–5 inquires as to her risks in pregnancy, and what can be done to mitigate those risks. Which statement is least accurate?

- **a.** She is likely to remain seizure-free
- **b.** She is at increased risk of fetal anomalies
- **c.** Blood levels of antiepileptics may go down
- **d.** She is likely to experience an increase in seizure activity

60–7. The patient in Question 60–5 inquires as to her pregnancy risks. Which of the following pregnancy complications is increased in women diagnosed with epilepsy as compared to the general population?

- **a.** Maternal death
- **b.** Spontaneous abortion
- **c.** Fetal-growth restriction
- **d.** All of the above

60–8. Many antiepileptic drugs are associated with fetal anomalies. Which of the following pairings between a medication and its associated fetal anomaly is correct?

- **a.** Valproate—cardiac anomalies
- **b.** Phenytoin—neural tube defects
- **c.** Carbamazepine—cardiac anomalies
- **d.** All of the above

60–9. A 32-year-old G2P1 at 10 weeks' gestation with a seizure disorder presents for prenatal care. In addition to aneuploidy screening, you recommend which of the following?

- **a.** Targeted sonogram at 18–20 weeks
- **b.** Fetal echocardiogram at 18–20 weeks
- **c.** Initiation of weekly biophysical profiles at 34 weeks
- **d.** All of the above

60–10. When do the majority of pregnancy-related strokes occur?

- **a.** Antepartum
- **b.** Intrapartum
- **c.** Postpartum
- **d.** The risk in unchanged throughout pregnancy

60–11. In normal pregnancy, cerebral blood flow decreases by 20% from mid-pregnancy until term. In a woman with gestational hypertension, how is cerebral blood flow altered?

- **a.** Increases
- **b.** Remains unchanged
- **c.** Decreases, but less than 20%
- **d.** The same as normal pregnancy

60–12. A 32-year-old G3P2 at 18 weeks' gestation has a history of migraine headaches controlled with Midrin. She presents complaining of a severe migraine, the worst she has ever experienced. She describes a severe, frontal headache with one episode of emesis and photophobia. She took one Midrin prior to arrival without relief. Her neurological exam is unremarkable other than possible up-going Babinski. Her blood pressure is 138/78 mm Hg. You administer one dose of Midrin, but the headache is not alleviated. What is the best next step in evaluation and treatment?

- **a.** Administer third dose of Midrin
- **b.** Computed tomography of the head
- **c.** Magnetic resonance imaging of the brain
- **d.** Administer morphine and ondansetron and continue to monitor

60–13. The patient in Question 60–12 undergoes imaging as shown below. What is the most likely diagnosis?

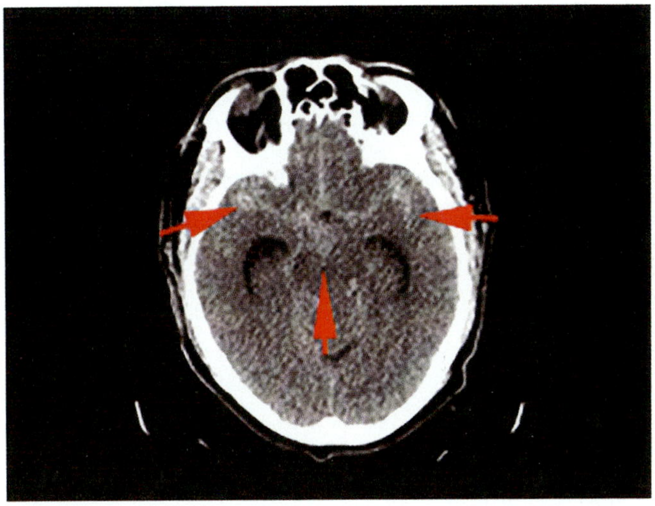

Used with permission from Dr. Ankur Patel.

- **a.** Migraine headache
- **b.** Subdural hematoma
- **c.** Intracerebral hemorrhage
- **d.** Subarachnoid hemorrhage

60–14. The patient described in Question 60–12 undergoes surgical repair of her aneurysm and does well. She presents at 37 weeks' gestation in active labor. What is the recommended mode of delivery?

- **a.** Cesarean delivery
- **b.** Spontaneous vaginal delivery
- **c.** Vaginal with an assisted second stage
- **d.** The optimal mode of delivery is unclear

60–15. During an imaging study for chronic headaches a woman is diagnosed with an intracranial aneurysm measuring 12 mm. She inquires as to the risk of rupture, and whether pregnancy will alter this risk. What is the best estimate of her risk prior to and during pregnancy?

- **a.** 0.1% risk of rupture, increased in pregnancy
- **b.** 0.1% risk of rupture, unchanged in pregnancy
- **c.** 1.0% risk of rupture, increased in pregnancy
- **d.** 1.0% risk of rupture, unchanged in pregnancy

60–16. A 26-year-old primigravida woman presents for prenatal care at 6 weeks' gestation. She has a history of relapsing, remitting multiple sclerosis with the magnetic resonance imaging findings shown below (arrows point to white matter lesions). You counsel her that disease activity as it pertains to pregnancy is best described by which statement below?

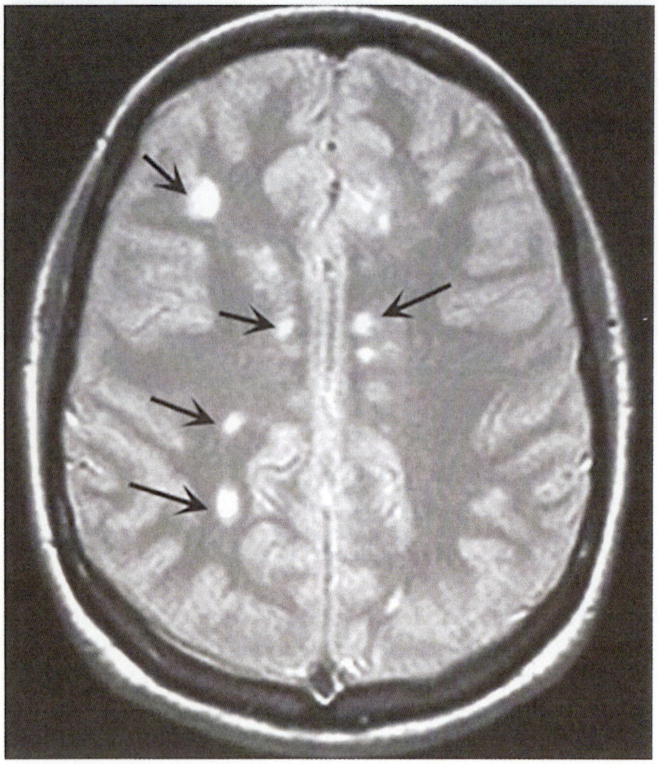

Reproduced with permission from Cunningham FG, Leveno KJ, Bloom SL, et al (eds): Neurological disorders. In Williams Obstetrics, 25th ed. New York, McGraw-Hill, 2018, Figure 60-4.

a. Unchanged by pregnancy

b. Worsened during pregnancy with a relapse postpartum

c. Worsened during pregnancy and improved postpartum

d. 30% of women improve, 30% are unchanged, 30% worsen

60–17. The patient in Question 60–16 inquires as to acceptable multiple sclerosis therapies. You counsel her that available data are limited, but it appears that all of the below medications are acceptable in pregnancy except which drug?

a. Prednisone

b. Fingolimod

c. Glatiramer acetate

d. Intravenous immunoglobulin

60–18. A 34-year-old G2P2 presents for preconception counseling. She was diagnosed with myasthenia gravis 6 months ago. She asks whether or not it is safe to become pregnant. You inform her that women with myasthenia gravis are at increased risk of multiple pregnancy complications including which of the following?

a. Preeclampsia

b. Preterm birth

c. Respiratory compromise

d. All of the above

60–19. When counseling the patient in Question 60–18, you include that certain medications often administered in pregnancy will need to be avoided due to possible exacerbation of her disease. Which of the below medications should be avoided in women with myasthenia gravis?

a. Narcotics

b. Gentamicin

c. Magnesium sulfate

d. All of the above

60–20. A 24-year-old G1 with myasthenia gravis presents for rate of growth sonogram with the findings shown below. Other than mild ptosis and generalized weakness she is doing well on pyridostigmine. Her prenatal care has been uncomplicated with normal aneuploidy screening and normal anatomy ultrasound. Which of the following is the most likely cause of her symptoms?

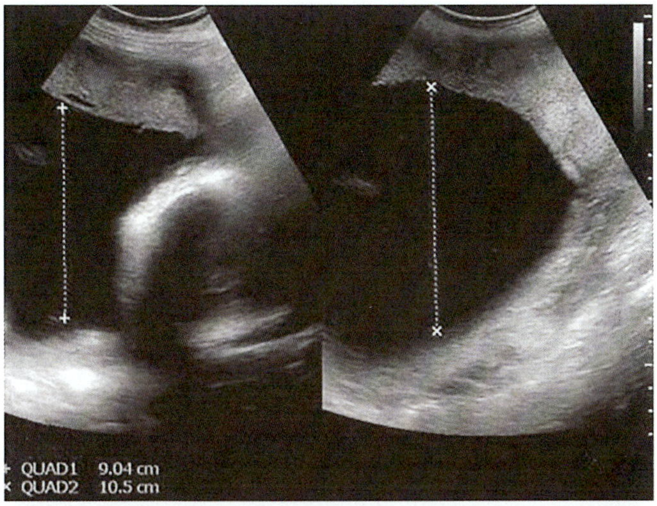

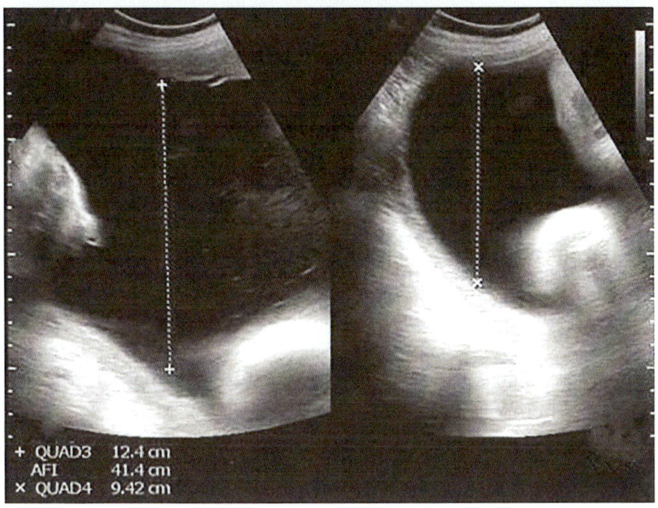

a. Hyperglycemia
b. Fetal trisomy 21
c. Anti-MuSK antibodies
d. Anti-acetylcholine-receptor antibodies

60–21. When counseling the patient in Question 60–20 regarding neonatal outcomes, you inform of which of the following?

a. Neonatal hypoglycemia is transient and treatable.
b. The infant will likely have permanent neurological issues.
c. Confirmation of the aneuploidy can be established postnatally.
d. The effect on the infant should be transient and resolve with clearance of maternal antibodies.

60–22. A 24-year-old G2P1 at 34 weeks' gestation presents to the clinic complaining of 24 hours of left-sided facial droop as shown below. Which intervention is least important?

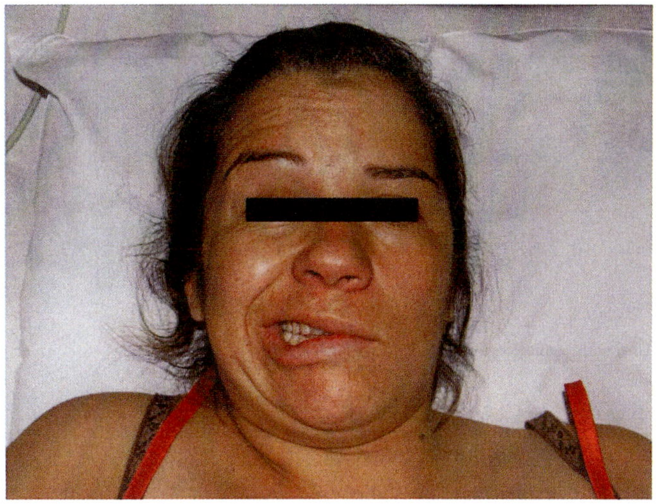

Reproduced with permission from Cunningham FG, Leveno KJ, Bloom SL, et al (eds): Neurological disorders. In Williams Obstetrics, 25th ed. New York, McGraw-Hill, 2018, Figure 60-5.

a. Prednisone
b. Valacyclovir
c. Eye protection to prevent drying and corneal abrasion
d. Neurological exam to rule out other causes such as stroke

60–23. A 34-year-old primigravida has a history of spinal cord injury at the T4 level resulting in paraplegia. She presents at 36 weeks' gestation with complaints of a new headache and flushing and sweating. Her blood pressure is 192/106 mmHg and her heart rate is 56 beats per minute. On exam her cervix is noted to be 8 cm dilated. Based on the patient's history what is her most likely diagnosis?

a. Anxiety
b. Autonomic dysreflexia
c. Normal reaction to labor pain
d. Pre-eclampsia with severe features

60–24. Regarding the patient in Question 60–23, below is a graph of her vital signs. What intervention led to the improvement in her blood pressure profile (lime green), narrowing of her pulse pressure, and stabilization of the maternal heart rate (black)?

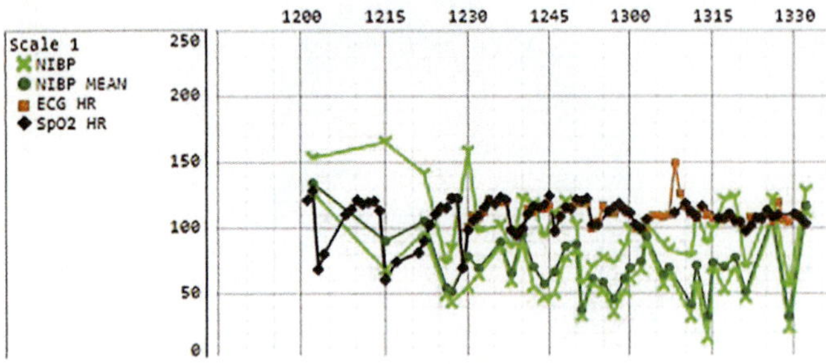

Used with permission from Dr. Santiago-Munoz.

a. Cesarean delivery
b. Epidural placement
c. Intravenous labetalol
d. Magnesium sulfate for seizure prophylaxis

60–25. Why is magnetic resonance imaging a preferred modality in the diagnosis of neurovascular disorders in pregnancy?

a. It is cost effective.
b. It does not involve ionizing radiation.
c. It is excellent for detecting recent hemorrhage.
d. None of the above

60–26. Which of the following medications is associated with an increased risk of this congenital anomaly shown on the below magnetic resonance imaging, when taken in early pregnancy?

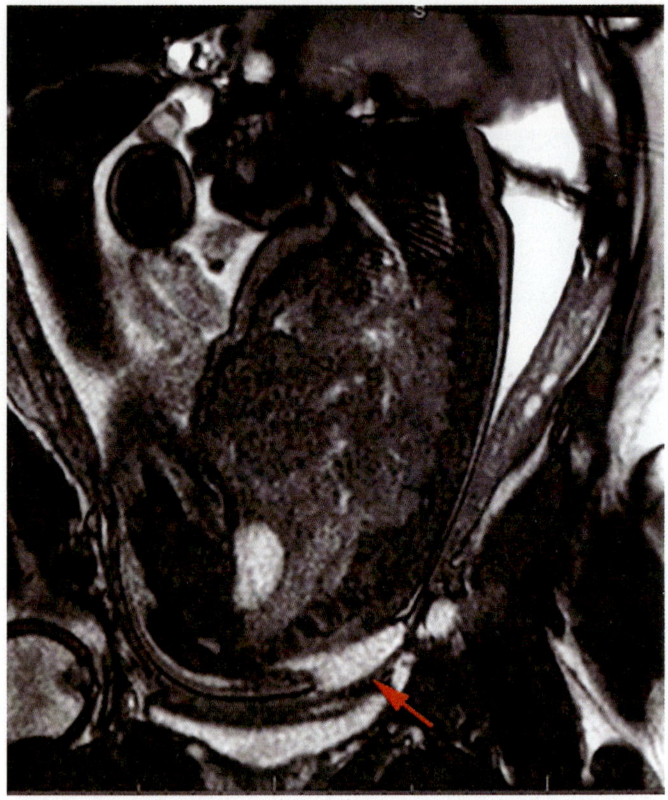

a. Valproate
b. Prednisone
c. Topiramate
d. Lamotrigine

60–27. What is the most common cause of subarachnoid hemorrhage?

a. Trauma
b. Cerebral venous thrombosis
c. Ruptured saccular aneurysm
d. Ruptured arteriovenous malformation

60–28. Serum levels of antiepileptic medications are unreliable in pregnancy for which of the following reasons?

a. Altered protein binding
b. Increased glomerular filtration
c. Levels are not available for new medications
d. None of the above

60–29. What is the most common etiology for ischemic stroke in pregnancy?

a. Cocaine use
b. Hypertension
c. Saccular aneurysm
d. Arteriovenous malformation

60–30. Which of the following is not an accurate statement regarding maternal middle cerebral artery embolism during pregnancy?

a. May be caused by paradoxical embolism
b. Occurs more commonly in the first trimester
c. Must exclude thrombosis and hemorrhage prior to diagnosis
d. Treatment may include antiplatelet therapy during pregnancy

60–31. Neurovascular disorders account for what percent of maternal deaths in the United States?

a. 1%
b. 5%
c. 10%
d. 20%

60–32. Which of the following medications used to treat migraine headaches should be avoided in pregnancy?

a. Ibuprofen
b. Metoprolol
c. Sumatriptan
d. Ergotamine derivatives

CHAPTER 60 ANSWER KEY

Question number	Letter answer	Page cited	Header cited
60–1	b	p. 1157	Headache
60–2	c	p. 1157	Headache
60–3	d	p. 1158	Headache
60–4	b	p. 1159	Seizure Disorders
60–5	b	p. 1159	Seizure Disorders
60–6	d	p. 1159	Seizure Disorders
60–7	d	p. 1159	Seizure Disorders
60–8	b	p. 1160	Table 60-2
60–9	a	p. 1160	Seizure Disorders
60–10	c	p. 1161	Cerebrovascular Diseases
60–11	a	p. 1161	Cerebrovascular Diseases
60–12	b	p. 1162	Cerebrovascular Diseases
60–13	d	p. 1163	Cerebrovascular Diseases
60–14	d	p. 1163	Cerebrovascular Diseases
60–15	d	p. 1163	Cerebrovascular Diseases
60–16	b	p. 1164	Demyelinating or Degenerative Disorders
60–17	b	p. 1164	Demyelinating or Degenerative Disorders
60–18	c	p. 1165	Demyelinating or Degenerative Disorders
60–19	d	p. 1165	Demyelinating or Degenerative Disorders
60–20	d	p. 1166	Demyelinating or Degenerative Disorders
60–21	d	p. 1167	Demyelinating or Degenerative Disorders
60–22	b	p. 1167	Neuropathies
60–23	b	p. 1167	Spinal Cord Injury
60–24	b	p. 1167	Spinal Cord Injury
60–25	b	p. 1156	Central Nervous System Imaging
60–26	a	p. 1160	Seizure Disorders
60–27	c	p. 1163	Cerebrovascular Diseases
60–28	a	p. 1160	Seizure Disorders
60–29	b	p. 1162	Cerebrovascular Disease
60–30	b	p. 1162	Cerebrovascular Disease
60–31	c	p. 1156	Introduction
60–32	d	p. 1158	Headache

CHAPTER 61

Psychiatric Disorders

61–1. Which of the following is not associated with psychiatric disorders in pregnancy?

a. Substance abuse

b. Poor neonatal outcomes

c. Increased number of prenatal care visits

d. Increased rate of postpartum psychiatric illness

61–2. What percent of pregnancy-associated suicides involve intimate-partner conflict?

a. 5%

b. 10%

c. 50%

d. 100%

61–3. A 25-year-old G1P1 presents for her postpartum visit 4 weeks after delivery. She reports that the first week at home was really rough. She's thrilled to be a mom, but she was amazed at how much she cried the first week. She also states that the exhaustion didn't help. She didn't call the office, because it wasn't "all day long." She is now feeling well, other than being tired. What the patient described is most likely:

a. Substance abuse

b. Postpartum blues

c. Personality disorder

d. Postpartum depression

61–4. How many times at minimum does the American College of Obstetricians and Gynecologists recommend patients be screened for depression and anxiety?

a. One

b. Two

c. Three

d. Seven

61–5. What percentage of depressed women are identified by their obstetricians and gynecologists in clinical practice?

a. 20%

b. 40%

c. 60%

d. 80%

61–6. According to the National Institute of Mental Health, what is the lifetime prevalence of depressive disorders in the United States?

a. 10%

b. 20%

c. 30%

d. 50%

61–7. Which of the following is not associated with postpartum depression?

a. Older maternal age

b. Antenatal depression

c. Physical or verbal abuse

d. Hyperemesis gravidarum

61–8. Which of the following medications for treatment of mood disorders was historically linked to fetal heart defects?

a. Fluoxetine

b. Duloxetine

c. Haloperidol

d. Amitriptyline

61–9. A 34-year-old multigravida presents at 18 weeks' gestation for prenatal care. The patient has a long history of mental illness and developmental delay. She has been maintained on lithium for the better part of 10 years, and she has been taking it regularly this pregnancy. The patient undergoes a targeted ultrasound with fetal echocardiogram. An image from the study is provided below. What is the most likely diagnosis for the fetus?

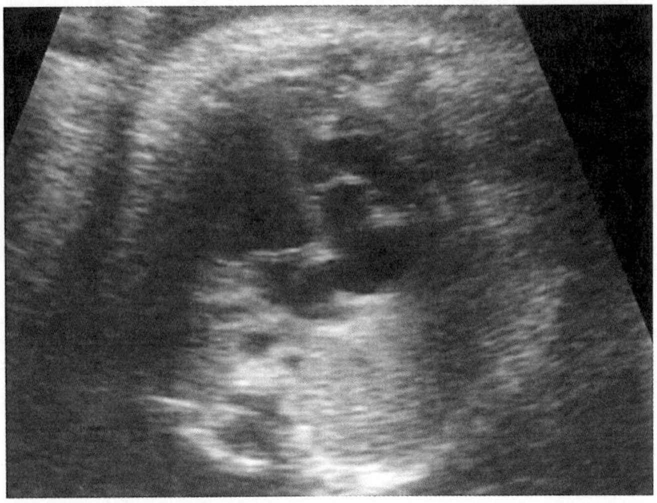

Used with permission from Dr. Jodi Dashe.

- **a.** Ebstein anomaly
- **b.** Neural-tube defect
- **c.** Tetralogy of Fallot
- **d.** Pulmonary hypertension

61–10. The fetal malformation in the ultrasound image below would most likely result from first-trimester exposure to which of the following psychiatric medications?

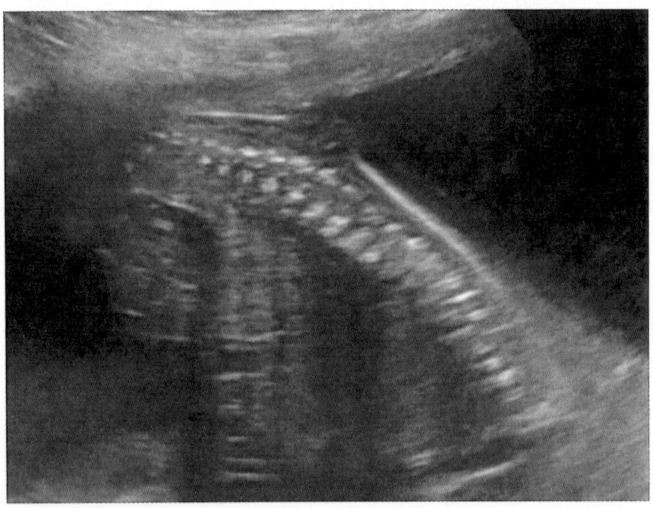

- **a.** Fluoxetine
- **b.** Haloperidol
- **c.** Valproic acid
- **d.** Amitriptyline

61–11. The fetal malformation in the ultrasound image below has been loosely associated with first-trimester exposure to which of the following psychiatric medications?

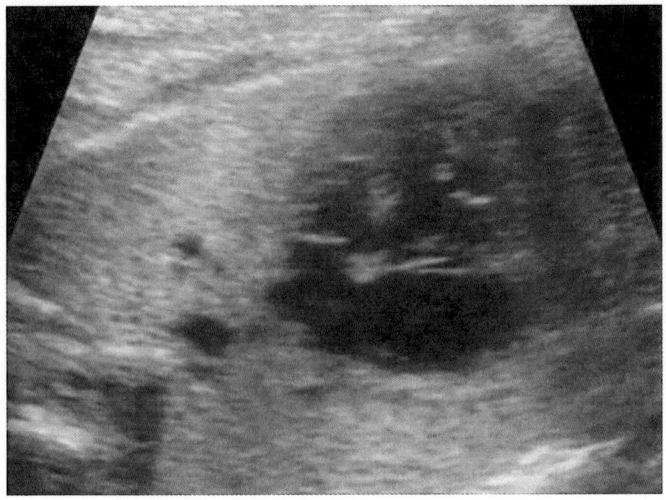

- **a.** Paroxetine
- **d.** Bupropion
- **c.** Haloperidol
- **d.** Amitriptyline

61–12. A 27-year-old G1P0 presents at 15 weeks' gestation for prenatal care. She has no significant past medical history. On interview, she reports symptoms of depression including sadness, crying, and a sleep disturbance. She denies suicidal/homicidal ideation. It does not appear that her depression is severe. What is the next step in your management?

- **a.** Begin treatment with lithium
- **b.** Routine care for now with reevaluation postpartum
- **c.** Psychotherapy and, if no response, antidepressant medication
- **d.** Immediate referral to psychiatric emergency department

61–13. What percentage of women with postpartum depression will remain depressed 1 year later if not treated?

- **a.** 5%
- **b.** 10%
- **c.** 25%
- **d.** 50%

61–14. Which of the following classes of drugs for the treatment of depression is most likely to be used in a reproductive-age woman?

- **a.** Typical antipsychotic
- **b.** Tricyclic antidepressant
- **c.** Monoamine oxidase inhibitor
- **d.** Selective serotonin-reuptake inhibitor

61–15. A 24-year-old G1P1 presented to your office for her postpartum checkup 6 weeks after giving birth. You diagnose her with depression and start a selective serotonin-reuptake inhibitor. The patient re-presents 2 months later, and she is feeling much improved. She asks for how long she needs to take this medication. She does not want to relapse, but she would prefer to not take medications as well. What is your response?

a. One month

b. Three months

c. Six months or more

d. She can stop the medication now

61–16. A 20-year-old G1P0 presents at 18 weeks' gestation for prenatal care. She has a history of major depression for which she was prescribed fluoxetine. This worked well for her. The patient stopped the medication at 12 weeks when she found out she was pregnant. She is now suffering from symptoms of depression which are impacting her life significantly. She is not suicidal or homicidal. What is your best next step in her care?

a. Start her on amitriptyline.

b. Order electroconvulsive therapy.

c. Start omega-3 fatty acid supplements

d. Restart her fluoxetine and refer her back to her psychiatrist.

61–17. Which of the following is associated with fetal exposure to serotonin-reuptake inhibitors after 20 weeks' gestation?

a. Ebstein anomaly

b. Neural tube defect

c. Ventricular septal defect

d. Persistent pulmonary hypertension

61–18. What percent of exposed neonates exhibit withdrawal from serotonin-reuptake inhibitors?

a. 10%

b. 20%

c. 30%

d. 40%

61–19. What is the perinatal complication rate of electroconvulsive therapy during pregnancy?

a. 1%

b. 3%

c. 5%

d. 10%

61–20. What is the lifetime prevalence of bipolar disorder?

a. 3.9%

b. 6.9%

c. 9.9%

d. 15.9%

61–21. If a person has bipolar disorder, what is the risk that their monozygotic twin will also have it?

a. 5–10%

b. 15–25%

c. 30–35%

d. 40–70%

61–22. Which of the following is not a treatment for bipolar disorder?

a. Lithium

b. Valproic acid

c. Amitriptyline

d. Carbamazepine

61–23. Which of the following statements about postpartum psychosis is true?

a. Incidence is 1/500 deliveries

b. It is more common in multiparous patients

c. It usually manifests itself 2 months after delivery

d. The most important risk factor is a history of bipolar disease

61–24. Which of the following is not a symptom of mania?

a. Confusion

b. Somnolence

c. Feeling excited

d. Being loquacious

61–25. A 27-year-old G2P1 presents at term in active labor. The patient has a history significant for postpartum psychosis in her last pregnancy 1 year ago. At that time, the patient required multiple medications and hospitalization. That baby has since been put up for adoption. Which of the following is the most appropriate plan of care for this pregnancy?

a. Initiate lithium therapy immediately after delivery

b. Schedule outpatient postpartum psychotherapy at discharge

c. Preemptively start a selective serotonin-reuptake inhibitor now

d. Counsel the patient that she has a 50–50 chance of this happening again, so she should plan to stay with a responsible family member postpartum in case she develops symptoms.

61–26. Which of the following is a fetal/neonatal complication of maternal ingestion of benzodiazepines?

a. Cleft lip

b. Neural tube defect

c. Ventricular septal defect

d. Neonatal withdrawal syndrome

61–27. A couple presents for counseling. They are pregnant with their first child at 20 weeks' gestation. The father of the baby has a history of schizophrenia. He was diagnosed 6 years ago, and he is well controlled on medication. They ask what the chances are that the child will have this mental illness. What number do you quote them?

a. 1%

b. 5–10%

c. 25%

d. 50–75%

61–28. Which of the following statements about schizophrenia is false?

a. It is a degenerative brain disorder.

b. It has a major genetic component.

c. There is a 50% concordance in monozygotic twins.

d. The association with maternal influenza A infection has been proven in multiple large studies.

61–29. A 26-year-old G1P0 at 22 weeks presents for consultation. She has a 4-year history of schizophrenia. She is fairly well controlled on haloperidol. She wants to know what she should do about her medication while pregnant. What is the best advice?

a. Stop the medication until after pregnancy.

b. Change to an atypical antipsychotic because it is safer in pregnancy.

c. Continue the current medication at the current dose because it is effective for this patient.

d. Reduce the dose until symptoms occur and then increase it just slightly from there so as to reduce the risk of fetal malformations.

61–30. What is the lifetime prevalence of anorexia?

a. 0.5–1%

b. 2–3%

c. 4–5%

d. 5–10%

61–31. Which of the following eating disorders carries the highest risk of large-for-gestational age neonates?

a. Bulimia

b. Anorexia

c. Binge-eating disorder

d. All have an equal risk

61–32. Which of the following eating disorders carries the highest risk of low-birthweight neonates?

a. Bulimia

b. Anorexia

c. Binge-eating disorder

d. All have an equally high risk

61–33. What is an example of a personality disorder characterized by dramatic presentations along with self-centeredness and erratic behavior?

a. Schizoid

b. Avoidant

c. Borderline

d. Schizotypal

CHAPTER 61 ANSWER KEY

Question number	Letter answer	Page cited	Header cited
61–1	**c**	p. 1173	Psychiatric Disorders
61–2	**c**	p. 1173	Psychiatric Disorders
61–3	**b**	p. 1174	Maternity Blues
61–4	**a**	p. 1174	Perinatal Evaluation and Screening
61–5	**b**	p. 1174	Perinatal Evaluation and Screening
61–6	**b**	p. 1175	Mood Disorders
61–7	**a**	p. 1176	Postpartum Depression
61–8	**a**	p. 1176	Table 61-3
61–9	**a**	p. 1176	Table 61-3
61–10	**c**	p. 1176	Table 61-3
61–11	**b**	p. 1176	Table 61-3
61–12	**c**	p. 1177	Figure 61-1
61–13	**c**	p. 1177	Postpartum Depression
61–14	**d**	p. 1177	Depression Treatment
61–15	**c**	p. 1177	Depression Treatment
61–16	**d**	p. 1178	Depression Treatment
61–17	**d**	p. 1178	Fetal and Neonatal Effects of Therapy
61–18	**c**	p. 1178	Fetal and Neonatal Effects of Therapy
61–19	**b**	p. 1178	Electroconvulsive Therapy
61–20	**a**	p. 1179	Bipolar and Related Disorders
61–21	**d**	p. 1179	Bipolar and Related Disorders
61–22	**b**	p. 1179	Bipolar Disorder in Pregnancy
61–23	**d**	p. 1179	Postpartum Psychosis
61–24	**b**	p. 1179	Postpartum Psychosis
61–25	**a**	p. 1179	Postpartum Psychosis
61–26	**d**	p. 1180	Anxiety Disorder Treatment
61–27	**a**	p. 1180	Schizophrenia Spectrum Disorders
61–28	**d**	p. 1180	Schizophrenia Spectrum Disorders
61–29	**c**	p. 1180	Schizophrenia Spectrum Disorders
61–30	**b**	p. 1180	Eating Disorders
61–31	**c**	p. 1180	Eating Disorders
61–32	**b**	p. 1180	Eating Disorders
61–33	**c**	p. 1181	Personality Disorders

CHAPTER 62

Dermatological Disorders

62–1. What percentage of women are diagnosed with a pregnancy-specific dermatosis?

a. 5%

b. 10%

c. 25%

d. 50%

62–2. What is the most common type of rash seen in cholestasis of pregnancy?

a. Papules

b. Plaques

c. Vesicles

d. There are generally no skin lesions

62–3. What part of the body is usually spared in cases of pemphigoid gestationis?

a. Face

b. Back

c. Arms

d. Abdomen

62–4. What is the etiology of pemphigoid gestationis?

a. Coxsackie virus

b. Herpes simplex virus

c. Maternal IgE antibodies targeting collagen IV

d. Maternal IgG antibodies targeting collagen XVII

62–5. A 25-year-old G1P0 at 24 weeks' gestation is diagnosed with pemphigoid gestationis. Two photographs are provided below. How do you counsel her?

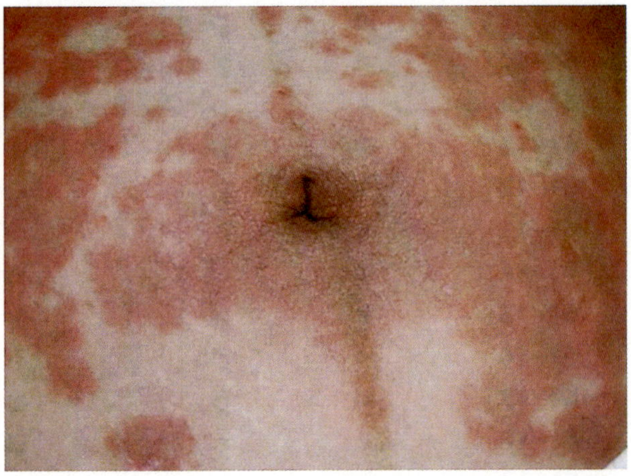

Reproduced with permission from Ehlers K, Santiago-Munoz P, Hoffman BL: Pemphigoid gestationis (update in) Cunningham FG, Leveno KJ, Bloom SL, et al (eds): Williams Obstetrics, 24th ed. New York, McGraw-Hill, 2014. Available at: http://accessmedicine.mhmedical.com/MultimediaPlayer.aspx?MultimediaID=7918794&SearchTerm=pemphigoid%20gestationis.

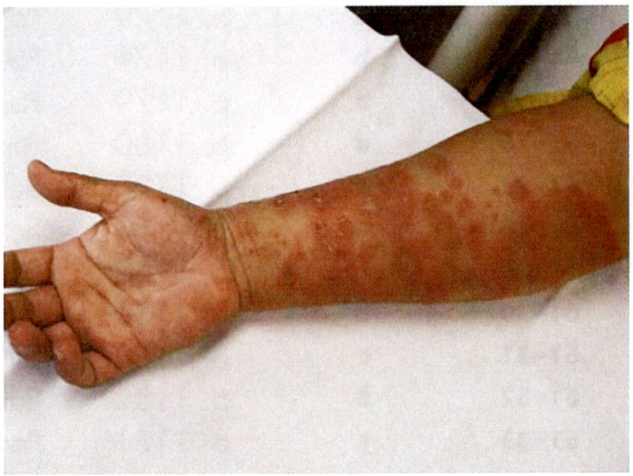

Reproduced with permission from Ehlers K, Santiago-Munoz P, Hoffman BL: Pemphigoid gestationis (update in) Cunningham FG, Leveno KJ, Bloom SL, et al (eds): Williams Obstetrics, 24th ed. New York, McGraw-Hill, 2014. Available at: http://accessmedicine.mhmedical.com/MultimediaPlayer.aspx?MultimediaID=7918794&SearchTerm=pemphigoid%20gestationis.

a. This won't happen in subsequent pregnancies.

b. Once the pregnancy is over, she will be flare-free.

c. The newborn is never affected with the same skin lesions.

d. Blistering is associated with preterm birth and intrauterine growth restriction.

62–6. Which of the following is considered rare?

a. Prurigo of pregnancy
b. Cholestasis of pregnancy
c. Pruritic folliculitis of pregnancy
d. Pruritic urticarial papules and plaques of pregnancy

62–7. All of the following are on the differential when assessing a patient for pemphigoid gestationis, but which is most important to rule out?

a. Allergic contact dermatitis
b. Stevens-Johnson syndrome
c. Atopic eruption of pregnancy
d. All of the above conditions are life threatening, making each important to rule out.

62–8. What is the gold standard for the diagnosis of pemphigoid gestationis?

a. Serum C3 levels
b. IgG antibodies to collagen IV
c. Culture for herpes simplex virus
d. Immunofluorescent staining of a skin punch biopsy

62–9. What is the first-line treatment for pemphigoid gestationis?

a. Acyclovir
b. Emollients
c. Cyclosporine
d. Steroids and antihistamines

62–10. A 21-year-old G1P0 at 33 weeks' gestation with diamnionic/dichorionic twins presents complaining of a pruritic rash for 4 days. It is mostly on her abdomen and thighs. A photo is provided below. She denies fever and sick contacts. You diagnose her with pruritic urticarial papules and plaques of pregnancy. All except which of the following is included in your counseling?

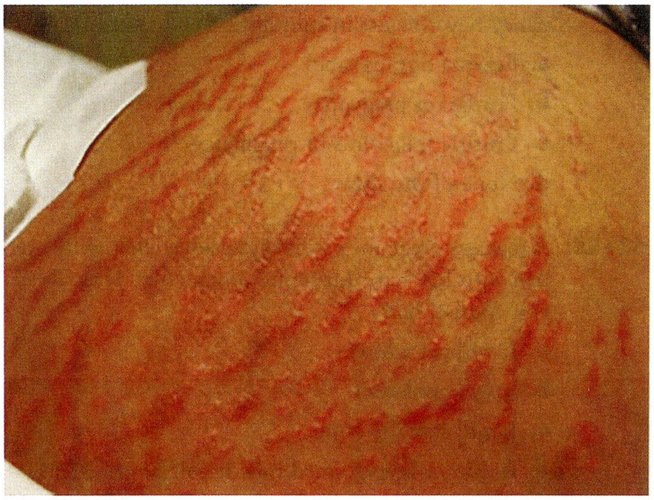

a. It will resolve postpartum.
b. It seldom recurs in other pregnancies.
c. It should respond to emollients, oral antihistamines, and steroids.
d. It is autoimmune in nature, and it is expected that the fetus will be affected 5–10% of the time.

62–11. Which of the following atopic eruptions of pregnancy is characterized by thickened, scaly, red patches involving extremity flexures?

a. Eczema of pregnancy
b. Prurigo of pregnancy
c. Pruritic folliculitis of pregnancy
d. None of the above

62–12. Which of the following atopic eruptions of pregnancy is characterized by 5- to 10-mm itchy papules or nodules?

a. Eczema of pregnancy
b. Prurigo of pregnancy
c. Pruritic folliculitis of pregnancy
d. None of the above

62–13. Which of the following atopic eruptions of pregnancy is characterized by sterile pustules?

a. Eczema of pregnancy
b. Prurigo of pregnancy
c. Pruritic folliculitis of pregnancy
d. None of the above

62–14. Which of the following atopic eruptions of pregnancy never recurs in subsequent pregnancies?

a. Eczema of pregnancy
b. Prurigo of pregnancy
c. Pruritic folliculitis of pregnancy
d. None of the above

62–15. A teenage pregnant patient is curious what will happen with her acne during her pregnancy. How do you counsel her?

a. It will get worse.
b. It will get better.
c. It will stay the same.
d. It cannot be predicted how it will be affected by pregnancy.

62–16. Which of the following treatments for acne vulgaris is contraindicated in pregnancy?

a. Azelaic acid
b. Benzoyl peroxide
c. Topical tazarotene
d. Over-the-counter topical salicylic acid

62–17. Which of the following oral antibiotics is not recommended for treatment of acne vulgaris in pregnancy?

a. Cephalexin
b. Amoxicillin
c. Doxycycline
d. Azithromycin

62–18. A 24-year-old primigravida presents at 15 weeks' gestation with a rash characterized by plaques. You diagnose her with psoriasis. Which of the following is first-line treatment?

a. Emollients
b. Cyclosporine
c. Ultraviolet phototherapy
d. High-potency topical corticosteroids

62–19. A 25-year-old G2P1 presents at 30 weeks' gestation. She is complaining of pruritic plaques and pustules on her abdomen. A photo is provided below. Which of the following lab values would you not expect to see?

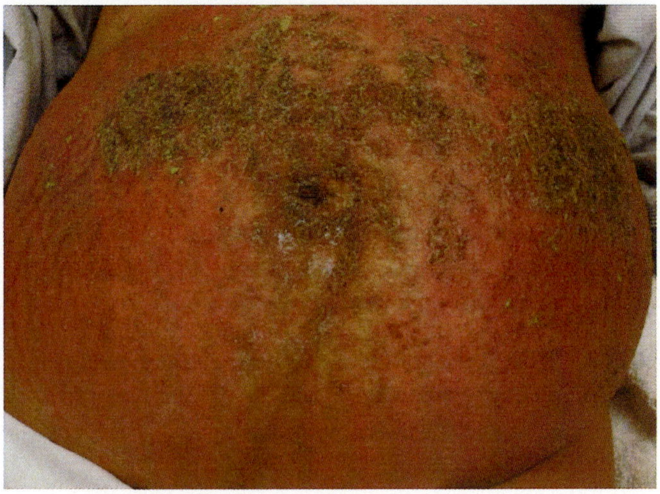

Used with permission from Dr. Paul Slocum.

a. Leukocytosis
b. Hypercalcemia
c. Hypoalbuminemia
d. Elevated erythrocyte sedimentation rate

62–20. For the patient in Question 62–19, which of the following complications would be of most concern to you?

a. Sepsis
b. Hypovolemia
c. Placental insufficiency
d. All of the above

62–21. What is the best initial choice of treatment for the patient in Question 62–19?

a. Emollients
b. Cephalexin
c. Oral steroids
d. Cyclosporine and phototherapy

62–22. For the patient in Question 62–19, at what time may she have a recurrence of this condition?

a. Menstruation
b. Subsequent pregnancy
c. While taking oral contraceptives
d. All of the above

62–23. What is the affected tissue in erythema nodosum?

a. Skin
b. Muscle
c. Hair follicle
d. Subcutaneous fat

62–24. Which of the following can trigger erythema nodosum?

a. Pregnancy
b. Sarcoidosis
c. Inflammatory bowel disease
d. All of the above

62–25. What is the characteristic rash seen with erythema nodosum?

a. Sterile pustules of the trunk
b. Erythematous papules and bullae of the abdomen
c. Nontender hypopigmented plaques of flexor surfaces of the arms and legs
d. Tender, red, warm nodules and plaques of extensor surfaces of the arms and legs

62–26. A 19-year-old G1P0 at 22 weeks' gestation presents for a lesion on her gum. A photo is provided below. She reports that it grew quickly, which really worried her. It has also been bleeding. What is the diagnosis?

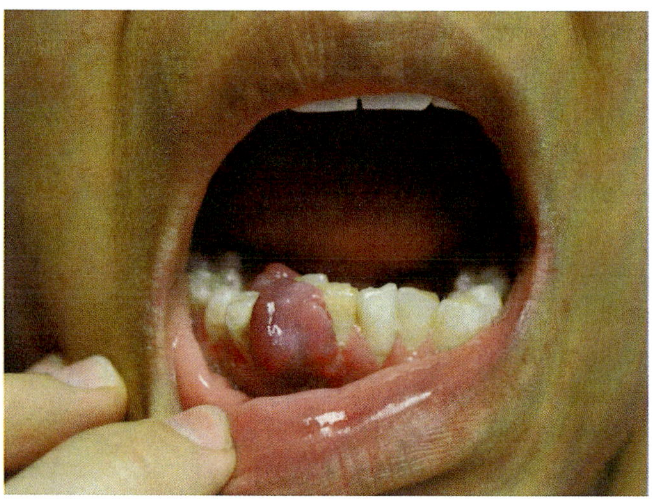

Used with permission from Dr. Sarah White.

a. Malignancy
b. Neurofibromatosis
c. Pyogenic granuloma
d. Human papilloma virus

62–27. The patient in Question 62–26 comes back to see you two weeks later. She reports that it is getting bigger and bleeds often. She is now finding it uncomfortable to eat. Which of the following is an acceptable treatment option?

a. Excision
b. Acyclovir
c. Podophyllin resin
d. Trichloroacetic acid 80–90% solution

62–28. What is the natural course of neurofibromas in pregnancy?

a. Increase in number and size
b. Increase in size but not in number
c. Increase in number but not in size
d. Increase in number but decrease in size

62–29. Which of the following complications is increased in patients with neurofibromatosis type 2?

a. Stillbirth
b. Preeclampsia
c. Intrauterine growth restriction
d. Preterm premature rupture of membranes

62–30. What dermatological disorder is characterized by facial pustules and coalescing draining sinuses?

a. Rosacea fulminans
b. Eczema of pregnancy
c. Pruritic folliculitis of pregnancy
d. Pruritic urticarial papules and plaques of pregnancy

62–31. Which of the following is an ultrapotent topical steroid?

a. 1% hydrocortisone
b. 0.05% clobetasol propionate
c. 0.1% triamcinolone acetonide
d. 0.05% betamethasone dipropionate

62–32. Although less of a risk than seen with systemic corticosteroids, which of the following complications is increased with the use of high and ultrapotent topical steroids in pregnancy?

a. Abruption
b. Preterm birth
c. Intrauterine growth restriction
d. Preterm premature rupture of membranes

CHAPTER 62 ANSWER KEY

Question number	Letter answer	Page cited	Header cited
62–1	**a**	p. 1184	Pregnancy-Specific Dermatoses
62–2	**d**	p. 1184	Intrahepatic Cholestasis of Pregnancy
62–3	**a**	p. 1184	Pemphigoid Gestationis
62–4	**d**	p. 1184	Pemphigoid Gestationis
62–5	**d**	p. 1184	Pemphigoid Gestationis
62–6	**c**	p. 1184–1185	Table 62-1
62–7	**b**	p. 1184–1185	Diagnosis and Treatment
62–8	**d**	p. 1186	Diagnosis and Treatment
62–9	**d**	p. 1186	Diagnosis and Treatment
62–10	**d**	p. 1186	Pruritic Urticarial Papules and Plaques of Pregnancy
62–11	**a**	p. 1186	Atopic Eruption of Pregnancy
62–12	**b**	p. 1186	Atopic Eruption of Pregnancy
62–13	**c**	p. 1186	Atopic Eruption of Pregnancy
62–14	**d**	p. 1186	Atopic Eruption of Pregnancy
62–15	**d**	p. 1187	Acne Vulgaris
62–16	**c**	p. 1187	Acne Vulgaris
62–17	**c**	p. 1187	Acne Vulgaris
62–18	**a**	p. 1187	Psoriasis and Pustular Psoriasis
62–19	**b**	p. 1187	Psoriasis and Pustular Psoriasis
62–20	**d**	p. 1187	Psoriasis and Pustular Psoriasis
62–21	**c**	p. 1187	Psoriasis and Pustular Psoriasis
62–22	**d**	p. 1187	Psoriasis and Pustular Psoriasis
62–23	**d**	p. 1187	Erythema Nodosum
62–24	**d**	p. 1187	Erythema Nodosum
62–25	**d**	p. 1187	Erythema Nodosum
62–26	**c**	p. 1188	Pyogenic Granuloma
62–27	**a**	p. 1188	Pyogenic Granuloma
62–28	**a**	p. 1188	Neurofibromatosis
62–29	**b**	p. 1188	Neurofibromatosis
62–30	**a**	p. 1188	Miscellaneous Conditions
62–31	**b**	p. 1188	Dermatological Treatment
62–32	**c**	p. 1188	Dermatological Treatment

CHAPTER 63

Neoplastic Disorders

63–1. What is the most common cancer diagnosed during pregnancy?

- **a.** Lymphoma
- **b.** Breast cancer
- **c.** Thyroid cancer
- **d.** Cervical cancer

63–2. What is the threshold radiation dose for intellectual disability at 8–15 weeks' gestation?

- **a.** 0.06 Gy
- **b.** 0.10 Gy
- **c.** 0.20 Gy
- **d.** 0.25 Gy

63–3. You are caring for a pregnant woman with invasive ductal carcinoma of the left breast who is undergoing chemotherapy and is currently 28 weeks. How many weeks in advance of her planned delivery would you recommend holding her chemotherapy?

- **a.** 1 week
- **b.** 2 weeks
- **c.** 3 weeks
- **d.** There is no reason to hold her chemotherapy prior to delivery.

63–4. A pregnant woman transfers to you at 20 weeks' gestation. She was diagnosed with lymphoma in the first trimester and is currently receiving chemotherapy. Due to severe anemia, her hematologist-oncologist is administering erythropoietin alfa. What side effect should you be most careful to watch for during her prenatal care course?

- **a.** Hypertension
- **b.** Oligohydramnios
- **c.** Gestational diabetes
- **d.** Fetal-growth restriction

63–5. A 32-year-old G0 who was recently diagnosed with cervical cancer and is preparing to start chemotherapy and radiation presents to your office to discuss fertility-sparing options. Which of the following options would you not recommend as a well-established fertility-preserving option?

- **a.** Cryopreservation
- **b.** Surgical transposition of the ovaries
- **c.** Gonadotropin-releasing hormone agonist administration
- **d.** All of the above should be recommended

63–6. Which of the following cancer treatment modalities has a clear and consistent link with adverse obstetrical outcomes?

- **a.** Abdominopelvic radiation
- **b.** Chemotherapy administered in childhood
- **c.** Chemotherapy administered in adulthood
- **d.** All of the above

63–7. A 25-year-old G1 presents at 28 weeks' gestation complaining of vaginal spotting. You perform a speculum exam for further evaluation and note the findings shown in the image. What is the risk of malignant transformation in this lesion?

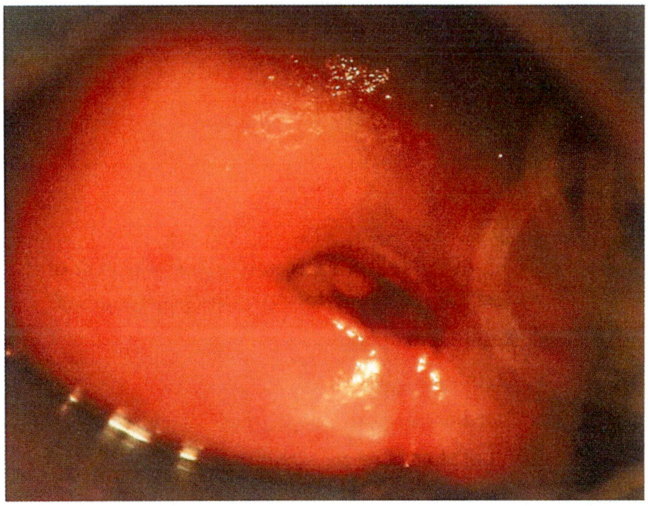

- **a.** 0.05%
- **b.** 0.10%
- **c.** 0.50%
- **d.** 1.0%

63–8. You are caring for a pregnant 35-year-old G1 with the condition shown in the photo. She is very concerned about transmission of the associated virus to the baby if she proceeds with a vaginal delivery. Which of the following statements would be the most appropriate counseling for your patient?

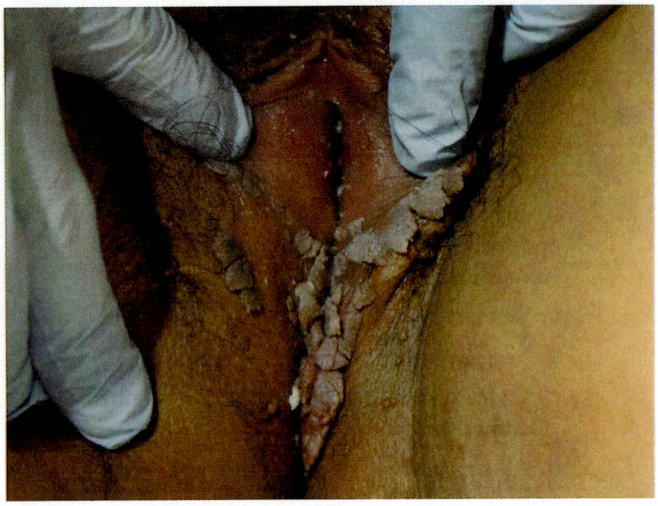

a. Congenital HPV infection does not occur due to vertical transmission
b. Cesarean delivery reduces the risk of neonatal laryngeal papillomatosis
c. Laryngeal warts present in the neonate at birth are most likely due to perinatal exposure
d. None of the above is true

63–9. You perform a Pap smear on a new obstetric patient at 9 weeks' gestation. The Pap cytology is low-grade squamous intraepithelial lesion. You perform a colposcopy, which is consistent with a cervical intraepithelial neoplasia 2 lesion. What is the chance of lesion regression upon reevaluation in the postpartum period?

a. 40–50%
b. 50–60%
c. 60–70%
d. 70–80%

63–10. Which of the following is not a significant risk of cervical conization performed during pregnancy?

a. Residual neoplasia
b. Membrane rupture
c. Bleeding requiring transfusion
d. All of the above are significant risks

63–11. Which of the following physiological changes that occur in pregnancy may result in an underestimation of cervical cancer spread and therefore impede accurate staging?

a. Urinary tract dilation
b. Broad ligament softening
c. Lymph node enlargement
d. All of the above

63–12. A 23-year-old G1 who is currently 28 weeks pregnant is diagnosed with stage IA1 cervical cancer. How would you advise her concerning the remainder of her care?

a. Vaginal delivery is contraindicated.
b. Early delivery at 34 weeks is recommended.
c. Definitive therapy is reserved until 12 weeks postpartum.
d. None of the above

63–13. You are caring for a 28-year-old G1 at 25 weeks' gestation who is diagnosed with stage IB1 cervical cancer. Which of the following is not a reasonable treatment option in light of her viable pregnancy?

a. Immediate radiotherapy
b. Immediate radical trachelectomy
c. Radical hysterectomy at time of delivery
d. None of the above

63–14. Which of the following hormones can stimulate growth of leiomyomas?

a. Estrogen
b. Progesterone
c. Estrogen and progesterone
d. Neither stimulates leiomyoma growth

63–15. While you are covering emergency room admissions, a 26-year-old woman presents with acute, new-onset midline abdominal pain. Her temperature in the emergency room is 99.6°F, blood pressure is 110/70 mm Hg, and pulse is 102 beats per minute. Her urine pregnancy test is positive. She has no significant medical history, but does report a history of heavy, cyclic menses. Her white count returns as 15,000, but the remainder of her chemistry and liver analytes appear normal. On your examination, she has focal midline lower abdominal tenderness, but no rebound or guarding is noted. An abdominal ultrasound is performed, and the image is shown. What is the best course of treatment for the likely underlying cause of her symptoms?

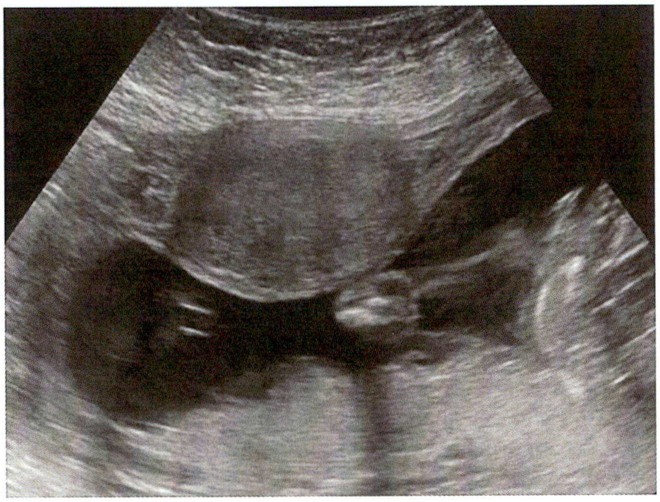

a. Observation only
b. Narcotic analgesia
c. Non-narcotic analgesia
d. Exploratory laparotomy

63–16. Which of the following pregnancy complications is not increased in the presence of uterine leiomyomas?

a. Preterm labor
b. Oligohydramnios
c. Placental abruption
d. Postpartum hemorrhage

63–17. You are seeing a 36-year-old G3P2A1 who recently suffered an early miscarriage at 6 weeks' gestation. She is interested in trying to conceive again. She reports normal, cyclic menses with light to moderate flow. Her ultrasound image is shown. What treatment would you recommend prior to her attempting pregnancy again?

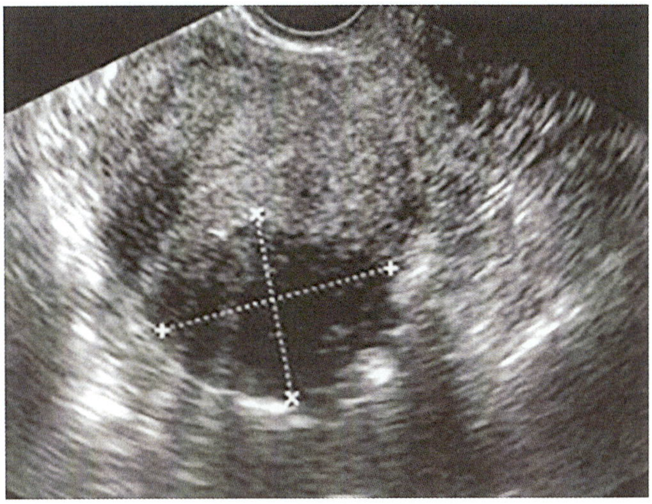

a. Uterine artery embolization
b. Hysteroscopic myomectomy
c. Repeat ultrasound in 8 weeks
d. No further treatment is needed

CHAPTER 63

63–18. A 34-year-old woman comes to see you for abnormal uterine bleeding. During the course of your work-up, you obtain the ultrasound images that are pictured. She subsequently becomes pregnant. What complication is she at increased risk for based on her ultrasound findings?

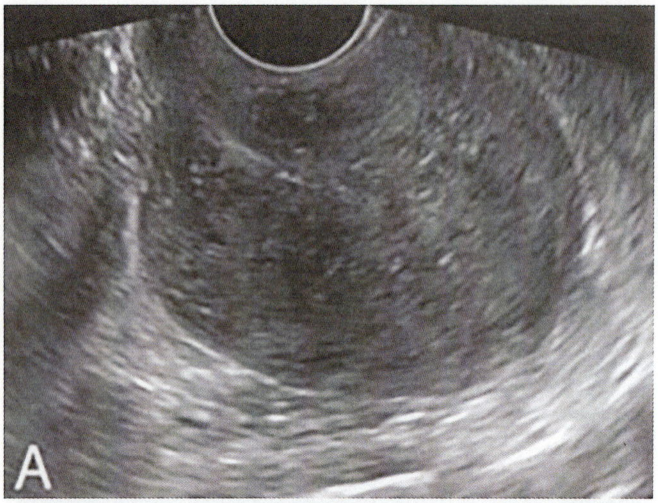

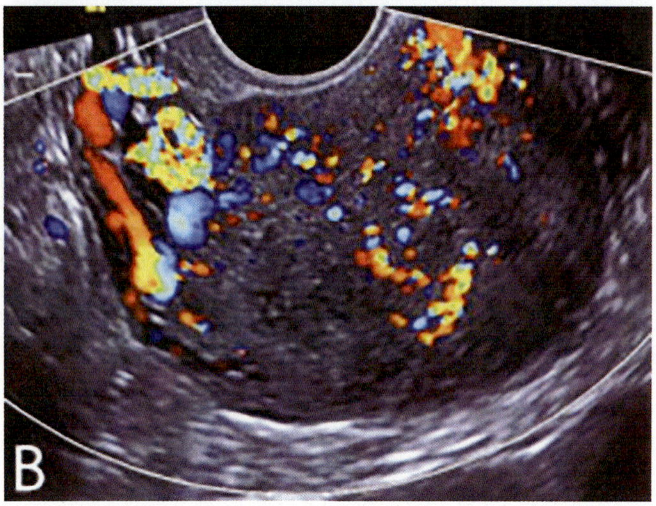

a. Preeclampsia
b. Gestational diabetes
c. Fetal-growth restriction
d. Postpartum hemorrhage

63–19. During a routine prenatal ultrasound, a 35-year-old woman with an otherwise uncomplicated pregnancy is noted to have the ultrasound findings shown. What do you tell her the risk of frank malignancy is with such findings?

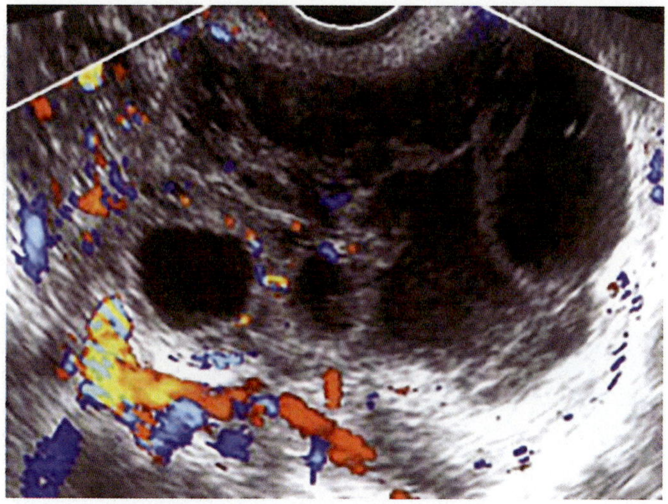

a. 0.5%
b. 1.0%
c. 1.5%
d. 2.0%

63–20. What pregnancy-specific condition is associated with abnormally elevated cancer antigen 125 levels?
a. Placenta previa
b. Placental abruption
c. Severe preeclampsia
d. All of the above

63–21. A pregnant patient at 21 weeks' gestation complains of intermittent left lower quadrant pain and nausea and vomiting. She undergoes exploratory laparotomy with the intraoperative images as shown. Which of the following is true, in general, of patients with this diagnosis?

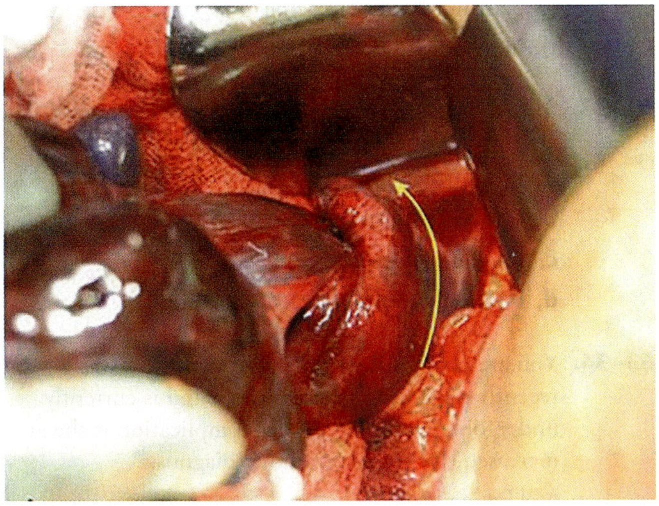

Reproduced with permission from Hoffman BL: Pelvic mass. In Hoffman BL, Schorge JO, Bradshaw KD, et al (eds): Williams Gynecology, 2nd ed. New York, McGraw-Hill Education, 2016, Figure 9-21A.

- **a.** Excision of the adnexa is always required
- **b.** All patients require progesterone supplementation
- **c.** Oophoropexy could prevent a recurrence of this complication
- **d.** All of the above

63–22. If the patient in Question 63–21 was only 7 weeks pregnant, which progesterone regimen would be acceptable for pregnancy maintenance postoperatively?

- **a.** Progesterone 300 mg daily for 3 weeks
- **b.** No additional supplementation is needed
- **c.** One injection of 17-hydroxyprogesterone caproate 150 mg
- **d.** 8-percent progesterone vaginal gel plus progesterone 100 mg daily for 3 weeks

63–23. A 20-year-old G1 at 18 weeks' gestation is noted to have an asymptomatic 10-cm complex adnexal mass with thick septa and solid components on a routine prenatal ultrasound. What management would you recommend for this patient?

- **a.** Expectant management
- **b.** Magnetic resonance imaging
- **c.** Immediate laparoscopic removal
- **d.** Emergent exploratory laparotomy

63–24. A 37-year-old G1 presents to your office at 13 weeks' gestation complaining of excessive coarse hair growth on her upper lip and chin as well as a deepening of her voice. An ultrasound reveals a 6 cm mostly solid right adnexal mass. Her total testosterone levels are found to be elevated for pregnancy. What would you recommend for this patient?

- **a.** Expectant management
- **b.** Magnetic resonance imaging
- **c.** Immediate laparoscopic removal
- **d.** Emergent exploratory laparotomy

63–25. A 26-year-old otherwise healthy woman presents to the emergency department complaining of peripheral swelling, abdominal pain, nausea, and difficulty breathing. She reports that she is currently undergoing fertility treatments with injectable medications. Which of the following would not be a concern given her clinical presentation?

- **a.** Virilization
- **b.** Ovarian rupture
- **c.** Renal dysfunction
- **d.** Venous thromboembolism

63–26. What is the most common type of ovarian cancer diagnosed in pregnancy?

- **a.** Epithelial tumor
- **b.** Germ cell tumor
- **c.** Sex cord-stromal tumor
- **d.** Low-malignant-potential tumor

63–27. You palpate a 2-cm, mobile, nontender breast mass in one of your pregnant patients. After further evaluation, her triple test is found to be concordant. What do you recommend for further management?

- **a.** Serial physical examination
- **b.** Immediate surgical excision
- **c.** Magnetic resonance imaging
- **d.** No additional exams or testing

63–28. You are caring for a 38-year-old G2P1 at 28 weeks' gestation who was recently diagnosed with intraductal carcinoma of the left breast based on a biopsy specimen. All except which of the following tests are indicated for metastasis evaluation?

- **a.** Liver ultrasound
- **b.** Chest sonography
- **c.** Head computed tomography
- **d.** Skeletal magnetic resonance imaging

CHAPTER 63

63–29. Which of the following breast cancer treatment options is contraindicated for use during pregnancy?

a. Cisplatin
b. Doxorubicin
c. Trastuzumab
d. Cyclophosphamide

63–30. A 34-year-old G3P2 presents for her new obstetrical visit at 9 weeks' gestation, during which you notice a thyroid nodule. Subsequent biopsy demonstrates malignancy. How should she be counseled regarding optimal management?

a. Termination should be considered.
b. Treatment can be delayed until postpartum.
c. She should undergo chemotherapy during the second trimester.
d. She should undergo thyroidectomy during the second trimester.

63–31. Reed-Sternberg cells, such as the one shown here, are consistent with which of the following lymphoid cell malignancies?

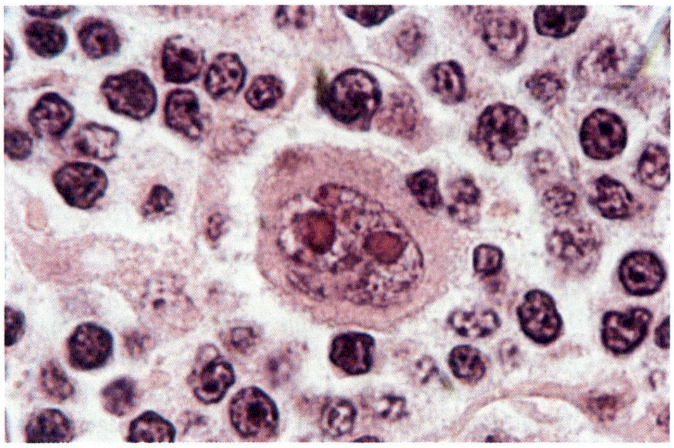

Reproduced with permission from Gascoyne RD, Skinnider BF: Pathology of malignant lymphomas. In Lichtman MA, Kipps TJ, Seligsohn U (eds): Williams Hematology, 8th ed. New York, McGraw-Hill, 2010, Figure 98-34.

a. Hairy cell leukemia
b. Hodgkin lymphoma
c. Acute myeloid leukemia
d. T cell derived lymphoma

63–32. What is the optimal treatment of a pregnant woman diagnosed with advanced-stage Hodgkin disease at 26 weeks' gestation?

a. Treatment with vinblastine alone
b. Delay treatment until after delivery at 34 weeks
c. Administration of doxorubicin, bleomycin, vinblastine, and dacarbazine
d. None of the above

63–33. All except which of the following viruses are associated with a non-Hodgkin lymphoma?

a. Hepatitis B virus
b. Epstein-Barr virus
c. Human herpes virus 8
d. Human immunodeficiency virus

63–34. You are caring for a laboring woman who was recently diagnosed with leukemia and is currently undergoing treatment. What complication is she at increased risk for based on her diagnosis?

a. Hemorrhage
b. Preeclampsia
c. Placental abruption
d. Small-for-gestational-age infant

63–35. What percentage of pregnant women with melanoma present with advanced stage disease (III or IV)?

a. 25%
b. 50%
c. 75%
d. 95%

63–36. What is the most common site of gastrointestinal cancer diagnosed during pregnancy?

a. Ileum
b. Rectum
c. Stomach
d. Descending colon

CHAPTER 63 ANSWER KEY

Question number	Letter answer	Page cited	Header cited
63–1	**b**	p. 1190	Introduction
63–2	**a**	p. 1191	Radiation Therapy
63–3	**c**	p. 1191	Chemotherapy
63–4	**a**	p. 1191	Molecular Therapy
63–5	**c**	p. 1192	Fertility and Pregnancy after Cancer
63–6	**a**	p. 1192	Fertility and Pregnancy after Cancer
63–7	**b**	p. 1192	Endocervical Polyp
63–8	**c**	p. 1193	Human Papillomavirus
63–9	**c**	p. 1193	Abnormal Cytology and Histology
63–10	**d**	p. 1193	Cervical Conization
63–11	**b**	p. 1194	Invasive Cervical Cancer
63–12	**d**	p. 1195	Management and Prognosis
63–13	**a**	p. 1195	Management and Prognosis
63–14	**c**	p. 1196	Leiomyomas
63–15	**c**	p. 1196	Symptoms
63–16	**b**	p. 1196	Pregnancy Complications
63–17	**d**	p. 1197	Fertility Considerations
63–18	**a**	p. 1197	Endometrial Lesions
63–19	**b**	p. 1198	Ovary
63–20	**c**	p. 1198	Diagnosis
63–21	**c**	p. 1198	Complications
63–22	**d**	p. 1198	Complications
63–23	**c**	p. 1199	Asymptomatic Adnexal Mass During Pregnancy
63–24	**a**	p. 1199	Pregnancy-Related Ovarian Tumors
63–25	**a**	p. 1199	Ovarian Hyperstimulation Syndrome
63–26	**b**	p. 1200	Ovarian Cancer
63–27	**a**	p. 1200	Diagnosis
63–28	**c**	p. 1201	Management
63–29	**c**	p. 1201	Management
63–30	**d**	p. 1201	Thyroid Cancer
63–31	**b**	p. 1202	Hodgkin Disease
63–32	**c**	p. 1202	Hodgkin Disease
63–33	**a**	p. 1202	Non-Hodgkin Disease
63–34	**a**	p. 1203	Leukemias
63–35	**b**	p. 1203	Melanoma
63–36	**b**	p. 1204	Gastrointestinal Cancers

CHAPTER 64

Infectious Diseases

64–1. Providing passive immunity to the fetus, what immunoglobulin is transferred across the placenta?

a. IgA

b. IgE

c. IgG

d. IgM

64–2. What is the most common perinatal infection in the developed world?

a. Toxoplasmosis

b. Cytomegalovirus

c. Varicella-zoster virus

d. Human parvovirus B19

64–3. Which of the following statements about cytomegalovirus (CMV) is true?

a. Pregnancy increases the severity of maternal CMV infection.

b. Women who become infected with CMV during pregnancy are at the greatest risk of having an infected fetus.

c. Anti-CMV IgG antibodies render a woman immune and thus safe from recurrence, reinfection, or reactivation.

d. Women of higher income groups are more likely to be immune than women of lower socioeconomic backgrounds.

64–4. A 22-year-old G1P0 at 20 weeks' gestation presents for consultation. Her anatomy ultrasound performed at an outside facility showed periventricular calcifications. The patient is a day-care worker with no significant medical history. She does not recall being unusually sick, but she states that she does not infrequently have a cold given her line of work. An image from the ultrasound is provided below. What is the most likely diagnosis?

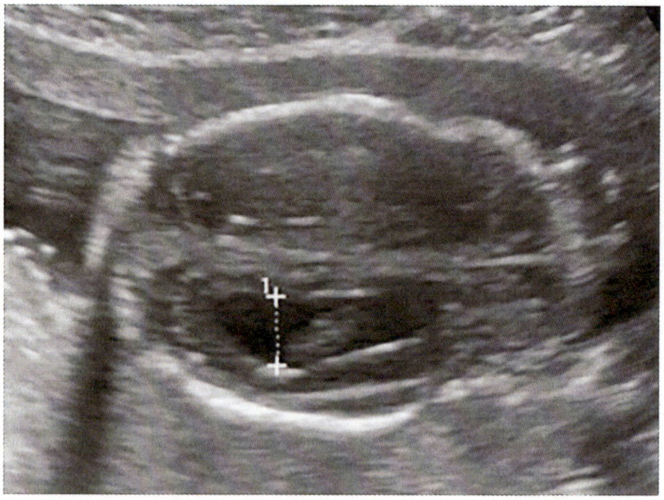

Used with permission from Dr. Jodi Dashe.

a. Congenital rubella

b. Congenital varicella

c. Congenital influenza

d. Congenital cytomegalovirus

64–5. A 30-year-old G1P0 presents at 18 weeks' gestation. Her primary physician decided to send testing for cytomegalovirus (CMV) because the patient reported a mononucleosis-like illness a month before. The testing revealed CMV IgG positive and CMV IgM positive. The patient is very concerned that her illness was primary CMV, and this baby will be affected. What is the best next step in your management?

a. Amniocentesis

b. CMV IgG avidity testing

c. Periumbilical blood sampling

d. No further evaluation is warranted

64–6. When there are abnormal sonographic findings and positive findings in fetal blood or amnionic fluid, what is the risk of symptomatic congenital CMV infection?

- **a.** 25%
- **b.** 50%
- **c.** 75%
- **d.** 100%

64–7. What is the best accepted way to prevent maternal primary cytomegalovirus (CMV) infection?

- **a.** Vaccination
- **b.** Hand washing
- **c.** Prophylaxis with valacyclovir
- **d.** CMV-specific hyperimmune globulin treatments for women at risk for primary infection

64–8. A 29-year-old G2P1 presents at 19 weeks' gestation. She reports a 2-day history of fever, runny nose, and myalgias. She now has a pruritic rash. A photograph is provided below. What is the most likely diagnosis?

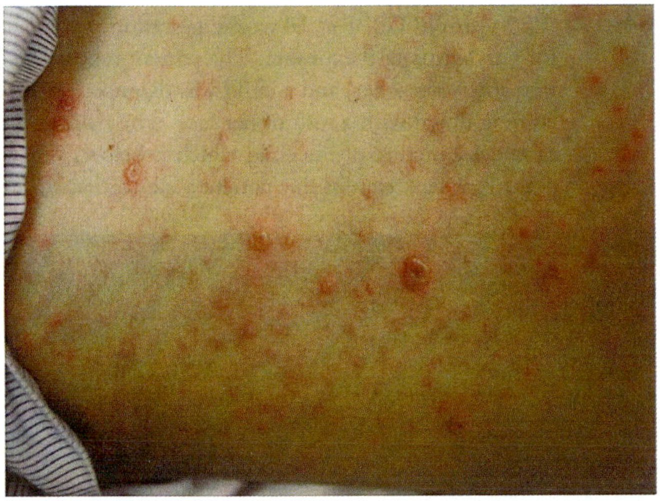

- **a.** Mumps
- **b.** Varicella
- **c.** Influenza
- **d.** Toxoplasmosis

64–9. Which of the following statements about varicella pneumonia in pregnancy is false?

- **a.** Maternal mortality rates are 1–2%.
- **b.** Only 2–5% of pregnant woman infected with varicella develop pneumonia.
- **c.** Having fewer than 100 cutaneous lesions is a risk factor for varicella pneumonia.
- **d.** Symptoms of varicella pneumonia usually appear 3–5 days into the illness course.

64–10. Which of the following statements about the infection shown in the photograph below is true?

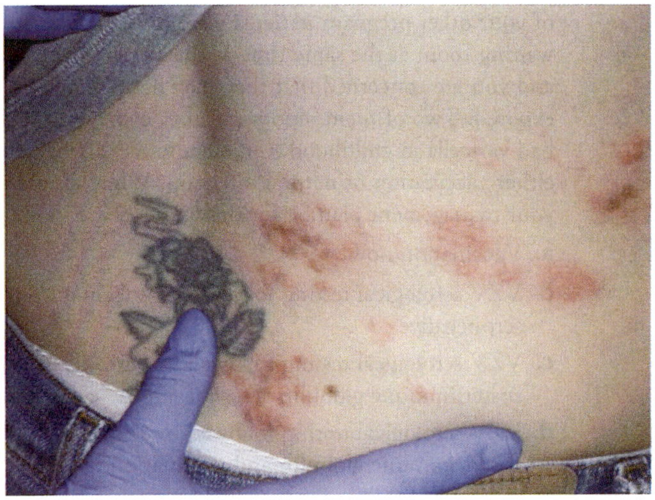

Used with permission from Dr. Mary Jane Pearson.

- **a.** It is painless
- **b.** It is more contagious than primary varicella
- **c.** Congenital varicella syndrome rarely develops
- **d.** It is more frequent and more severe in pregnancy

64–11. An infant is born with congenital varicella. A photograph is provided below. At what gestational age did the maternal infection most likely occur?

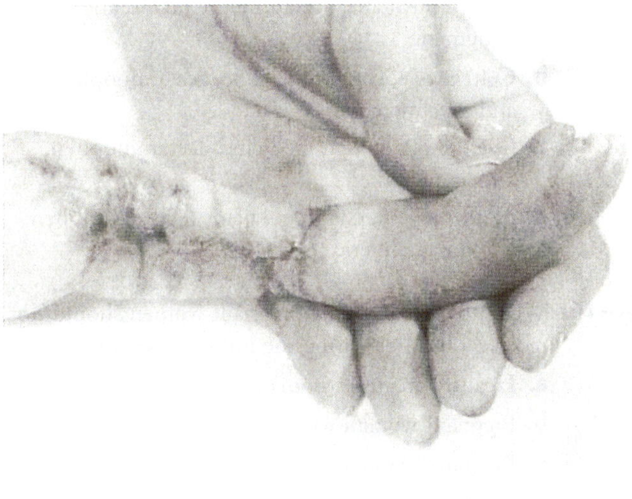

Reproduced with permission from Cunningham FG, Leveno KJ, Bloom SL, et al (eds): Infectious diseases. In Williams Obstetrics, 25th ed. New York, McGraw-Hill, 2018, Figure 64-3.

- **a.** 6 weeks' gestation
- **b.** 16 weeks' gestation
- **c.** 26 weeks' gestation
- **d.** 36 weeks' gestation

64–12. A 27-year-old multigravida presents at 6 weeks' gestation complaining of fever and a pruritic rash. You diagnose her with varicella-zoster virus (VZV). Three of your other pregnant patients were in the office waiting room at the same time as the sick patient, and you are concerned that they may have been exposed. Two of them report a history of having had varicella in childhood. One reports no history of either vaccination or natural infection. What should your management plan be for that patient?

- **a.** Vaccination now
- **b.** VZV serological testing followed by vaccination if seronegative
- **c.** VZV serological testing followed by varicella-zoster immune globulin if seronegative
- **d.** VZV serological testing followed by varicella-zoster immune globulin and vaccination if seronegative

64–13. A 17-year-old G1P0 at 24 weeks' gestation presents with a 2-day history of coughing, sneezing, vomiting, myalgias, and headache. Her family that she lives with is also sick. On exam, she is tachycardic to 123 beats per minute. Her blood pressure is normal, and she is febrile to 38.7°C. Her lungs are clear on exam. You order a chest radiograph, and you swab her for influenza because it is flu season. The chest radiograph and flu swab are both negative. What should you give this patient for her illness?

- **a.** Cough medicine, acetaminophen, and an antiemetic
- **b.** Ceftriaxone, cough medicine, acetaminophen, and an antiemetic
- **c.** Oseltamivir, cough medicine, acetaminophen, and an antiemetic
- **d.** Azithromycin, cough medicine, acetaminophen, and an antiemetic

64–14. Which of the following pregnant women should not receive a flu shot during the influenza season?

- **a.** Healthy pregnant woman
- **b.** Pregnant woman with asthma
- **c.** Pregnant woman with well-controlled HIV
- **d.** All women who will be pregnant during the influenza season should receive the flu shot

64–15. High-avidity IgG antibodies to rubella indicate that infection was at least how many months in the past?

- **a.** 2 months
- **b.** 4 months
- **c.** 6 months
- **d.** 8 months

64–16. Which of the following is not an ultrasound finding in cases of congenital rubella?

- **a.** Macrocephaly
- **b.** Hepatomegaly
- **c.** Microphthalmia
- **d.** Cardiac septal defects

64–17. Which of the following vaccinations should not be offered in pregnancy?

- **a.** Influenza
- **b.** Hepatitis B
- **c.** Measles, mumps, rubella
- **d.** Tetanus, diphtheria, and pertussis

64–18. What is the most frequent infectious agent of nonimmune hydrops in autopsied fetuses?

- **a.** Syphilis
- **b.** Chlamydia
- **c.** Toxoplasmosis
- **d.** Parvovirus B19

64–19. A 25-year-old G2P1 at 18 weeks' gestation presents for parvovirus B19 exposure. The patient reports that she is a teacher, and a child was diagnosed after coming down with a rash of her face. The patient provides a picture of the child which is below. What is the best next step in this patient's management?

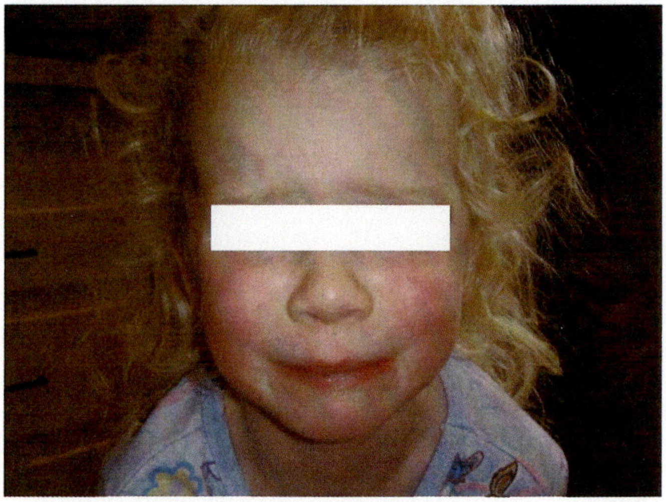

Used with permission from Dr. Gary Cunningham.

- **a.** Cordocentesis to assess for fetal anemia
- **b.** Parvovirus B19 immunoglobulin treatment
- **c.** Serial ultrasounds every two weeks for the next ten weeks
- **d.** Maternal serological testing for IgG and IgM antibodies

64–20. A 29-year-old G3P0 at approximately 35 weeks' gestation presents for her first prenatal visit. She reports previously uncomplicated prenatal care in Mexico. You send her routine prenatal labs and order an ultrasound for evaluation of anatomy and dating. The fetal abdominal circumference and femur length confirm her dating. However, the fetal head is lagging in size with thinned cerebral cortex and unilateral ventriculomegaly, although visualization is limited due to advanced gestational age. Postnatal magnetic resonance imaging of the neonatal head demonstrates thinned cerebral white matter, and thinning of the corpus callosum, as well as foci of cystic volume loss in the subcortical white matter. These findings make you concerned for which of the following?

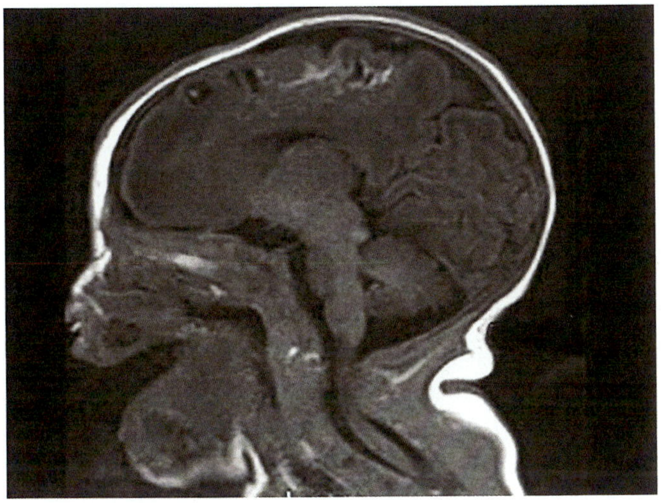

Used with permission from Dr. Emily Adhikari.

a. Zika
b. Ebola
c. Rubella
d. West Nile

64–21. In which of the following cases is intrapartum prophylaxis against group B streptococcus (GBS) not indicated?

a. Prior infant with invasive GBS disease
b. GBS bacteriuria during the current pregnancy
c. Unknown GBS status in a pregnant woman in active labor at 36 weeks' gestation
d. Negative GBS screening culture this pregnancy, but a positive GBS screening culture in the last pregnancy

64–22. A 26-year-old multigravida at 35 weeks' gestation presents in active labor. She's had very limited prenatal care. She thinks her water may have broken yesterday morning. At presentation, she has a temperature of 38.3°C with no identifiable source. How many identifiable risk factors does she have for group B streptococcus sepsis?

a. Zero
b. One
c. Two
d. Three

64–23. Women with a reported penicillin allergy but no history of anaphylaxis should be given which of the following antibiotics for intrapartum prophylaxis against perinatal group B streptococcus disease?

a. Cefazolin
b. Penicillin
c. Vancomycin
d. Erythromycin

64–24. A 25-year-old G1P0 presents at 36 weeks' gestation with scotomata and elevated blood pressures. She had uncomplicated prenatal care, and her group B streptococcus screening at 35 weeks' gestation was positive. She is found to have severe preeclampsia, and the fetus is breech. The decision is made that she needs a cesarean delivery. The patient reports a childhood allergy to penicillin. She recalls a rash, but nothing else. What should the patient receive for intrapartum GBS prophylaxis?

a. Cefazolin
b. Ampicillin
c. Vancomycin
d. The patient does not need GBS prophylaxis

64–25. A 30-year-old G3P2 presents for a small abscess on her neck (see photograph below). She undergoes incision and drainage with culture. The patient is found to have methicillin-resistant *Staphylococcus aureus* (MRSA) on culture. Which of the following antibiotics is the most appropriate choice for this pregnant patient with an MRSA skin infection?

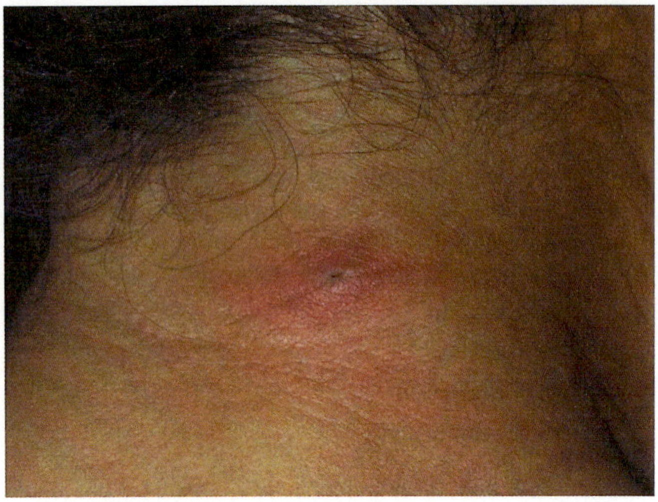

a. Rifampin
b. Linezolid
c. Doxycycline
d. Trimethoprim-sulfamethoxazole

64–26. A pale placenta with multiple microabscesses (see photo below) is consistent with which of the following infections?

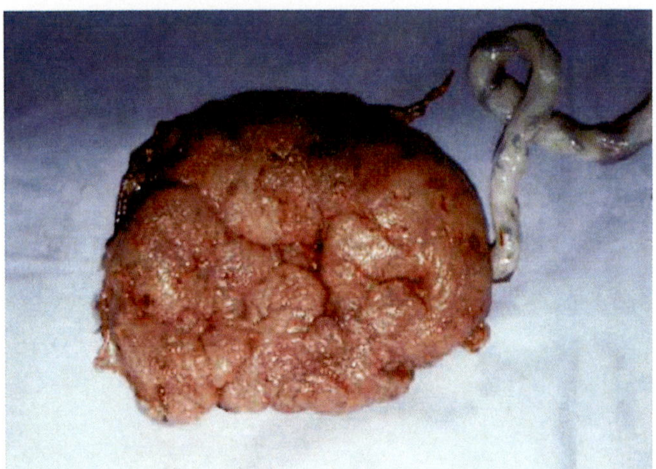

Reproduced with permission from Cunningham FG, Leveno KJ, Bloom SL, et al (eds): Infectious diseases. In Williams Obstetrics, 25th ed. New York, McGraw-Hill, 2018, Figure 64-9A.

a. Rubella
b. Listeriosis
c. Salmonellosis
d. Parvovirus B19

64–27. Which of the following is the best treatment choice for listeriosis in pregnancy?

a. Doxycycline
b. Clindamycin
c. Azithromycin
d. Ampicillin and gentamicin

64–28. Which of the following statements about toxoplasmosis in pregnancy is true?

a. The risk of fetal infection decreases as gestation progresses
b. The severity of fetal infection increases as gestation progresses
c. Most infected fetuses are born with obvious stigmata of toxoplasmosis
d. Maternal infection is associated with a fourfold increased preterm delivery rate before 37 weeks

64–29. A 32-year-old primigravida at 22 weeks' gestation is diagnosed with toxoplasmosis. Findings on the fetal ultrasound include intracranial calcifications, placental thickening, and hyperechoic bowel. Testing confirms fetal infection. Which of the following is the best treatment for this patient?

a. Spiramycin
b. There is no treatment
c. Trimethoprim-sulfamethoxazole
d. Pyrimethamine-sulfadiazine with folinic acid

64–30. A pregnant woman with uncomplicated malaria caused by *Plasmodium vivax* should be treated with which of the following?

a. Primaquine
b. Doxycycline
c. Chloroquine
d. Artemether-lumefantrine

64–31. Which of the following is an acceptable choice for malaria prophylaxis in a pregnant woman?

a. Primaquine
b. Doxycycline
c. Chloroquine
d. Atovaquone/proguanil

64–32. Which of the following statements about postexposure anthrax prophylaxis in asymptomatic pregnant and lactating women is false?

a. Ciprofloxacin is first line.
b. Regimens are given for 3 months.
c. Amoxicillin can be used if the strain is sensitive to it.
d. In cases of allergy to ciprofloxacin and penicillin, doxycycline is given because the risks of anthrax outweigh the risks of doxycycline to the fetus.

CHAPTER 64 ANSWER KEY

Question number	Letter answer	Page cited	Header cited
64–1	**c**	p. 1209	Fetal and Newborn Immunology
64–2	**b**	p. 1210	Cytomegalovirus
64–3	**b**	p. 1210	Maternal Infection
64–4	**d**	p. 1211	Figure 64-1
64–5	**b**	p. 1211	Figure 64-2
64–6	**c**	p. 1212	Prenatal Diagnosis
64–7	**b**	p. 1212	Management and Prevention
64–8	**b**	p. 1212	Maternal Infection
64–9	**c**	p. 1212	Maternal Infection
64–10	**c**	p. 1212	Maternal Infection
64–11	**b**	p. 1213	Figure 64-3
64–12	**c**	p. 1213	Management
64–13	**c**	p. 1214	Maternal and Fetal Infection
64–14	**d**	p. 1214	Vaccination
64–15	**a**	p. 1215	Diagnosis
64–16	**a**	p. 1215	Fetal Effects
64–17	**c**	p. 1215	Management and Prevention
64–18	**d**	p. 1217	Fetal Infection
64–19	**d**	p. 1217	Diagnosis and Management
64–20	**a**	p. 1219	Figure 64-5
64–21	**d**	p. 1221	Figure 64-6
64–22	**d**	p. 1221	Figure 64-6
64–23	**a**	p. 1222	Table 64-3
64–24	**d**	p. 1222	Intrapartum Antimicrobial Prophylaxis
64–25	**d**	p. 1223	Management
64–26	**b**	p. 1224	Maternal and Fetal Infection
64–27	**d**	p. 1224	Maternal and Fetal Infection
64–28	**d**	p. 1225	Maternal and Fetal Infection
64–29	**d**	p. 1226	Management
64–30	**c**	p. 1227	Diagnosis and Management
64–31	**c**	p. 1227	Prevention and Chemoprophylaxis
64–32	**b**	p. 1228	Anthrax

CHAPTER 65

Sexually Transmitted Infections

65–1. What is the incubation period for syphilis?

a. 3–4 days
b. 7–10 days
c. 3–4 weeks
d. 7–10 weeks

65–2. A 29-year-old G3P2 presents at 22 weeks' gestation for prenatal care. She has a past history of chlamydia and asthma. On her initial prenatal labs, her RPR returns 1:128. Her treponemal-specific test is positive. She denies a history of syphilis. Exam findings are depicted in the photo below. What is her stage?

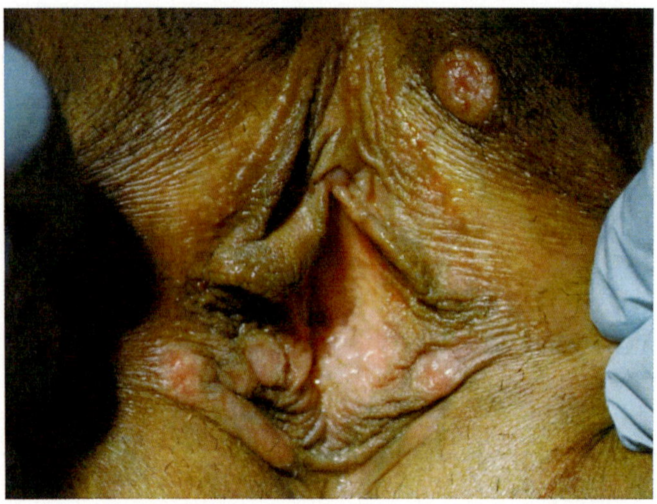

a. Primary
b. Secondary
c. Late latent
d. Early latent

65–3. If the patient in Question 65–2 were to go untreated, how long would it take for the lesion depicted in the picture to resolve?

a. 5–7 days
b. 1–2 weeks
c. 2–8 weeks
d. It would not resolve without treatment

65–4. The patient in Question 65–2 declined treatment the day you saw her. She was upset by the news she had syphilis, and she insisted on leaving. Your staff attempts to get her to stay, but she does not. She returns to the office 2 months later. She is no longer with her husband, and she would like treatment. A photo of her perineum is provided below. What is her stage now?

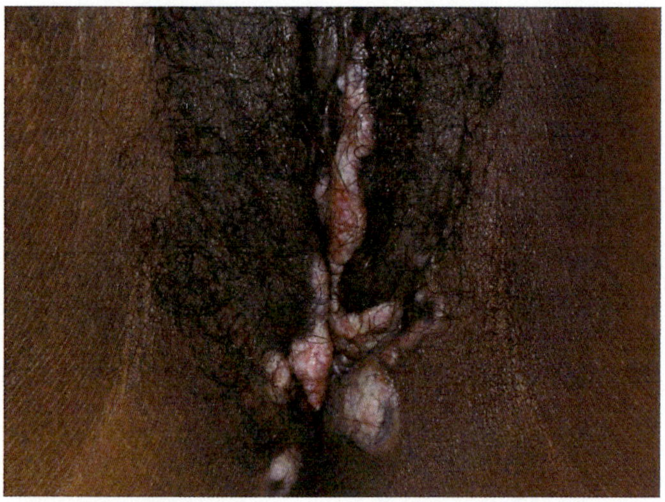

a. Primary
b. Secondary
c. Late latent
d. Early latent

65–5. A 22-year-old primigravida presents for prenatal care. She has an RPR of 1:64 and her treponemal-specific test is positive. On your exam, you note the findings depicted in the photographs below. What stage of syphilis does the patient have?

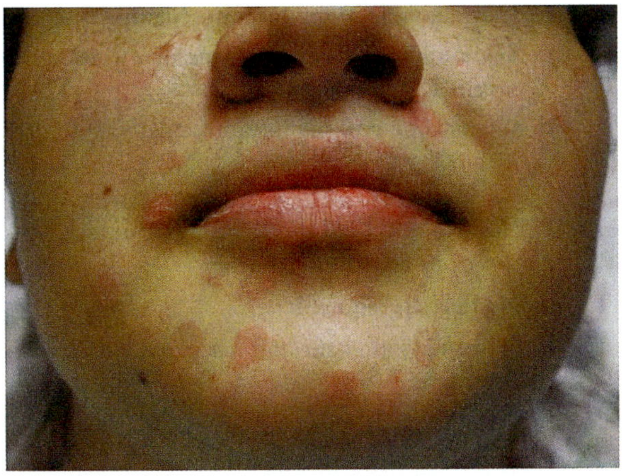

Reproduced with permission from Cunningham FG, Leveno KJ, Bloom SL, et al (eds): Sexually transmitted infections. In Williams Obstetrics, 25th ed. New York, McGraw-Hill, 2018, Figure 65-2a.

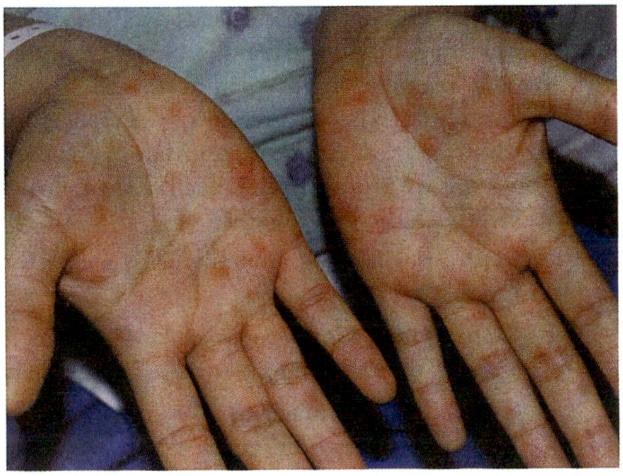

Reproduced with permission from Cunningham FG, Leveno KJ, Bloom SL, et al (eds): Sexually transmitted infections. In Williams Obstetrics, 25th ed. New York, McGraw-Hill, 2018, Figure 65-2b.

a. Primary
b. Secondary
c. Late latent
d. Early latent

65–6. A 20-year-old multigravida presents at 17 weeks' gestation. Her RPR is 1:8 and treponemal-specific testing is positive. She denies a history of syphilis, and her physical exam reveals no evidence of syphilis. In review of her records, you note that she had her last baby 6 months ago, and at that time her RPR was nonreactive. What stage is she?

a. Primary
b. Secondary
c. Late latent
d. Early latent

65–7. A 25-year-old G7P2 presents in active labor. The patient has no prenatal care. She has a history of drug use, mental illness, and prostitution. A bedside ultrasound confirms a fetal demise with an estimated fetal weight of 2500 grams. Her vital signs are normal, and she is 6 cm dilated. Prenatal labs are sent on the patient. Her random glucose is 100 mg/dL. Her hemoglobin is 11 g/dL. Her tests for human immunodeficiency virus and hepatitis B are negative. Her RPR is 1:32 and treponemal-specific testing is positive. Her urine toxicology is positive only for marijuana. After delivery of the stillborn, a fetogram is performed. An image of that is provided below. A picture of her placenta is also provided. What is the most likely cause of the stillbirth?

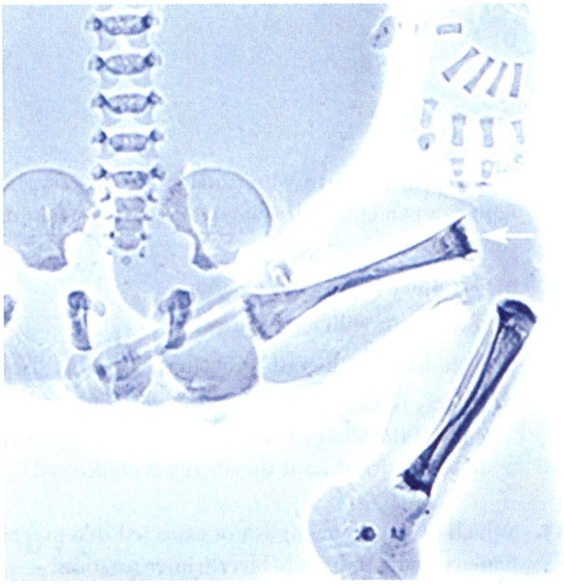

Reproduced with permission from Cunningham FG, Leveno KJ, Bloom SL, et al (eds): Sexually transmitted infections. In Williams Obstetrics, 25th ed. New York, McGraw-Hill, 2018, Figure 65-4a.

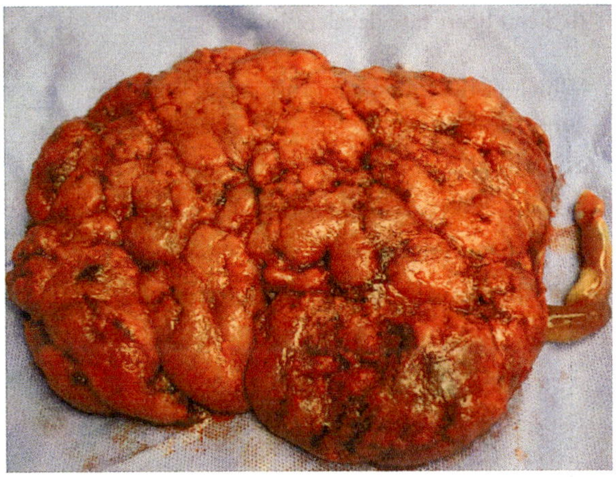

Used with permission from Dr. Ed Wells.

a. Preeclampsia
b. Marijuana use
c. Congenital syphilis
d. Untreated gestational diabetes

CHAPTER 65

65–8. Which of the following statements about testing for syphilis is true?

a. The RPR remains positive forever regardless of treatment.

b. The treponemal antibody test reverts to negative with treatment.

c. The RPR reverts to negative in most patients after treatment.

d. If the RPR is reactive, then the treponemal antibody test is not required.

65–9. If a pregnant woman is diagnosed with syphilis, and her stage cannot be determined, how many weekly doses of penicillin should she receive?

a. 1

b. 2

c. 3

d. 4

65–10. If a pregnant woman who is diagnosed with syphilis reports a penicillin allergy, what is the best plan of care?

a. Treatment with doxycycline

b. Treatment with azithromycin

c. Treatment with erythromycin

d. Allergy testing followed by treatment with penicillin if the allergy is not confirmed, and penicillin desensitization if the allergy is confirmed,

65–11. Which of the following is not expected in a pregnant patient having a Jarisch-Herxheimer reaction?

a. Hypothermia

b. Uterine contractions

c. Decreased fetal movement

d. Fetal heart rate decelerations

65–12. Which of the following is not a risk factor for gonorrhea?

a. Drug abuse

b. Age >25 years

c. Hispanic ethnicity

d. Other sexually transmitted infections

65–13. A 17-year-old primigravida presents for prenatal care at 10 weeks' gestation. Her test for gonorrhea is positive. She has no allergies. Which of the following is the best choice for her treatment?

a. Cefixime 400 mg by mouth

b. Ceftriaxone 250 mg intramuscularly

c. Gentamicin 240 mg intramuscularly and azithromycin 1 g by mouth

d. Ceftriaxone 250 mg intramuscularly and azithromycin 1 g by mouth

65–14. For how long should the patient in Question 65–13 refrain from sexual intercourse?

a. No delay is required

b. Three days after she and her partner complete treatment

c. Seven days after she and her partner complete treatment

d. Fourteen days after she and her partner complete treatment

65–15. A 19-year-old G2P1 presents at 15 weeks' gestation complaining of arthralgias and subjective fever for 1 week. She notes that the pain is worse on the dorsal side of her wrists. On review of her prenatal labs sent last visit, you see she is positive for gonorrhea. You suspect septic arthritis. Which of the following is the best choice for treatment?

a. Ceftriaxone 250 mg intramuscularly and azithromycin 1 g by mouth

b. Ceftriaxone 1 g intravenously every 12 hours for 4 weeks and azithromycin 1 g by mouth one time

c. Ceftriaxone 2 g intravenously every 12 hours for 10–14 days and azithromycin 1 g by mouth one time

d. Ceftriaxone 1 g intramuscularly every 24 hours, continued until there is clinical improvement for 24–48 hours, and azithromycin 1 go by mouth one time, followed by oral antibiotics to complete 1 week of therapy

65–16. In regard to the patient in Question 65–15, treating for potential co-infection with which of the following is the purpose of adding azithromycin to the regimen?

a. *Escherichia coli*

b. *Toxoplasma gondii*

c. *Chlamydia trachomatis*

d. Group B *Streptococcus*

65–17. Which of the following organisms has been associated with delayed postpartum metritis?

- **a.** *Neisseria gonorrhoeae*
- **b.** Herpes simplex virus
- **c.** *Chlamydia trachomatis*
- **d.** Group B *Streptococcus*

65–18. Screening for which of the following infections is recommended by the American College of Obstetrics and Gynecology for all women at their first prenatal visit?

- **a.** Chlamydia
- **b.** Gonorrhea
- **c.** Chlamydia and gonorrhea
- **d.** Chlamydia, gonorrhea, and herpes

65–19. When should a pregnant woman who has been treated for chlamydia be rescreened?

- **a.** 3 months after treatment
- **b.** 3–4 weeks after treatment
- **c.** Rescreening is not necessary
- **d.** 3–4 weeks after treatment and again 3 months after treatment

65–20. Which of the following statements about expedited partner treatment (EPT) is false?

- **a.** It is not recommended for syphilis
- **b.** EPT is acceptable for treatment of sexual contacts in the case of chlamydia
- **c.** Because treatment guidelines now recommend ceftriaxone intramuscularly, EPT is a less desirable choice for gonorrhea
- **d.** EPT involves the obstetrical provider seeing the male partner, providing counseling, and then treating him as opposed to referring the male partner to his own health care provider

65–21. What percentage of pregnant women seronegative for herpes simplex virus (HSV) will acquire HSV-1 or -2 during pregnancy?

- **a.** 4–5%
- **b.** 9–10%
- **c.** 14–15%
- **d.** 19–20%

65–22. A 22-year-old G1P0 at 6 weeks' gestation presents for pain of her perineum, subjective fever, and body aches. She noticed that her perineum was itchy several days ago, but then it became painful. She thought the pain was from scratching, but the tender area has spread. This has never happened to her before. A photo of her perineum is provided below. What is the most likely diagnosis?

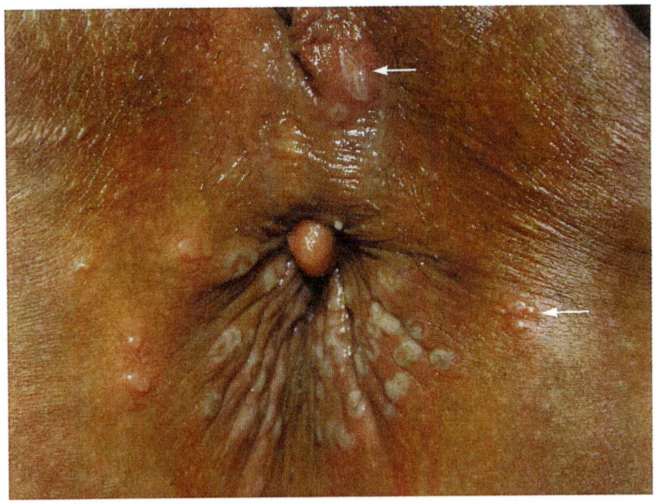

Reproduced with permission from Cunningham FG, Leveno KJ, Bloom SL, et al (eds): Sexually transmitted infections. In Williams Obstetrics, 25th ed. New York, McGraw-Hill, 2018, Figure 65-8.

- **a.** HSV
- **b.** Syphilis
- **c.** Varicella
- **d.** Molluscum contagiosum

65–23. You send a sexually transmitted disease panel on the patient in Question 65–22. You also send herpes simplex virus (HSV) PCR after swabbing her lesions. Human immunodeficiency virus and hepatitis B are negative. Her serum HSV-1 and -2 antibodies are also negative. The swab of the lesion is positive for HSV-2. What is her diagnosis?

- **a.** Recurrent HSV infection
- **b.** First episode primary infection
- **c.** First episode nonprimary infection
- **d.** Asymptomatic HSV viral shedding

65–24. What is the most frequent route of herpes simplex virus infection to the fetus/neonate?

- **a.** Postnatal
- **b.** Peripartum
- **c.** Intrauterine
- **d.** All routes occur with equal frequency

65–25. Which of the following statements about testing for herpes simplex virus is true?

- **a.** Culture results return faster than PCR results
- **b.** IgM antibody detection is useful for timing the infection
- **c.** A negative culture or PCR excludes infection with HSV
- **d.** IgG antibodies develop 1–2 weeks after the primary infection and then persist

65–26. Which of the following is not a recommended medication regimen for symptomatic recurrent herpes simplex virus infection?

- **a.** Acyclovir 800 mg by mouth twice per day for 5 days
- **b.** Valacyclovir 500 mg by mouth twice per day for 3 days
- **c.** Valacyclovir 1 g by mouth twice per day for 10 days
- **d.** Acyclovir 400 mg by mouth three times per day for 5 days

65–27. The American College of Obstetricians and Gynecologists recommends starting herpes simplex virus suppression to prevent cesarean section for outbreaks at what gestational age?

- **a.** 32 weeks
- **b.** 34 weeks
- **c.** 36 weeks
- **d.** 38 weeks

65–28. A 19-year-old G1P0 at 39 weeks' gestation presents to triage in active labor at 4 cm dilation. Membranes are intact. She has a history of herpes simplex virus for which she has not been taking suppression. You examine her and determine she has no lesions. She is, however, complaining of a 2-day history of prodromal symptoms including tingling and itching. What is the best management plan?

- **a.** Cesarean section
- **b.** Allow her to labor, but avoid placing a fetal scalp electrode
- **c.** Load with intravenous acyclovir and then proceed with cesarean section
- **d.** Load with intravenous acyclovir, allow her to labor, but assist with the second stage

65–29. Which of the following is not recommended for the treatment of genital warts in pregnancy?

- **a.** Cryotherapy
- **b.** Surgical excision
- **c.** Podophyllin resin
- **d.** TCA 80–90% solution

65–30. Which of the following statements about juvenile-onset recurrent respiratory papillomatosis is true?

- **a.** Precipitous labor is a risk factor for this disease.
- **b.** It is a common cause of respiratory distress in children.
- **c.** It is most often caused by human papillomavirus 16 and 18.
- **d.** Cesarean section is not recommended in patients with genital warts to prevent transmission of human papillomavirus.

65–31. Which of the following is not a component of the diagnostic criteria for the infection demonstrated in the photo below?

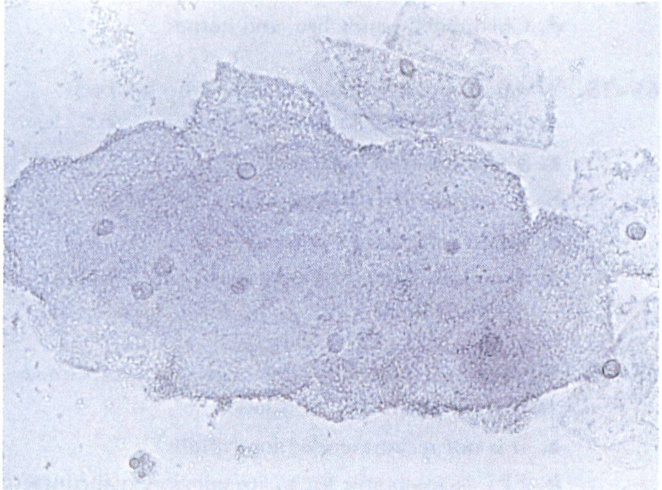

- **a.** Vaginal pH >4.5
- **b.** >50% clue cells seen microscopically
- **c.** Thin, milky, noninflammatory vaginal discharge
- **d.** Fishy odor after addition of 10% potassium hydroxide to a sample of vaginal secretions

65–32. You are seeing a 25-year-old G3P0 at 17 weeks' gestation for her second prenatal appointment. You note on the results of her Pap test that trichomonads were seen. She has noticed mild discharge that she assumes is normal for pregnancy. Which of the following is the best next step in management?

- **a.** Metronidazole 2 g by mouth one time
- **b.** Perform a wet prep microscopy to confirm
- **c.** Clindamycin 2% cream at bedtime for 3 days
- **d.** Disregard the Pap test results and reassure the patient

65–33. How long can it take after a person is infected with human immunodeficiency virus for them to have a positive antibody serotest?

- **a.** Seven days
- **b.** Two weeks
- **c.** Three weeks
- **d.** One month

65–34. Which of the following statements about vertical transmission of human immunodeficiency virus (HIV) is true?

a. Neonatal infection rates are directly related to viral burden.

b. HIV vertical transmission does not occur in the first half of pregnancy.

c. Comorbid sexually transmitted diseases reduce vertical transmission rates.

d. Vertical transmission rates from breastfeeding do not correlate with viral load.

65–35. A 30-year-old multigravida at 6 weeks' gestation presents for prenatal care. She was diagnosed with human immunodeficiency virus (HIV) 4 years ago, and she has been on and off medication since. She is not taking any medications for HIV at this time. Which of the following statements about her HIV care in this pregnancy is false?

a. She needs to have resistance testing sent.

b. She needs a treatment regimen with at least three antiviral agents.

c. She should not be treated until resistance testing results come back.

d. Treatment will reduce perinatal transmission regardless of CD4 or viral load.

65–36. At what viral load should a pregnant woman with human immunodeficiency virus be offered an elective cesarean section, and at what gestational age should that cesarean section be performed?

a. >500 copies/mL and 39 weeks' gestation

b. >750 copies/mL and 37 weeks' gestation

c. >1000 copies/mL and 38 weeks' gestation

d. >10,000 copies/mL and 36 weeks' gestation

65–37. Which of the following medications used for the treatment of postpartum hemorrhage should be avoided in human immunodeficiency virus positive pregnant women on reverse transcriptase and protease inhibitors?

a. Oxytocin

b. Misoprostol

c. Methylergonovine

d. Carboprost tromethamine

65–38. A 29-year-old multigravida with no prenatal care and a history of three prior vaginal deliveries presents in active labor. Her cervical exam is 6 cm dilated, 75% effacement, and –1 station. Membranes ruptured spontaneously approximately 3 hours prior to presentation. She reports that she is human immunodeficiency virus positive, but you have no labs on her for the past 2 years. What is the best delivery plan for this patient?

a. Load intravenous zidovudine and proceed with vaginal delivery

b. Proceed with urgent cesarean section, not delaying for intravenous zidovudine

c. Load intravenous zidovudine over 3 hours and proceed with urgent cesarean section

d. Load intravenous zidovudine over 30 minutes and proceed with urgent cesarean section

CHAPTER 65 ANSWER KEY

Question number	Letter answer	Page cited	Header cited
65–1	**c**	p. 1235	Pathogenesis and Transmission
65–2	**a**	p. 1236	Figure 65-1
65–3	**c**	p. 1236	Maternal Syphilis
65–4	**b**	p. 1236	Figure 65-3
65–5	**b**	p. 1236	Figure 65-2
65–6	**d**	p. 1237	Maternal Syphilis
65–7	**c**	p. 1237	Figure 65-4
65–8	**c**	p. 1237	Diagnosis
65–9	**c**	p. 1238	Table 65-1
65–10	**d**	p. 1239	Penicillin Reactions
65–11	**a**	p. 1239	Penicillin Reactions
65–12	**b**	p. 1239	Screening and Treatment
65–13	**d**	p. 1240	Screening and Treatment
65–14	**c**	p. 1240	Screening and Treatment
65–15	**d**	p. 1240	Disseminated Gonococcal Infections
65–16	**c**	p. 1240	Disseminated Gonococcal Infections
65–17	**c**	p. 1240	Chlamydial Infections
65–18	**a**	p. 1240	Screening and Treatment
65–19	**d**	p. 1241	Screening and Treatment
65–20	**d**	p. 1241	Expedited Partner Treatment
65–21	**a**	p. 1242	Adult Disease
65–22	**a**	p. 1242	Figure 65-5
65–23	**b**	p. 1242	Clinical Manifestations
65–24	**b**	p. 1242	Vertical Transmission
65–25	**d**	p. 1243	Diagnosis
65–26	**c**	p. 1244	Table 65-4
65–27	**c**	p. 1244	Peripartum Shedding Prophylaxis
65–28	**a**	p. 1244	Peripartum Shedding Prophylaxis
65–29	**c**	p. 1245	Condyloma Acuminata Treatment
65–30	**d**	p. 1245	Neonatal Infection
65–31	**b**	p. 1245	Diagnosis
65–32	**b**	p. 1246	Diagnosis
65–33	**d**	P. 1248	Prenatal HIV Screening
65–34	**a**	p. 1248	Vertical Transmission
65–35	**c**	p. 1249	Antiretroviral Therapy
65–36	**c**	p. 1249	Delivery Planning
65–37	**c**	p. 1249	Delivery Planning
65–38	**a**	p. 1250	Table 65-5

INDEX

Note: Page numbers followed by *f* represent figures.